Clinical Pharmacokinetics:

Concepts and Applications

Clinical Pharmacokinetics: Concepts and Applications

Malcolm Rowland, PhD.

Department of Pharmacy
University of Manchester
Manchester, England

Thomas N. Tozer, PhD.

School of Pharmacy
University of California
San Francisco, California

Second Edition

Lea & Febiger   Philadelphia • London • 1989

Lea & Febiger
600 Washington Square
Philadelphia, PA   19106-4198
U.S.A.
(215) 922-1330

First Edition, 1980
   Reprinted, 1982, 1983, 1984, 1986

Library of Congress Cataloging-in-Publication Data

Rowland, Malcolm.
   Clinical pharmacokinetics.

   Bibliography: p.
   Includes index.
   1. Pharmacokinetics. 2. Chemotherapy. I. Tozer,
Thomas N.   II. Title. [DNLM: 1. Drug Therapy.
2. Pharmacokinetics.   QV 38 R883c]
RM301.5.R68   1988   615.5′8   88-8993
ISBN 0-8121-1160-5

Printed in the United States of America

Print Number 5   4   3   2   1

To Margaret and Dawn

PREFACE

In the eight years since the introduction of the first edition of this book the subject of pharmacokinetics, and particularly its clinical application, has grown enormously. Although notable gains have been made in our basic understanding of the area, it is at the clinical level that the greatest impact has occurred. Increasingly, pharmacokinetics has been identified as a major source of variability in response to drugs, so that even during development of a medicine pharmacokinetic studies are performed on patient populations likely to receive the drug. In the hospital, one has seen the rise of clinical pharmacokinetic services, with monitoring and interpretation of plasma concentrations of drugs used as a guide to therapy. For us, as teachers of the subject, not only are these changes most satisfying, but the findings in the associated research provide an ever richer source of instructional material.

This book continues to be directed to all concerned with the development, evaluation, and the use of medicines. Such persons include not only students in the professions of pharmacy and medicine but also pharmaceutical scientists, toxicologists, veterinarians, veterinary scientists, analytical chemists, biochemists, and clinical chemists.

This second edition continues the central theme of the first one. The book is a primer on pharmacokinetics with clinical applications. Each chapter has a stated set of objectives, identifying the major aspects to be learned, and a series of problems, allowing the reader to test his or her understanding of the material. Also, there is a list of suggested further reading located in the back of the book.

The major changes between the current and first editions of the book are in organization and size. The book is now divided into five sections: Absorption and Disposition Kinetics, Therapeutic Regimens, Physiologic Concepts and Kinetics, Individualization, and Selected Topics. The section on Therapeutic Regimens has been moved forward as this, for many, is the major focus and application of clinical pharmacokinetics. Indeed, those wishing to gain a general overview of the subject need only study Sections One and Two, together with Chapter 13, Variability, and Chapter 18, Monitoring. Section Three deals with the physiologic concepts relevant to an understanding of the processes of absorption, distribution, and elimination. This section forms the basis for an appreciation of the material in Section Four, which is concerned with the identification, description, and accounting of variability in drug response. Covered here are genetics, age and weight, disease, interacting drugs, and therapeutic drug monitoring.

Section Five contains selected topics. These are intended for those readers who wish to gain a more detailed insight into various aspects of clinical pharmacokinetics. The topics are distribution kinetics, pharmacologic response, metabolite kinetics, dose and time dependencies, turnover concepts, and dialysis. Also included is a chapter considering drugs with a small volume of distribution. Each topic is self-contained; they have not been arranged in any particular sequence. It was our original intention that the material covered in Section Five, together with chapters dealing with clinical pharmacokinetics of specific drugs, would form a sequel to the first edition of this book. It was to have been entitled "Clinical Pharmacokinetics: Specialized Topics and Selected Drugs." We decided to incorporate the selected topics into the current book. This decision was primarily a consequence of the appearance of several excellent monographs on the clinical pharmacokinetics of specific drugs during the intervening years.

We continue to adopt a uniform set of symbols and to use milligrams/liter as the standard measure of concentration. We do recognize, however, the increasing trend toward the adoption of molar units and have provided a factor for conversion between the two units of measurement in the pertinent figure legends. We shall only be convinced of the virtue of solely using the molar system of measurement when drugs are prescribed in such units. We have adopted the convention of using the term *log* to denote the logarithm to the natural base *e*.

Although we feel that all equations given are important to the understanding and application of pharmacokinetics, some are more important and have wider application than others. For ease of reference we have indicated these more important equations with this symbol ★.

We would especially like to thank Mandy North, Manchester, England, for drawing all the illustrations new to this second edition.

We have been enormously gratified by the wide and diverse readership of the first edition of the book and by the many encouraging comments we have received. We would like to believe that it has been instrumental in furthering the rational management of drug therapy. We sincerely hope that the second edition will continue to do so.

Manchester, England   Malcolm Rowland
San Francisco, California   Thomas N. Tozer

PREFACE TO FIRST EDITION

For eight years we jointly shared responsibility for teaching basic courses in pharmacokinetics at the University of California. The students were from a variety of persuasions, including professional students in pharmacy, clinical pharmacology fellows, and graduate academic students. Their feedback on the course resulted in our making a dramatic shift in the way we presented the material. Over the years the emphasis shifted from kinetics and modeling to providing a conceptual base for applying pharmacokinetics to rational drug therapy. We firmly believe that the reoriented content of these courses goes much further in relating to the needs of students and of practitioners of pharmacotherapeutics. One of the major difficulties in teaching the subject has been the lack of a book that teaches the application of pharmacokinetics in drug therapy. This deficiency prompted the writing of this book.

The title of the book was chosen because it emphasizes the bedside application of pharmacokinetics. The book, in fact, is a primer on pharmacokinetics with clinical applications. It should be useful to any student, practitioner, or researcher who is interested or engaged in the development, evaluation, or use of drugs in man. It is an introductory text and therefore presumes that the reader has had little or no experience or knowledge in the area. Previous exposure to certain aspects of physiology and pharmacology would be helpful, but is not essential. Some knowledge of calculus is also desirable.

In our experience, the average student has felt very uncomfortable with kinetic principles and mathematics. Indeed, in many cases there is a strong mental block. Our desire is to teach the application of pharmacokinetics in therapeutics. We believe we are achieving this goal by applying the essential concepts through problem solving with only the essence of required mathematics. This approach is a theme throughout the book. In this respect this book is a programmed learning text. Every attempt is made at the beginning of each chapter to present objectives that identify the more important points to be learned. To further aid in the learning process, examples are worked out in detail in the text. At the end of many chapters there are two kinds of problems. The first is study problems, which allow the reader to test his grasp of the material in the chapter. The second kind is unifying problems, which build upon the material of previous chapters. For the interested reader there is a list of suggested further reading located at the back of the book.

An attempt has been made to establish uniformity for symbols and units throughout the book; definitions of symbols begin on p. 280. The liter is used as the standard measure of volume and hour as the standard unit of time. A special comment should be made on the choice of mg/liter for the units of drug concentration. Although molarity has considerable utility and has been strongly advocated for common use, the dosage of drugs is most often expressed in milligrams. Until doses are given in molar units, we feel that mg/liter is the more convenient unit for concentration.

The book is divided into four sections: Concepts, Disposition and Absorption

Kinetics, Therapeutic Regimens, and Individualization. Section I contains the fundamental concepts in drug absorption, distribution and elimination. Section II covers the kinetics of drug and metabolites following drug administration and integrates kinetics with the fundamental concepts. Section III deals with the basic elements of the design and evaluation of therapeutic regimens, while Section IV examines the causes of variability in human drug response, the adjustment of dosage based on age, weight, and renal function, explores the kinetic consequences of drug interactions, and presents principles for the monitoring of drug therapy using plasma concentrations. The sequence is intended to give the reader the basic underlying concepts, the quantitative tools, and the essence of the kinetic basis for variability in human drug response.

The content of the book, by design, has been limited. There are many important areas of pharmacokinetics either touched on only lightly or not covered at all. Most of these areas are more specialized, dealing with such topics as distribution dynamics, including multicompartment systems, dose and time dependencies, turnover concepts, dialysis, and kinetic considerations in the treatment of drug overdose. These and other specialized topics and a more detailed examination of the clinical pharmacokinetics of selected drugs, including digoxin, theophylline, and phenytoin, form the basis of a sequel to this book entitled Clinical Pharmacokinetics: Specialized Topics and Selected Drugs.

We wish to express our gratitude to Jere E. Goyan, Dean, and Sidney Riegelman, Associate Dean for Research Services, School of Pharmacy, University of California, for their encouragement. We also wish to acknowledge Paul Bailey of Manchester, England, for his preparation of the illustrations. We particularly wish to thank our past students whose comments have been so useful in formulating our ideas.

To the reader of the book we hope that we have succeeded in helping you develop kinetic reasoning that will be of personal value in your practice. In general perspective, we hope we have made some contribution to the development of a more rational management of drug therapy.

Manchester, England   Malcolm Rowland
San Francisco, California   Thomas N. Tozer

CONTENTS

1

Why Clinical Pharmacokinetics?

Those patients who suffer from chronic ailments such as diabetes and epilepsy may have to take drugs every day for the rest of their lives. At the other extreme are those who take a single dose of a drug to relieve an occasional headache. The duration of drug therapy is usually between these extremes. The manner in which a drug is taken is called a *dosage regimen*. Both the duration of drug therapy and the dosage regimen depend on the therapeutic objectives, which may be either the cure, the mitigation, or the prevention of disease. Because all drugs exhibit undesirable effects, such as drowsiness, dryness of the mouth, gastrointestinal irritation, nausea, and hypotension, successful drug therapy is achieved by optimally balancing the desirable and the undesirable effects. To achieve optimal therapy, the appropriate "drug of choice" must be selected. This decision implies an accurate diagnosis of the disease, a knowledge of the clinical state of the patient, and a sound understanding of the pharmacotherapeutic management of the disease. Then the questions: How much?, How often?, and How long?, must be answered. The question "how much" recognizes that the magnitudes of the therapeutic and toxic responses are functions of the dose given. The question "how often" recognizes the importance of time, in that the magnitude of the effect eventually declines with time following a single dose of drug. The question "how long" recognizes that there is a cost (in terms of side effects, toxicity, economics) incurred with continuous drug administration. In practice, these questions cannot be divorced from one another. For example, the convenience of giving a larger dose less frequently may be more than offset by an increased incidence of toxicity.

In the past, the answers to many important therapeutic questions were obtained by trial and error. The clinical investigator selected the dose, the interval between doses, and the route of administration and followed the patient's progress. The desired effect and any signs of toxicity were carefully noted, and if necessary, the dosage regimen was adjusted empirically until an acceptable balance between the desired effect and toxicity was achieved. Eventually, after considerable experimentation on a large number of patients, reasonable dosage regimens were established (Table 1–1), but not without some regimens producing excessive toxicity or proving ineffective. Moreover, the above empirical approach left many questions unanswered. Why, for example, does theophylline have to be given every 6 to 8 hours to be effective, while digoxin can be given daily? Why must oxytocin be infused intravenously? Why is morphine more effective given intramuscularly than when given orally? Furthermore, this empirical approach contributes little, if anything, toward establishing a safe, effective dosage regimen of another drug. That is, our basic understanding of drugs has not been increased.

**Table 1–1. Empirically Derived Usual Adult Dosage Regimens of Some Representative Drugs
Before the Introduction of Clinical Pharmacokinetics**[a]

Drug	Indicated Use	Route	Dosage Regimen
Theophylline	Relief of asthma	Oral	160 milligrams every 6 hours
Digoxin	Amelioration of conges-tive cardiac failure	Oral	1.5–2 milligrams initially over 24 hours, thereafter 0.25–0.5 milligram once a day
Oxytocin	Induction and mainte-nance of labor	Intravenous	0.2–4 milliunits/minute infusion
Morphine sulfate	Relief of severe pain	Intramuscular Oral	10 milligrams when needed Not recommended because of reduced effectiveness

[a]Taken from American Medical Association: Drug Evaluations. 2nd Ed., Publishers Science Group, Acton, MA, 1973.

To overcome some of the limitations of the empirical approach and to answer some of the questions raised, it is necessary to delve further into the events that follow drug administration. *In vitro* and *in vivo* studies show that the magnitude of the response is a function of the concentration of drug in the fluid bathing the site(s) of action. From these observations the suggestion might be made that the therapeutic objective can be achieved by maintaining an adequate concentration of drug at the site(s) of action for the duration of therapy. However, rarely is a drug placed at its site of action. Indeed, most drugs are given orally, and yet they act in the brain, on the heart, at the neuromuscular junction, or elsewhere. A drug must therefore move from the site of administration to the site of action. Simultaneously, however, the drug distributes to all other tissues including those organs, notably the liver and the kidneys, that eliminate it from the body.

Figure 1–1 illustrates the events occurring after an oral dose of drug is administered. The rate at which drug initially enters the body exceeds its rate of elimination; the concentrations of drug in blood and in tissue rise, often sufficiently high to elicit the desired therapeutic effects and sometimes even to produce toxicity. Eventually, the rate of drug elimination exceeds the rate of its

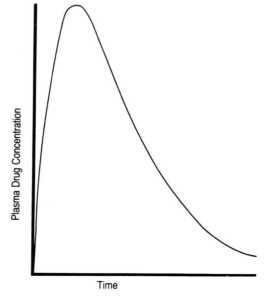

Fig. 1–1. Plasma concentration of drug following an oral dose of a drug. Before the peak is reached, the rate of absorption exceeds that of elimination. At the peak, the two rates are equal and thereafter the rate of elimination exceeds that of absorption.

absorption, and thereafter, the concentration of drug in both blood and tissues declines and the effect(s) subsides. To administer drugs optimally, therefore, knowledge is needed not only of the mechanisms of drug absorption, distribution, and elimination but also of the kinetics of these processes, that is, *pharmacokinetics*. The application of pharmacokinetic principles to the therapeutic management of patients is *clinical pharmacokinetics*.

Drug administration can be divided into two phases, a *pharmacokinetic phase* in which dose, dosage form, frequency, and route of administration are related to drug level–time relationships in the body, and a *pharmacodynamic phase* in which the concentration of drug at the site(s) of action is related to the magnitude of the effect(s) produced (Fig. 1–2). Once both of these phases have been defined, a dosage regimen can be designed to achieve the therapeutic objective. Despite the greater amount of information required with this approach, it has several advantages over the empirical approach. First, and most obvious, distinction can be made between pharmacokinetic and pharmacodynamic causes of an unusual drug response. Second, the basic concepts of pharmacokinetics are common to all drugs; information gained about the pharmacokinetics of one drug can help in anticipating the pharmacokinetics of another. Third, understanding the pharmacokinetics of a drug often explains the manner of its use; occasionally such an understanding has saved a drug that otherwise may have been discarded or has suggested a more appropriate dosage regimen. Lastly, knowing the pharmacokinetics of a drug aids the clinician in anticipating the optimal dosage regimen for an individual patient and in predicting what happens when a dosage regimen is changed.

A basic tenet of clinical pharmacokinetics is that the magnitudes of both the desired response and toxicity are functions of the drug concentration at the site(s) of action. Accordingly, therapeutic failure results when either the concentration is too low, giving ineffective therapy, or is too high, producing unacceptable toxicity. Between these limits of concentration lies a region associated with therapeutic success; this region may be regarded as a "therapeutic window." Rarely can the concentration of the drug at the site of action be measured directly; instead the concentration is measured at an alternative and more accessible site, *the plasma*.

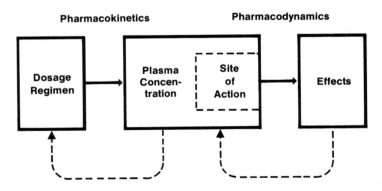

Fig. 1–2. An alternative approach to the design of a dosage regimen. The pharmacokinetics and the pharmacodynamics of the drug are first defined. Then, either the plasma drug concentration-time data or the effects produced, via pharmacokinetics, are used as a feedback (dashed lines) to modify the dosage regimen to achieve optimal therapy.

Based on the foregoing considerations, an optimal dosage regimen might be defined as one that maintains the plasma concentration of a drug within the therapeutic window. For many drugs, this therapeutic objective is met by giving an initial dose to achieve a plasma concentration within the therapeutic window and then maintaining this concentration by replacing the amount of drug lost with time. One popular and convenient means of maintenance is to give a dose at discrete time intervals. Figure 1–3 illustrates the basic features associated with this approach by depicting the concentrations that follow the administration of two regimens, A and B; the dosing interval is the same but the dose given in regimen B is twice that given in regimen A. Because some drug always remains in the body from the preceding dose, accumulation occurs until, within a dosing interval, the amount lost equals the dose given; a characteristic saw-toothed plateau is then achieved. With regimen A, several doses had to be given before drug accumulation was sufficient to produce a therapeutic concentration. Had therapy been stopped before then, the drug might have been thought ineffective and perhaps abandoned prematurely. Alternatively, larger doses might have been tried, e.g., regimen B, in which case, although a therapeutic response would have been achieved fairly promptly, toxicity would have ensued with continued administration.

The synthetic antimalarial agent, quinacrine, developed during World War II to substitute for the relatively scarce quinine, is an example. Quinacrine was either ineffective acutely against malaria or eventually produced unacceptable toxicity when a dosing rate sufficiently high to be effective acutely was maintained. Only after its pharmacokinetics had been defined was this drug used successfully. Quinacrine is eliminated slowly and accumulates extensively with repeated daily administration. The answer was to give large doses over the first few days to rapidly achieve therapeutic success, followed by small daily doses to maintain the concentration within the therapeutic window.

The plateau situation in Figure 1–3 shows that both the width of the therapeutic window and the speed of drug elimination govern the size of the maintenance dose and the frequency of administration. When the window is narrow and the drug is eliminated rapidly, small doses must be given often to achieve therapeutic success. Both theophylline and digoxin have a narrow therapeutic window, but because theophylline is eliminated much more rapidly than digoxin, it has to be given more frequently. Oxytocin is an extreme example; it also has a narrow therapeutic window but is eliminated within minutes. The only means

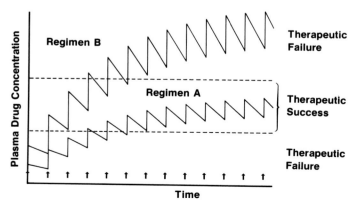

Fig. 1–3. When a drug is given in a fixed dose and at fixed time intervals (denoted by the arrows), it accumulates within the body until a plateau is reached. With regimen A, therapeutic success is achieved although not initially. With regimen B, the therapeutic objective is achieved more quickly but the plasma drug concentration is ultimately too high.

of adequately ensuring a therapeutic concentration of oxytocin therefore is to infuse it at a precise and constant rate directly into the blood. This degree of control is not possible with other modes of administration. Besides, had oxytocin been given orally, this polypeptide hormone would have been destroyed by the proteolytic enzymes in the gastrointestinal fluids. Morphine, given orally, is also destroyed substantially before entering the general circulation, but for a reason different from that of oxytocin. Morphine is rapidly metabolized in the liver, an organ lying between the gastrointestinal tract and the general circulation.

Figure 1–4 illustrates an important problem in drug therapy, variability. There is a wide range of daily dose requirements of the oral anticoagulant, warfarin, needed to produce a similar prothrombin time (an index of blood coagulability). Sources of variability in drug response include the patient's age, weight, degree of obesity, type and degree of severity of the disease, the patient's genetic make-up, other drugs concurrently administered, and environmental factors. The result is that a standard dosage regimen of a drug may prove therapeutic in some patients, ineffective in others, and toxic in still others. The need to adjust the dosage regimen of a drug for an individual patient is evident; this need is clearly greatest for drugs that have a narrow therapeutic window, that exhibit a steep concentration-response curve, and that are critical to drug therapy. Examples are digoxin, used to treat some cardiac disorders; phenytoin, used to prevent epileptic convulsions; theophylline, used to diminish chronic airway resistance in asthmatics; and lidocaine, used to suppress ventricular arrhythmias. With these drugs, and with many others, variability in pharmacokinetics is a major source of total variability in drug response. Accounting for the variability in pharmacokinetics more readily permits improved individual dosage adjustment.

Coadministration of several drugs to a patient, prevalent in clinical practice, is fraught with problems. Each agent may have been chosen rationally, but when coadministered, the outcome can be unpredictable. Cimetidine, for example, devoid of anticoagulant activity, potentiates the hypoprothrombinemic effect of the oral anticoagulant, warfarin. Possible causes of this kind of effect are many. Often, such drug interactions involve a change in pharmacokinetics. Some drugs stimulate drug-metabolizing enzymes and hasten drug loss; others inhibit these enzymes and slow elimination. Many others displace a drug from plasma and tissue binding sites or interfere with its absorption. Such interactions

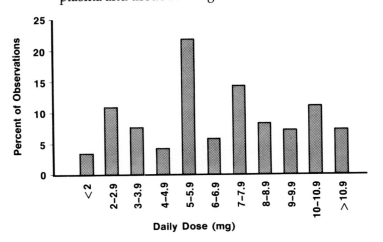

Fig. 1–4. The daily dose of warfarin, required to produce similar prothrombin times in 200 adult patients, varies widely. (Redrawn from Koch-Weser, J.: The serum level approach to individualization of drug dosage. Eur. J. Clin. Pharmacol., 9:1–8, 1975.)

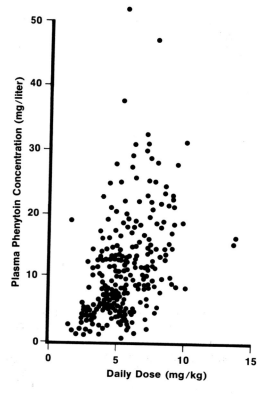

Fig. 1–5.   Although the average plateau plasma concentration of phenytoin tends to increase with the dosing rate, there is considerable variation in the individual values. (One mg/liter = 3.97 micromolar.) (Redrawn from Lund, L.: Effects of phenytoin in patients with epilepsy in relation to its concentration in plasma. *In* Biological Effects of Drugs in Relation to Their Plasma Concentration. Edited by D.S. Davies and B.N.C. Prichard. Macmillan, London and Basingstoke, 1973, pp. 227–238.)

are graded; the change in the pharmacokinetics of a drug varies continuously with the plasma concentration of the interacting drug and hence with time. Indeed, given in sufficiently high doses, any drug will probably interact with another drug. It is always a question of degree. Understanding the quantitative elements of interactions ensures the more rational use of drugs that may have to be coadministered.

Figure 1–5 illustrates a situation in which monitoring of the drug concentration may be beneficial. Over the narrow range of the daily dose of the antiepileptic drug, phenytoin, the plateau plasma drug concentration varies markedly within the patient population. Yet the therapeutic window of phenytoin is very narrow, 7 to 20 milligrams/liter; beyond 20 milligrams/liter, the frequency and the degree of toxicity increase progressively with concentration. Here again, pharmacokinetics is the major source of variability. A pragmatic approach to this problem would be to adjust the dosage until the desired objective is achieved. Control on a dosage basis alone, however, has proved difficult. Control is achieved more readily and accurately when plasma drug concentration data and the pharmacokinetics of the drug are known.

Drug selection and therapy have traditionally been based solely upon observations of the effects produced. In this chapter, the application of pharmacokinetics principles to decision making in drug therapy has been illustrated. Both approaches are needed to achieve optimal drug therapy. This book emphasizes the pharmacokinetic approach. It begins with a consideration of kinetic concepts basic to pharmacokinetics and ends with a section containing selected topics.

Absorption and Disposition Kinetics

2

Basic Considerations

Pharmacokinetics has many useful applications that stem from basic concepts. These concepts are developed in this section of the book. This chapter specifically defines terms and describes a basic model for drug absorption and disposition.

ANATOMIC AND PHYSIOLOGIC CONSIDERATIONS

Measurement of a drug in the body is limited usually to the blood or the plasma. Nonetheless, the limited information obtained has proved very useful. Such usefulness can be explained by the anatomic and physiologic features of the body that affect a drug following its administration.

Blood or plasma, in addition to being a practical and convenient site of measurement, is the most logical one for determining drug in the body. Blood both receives a drug from the site of administration and carries it to all the tissues including those in which the drug acts and those in which it is eliminated from the body. This movement of a drug is depicted schematically in Figure 2–1.

Absorption

There are several sites at which drugs are commonly administered. These sites may be classified as either intravascular or extravascular. *Intravascular* admin-

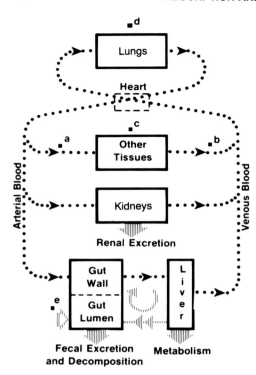

Fig. 2–1. Once absorbed from any of the many sites of administration, a drug is distributed by blood to all sites within the body including the eliminating organs. Sites of administration are: *a*, artery; *b*, peripheral vein; *c*, muscle and subcutaneous tissue; *d*, lung; and *e*, gastrointestinal tract. The dotted (•➤•) and shaded (⸱⫴⸱) lines with arrows refer to the mass movement of drug in blood and in bile, respectively. The movement of virtually any drug can be followed from site of administration to site of elimination.

istration refers to the placement of a drug directly into the blood, either intravenously or intra-arterially.

Extravascular modes of administration include the oral, sublingual, buccal, intramuscular, subcutaneous, dermal, pulmonary, and rectal routes. To enter the blood, drug administered extravascularly must be absorbed: No absorption step is required when a drug is administered intravascularly.

Drug may also be administered regionally, e.g., into the pleural or peritoneal cavities or into the cerebrospinal fluid. Regional administration includes intra-arterial injection into the vessel leading to a tissue, to be treated, e.g., one containing a cancerous tumor. It is a potential means of gaining a selective therapeutic advantage. This advantage, in comparison with other routes of administration, comes about by increasing drug exposure locally, where it is needed, and decreasing or producing little or no change in drug throughout the rest of the body, where it is not wanted.

Distribution

Once absorbed, a drug is distributed to the various tissues of the body. Both rate and extent of distribution are determined by how well each tissue is perfused with blood, tissue size, binding of drug to plasma proteins and tissue components, and permeability of tissue membranes.

Elimination

The two principal organs of elimination, the liver and the kidneys, are shown separately. The kidneys are the primary site for excretion of the chemically unaltered, or unchanged, drug. The liver is the usual organ for drug metabolism; however, the kidneys and other organs can also play an important metabolic role for certain drugs. The metabolites so formed are either further metabolized or excreted unchanged. The liver may also secrete unchanged drug into the bile. The lungs are, or may be, an important route for eliminating volatile substances, for example, the gaseous anesthetics. Another potential route of elimination is via a mother's milk. Although an insignificant route of elimination in the mother, the drug may be consumed in sufficient quantity to affect the suckling infant.

DEFINITIONS

Although the processes of absorption and elimination are descriptive and their meanings are apparent at first glance, it is only within the context of experimental observation that they can be quantified (Chaps. 3, 4, and 6).

Chemical Purity and Analytic Specificity

Before considering each process, a general statement is needed about the chemical purity of prescribed medicines and the specificity of chemical assays.

Over the years, a major thrust of the pharmaceutical industry has been to produce therapeutic agents that are not only as safe and effective as possible but also are well characterized to ensure reproducible qualities. The majority of administered drugs today are therefore essentially pure materials, and coupled with specific analytic techniques for their determination in biologic fluids, definitive information about their pharmacokinetics can be gained. However, a large number of drug substances are not single chemical entities but rather mixtures. This particularly applies to stereoisomers. The most common stereoisomers found together in medicines are optical isomers, or compounds for which their structures are mirror images; the drug substance is usually a racemate, a 50:50 mixture of the l- and d-isomers. Some drug substances contain geometric isomers and still others, especially those of high molecular weight derived from natural products or through fermentation, may be a mixture of structurally related, but chemically distinct, compounds. Each chemical entity within the drug substance can have a different pharmacologic, toxicologic and pharmacokinetic profile. Sometimes these differences are small and inconsequential, other times the differences can be therapeutically important. For example, d-amphetamine is a potent central nervous stimulant whereas l-amphetamine is almost devoid of such activity. Despite such differences, many commonly employed chemical assays do not distinguish between stereoisomers. Obviously, under these circumstances, attempting to quantify the various processes and to relate plasma concentration to response is fraught with problems that are without simple solutions. Notwithstanding these problems, specific information about each chemical entity should be sought whenever possible.

An added problem exists following drug administration, namely the formation of metabolites. To be of value, an analytic procedure must distinguish between drug and metabolite(s). Nowadays, most assays have this desired specificity. A potential problem exists, however, when using radiolabeled drugs. Incorporation of one or more radionuclides, usually ^{14}C and ^{3}H, into the molecular structure allows for simple and ready detection within a complex biologic milieu, but not necessarily of the administered drug. Complete recovery of all of a radiolabeled dose in urine, following oral drug administration, is useful in identifying the ultimate location of drug-related material but may provide little to no information about the drug. For example, almost all of an orally administered drug may have been destroyed in the gastrointestinal tract, from which the degradation products enter the body and are eventually excreted in urine. A basic lesson is learned here. Distinguish carefully between the drug and its metabolite(s). Many metabolites are of interest, especially if they are active or toxic. Each chemical entity must be considered separately.

Absorption

Absorption is defined as the process by which the unchanged drug proceeds from the site of administration to the site of measurement within the body. To illustrate why absorption is defined in this way, consider the events depicted in Figure 2–2, as a drug, given orally, moves from the site of administration to the general circulation. There are several possible sites of loss. One site is the

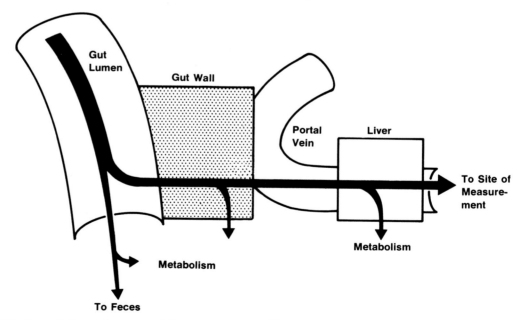

Fig. 2–2. A drug, given as a solid, encounters several barriers and sites of loss in its sequential movement during gastrointestinal absorption. Incomplete dissolution or metabolism in the gut lumen or by enzymes in the gut wall is a cause of poor absorption. Removal of drug as it first passes through the liver further reduces absorption.

gastrointestinal lumen where decomposition may occur. Suppose, however, that a drug survives destruction in the lumen only to be completely metabolized as it passes through the membranes of the gastrointestinal tract. One would ask, Is the drug absorbed? Even though the drug leaves the gastrointestinal tract, it would not be detected in the general circulation. Hence, the drug is not absorbed. Taking this argument one step further, Is the drug absorbed if all of the orally administered drug were to pass through the membranes of the gastrointestinal tract into the portal vein only to be metabolized completely on passing through the liver? In an experiment performed *in vitro* in which the passage of a drug across the intestinal membranes is studied separately, the answer would be positive. If, however, as is common, blood or plasma in an arm vein is the site of measurement, then, because no drug would be detected, the answer would be negative. Indeed, loss at any site prior to the site of measurement contributes to a decrease in the apparent absorption of the drug. The gastrointestinal tissues and the liver, in particular, are often sites of elimination. The requirement for an orally administered drug to pass through these tissues, prior to reaching the site of measurement, makes the extent of absorption dependent on elimination. The loss of drug as it passes, for the first time, through organs of elimination, such as the gastrointestinal membranes and the liver, during the absorption process is known as the *first-pass effect*.

Absorption is not restricted to oral administration. It is equally applicable to events following other routes, for example, intramuscular and subcutaneous, of administration. Monitoring intact drug in blood or plasma offers a useful means of assessing the entry of drug into the body from any site of administration.

Disposition

As absorption and elimination of drugs are interrelated for physiologic and anatomic reasons, so too are distribution and elimination. Once absorbed, a drug is delivered simultaneously by arterial blood to all tissues, including organs of elimination. Viewed from blood or plasma, distinction between elimination and distribution is often difficult. Disposition is the term used when distinction is not desired or is difficult to obtain. *Disposition* may be defined as all the processes that occur subsequent to the absorption of a drug. By definition, the components of disposition are distribution and elimination.

Distribution. Distribution is the process of reversible transfer of a drug to and from the site of measurement, usually the blood or plasma. Any drug that leaves the site of measurement and does not return has undergone elimination, not distribution. For example, once secreted into the bile, a drug may be reabsorbed from the gallbladder or from the intestinal tract. By doing so, the drug completes a cycle, the *enterohepatic cycle* (see Fig. 2–1). If all the drug is reabsorbed in this manner, biliary secretion is not a route of elimination; the cycling is then a component of distribution. The situation is analogous to one in which water is pumped from one reservoir into another, only to drain back into the original reservoir. Biliary secretion is truly a route of elimination only to the extent that the drug fails to be reabsorbed. This failure may result from decomposition in the intestinal lumen, from poor absorption characteristics, or from other complications. Unchanged drug that is neither reabsorbed nor decomposed is excreted in the feces.

Elimination. Elimination is the irreversible loss of drug from the site of measurement. Elimination occurs by two processes, excretion and metabolism. *Excretion* is the irreversible loss of the chemically unchanged drug. *Metabolism* is the conversion of one chemical species to another. Occasionally, drug metabolites are converted back to the drug. As with enterohepatic cycling, this *metabolic interconversion* is a route of elimination only to the extent that the metabolite is excreted or otherwise irreversibly lost from the body.

BASIC MODEL FOR DRUG ABSORPTION AND DISPOSITION

The complexities of human physiology would appear to make it difficult, if not impossible, to model how the body handles a drug. Perhaps surprisingly then, it is a simple pharmacokinetic model, depicted in Figure 2–3, which has proved useful in most applications and is emphasized throughout the majority of this book. More complex models are necessary to describe the pharmacokinetics of some drugs. Examples of such models are described in Chapters 19, 22, and 25.

The boxes in Figure 2–3 can be thought of as *compartments* that logically fall into two classes, transfer and chemical. The site of administration, the body, and the excreta are clearly different places. Each place may be referred to as a location or transfer compartment. In contrast, metabolism involves a chemical conversion, and the metabolite is therefore in a chemical compartment.

The model is based on amounts of drug. However, only the amount of drug in the urine can be measured directly. The amount of drug metabolized includes metabolites in, as well as eliminated from, the body. The amount in the body is usually determined from measurement of the blood or plasma concentration. Estimates of drug in the absorption compartment are also made indirectly from either blood or urine data. Drug at the absorption site includes drug that is

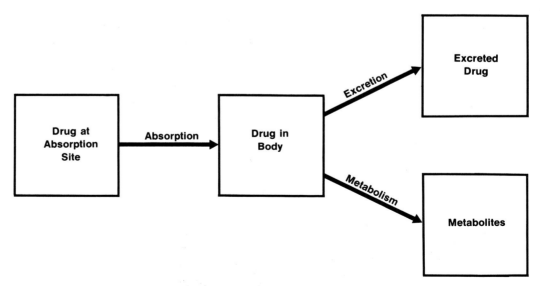

Fig. 2–3. A drug is simultaneously absorbed into and eliminated from the body. The processes of absorption, excretion, and metabolism are indicated with arrows and the compartments with boxes.

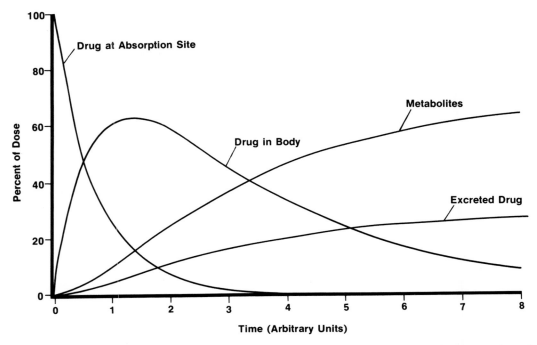

Fig. 2–4. Time course of drug in each of the compartments shown in Figure 2–3. The amount in each compartment is expressed as a percentage of the dose administered. In this example, all the dose is absorbed.

never absorbed, for example, drug that is decomposed in the gastrointestinal tract or lost in the feces.

The model is readily visualized from mass balance considerations. The dose is accounted for at any one time by the molar amount of substance in each of the compartments:

$$\text{Dose} = \frac{\text{Amount at}}{\text{absorption site}} + \frac{\text{Amount in}}{\text{body}} + \frac{\text{Amount}}{\text{metabolized}} + \frac{\text{Amount}}{\text{excreted}} \qquad 1$$

The mass balance of drug and related material with time is shown in Figure 2–4. Since the sum of the molar amounts of drug in transfer and chemical compartments is equal to the dose, the sum of the rates of change of the drug in these compartments must be equal to zero so that:

$$\frac{\text{Rate of change of}}{\text{drug in body}} = \frac{\text{Rate of}}{\text{absorption}} - \frac{\text{Rate of}}{\text{elimination}} \qquad 2$$

The relationships expressed in Equations 1 and 2 apply under all circumstances regardless of the nature of the absorption and the elimination processes. They are particularly useful in developing more complex models for quantifying drug absorption and disposition. *Pharmacokinetics* is the quantitation of the time course of a drug and its metabolites in the body and the development of appropriate models to describe the observations.

Study Problems

(Answers to Study Problems are in Appendix G.)

1. Define the terms listed in the objectives at the beginning of this chapter.

2. Answer each of the following questions, which relate to Figure 2–4 and Equations 1 and 2.

   (a) Does a 100 percent recovery of unchanged drug in the urine following oral administration indicate that the drug is completely absorbed and not metabolized?

   (b) When does drug in the body reach a peak following administration of an oral dose?

   (c) Can the amount of drug absorbed up to a given time be determined?

   (d) When is the rate of change of drug in the body equal to the rate of drug elimination?

   (e) When does the rate of change of drug in the body approach the rate of absorption?

3. Following oral administration of a drug labeled with a radioactive atom, all of the radioactivity was recovered in urine. Can you conclude that the drug was completely absorbed?

3

Intravenous Dose

Objectives

The reader will be able to:

1. **Define the meaning of half-life, elimination rate constant, first-order process, volume of distribution, clearance, renal clearance, and fraction excreted unchanged.**

2. **Estimate the values of half-life, elimination rate constant, volume of distribution, and clearance from plasma or blood concentrations of a drug following an intravenous dose.**

3. **Estimate the values of half-life, elimination rate constant, and fraction excreted unchanged from urinary excretion data following an intravenous dose.**

4. **Estimate the value of the renal clearance of a drug from combined plasma and urine data.**

5. **Calculate the concentration of drug in the plasma and the amount of drug in the body with time following an intravenous dose, given values for the pharmacokinetic parameters.**

Administering a drug intravascularly ensures that all of the dose enters the general circulation. By rapid injection, elevated concentrations of drug in the blood can be promptly achieved; by infusion at a controlled rate, a constant concentration can be maintained. With no other route of administration can such control be as promptly and efficiently achieved. Of the two intravascular routes, the intravenous one is the most frequently employed. Intra-arterial administration, which has greater inherent manipulative dangers, is reserved for situations requiring drug localization in a specific organ or tissue.

The disposition characteristics of a drug are defined by analyzing the temporal changes of drug and metabolites in blood, plasma, and occasionally urine following intravenous administration.

How this information is obtained following a rapid injection of the drug forms the basis of this chapter. The remaining chapter in this section deals with events following an extravascular dose. The pharmacokinetic information so derived forms a basis for making rational decisions in therapeutics, the subject of subsequent sections.

CONCEPT OF A BOLUS

Intravenous administration is most commonly accomplished by infusion. Both rate of infusion and the total amount of drug administered must be considered. For a given dose the shorter the duration of an infusion, the earlier and the higher is the maximum concentration in the body fluids. Usually the onset of pharmacologic response(s) is more rapid and the intensity is greater as well. Maximum concentrations are achieved when the dose is placed instantaneously into the blood as a slug or bolus, but the resulting extremely high concentrations may produce adverse effects. These effects may be circumvented by infusing the drug, but then some time may be required for the effect to appear.

Whenever the intent is to administer a drug as rapidly as possible, even though it is infused, it is often said to be given as a bolus dose. A study with procainamide illustrates this point.

Procainamide is usually given orally and in emergencies intramuscularly for the treatment of cardiac arrhythmias. Procainamide hydrochloride, one gram corresponds to 886-milligrams of the base, can be injected intravenously to define its disposition kinetics. Injecting such a dose within a few seconds would achieve this objective, but the extremely high plasma concentrations produced in these early moments almost certainly would cause a severe lowering of blood pressure. The problem can be avoided by infusing procainamide hydrochloride at a constant rate of 100 milligrams/minute for 10 minutes (Fig. 3–1). Administered in this manner, the peak plasma concentration is below that which produces significant hypotension, while the amount of drug eliminated during the 10-minute infusion is a small fraction of the dose administered. Consequently, from the intent and the lack of elimination, it is said that an intravenous bolus dose of procainamide has been given.

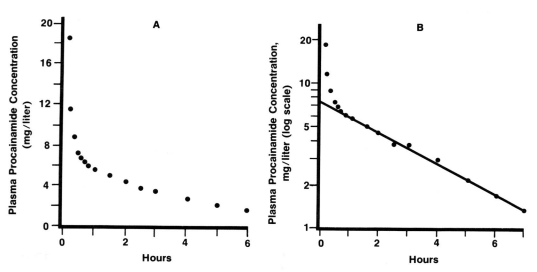

Fig. 3–1. *A*, Concentration of procainamide, expressed as procainamide hydrochloride, in plasma after an intravenous infusion of 1 gram procainamide hydrochloride at the rate of 100 milligrams/minute for 10 minutes into a 70-kilogram volunteer. *B*, The data shown in *A* replotted on semilogarithmic graph paper. Note the short distribution phase. (One mg/liter = 3.7 micromolar.) (Modified from the data of Koch-Weser, J.: Pharmacokinetics of procainamide in man. Ann. N.Y. Acad. Sci., *179*:370–382, 1971.)

DISPOSITION VIEWED FROM PLASMA

Several methods are employed for graphically displaying plasma concentration-time data. One common method, shown with procainamide in Figure 3–1A, is to plot concentration against time on regular (Cartesian) graph paper. Depicted in this manner, the plasma concentration is observed to fall rapidly immediately after giving the bolus, in this case from 18 to 6 milligrams procainamide/liter within 20 minutes. Thereafter, the rate of decline becomes much slower, taking almost another 3 hours before the concentration falls 50 percent to 3 milligrams/liter. Another method of display is a plot of the same data on semilogarithmic paper (Fig. 3–1B). The time scale is the same as before, but now the ordinate (concentration) scale is logarithmic. Notice the sharp break at about 45 minutes when the plasma concentration is about 6 milligrams/liter. Before this time, the fall is rapid. Thereafter, the decline is slower and, on this semilogarithmic plot, appears to continue linearly. The early phase is commonly called the *distribution phase* and the latter, the *elimination phase*. This distinction is sometimes not clear-cut, an aspect more completely discussed in Chapter 19.

Distribution Phase

The distribution phase is so called because distribution primarily determines the early rapid decline in plasma concentration. For procainamide, distribution is extremely rapid and occurs significantly even over the 10-minute period of drug administration. This must be so because the amount of procainamide hydrochloride in plasma at the end of this period is only 48 milligrams. This value is calculated by multiplying the peak plasma concentration, 16 milligrams/liter, by the plasma volume, 3 liters. The majority, 952 milligrams or 95 percent of the total dose (1 gram), must have already left the plasma and been distributed into other tissues. Among these tissues are the liver and the kidneys, which also clear drug from the body. However, for procainamide and for many other drugs, the fraction of the administered dose lost during the distribution phase is small.

Elimination Phase

During the distribution phase, changes in the concentration of drug in plasma reflect primarily movement of drug within, rather than loss from, the body. However, with time, distribution equilibrium of drug in tissue with that in plasma is established in more and more tissues, and eventually, changes in plasma concentration reflect a proportional change in the concentrations of drug in all other tissues and, hence, in the amount of drug in the body. During this proportionality phase, the body acts kinetically as a single container or compartment. As the decline of the plasma concentration is now due only to elimination of drug from the body, this phase is often called the elimination phase.

Elimination Half-life. The elimination phase is characterized by two parameters, the *elimination half-life ($t_{1/2}$) and the apparent volume of distribution (V)*. The elimination half-life is the time taken for the plasma concentration, as well as the amount of the drug in the body, to fall by one-half. The half-life of procainamide, determined by the time taken to fall from 6 to 3 milligrams/liter, is

2.7 hours (Fig. 3–1B). This is the same time that it takes for the concentration to fall from 4 to 2 milligrams/liter or from 2 to 1 milligram/liter. In other words, for procainamide at the dose administered, the elimination half-life is independent of the amount of drug in the body. It follows, therefore, that less drug is eliminated in each succeeding half-life. Initially there is 1 gram in the body. After 1 half-life (2.7 hours), 500 milligrams remain. After 2 half-lives (5.4 hours), 250 milligrams remain, and after 3 half-lives (8.1 hours), 125 milligrams remain. In practice, all the drug (97 percent) may be regarded as having been eliminated by 5 half-lives (13.5 hours).

Volume of Distribution. The concentration achieved after distribution is complete is a result of the dose and the extent of distribution of drug into the tissues. This extent of distribution can be determined by relating the concentration obtained with a known amount of drug in the body. This is analogous to the determination of the volume of a reservoir by dividing the amount of dye added to it by the resultant concentration, after thorough mixing. The volume measured is, in effect, a dilution space.

The apparent volume into which a drug distributes in the body at equilibrium is called the *(apparent) volume of distribution.* Plasma, rather than blood, is usually measured. Consequently, the volume of distribution, V, is the volume of plasma at the drug concentration, C, required to account for all the drug in the body, A.

★

$$V = A/C$$

1

$$\frac{\text{Volume of}}{\text{distribution}} = \frac{\text{Amount in body}}{\text{Plasma drug concentration}}$$

The volume of distribution is useful in estimating the plasma concentration when a known amount of drug is in the body or, conversely, in estimating the dose required to achieve a given plasma drug concentration.

Calculation of the volume of distribution requires that distribution equilibrium be achieved between drug in tissues and that in plasma. The amount of drug in the body is known immediately after an intravenous bolus; it is the dose administered. However, distribution equilibrium has not yet been achieved. An estimate is needed of the plasma concentration that would have resulted had all the drug spontaneously distributed into its final volume of distribution. To do this, use is made of the linear decline during the elimination phase seen in the semilogarithmic plot (Fig. 3–1B).

The decline in plasma concentration during the elimination phase can be characterized by the linear equation

$$\log C = \log C(0) - kt$$

2

where k is the slope of the line in Figure 3–1B and $C(0)$ is the concentration one would determine from this equation at zero time. The negative sign arises because the concentration declines with time. The term $C(0)$ is an extrapolated value and is an estimate of the concentration which when multiplied by the volume term, V, accounts for the dose administered, i.e.,

$$\text{Dose} = V \cdot C(0)$$

3

In practice, $C(0)$ is estimated by extrapolating the straight line in Figure 3–1B back to zero time. In the example with procainamide, $C(0)$ is 7.7 milligrams/liter. Since 1 gram was administered to the patient, the volume of distribution of procainamide is 130 liters. Knowing the volume of distribution, the amount of drug in the body can now be estimated at any time during the elimination phase. For example, when the concentration of procainamide in plasma is 2 milligrams/liter, there are 260 milligrams in the body.

The volume of distribution is a direct measure of the extent of distribution. It rarely, however, corresponds to a real volume, such as plasma volume (3 liters), extracellular water (16 liters), or total body water (42 liters). Drug distribution may be to any one or a combination of the tissues and fluids of the body. Furthermore, the binding to tissue components may be so great that the volume of distribution is many times the total body size. This must be the case for procainamide as its volume of distribution of 130 liters well exceeds body size, approximately 70 liters.

To appreciate the effect of tissue binding, consider the distribution of 100 milligrams of a drug in a 1-liter system composed of water and 10 grams of activated charcoal, and where 99 percent of the drug is adsorbed onto the charcoal. When the charcoal has settled, the concentration of drug in the water phase would be 1 milligram/liter; thus, 100 liters of the aqueous phase would be required to account for all the drug in the system, a volume much greater than that of the total system. Values of the volumes of distribution for selected drugs are shown in Figure 3–2. The causes for this wide range of values are discussed in Chapter 10.

First-Order Elimination. Why the elimination for procainamide (and for most other drugs) is linear when plotted on semilogarithmic paper can be appreciated as follows. Taking the antilogarithm of both sides of Equation 2 yields

$$C = C(0) \cdot e^{-kt} \qquad \bigstar \; 4$$

And multiplying both sides by V, gives

$$A = \text{Dose} \cdot e^{-kt} \qquad \bigstar \; 5$$

since $C \cdot V$ and $C(0) \cdot V$ are the amount of drug in the body and the dose administered, respectively. Equations 4 and 5 enable the concentration and amount of drug in the body at any time to be estimated. When the decline in the plasma concentration or amount of drug in the body can be described by a single exponential term as given by Equations 4 and 5, it is said to be (mono)exponential. Since the elimination half-life ($t_{1/2}$) is the time taken for the concentration and the amount of drug in the body to fall by one-half, e.g., from $C(0)$ to $\frac{1}{2} C(0)$, it follows from Equation 4 that:

$$0.5 = e^{-kt_{1/2}} \qquad 6$$

or

$$e^{-kt_{1/2}} = 2$$

Taking the logarithm of both sides,

$$k \cdot t_{1/2} = \log 2 = 0.693$$

one obtains the important relationship,

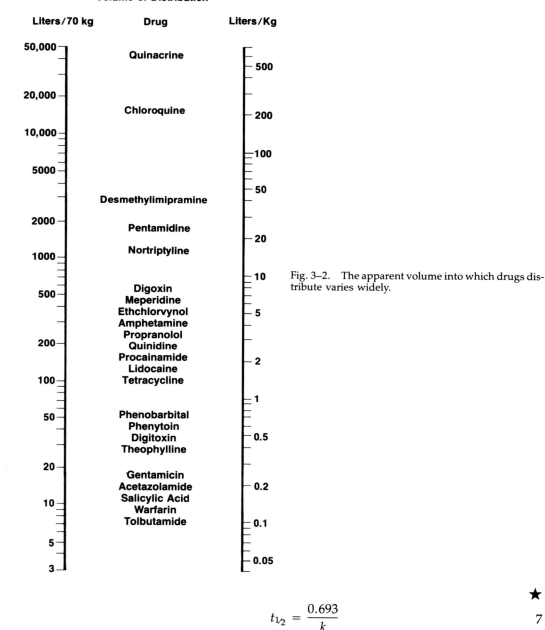

Fig. 3–2. The apparent volume into which drugs distribute varies widely.

$$t_{1/2} = \frac{0.693}{k}$$

★

7

Although the constant k is in the exponent in Equation 4 and can be calculated from Equation 7, its meaning may be better understood by examining the rate at which the amount of drug in the body, A, is changing with time. This is obtained by differentiating Equation 5,

$$\frac{dA}{dt} = -k \cdot \text{Dose} \cdot e^{-kt}$$

8

but since $A = \text{Dose} \cdot e^{-kt}$, it follows that

$$\frac{dA}{dt} = -k \cdot A \qquad\qquad 9$$

The term on the left-hand side of Equation 9 is the rate of change of the amount of drug in the body. During distribution equilibrium, this is also the rate of elimination of drug from the body. Processes such as this, in which the rate of reaction is proportional to the amount present, are known as *first-order processes*. The proportionality constant is known as the *first-order rate constant* with dimensions of time^{-1}. Because k characterizes the elimination process, it is known as the *elimination rate constant*. Since the rate constant can also be defined by rearranging Equation 9 to yield

★

$$k = \frac{\text{Rate of elimination}}{\text{Amount in body}} \qquad\qquad 10$$

the elimination rate constant may simply be regarded as the *fractional rate of drug removal*. For example, since the half-life of procainamide is 2.7 hours, the value of its elimination rate constant is 0.25 hour^{-1}. Hence, the speed of the elimination process of procainamide can be characterized either by its half-life, 2.7 hours, or by saying that the fractional rate of elimination is 0.25 (or 25 percent) of the drug in the body per hour.

It is important to realize that k refers to the fractional rate of elimination and not to the actual amount eliminated per unit time. Consider, for example, that the time scale in Figure 3–1B was in days rather than in hours. The half-life would then be expressed as 0.11 days and the corresponding value for k would be 6.3 days^{-1}. Clearly 6.3 times the amount in the body cannot be eliminated in one day. What is meant is that the fractional rate of elimination, at any moment, is 6.3 times the amount of drug in the body per day. However, because levels in the body decline rapidly, the amount eliminated during the day is, of necessity, less than the dose. To avoid confusion, a unit of time may be selected so that the value of k is much less than 1.

Fraction of Dose Remaining. Another view of the kinetics of drug elimination may be gained by examining how the fraction of the dose remaining in the body varies with time. The fraction remaining is obtained by dividing the amount in the body by the dose administered, which, upon appropriate substitution, yields the following:

★

$$\begin{matrix}\text{Fraction of dose}\\\text{remaining in the body}\end{matrix} = \frac{A}{\text{Dose}} = e^{-kt} \qquad\qquad 11$$

The fraction of the dose remaining is, therefore, given by e^{-kt}. It is useful, however, to express time relative to the half-life. The value of doing so is seen by letting n be the number of half-lives elapsed after the bolus dose ($n = t/t_{1/2}$). Then, as $k = 0.693/t_{1/2}$,

$$\begin{matrix}\text{Fraction of dose}\\\text{remaining in the body}\end{matrix} = e^{-kt} = e^{-0.693n} \qquad\qquad 12$$

Since $e^{-0.693} = \frac{1}{2}$, it follows that

$$\begin{matrix}\text{Fraction of dose}\\\text{remaining in the body}\end{matrix} = (\tfrac{1}{2})^n \qquad\qquad 13$$

Thus, $\frac{1}{2}$ or 50 percent of the dose remains after 1 half-life, and $\frac{1}{4}$ ($\frac{1}{2} \times \frac{1}{2}$) or 25 percent remains after 2 half-lives, and so on.

Total Clearance. Just as the parameter, volume of distribution, is needed to relate the concentration to the amount of drug in the body, so there is a need to have a parameter to relate the concentration to the rate of drug elimination. Clearance (total) denoted by CL, is that proportionality factor. Thus,

★

$$\text{Rate of elimination} = CL \cdot \text{Concentration} \qquad 14$$

The units of clearance, like those of flow, are volume per unit time. For example, if the clearance value is 1 liter/hour, then at a concentration of 1 milligram/liter, the rate of drug elimination is 1 milligram/hour. Ordinarily, as the concentration of a drug increases, so does its rate of elimination; clearance remains the same. From Equation 9, the rate of elimination = $k \cdot A$. Since $A = V \cdot C$; from Equation 1, it follows that

$$\text{Rate of elimination} = k \cdot V \cdot C \qquad 15$$

Comparison of Equations 14 and 15 leads to the relationship

$$\text{Clearance} = k \cdot V \qquad 16$$

Using Equation 16, the (total) clearance of procainamide is calculated to be 33 liters/hour or 0.5 liter/minute. So that at a plasma concentration of 1 milligram/liter, for example, the rate of elimination of procainamide from the body is 0.5 milligram/minute.

Clearance and Elimination Half-life. It is more common to refer to the half-life rather than to the elimination rate constant of a drug. Recall that $t_{1/2} = 0.693/k$, so that half-life is related to clearance by:

★

$$t_{1/2} = \frac{0.693 \cdot \text{Volume of distribution}}{\text{Clearance}} \qquad 17$$

Equation 17 is purposely arranged in the above manner to stress that half-life (and elimination rate constant) reflects rather than controls volume of distribution and clearance. One can independently alter the volume of distribution or clearance and hence change the half-life but not vice versa. In some instances, the volume of distribution and clearance can change by essentially the same extent, in which case the half-life remains unaltered. To show the application of Equation 17 consider the use of creatinine, a product of muscle catabolism, as a marker of renal function. Creatinine has a clearance of 125 milliliters/minute and is evenly distributed throughout the 42 liters of total body water. As expected by calculation using Equation 17, its half-life is 4 hours. Inulin, a polysaccharide also used to assess renal function, has the same clearance as creatinine. However, inulin has a half-life of only 1.5 hours because it is restricted to the 16 liters of extracellular water.

Clearance, Area, and Volume of Distribution. Thus far, clearance has been estimated from the half-life and the volume of distribution of a drug. Clearance can be estimated in another way. By rearranging Equation 14, it can be seen that during a small interval of time, dt,

$$\text{Amount eliminated in interval } dt = \text{Clearance} \cdot C \cdot dt \qquad 18$$

where the product $C \cdot dt$ is the corresponding small area under the plasma drug concentration-time curve. For example, if the clearance of a drug is 1 liter/minute and the area under the curve between 60 and 61 minutes is 1 milligram-minute/liter, then the amount of drug eliminated in that minute is 1 milligram. The total amount of drug eventually eliminated, which for an intravenous dose equals the dose administered, is assessed by adding up or integrating the amount eliminated in each time interval, from time zero to infinite time, and therefore,

★

$$\text{Dose} = \text{Clearance} \cdot AUC \qquad\qquad 19$$

where AUC is the total area under the concentration-time curve. Thus, once the total area under the plasma concentration-time curve is known (Appendix A), clearance is readily calculated. Note that there is no need to know the half-life or volume of distribution to calculate clearance. Furthermore, this calculation of clearance is independent of the shape of the concentration-time profile.

The volume of distribution (V) is used to relate the plasma concentration to the amount of drug in the body during the elimination phase. Often the value obtained by the method of extrapolation (Eq. 3) is a reasonable estimate of this volume term. Occasionally it is not. The best method of calculating the volume of distribution is to divide the clearance by the elimination rate constant

★

$$V = \frac{CL}{k} = \frac{\text{Dose}}{AUC \cdot k} \qquad\qquad 20$$

Unlike the method of extrapolation, the present method of estimating V is not restricted to the intravenous bolus situation but can be obtained under a variety of conditions, e.g., long-term intravenous infusions. Consequently, the value of V, estimated using Equation 20, is applied throughout the remainder of this book, although other volume terms are examined in Chapter 19.

RENAL CLEARANCE

Elimination of drug occurs by renal excretion and extrarenal pathways, usually hepatic metabolism. Not only is renal excretion an important route of elimination for many drugs, but useful pharmacokinetic information can be obtained from analysis of urinary data. Central to this analysis is the concept of *renal clearance*.

Analogous to total clearance, renal clearance (CL_R) is defined as the proportionality term between urinary excretion rate and plasma concentration:

★

$$\text{Excretion rate} = CL_R \cdot C \qquad\qquad 21$$

Renal clearance, like total clearance, has units of flow, usually milliliters/minute or liters/hour.

Practical problems arise, however, in estimating renal clearance following an intravenous bolus dose of drug. Urine is collected over a finite period, e.g., 4 hours, during which the plasma concentration is changing continuously. Shortening the collection period permits one to better estimate the excretion rate at a particular concentration, but this procedure tends to increase error owing to incomplete bladder emptying. This is especially true for periods of urine collection of less than 15 minutes. Lengthening the collection interval, to avoid the problem of incomplete emptying, requires a modified approach to estimate renal clearance. This approach is analogous to that taken with total clearance. By rearranging Equation 21, during a very small interval of time, dt,

$$\text{Amount excreted} = CL_R \cdot C \cdot dt \qquad 22$$

where $C \cdot dt$ is the corresponding small area under the plasma drug concentration-time curve. The urine collection interval (denoted by Δt) is composed of many such very small increments of time, and the amount of drug excreted in a collection interval is the sum of the amounts excreted in each of these small increments of time, that is

$$\begin{array}{l}\text{Amount excreted in} \\ \text{collection interval}\end{array} = CL_R \cdot [AUC \text{ within interval}] \qquad 23$$

As the amount excreted in a collection period is known, the problem in calculating renal clearance rests with estimating the area under the plasma drug concentration-time profile within the time interval (see Appendix A). The average plasma drug concentration during the collection interval is given by (AUC within interval/Δt). This average plasma concentration is neither the value at the beginning nor at the end of the collection time but at some intermediate point. By assuming that the plasma concentration changes linearly with time, the appropriate concentration is that at the midpoint of the collection interval. Because the plasma concentration of drug is in fact changing exponentially with time, this assumption of linear change is reasonable only when drug loss during the interval is small. In practice, the interval should be less than an elimination half-life.

Extending Equation 23 over all time intervals, from zero to infinity, one obtains the useful relationship

$$\bigstar$$
$$\text{Renal clearance} = \frac{\text{Total amount excreted unchanged}}{AUC} \qquad 24$$

where AUC is the total area under the plasma drug concentration-time curve. To apply Equation 24 care must be taken to ensure that all urine is collected for a sufficient period of time to gain a good estimate of the total amount excreted unchanged. In practice, the period of time must be at least 5–6 elimination half-lives of the drug (see Appendix B). Thus, if the half-life of a drug is in the order of a few hours no practical difficulties exist in ensuring urine collections taken over an adequate period of time. Severe difficulties with compliance in urine collection occur, however, for drugs such as digitoxin and phenobarbital with a half-life of about a week, since all urine formed over a period of at least one month must be collected.

DISPOSITION VIEWED FROM URINE ONLY

Lack of sufficiently sensitive analytic techniques previously prevented measurement of the concentration of many drugs in plasma. In the absence of plasma measurements, neither volume of distribution nor clearance can be determined.

Nonetheless, useful information can still be obtained from urine data alone, when such is necessary.

Elimination and Excretion Rate Constant

The elimination half-life of the cardiac glycoside, digitoxin, was estimated from urine data before methods were available for measuring the extremely low concentrations in plasma. The approach was to plot the average excretion rate against the midpoint of the collection time on semilogarithmic paper and, from the slope of the straight line, obtain an estimate of the half-life. Intuitively, the approach is easy to see. Assuming that renal clearance is constant, the urinary excretion rate is proportional to plasma concentration, and plotting urinary excretion rate against time is like plotting plasma concentration against time. The half-life is then taken as the time for the urinary excretion rate (or plasma concentration) to fall by one-half. For digitoxin, this is 5 to 6 days in a healthy subject (Fig. 3–3). Conversely, when a straight line is obtained by plotting the urinary excretion rate against the midpoint time, constancy of renal clearance is inferred. The need for using midpoint time follows from the previous discussion; the measured urinary excretion rate reflects the average plasma concentration during the collection interval. Formal proof of the foregoing discussion is given in Appendix B.

Renal Excretion as a Fraction of Total Elimination

An important pharmacokinetic parameter is the fraction of the amount entering the general circulation that is excreted unchanged, fe. It is a quantitative measure of the contribution of renal excretion to overall drug elimination. Knowing the fraction aids in establishing appropriate modifications in the dosage regimen of a drug for patients with varying degrees of renal function. The value of fe among drugs ranges between 0 and 1.0. When the value is low, excretion is a minor pathway of drug elimination. Occasionally, renal excretion is the only route of elimination, in which case the value of fe is 1.0. By definition the

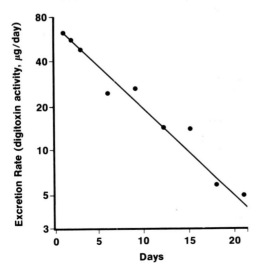

Fig. 3–3. Average daily rate of urinary excretion of digitoxin activity for 13 subjects after a single oral dose of 1.2 milligrams. (One mg = 1.3 micromoles.) (Redrawn from Swintosky, J.V.: Excretion equations and interpretation for digitoxin. Nature, 179:98, 1957.)

difference, $1 - fe$, is the fraction of the amount entering the circulation that is eliminated by extrarenal mechanisms, usually metabolism.

An estimate of fe is most readily obtained from cumulative urinary excretion data following intravenous administration, since by definition

$$fe = \frac{\text{Total drug excreted unchanged}}{\text{Dose}} \qquad 25$$

★

In practice, care should always be taken to ensure complete urinary recovery (i.e., collect urine for at least 5 elimination half-lives). In the case of digitoxin the reported value of fe ranges between 0.3 and 0.35 in patients with normal renal function. At any instant, the fraction fe may be defined as the ratio of the rate of excretion to the rate of elimination,

$$fe = \frac{\text{Rate of excretion}}{\text{Rate of elimination}} \qquad 26$$

Appropriately substituting for numerator and denominator in Equation 26, it is seen that

$$fe = \frac{CL_R \cdot C}{CL \cdot C} = \frac{CL_R}{CL} \qquad 27$$

Thus, fe may also be defined and estimated as the ratio of the renal to total clearance. This is particularly useful in those situations in which total urine collection is not possible.

In practice, estimates of CL and CL_R are obtained directly whereas extrarenal clearance is determined by difference. Thus, extrarenal clearance is $(1 - fe) \cdot CL$.

ESTIMATION OF PHARMACOKINETIC PARAMETERS

To appreciate how the pharmacokinetic parameters defining disposition are estimated consider the plasma and urine data in Table 3–1, obtained following an intravenous bolus dose of 50 milligrams of a drug.

Table 3–1. Plasma and Urine Data Obtained Following an Intravenous Bolus Dose

Observation					Treatment of Data		
Plasma Data		Urine Data			*AUC* Within Time Interval (mg-hour/ liter)	Amount Excreted in Time Interval (mg)	Cumulative Amount Excreted (mg)
Time (hours)	Concen- tration (mg/liter)	Time Interval of Collection (hours)	Volume of Urine (ml)	Concentration of Unchanged Drug in Urine (mg/liter)			
1	2.0	0–2	120	133	4.0	16	16.0
3	1.13	2–4	180	50	2.26	9	25.0
5	0.70	4–6	89	63	1.40	5.6	30.6
7	0.43	6–8	340	10	0.86	3.4	34.0
10	0.20	8–12	178	18	0.80	3.2	37.2
18	0.025	12–24	950	2	0.43	1.9	39.1

Plasma Data Alone

A plot of plasma concentration versus time indicates that the values are dropping progressively, but only after the data are plotted on semilogarithmic paper (Fig. 3–4) can the half-life and elimination rate constant be readily determined. The half-life, taken as the time for the concentration to fall in half (e.g., from 1.0 to 0.5 mg/liter, or 0.2 to 0.1 mg/liter), is 2.8 hours, so that k is 0.25 hour^{-1}. Clearance is determined by dividing dose by the area under the curve. The total area under the plasma concentration-time curve, estimated using the trapezoidal rule (Appendix A), is 10.2 milligrams-hour/liter and when divided into the dose yields a value of 4.9 liters/hour for clearance. The volume of distribution, estimated from CL/k (Eq. 20), is therefore 19.6 liters. This value is virtually identical to that calculated by dividing dose by the intercept concentration at zero time, because no distinct distribution phase is apparent.

Plasma and Urine Data

Both plasma and urine data are required to estimate the renal clearance of the drug. This parameter can be obtained from the slope of a plot of the amount excreted within a collection interval against the area under the plasma concentration-time curve within the same time interval (Fig. 3–5). The straight line implies that the renal clearance is constant and independent of the plasma concentration. The slope of the line indicates that the renal clearance of this drug is 4 liters/hour. Essentially the same value is obtained by multiplying the total clearance (5.0 liters/hour) by fe (0.78) (cf. Eq. 27). The cumulative amount excreted is 39.1 milligrams, so the fraction of the dose excreted unchanged, fe, is 39.1 milligrams/50 milligrams, or 0.78.

Urine Data Alone

The elimination half-life of the drug can be obtained from either excretion rate or cumulative excretion data. The appropriate methods are dealt with in Appendix B.

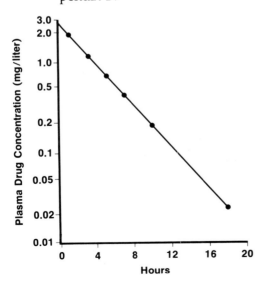

Fig. 3–4. Semilogarithmic plot of the plasma concentration-time data given in Table 3–1.

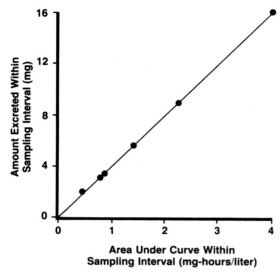

Fig. 3–5. The amount excreted is directly proportional to the area under the plasma concentration-time curve measured over the urine collection interval. Renal clearance is given by the slope of the line. Data from Table 3–1.

A Question of Precision

Had you, the reader, plotted the same data and calculated the pharmacokinetic parameters, you may have obtained answers that differ from those given. This is not unusual and will occur in many cases when you check your answers to the problems at the end of each chapter against those given in Appendix G. The reason lies in differences in the drawing of a line through the data, after they have been plotted, and in rounding-off errors. In addition, all measurements have error associated with analytic methods, conditions of storage, and handling of the sample prior to analysis.

Also, had the study just considered been repeated subsequently in the same individual the estimated half-life may have been 3.1 hours instead of 2.8 hours. For almost all clinical situations, this degree of variation is acceptable. To reflect the acceptable 5 to 10 percent variation, most answers here and throughout the remainder of the book are only given to two or three significant places.

Measurement Fluid

So far, the pharmacokinetics of the drug within the body have been defined with reference to drug in plasma. Sometimes the reference is drug in serum or whole blood. The major difference between plasma and serum is the removal of fibrinogen in the latter case by the clotting of blood, and as most drugs do not bind to fibrinogen, no difference between the concentrations of drug in plasma and serum is expected. Consequently, throughout the book the term plasma is taken to include serum.

Within blood, drug can bind to many constituents including plasma proteins and blood cells. Drug concentrations in whole blood and plasma can differ, thereby yielding different values for many pharmacokinetic parameters, an aspect discussed in some depth subsequently in the book. Accordingly, unlike serum and plasma, blood and plasma cannot be considered to be equivalent, although for many applications in pharmacokinetics the difference is relatively unimportant. Because of ease of clinical analysis, most measurements are made in plasma, rather than in blood.

Strictly speaking, one should use the terminology, *Concentration of drug in plasma (or blood, or plasma water)*. For expediency, throughout the rest of the book we often shorten this phrase to *plasma (or blood) drug concentration*. Indeed, this is sometimes even further shortened to *plasma concentration (or blood concentration)* in many contexts in which concentration of a drug is understood. Similarly, we often use the phrase *amount in body* to refer to the amount of drug in the body.

EFFECT OF DOSE

An adjustment in dose is often necessary to achieve optimal drug therapy. Adjustment is made more readily when the values of the pharmacokinetic parameters of a drug do not vary with dose or with concentration. The possibility for a change with dose exists, however, for many reasons and these are dealt with in Chapter 22 under the title of Dose and Time Dependencies. Throughout the majority of the book, however, the pharmacokinetic parameters are assumed not to change with either dose or time.

Study Problems

(Answers to Study Problems are in Appendix G.)

1. Assuming first-order elimination and intravenous bolus administration, calculate the following.

   (a) How much drug (fraction of initial amount) remains in the body at 4 half-lives?

   (b) The half-life of a drug is 6 hours. What fraction is left in the body at 20 hours?

   (c) Twenty percent of a dose remains in the body at 10 hours. What is the half-life of the drug?

2. Table 3–2 summarizes plasma data obtained after a bolus dose of ceftriazone, a semisynthetic cephalosporin antibiotic, in a newborn infant. (Adapted from Schaad, U.B., Hayton, W.L., and Stoeckel, K.: Clin. Pharmacol. Ther., 37:522–528, 1985.)

Table 3–2. Plasma Concentrations of Ceftriaxone After Intravenous Administration of a 184-milligram (50 milligrams/kilogram) Dose

Time (hours)	1	6	12	24	48	72	96	144
Concentration (mg/liter)	137	120	103	76	42	23	12	3.7

   (a) Plot the plasma concentration of ceftriaxone versus time on three-cycle semilogarithmic paper. Estimate the half-life of the drug.

   (b) Estimate the total area under the plasma ceftriaxone concentration-time curve.

   (c) Estimate the total clearance.

   (d) Calculate the volume of distribution.

3. Plot on linear and on semilogarithmic graph paper the following plasma concentration-time relationship:

$$C = 0.9e^{-0.347t}$$

where C is in milligrams/liter and time is in hours.

4. The data given in Table 3–3 are the plasma concentrations of cocaine hydrochloride as a function of time after intravenous administration of 33 milligrams cocaine hydrochloride to a subject. (Molecular weight of cocaine hydrochloride = 340; molecular weight of cocaine = 303.) (Adapted from Chow, M.J., Ambre, J.J., Ruo, T.I., Atkinson, A.J., Bowsher, D.J., and Fischman, M.W.: Clin. Pharmacol. Ther., *38*:318–324, 1985.)

Table 3–3. Plasma Concentrations of Cocaine Hydrochloride After a Single Intravenous Dose of 33 Milligrams

Time (hours)	0.16	0.5	1.0	1.5	2.0	2.5	3.0
Concentration (micrograms/liter)	170	122	74	45	28	17	10

(a) Prepare a plot of plasma concentration versus time on semilogarithmic paper.

(b) Estimate the half-life and total clearance of cocaine.

(c) Given that the body weight of the subject is 75 kilograms, calculate the volume of distribution of cocaine in liters/kilogram.

4

Extravascular Dose

Objectives

The reader will be able to:

1. Describe the characteristics of, and the differences between, first-order and zero-order absorption processes.

2. Determine whether absorption or disposition rate limits drug elimination, given plasma drug concentration-time data following different dosage forms or routes of administration.

3. Anticipate the effect of altering rate of absorption, extent of absorption, clearance, or volume of distribution on the plasma concentration and amount of drug in the body following extravascular administration.

4. Estimate the availability of a drug, given either plasma concentration or urinary excretion data following both extravascular and intravascular administration.

5. Estimate the relative availability of a drug, given either plasma concentration or urinary excretion data following different dosage forms or routes of administration.

6. Estimate the renal clearance of a drug from plasma concentration and urinary excretion data following extravascular administration.

7. Knowing the availability, estimate clearance, volume of distribution, and elimination half-life from plasma concentration data following extravascular administration.

For systemically acting drugs, absorption is a prerequisite for therapeutic activity when they are administered extravascularly. The factors that influence drug absorption are considered in Chapter 9. In this chapter the following aspects are examined: the impact of rate and extent of absorption on both plasma concentration and amount of drug in the body; the effect of alterations in absorption and disposition on body level-time relationships; and the methods used to assess pharmacokinetic parameters from plasma and urinary data following extravascular administration.

Throughout this book, the term *availability* is used to express the completeness of absorption. Thus, availability is defined as the fraction, or percent, of the administered dose of drug that is absorbed intact.

KINETICS OF ABSORPTION

The oral absorption of drugs in man often approximates first-order kinetics. The same holds true for the absorption of drugs from many other extravascular sites including subcutaneous tissue and muscle. As with other first-order processes, absorption is characterized by an absorption rate constant, ka, and a corresponding half-life. The half-lives for the absorption of drugs administered to man usually range from 15 minutes to 1 hour. Occasionally they are longer.

Sometimes, most of a drug is absorbed at essentially a constant (zero-order) rate. The absorption kinetics are then called *zero order*, because the rate of absorption is proportional to the amount remaining to be absorbed raised to the power of zero. Differences between zero-order and first-order kinetics are illustrated in Figure 4–1. Zero-order absorption, characterized by a constant rate of absorption, is essentially independent of the amount absorbed. A plot of the amount remaining to be absorbed against time on regular graph paper yields a straight line whose slope is the rate of absorption (Fig. 4–1A). Recall from Chapter 3 that the fractional rate of decline is constant for a first-order process; the amount declines linearly with time when plotted on semilogarithmic paper. In contrast, for a zero-order absorption process, the fractional rate of absorption increases with time, because the rate is constant but the amount remaining decreases. This is reflected in an ever-increasing gradient with time in a semilogarithmic plot of the amount remaining to be absorbed (Fig. 4–1B). A method of determining the kinetics of absorption following extravascular administration is given in Appendix C.

For the remainder of this chapter, and for much of the book, absorption is assumed to be first order. If absorption is zero order, then the equations developed in Chapter 6 (Constant-rate Regimens) apply.

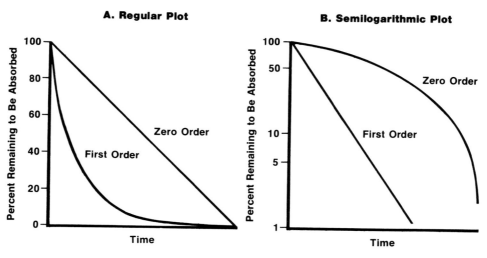

Fig. 4–1. A comparison of zero-order and first-order absorption processes. Depicted are: *A*, cartesian, and *B*, semilogarithmic plots of the percent remaining to be absorbed against time.

BODY LEVEL-TIME RELATIONSHIPS

Comparison with an Intravenous Dose

Absorption delays and reduces the *magnitude of the peak* compared to that seen following an equal intravenous bolus dose. These effects are portrayed for aspirin in Figure 4–2. The rise and fall of the drug concentration in plasma are best understood by remembering that at any time

$$\underbrace{\frac{dA}{dt}}_{\substack{\text{Rate of} \\ \text{change of} \\ \text{drug in} \\ \text{body}}} = \underbrace{\frac{dAa}{dt}}_{\substack{\text{Rate of} \\ \text{absorption}}} - \underbrace{k \cdot A}_{\substack{\text{Rate of} \\ \text{elimination}}} \qquad\qquad 1$$

where Aa is the amount of drug at the absorption site remaining to be absorbed. When absorption occurs by a first-order process, the rate of absorption is given by $ka \cdot Aa$.

Initially, with all drug at the absorption site and none in the body, the rate of absorption is maximal and the rate of elimination is zero. Thereafter, as drug is absorbed, its rate of absorption decreases, whereas its rate of elimination increases. Consequently, the difference between the two rates diminishes. However, as long as the rate of absorption exceeds the rate of elimination the plasma concentration continues to rise. Eventually, a time is reached when the rate of elimination matches the rate of absorption; the concentration is then at a maximum. Subsequently, the rate of elimination exceeds the rate of absorption and the plasma concentration declines.

The peak plasma concentration is always lower following extravascular administration than the initial value following an equal intravenous bolus dose. In the former case, at the peak time some drug remains at the absorption site and some has been eliminated, while the entire dose is in the body immediately

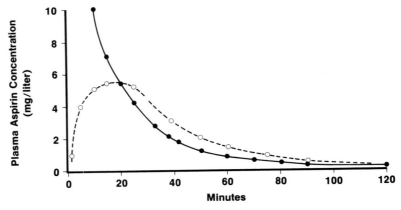

Fig. 4–2. Aspirin (650 mg) was administered as an intravenous bolus (●) and as an oral solution (○) on separate occasions to the same individual. Absorption causes a delay and a lowering of the peak concentration. (One mg/liter = 5.5 micromolar.) (Modified from the data of Rowland, M., Riegelman, S., Harris, P.A., and Sholkoff, S.D.: Absorption kinetics of aspirin in man following oral administration of an aqueous solution. J. Pharm. Sci., *61*:379–385, 1972. Adapted with permission of the copyright owner.)

following the intravenous dose. Beyond the peak time, the plasma concentration on extravascular administration exceeds that following the intravenous dose because of the continual entry of drug into the body.

Frequently, the rising portion of the plasma concentration-time curve is called the absorption phase and the declining portion the elimination phase. As will be seen, this description may be misleading. Also, if drug is not fully available its concentration may remain lower at all times than that observed after intravenous administration.

Lag time is the delay between drug administration and the beginning of absorption. The lag time can be anywhere from a few minutes to many hours. Long lag times have been observed following ingestion of enteric-coated tablets. The coating is resistant to the gastric environment to protect an acid-labile drug or to prevent one that produces gastric irritation from doing so. Contributing factors are the delay in gastric emptying and the time taken for the protective coating to dissolve or to swell and release the inner contents into the intestinal fluids. Once absorption begins, however, it may be as rapid as from uncoated tablets. Clearly, enteric-coated products should not be used when a prompt and predictble response is desired. A method for estimating the lag time is discussed in Appendix C.

Availability and *area* are also important factors. As discussed more fully in Chapters 7 and 9, the completeness of absorption is of primary importance in therapeutic situations. The availability, F, is proportional to the total area under the plasma concentration-time curve, irrespective of its shape. This must be so. Recall from Chapter 3 that:

Total amount eliminated $=$ Clearance $\cdot$ AUC   2

but the total amount eliminated is the amount absorbed, $F \cdot$ Dose, therefore:

$$F \cdot \text{Dose} = \text{Clearance} \cdot AUC$$

Amount   Total amount   3
absorbed   eliminated

Thus, knowing dose, clearance, and area, availability may be determined.

Changing Dose

Increasing the dose, unless this alters the absorption half-life or the availability, produces a proportional increase in the plasma concentration at all times. Hence, the time for the peak remains unchanged, but its magnitude increases proportionally with the dose. The explanation is readily apparent. Suppose, for example, that the dose is doubled. Then, at any given time, the amount absorbed is doubled and, with twice as much entering the body, twice as much is eliminated. Being the difference between the amounts absorbed and eliminated, the amount of drug in the body at any time is, therefore, also doubled. And so too is the total area under the curve. One arrives at the same conclusion by examining Equation 3.

Changing Absorption Kinetics

Alterations in either absorption or disposition produce changes in the time profiles of the amount of drug in the body and the plasma drug concentration.

This point can be illustrated if one considers the three situations depicted in semilogarithmic plots in Figure 4–3, involving changes only in the absorption half-life. All other factors (availability, clearance, and volume of distribution, and hence elimination half-life) remain constant.

In case A, the absorption half-life is much shorter than the elimination half-life. In this case, by the time the peak is reached, most of the drug has been absorbed and little has been eliminated. Thereafter, decline of drug from the body is determined primarily by the disposition of the drug, that is, *disposition is the rate-limiting step*. The half-life estimated from the decline phase is, therefore, the elimination half-life.

In case B, the absorption half-life is longer than in case A but still shorter than the elimination half-life. The peak occurs later because it takes longer for the amount in the body to reach the value at which the rate of elimination matches the rate of absorption; the peak amount is lower because less drug has been absorbed by that time. Even so, absorption is still essentially complete before the majority of the drug has been eliminated. Consequently, disposition remains the rate-limiting step.

Absorption Rate-limited Elimination

Occasionally, the absorption half-life is much longer than the elimination half-life and case C prevails (Fig. 4–3). The peak occurs later and is lower than in

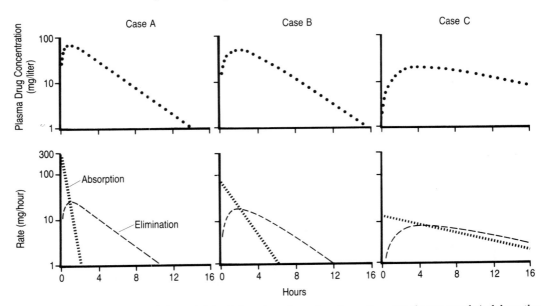

Fig. 4–3. A slowing (from left to right) of drug loss from the absorption site (lower graphs) delays the attainment and decreases the magnitude of the peak plasma drug concentration (top graphs). In Cases A and B (bottom two graphs), absorption (||||||) is a faster process than elimination (-----). In Case C (third graph on bottom), absorption (||||||) rate limits elimination so that decline of drug in plasma reflects absorption rather than elimination; because there is a net elimination of drug during the decline phase, the rate of elimination is slightly greater than the rate of absorption. In all three cases, availability is 1.0 and clearance is unchanged. Consequently, the areas under the plasma concentration-time curves (top three graphs) are identical. The areas under the curves in the bottom graphs are also equal because the integral of the rate of absorption, amount absorbed, equals the integral of the rate of elimination, amount eliminated.

the two previous cases. The half-life of the decline of drug in the body now corresponds to the absorption half-life for the following reason. During the rise to the peak, the rate of elimination increases and eventually, at the peak, equals the rate of absorption. However, in contrast to the previous situations, absorption is so slow that much of the drug remains to be absorbed well beyond the peak time. The drug is either at the absorption site or has been eliminated; little is in the body. In fact, during the decline phase, the drug is eliminated as fast as it is absorbed. *Absorption is now the rate-limiting step.* Under these circumstances, since the rate of elimination essentially matches the rate of absorption, the following approximation ($\approx$) can be written

$$\underset{\substack{\text{Rate of} \\ \text{elimination}}}{k \cdot A} \quad \approx \quad \underset{\substack{\text{Rate of} \\ \text{absorption}}}{ka \cdot Aa} \qquad\qquad 4$$

that is,

$$\underset{\substack{\text{Amount} \\ \text{in body}}}{} \approx \left(\frac{ka}{k}\right) \cdot \underset{\substack{\text{Amount at} \\ \text{absorption} \\ \text{site}}}{} \qquad\qquad 5$$

Accordingly, the amount in the body (and the plasma concentration) during the decline phase is directly proportional to the amount of drug at the absorption site. For example, when the amount at the absorption site falls by one-half, so does the amount in the body. However, the time for this to occur is the absorption half-life.

Absorption influences the kinetics of drug in the body; but what of the area under the plasma concentration-time curve? Because availability and clearance were held constant, it follows from Equation 3 that the area must be the same for cases A, B, and C.

Distinguishing Absorption from Disposition Rate-limited Elimination

Although disposition generally is rate-limiting, the preceding discussion suggests that caution may need to be exercised in interpreting the meaning of the half-life determined from the decline phase following extravascular administration. Confusion is avoided if the drug is given intravenously. In practice, however, intravenous dosage forms of many drugs do not exist for clinical use. An alternative solution to the problem of distinguishing between absorption and disposition rate-limitations is to alter the absorption kinetics of the drug. This is most readily accomplished by giving the drug either in different dosage forms or by different routes. To illustrate this point, two drugs are considered, theophylline and penicillin G.

Food and water influence the oral absorption kinetics of theophylline but not the half-life of the decline phase (Fig. 4–4). Here then, disposition rate-limits theophylline elimination. In contrast, for penicillin, with a very short elimination half-life, intramuscular absorption can become rate-limiting by formulation of a sparingly soluble salt (Fig. 4–5).

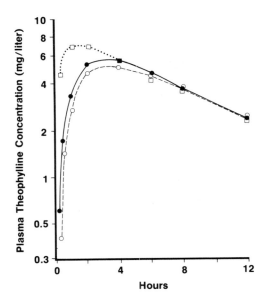

Fig. 4–4. Two tablets, each containing 130 milligrams theophylline, were taken by 6 healthy volunteers under various conditions, Absorption of the theophylline was most rapid when the tablets were dissolved in 500 milliliters water and taken on an empty stomach (□). Taking the tablets with 20 milliliters of water on an empty stomach (○) resulted in slower absorption than taking them with the same volume of water immediately following a standardized high carbohydrate meal (●). Despite differences in rates of absorption, however, the terminal half-life (6.3 hours) was the same and, therefore, it is the elimination half-life of theophylline. (One mg/liter = 5.5 micromolar.) (Modified from Welling, P.G., Lyons, L.L., Craig, W.A., and Trochta, G.A.: Influence of diet and fluid on bioavailability of theophylline. Clin. Pharmacol. Ther., 7:475–480, 1975.)

Changing Disposition Kinetics

What happens to the plasma concentration-time profile of a drug when the absorption kinetics remain constant, but modifications in disposition occur? When clearance is reduced, but availability remains constant, the area under the plasma concentration-time curve must increase; so must both the time and magnitude of the peak concentration. These events are depicted in Figure 4–6. With a reduction in clearance and, hence, elimination rate constant, a greater amount of drug must be absorbed, and the plasma concentration must be greater prior to the time when the rate of elimination equals the rate of absorption.

As shown in Figure 4–7, the events are different when an increased volume of distribution is responsible for a longer elimination half-life. Under these circumstances, if availability and clearance remain unchanged, so does the area under the curve. The peak occurs later and is lower, however. With a larger volume of distribution, more drug must be absorbed before the plasma concentration reaches a value at which the rate of elimination ($CL \cdot C$) equals the rate

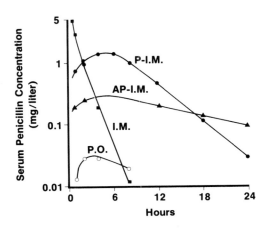

Fig. 4–5. Penicillin G (3 mg/kg) was administered to the same individual on different occasions. An aqueous solution was given intramuscularly (I.M.) and orally (P.O.); procaine penicillin was injected intramuscularly in oil (P-I.M.) and in oil with aluminum monostearate (AP-I.M.). The differing rates of decline of the plasma concentration of penicillin G point to an absorption rate-limitation when this antibiotic is given orally in aqueous solution and intramuscularly as with the procaine salt in oil. Distinction between rate-limited absorption and rate-limited disposition following intramuscular administration of the aqueous solution can only be made by giving penicillin G intravenously. (One mg/liter = 3.0 micromolar.) (Modified from Marsh, D.F.: Outline of Fundamental Pharmacology. Charles C Thomas, Springfield, IL, 1951.)

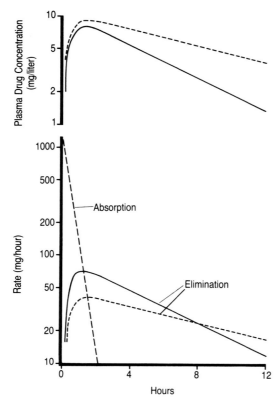

Fig. 4–6.   A twofold reduction in clearance increases the area under the plasma concentration-time (stippled line, top graph) twofold compared to that of the control (solid line) after a single extravascular dose. With no change in absorption kinetics (and hence absorption rate profile) (----, bottom graph), the rate of elimination is observed to be lower at first but to increase to a value greater than that of the control (solid line, bottom graph), as the area under these rate curves must be equal to the dose (see Fig. 4–3). The decrease in clearance causes the peak concentration to be greater and to occur at a later time (only slightly different here). The peak time occurs when the rate of elimination equals the rate of absorption (bottom graph). The terminal slope reflects the increased elimination half-life.

of absorption; the absorption rate is lower then and so is the plasma concentration.

Predicting Changes in Peak

Qualitative changes in peak concentration and the time of its occurrence, when absorption or disposition is altered, are difficult to predict. To facilitate this prediction, a memory aid has been found to be useful. The basic principle of the method (Fig. 4–8) is simple; absorption increases and elimination decreases the amount of drug in the body. The faster the absorption process (measured by absorption rate constant) the greater is the slope of the absorption line, and the converse. The faster the elimination process (elimination rate constant) the steeper is the decline of the elimination line.

If the absorption rate constant is increased, the new point of intersection indicates that the peak amount is increased and that it occurs at an earlier time. If the elimination rate constant is increased, the new point of intersection occurs at an earlier time, but at a lower amount.

The graph is designed for predicting changes in peak time and specifically in peak amount in the body. It applies as well to peak plasma concentration with the exception of when the volume of distribution is altered. An increase in the volume of distribution causes a decrease in the peak concentration, and the converse, as explained under Changing Disposition Kinetics.

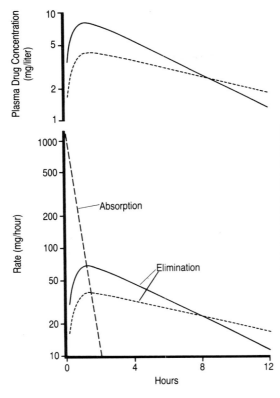

Fig. 4–7. A twofold increase in the volume of distribution causes an increase in the elimination half-life and delays the time at which the peak plasma concentration occurs (stippled line, top graph) compared to the control observation (solid line) after a single extravascular dose. With no change in clearance, the area is unchanged and the peak concentration is thereby reduced. Because of a lower concentration, the rate of elimination is initially slowed (stippled line, bottom graph), but since the amount eliminated is the same (the dose), the rate of elimination eventually is greater than that of the control (solid line, bottom graph).

ASSESSMENT OF PHARMACOKINETIC PARAMETERS

How some parameter values are estimated following extravascular administration can be appreciated by considering both the plasma concentration-time curves in Figure 4–9, obtained following intramuscular and oral administrations of 500 milligrams of a drug, and the additional information in Table 4–1.

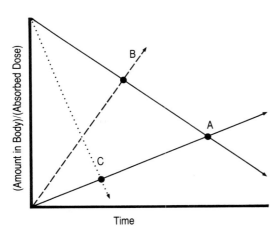

Fig. 4–8. Memory aid to assess changes in peak time and peak amount in the body after extravascular administration of a single dose when absorption or disposition is altered. The relative peak time and the relative peak amount are indicated by the intersection of the absorption and elimination lines (A) with slopes representing the absorption and elimination rate constants, respectively. The predictions for an increased absorption rate constant (dashed line, B) and an increased elimination rate constant (dotted line, C) are shown. (Modified from Øie, S. and Tozer, T.N.: A memory aid to assess changes in peak time and peak concentration with alteration in drug absorption or disposition. Am. J. Pharm. Ed., 46:154–155, 1982).

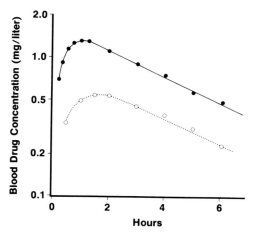

Fig. 4–9.   A 500-milligram dose was given intramuscularly (●—●) and orally (○· · ·○) to the same subject on separate occasions. The drug is less available and is absorbed more slowly from the gastrointestinal tract. A parallel decline, however, implies that in both instances disposition is rate-limiting.

Table 4–1. Data Obtained Following Administration of 500 milligrams of a Drug in Solution by Different Routes

	Plasma Data		Urine Data
Route	Area (mg-hour/ liter)	Half-life; Decay Phase (minutes)	Cumulative Amount Excreted Unchanged (mg)
Intravenous	7.6	190	152
Intramuscular	7.4	185	147
Oral	3.5	193	70

Plasma Data Alone

Availability. Supplemental data from intravenous administration allow calculation of the availability, F. The total area under the concentration-time curve following extravascular administration is divided by the area following an intravenous bolus, appropriately correcting for dose. The basis for this calculation, which assumes that *clearance remains constant,* is as follows:

Intravenous (i.v.) dose

$$\text{Dose}_{i.v.} = \text{Clearance} \cdot AUC_{i.v.} \qquad 6$$

Extravascular (e.v.) dose

$$F_{e.v.} \cdot \text{Dose}_{e.v.} = \text{Clearance} \cdot AUC_{e.v.} \qquad 7$$

which upon division yields

★

$$F_{e.v.} = \left(\frac{AUC_{e.v.}}{AUC_{i.v.}}\right)\left(\frac{\text{Dose}_{i.v.}}{\text{Dose}_{e.v.}}\right) \qquad 8$$

For example, appropriately substituting the area measurements in Table 4–1 into Equation 8 indicates that the intramuscular availability of the drug is 97 percent. This value is sufficiently close to 100 percent to conclude that all drug injected into muscle is absorbed. In contrast, only 46 percent is absorbed when it is given orally in solution.

An alternative method of estimating the availability, which gives the same answer, is to substitute the value for clearance directly into Equation 7. Clearance can be estimated from blood (or plasma) data following either an intravenous bolus dose or a constant-rate intravenous infusion (Chap. 6).

Relative availability is determined when there are no intravenous data. Cost, stability, solubility limitations, and potential hazards are major reasons for the lack of an intravenous preparation. Relative availability is determined by comparing different dosage forms, different routes of administration, or different conditions (e.g., diet, disease state). As with the calculation of availability, clearance is assumed to be constant.

Thus, taking the general case:

Dosage form A

$$F_A \cdot \text{Dose}_A = \text{Clearance} \cdot AUC_A$$
$$\begin{matrix} \text{Amount} \\ \text{absorbed} \end{matrix} \qquad \begin{matrix} \text{Total amount} \\ \text{eliminated} \end{matrix} \qquad\qquad 9$$

Dosage form B

$$F_B \cdot \text{Dose}_B = \text{Clearance} \cdot AUC_B \qquad\qquad 10$$

So that,

★

$$\begin{matrix} \text{Relative} \\ \text{availability} \end{matrix} = \frac{F_A}{F_B} = \left(\frac{AUC_A}{AUC_B}\right) \left(\frac{\text{Dose}_B}{\text{Dose}_A}\right) \qquad 11$$

The reference dosage form chosen is usually the one that is most available, that is, the one having the highest area-to-dose ratio. In the example considered, this would be the intramuscular dose; the relative availability of the oral dose would be 46 percent. If only two oral doses had been compared, they may have been equally, albeit poorly, available. It should be noted that all the preceding relationships hold, irrespective of route of administration, rate of absorption, or shape of the curve. Constancy of clearance is the only requirement.

Other Pharmacokinetic Parameters. Given only extravascular data, it is sometimes difficult to estimate pharmacokinetic parameters. Indeed, no pharmacokinetic parameter can be determined confidently from observations following only a single oral dose. Consider: Area can be calculated without knowing availability, but clearance cannot. Similarly, although a half-life can be ascribed to the decay phase, without knowing whether absorption or disposition is rate-limiting, the value cannot be assigned as the absorption or the elimination half-life. Without knowing any of the foregoing parameters, the volume of distribution clearly cannot be calculated.

Fortunately, there is a sufficient body of data to determine at least the elimination half-life of most drugs. Failure of food, dosage form, and, in the example in Figure 4–7, route of administration to affect the terminal half-life indicates that this must be the elimination half-life of the drug. Also, a drug is nearly always fully available ($F = 1$) from the intramuscular or the subcutaneous site. Hence, clearance can be calculated knowing area (Eq. 3), and the volume of distribution can be estimated once the elimination half-life is known. Consider, for example, just the intramuscular data in Table 4–1. Clearance, obtained by dividing dose (500 mg) by area (7.4 mg-hour/liter), is 1.1 liters/minute. Dividing clearance by the elimination rate constant (0.693/185 minutes) gives the volume of distribution, in this case 300 liters.

Previously, a range of likely absorption half-lives was quoted. The values were estimated indirectly from plasma concentration-time data. Direct measurements of absorption kinetics are impossible because plasma is the site of measurement for both absorption and disposition. To calculate the kinetics of absorption, a method must therefore be devised to separate these two processes. One simple, graphic method for achieving this separation is discussed in Appendix C.

Urine Data Alone

Given only urine data, neither clearance nor volume of distribution can be calculated. If the renal clearance of drug is constant, the rate of drug excretion is proportional to its plasma concentration, and under these circumstances, theoretically, excretion rate data can be treated in a similar manner to the plasma data. In practice, during the first collection of urine, usually 1 or 2 hours after drug administration, absorption of many well-absorbed drugs is complete. Urinary excretion rate data are then of little use in estimating the absorption kinetics of the drug.

Cumulative urine data can be used to estimate availability. The method assumes that the value of fe remains constant. Recall from Chapter 3 that fe is the ratio of the total amount excreted unchanged (Ae_∞) to the total amount absorbed.

★

$$fe = \frac{Ae_\infty}{F \cdot \text{Dose}}$$

12

Then, using the subscripts A and B to denote two treatments, it follows that

$$F_A \cdot \text{Dose}_A = Ae_{\infty,A}/fe$$

13

$$F_B \cdot \text{Dose}_B = Ae_{\infty,B}/fe$$

Amount   Total amount

14

absorbed   eliminated

which upon division gives:

★

$$\frac{F_A}{F_B} = \left(\frac{Ae_{\infty,A}}{Ae_{\infty,B}}\right) \cdot \left(\frac{\text{Dose}_B}{\text{Dose}_A}\right)$$

15

The ratio of the cumulative amount excreted unchanged is therefore the ratio of the availabilities. When dose B is given intravenously, the ratio is the availability of the drug. Otherwise the ratio gives the relative availability. For example, from the cumulative urinary excretion data in Table 4–1, it is apparent that the intramuscular dose is almost completely available; the corresponding value for the oral dose is only 46 percent [(70 mg/152 mg) × 100]. Notice that this value is the same as that estimated from plasma data.

Urine data alone can be particularly useful for estimation of availability when the fraction excreted unchanged approaches 1. Under this condition, changes in renal clearance (and hence total clearance) affect the AUC, but not the amount excreted, which is a direct measure of the amount absorbed. The major problem here is in ensuring complete urine collection for a sufficiently long period of time.

Plasma and Urine Data

When both plasma and urine data are available, in addition to the other pharmacokinetic parameters, the renal clearance of a drug can be estimated. The approach is identical to that taken for an intravenous dose (Chap. 3). Since no knowledge of availability is required, the estimate of renal clearance from combined plasma and urine data following extravascular administration is as accurate as that obtained following intravenous drug administration.

Study Problems

(Answers to Study Problems are in Appendix G.)

1. Depicted in Figure 4–10 are curves of the plasma concentration and of the amount in the body with time following the oral ingestion of a single dose of drug. Draw five pairs of curves identical to those in Figure 4–10. Draw another curve on each pair of these curves that shows the effect of each of the following alterations in pharmacokinetic parameters.

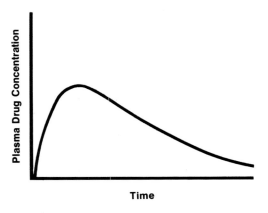
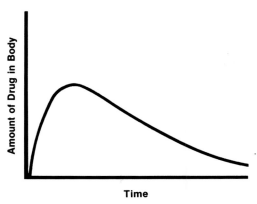

Fig. 4–10.

(a) *V* increased, *k* decreased

(b) *ka* increased

(c) *CL* increased, *k* increased

(d) *CL* decreased, *k* decreased

(e) *F* decreased

In each case, assume that the dose administered and all other parameters (among *F, ka, V, CL*, and *k*) remain unchanged.

2. Channer and Roberts (1985) studied the effect of delayed esophageal transit on the absorption of acetaminophen. Each of twenty patients awaiting cardiac catheterization swallowed a single 500-milligram tablet containing acetaminophen and barium sulfate. The first eleven subjects swallowed the tablet while lying down; in ten of these subjects transit of the tablet was delayed, as visualized by fluoroscopy. In the other nine subjects who swallowed the tablet while standing, it entered the

stomach immediately. In both groups the tablet was taken with a sufficient volume of water to ease swallowing. Table 4–2 lists the average plasma acetaminophen data obtained over 6 hours after swallowing the tablet.

Table 4–2[a]

Time (minutes)	Plasma Acetaminophen Concentration (mg/liter)[b]	
	Subjects standing	Subjects lying down
0	0	0
10	2.1	0.1
20	5.6	0.3
30	5.8	1.1
40	6.3	1.9
50	4.7	2.8
60	4.1	3.2
90	3.5	3.9
120	2.8	3.1
150	2.2	2.9
180	1.8	1.8
210	1.7	1.7
240	1.5	1.5
360	0.7	0.7

[a]Abstracted from Channer, K.S. and Roberts, C.J.C.: Clin. Pharmacol. Ther., *17*:72–76, 1985.
[b]One milligram/liter = 6.6 micromolar.

(a) What effect does delayed esophageal transit have on the speed and extent of absorption of acetaminophen?

(b) What process, absorption or disposition, rate limits the decline in plasma drug concentration?

(c) Acetaminophen is used for the relief of pain. Do the findings of this study affect the recommendation for the use of this drug?

3. Graffner *et al.* (Clin. Pharmacol. Ther., *17*:414–423, 1975) in evaluating different dosage forms of procainamide obtained the following *AUC* and cumulative urine excretion data listed in Table 4–3.

Table 4–3.

Route	Dose (mg)	AUC (mg-hour/liter)	Amount Excreted (0–48 hr) (mg)
i.v.	500	13.1	332
oral			
formulation 1	1000	20.9	586
formulation 2	1000	19.9	554

(a) Estimate both the absolute and relative availabilities of formulation 2 from both plasma and urine data. What are the assumptions made in your calculations?

(b) The half-life of procainamide found in this study was 2.7 hours. Was the urine collected over a long enough time interval to obtain a good estimate of the cumulative amount excreted at infinite time?

(c) Does the renal clearance of procainamide vary much among the three treatments?

4. Kostenbauder *et al.* (1975) measured the plasma phenytoin concentration after the administration of sodium phenytoin intramuscularly (500 mg) and intravenously (250 mg). The average data obtained in 12 subjects, each of whom received both treatments, are listed in Table 4–4.

Table 4–4.[a]

Time (hours)	Route	0	1	2	4	6	8	12	24	48	72	96	120
Plasma Phenytoin	Intramuscular	0	3.0	3.2	3.5	3.2	3.6	3.8	4.1	3.2	1.6	0.8	0.4
Concentration (mg/liter)[b]	Intravenous	5.6	5.4	5.2	4.9	—	3.9	3.2	2.2	0.88	0.42	—	—

[a]Abstracted from Kostenbauder, H.B., Rapp, R.P., McGovren, J.P., Foster, T.S., Perrier, D.G., Blacker, H.M., Hulon, W.C., and Kinkel, A.W.: Clin. Pharmacol. Ther., *18*:449–456, 1975.
[b]One milligram/liter = 4.0 micromolar.

(a) Estimate the completeness of absorption of phenytoin from the intramuscular site based on area comparisons.

(b) From an appropriate plot of the data, comment on the process limiting the decline of the plasma phenytoin concentration following intramuscular administration.

(c) The authors analyzed the plasma concentration-time data and found that, following intramuscular administration, 23 percent of the dose was absorbed within the first hour and thereafter absorption was much slower. The cumulative absorption data are shown in Table 4–5. After the rapid absorption in the first hour, is the subsequent absorption better characterized by a zero-order or a first-order process?

Table 4–5.

Time (hours)	1	6	19	40	65
Percent of available drug absorbed from intramuscular site	23	40	60	80	90

5. Rowland *et al.* (Rowland, M., Epstein, W., and Riegelman, S.: J. Pharm. Sci., *57*:984–989, 1968) gave griseofulvin orally, 0.5 gram of micronized drug, and, on another occasion intravenously, 100 milligrams, to human volunteers. The plasma concentration-time data obtained in one subject are given in Table 4–6 below.

Table 4–6.

Time (hours)	Route	0	1	2	3	4	5	7	8	12	24	28	32	35	48
Plasma Griseofulvin Concentration (mg/liter)[a]	Intravenous	0	1.4	1.1	0.98	0.90	0.80	—	0.68	0.55	0.37	—	0.24	—	0.14
	Oral		0	0.4	0.95	1.15	1.15	1.05	1.2	1.2	0.90	1.05	0.90	0.85	0.80 0.50

[a]One milligram/liter = 2.8 micromolar.

From appropriate plots and calculations, what can be concluded from these data with respect to:

(a) Rate of absorption of the drug with time on oral administration in this individual?

(b) Completeness of absorption?

SECTION TWO

Therapeutic Regimens

5

Therapeutic Response and Toxicity

Objectives

The reader will be able to:

1. **Explain why effect (desired or toxic) of a drug is often better correlated with plasma concentration than with dose.**

2. **Define the terms: graded response, all-or-none response, therapeutic concentration range, utility curve, and tolerance.**

3. **List the range of plasma concentrations associated with therapy for any of the drugs given in Table 5–2.**

4. **Discuss briefly situations in which poor plasma concentration-response relationships are likely to occur.**

The rational design of safe and efficacious dosage regimens is now examined. In this section, fundamental aspects of dosage regimens are covered from the point of view of treating a patient population with a given disease. It is realized, of course, that individuals vary in their response to drugs, and subsequently, in Section Four, attention is turned toward the establishment of dosage regimens in individual patients.

A therapeutic dosage regimen is basically derived from the kinds of information shown in Table 5–1. One consideration includes those factors that relate to both efficacy and safety of the drug, that is, its pharmacodynamics and toxicology. Another consideration is how the body acts on the drug and its dosage form, the essence of pharmacokinetics. A third consideration is that of the clinical state of the patient and his or her total therapeutic regimen. A fourth category includes all other factors such as genetic differences, tolerance, and drug interactions. All of these determinants are, of course, interrelated and interdependent.

Dosage regimens are designed to achieve therapeutic concentrations continuously or intermittently. Intermittent therapy is pertinent if therapeutic concentrations are required only periodically (this has been argued as a desirable condition for antibiotic treatment of some infectious diseases), if tolerance develops to the drug, or if the therapeutic effects of the drug persist and increase in intensity even though the drug rapidly disappears. The objective of most drug therapy is to produce and maintain a therapeutic response. In all cases, attempts

Table 5–1. Determinants of a Dosage Regimen

Activity-Toxicity		Pharmacokinetics
Therapeutic window		Absorption
Side effects		Distribution
Toxicity		Metabolism
Concentration-response		Excretion
relationships		

Dosage Regimen

Clinical Factors		Other Factors
State of patient	Management of therapy	Route of administration
		Dosage form
Age, weight	Multiple drug	Tolerance-dependence
Condition being	therapy	Pharmacogenetics-
treated	Convenience of	idiosyncrasy
Existence of	regimen	Drug interactions
other disease	Compliance of	Cost
states	patient	

are made to minimize undesirable and toxic effects and to prevent ineffective therapy by an appropriate adjustment in the dosage regimen. Optimization of drug therapy is commonly achieved empirically, sometimes at considerable expense, time, and occasional toxicity, by relating response to the dose administered. Evidence exists, however, indicating that response is often better correlated with either the plasma concentration or the amount of drug in the body than with the dose administered.

Accordingly, it would seem to be most appropriate to apply pharmacokinetic principles to the design of dosage regimens. Thus, given pharmacokinetic data following a single dose, the plasma concentration or amount of drug in the body following any dosing scheme can be estimated. Ultimately, however, the value of a dosage regimen must be assessed by the therapeutic and toxic responses produced. Pharmacokinetics simply facilitates the rapid achievement of an appropriate dosage regimen and serves as a useful means of evaluating existing dosage regimens.

In this chapter, various elements of the concentration-response relationship are explored. Principles for attaining and maintaining a therapeutic level of drug in the body are discussed in the subsequent two chapters of this section.

RESPONSE AND CONCENTRATION

Response may be as vague as a general feeling of improvement or as precise as a prothrombin time of 24 seconds in anticoagulant therapy.

Information relating concentration to response has been obtained at three levels: *in vitro* experiments, animal studies, and investigations in both human volunteers and patients. The last level is the most relevant to human drug therapy but, unfortunately, only limited information is obtainable here about the nature of the drug-receptor interaction. *In vitro* experiments, which include studies of the action of drugs on enzymes, on other proteins, on microorganisms, and on isolated tissues and organs, serve this purpose best. However, in isolating the variables, many of the complex interrelationships that exist *in vivo* are destroyed. Animal studies bridge the gap between *in vitro* experimentation and human investigation. Studies in animals introduce both the variable time, with all that it connotes, and the elements of absorption and disposition as well as the feedback control systems that operate to maintain homeostasis. Animal studies are most useful for evaluating the pharmacologic spectrum of activity of a potential therapeutic agent and for determining aspects of its toxicity profile. Irrespective of the level of information, however, the conclusion is the same: A relationship, although sometimes complex, exists between the concentration of drug at the site of measurement and the response.

The majority of drugs used clinically act reversibly in that the effect is reversed upon reducing their concentration at the site of action. Many responses produced are *graded*, so called because the magnitude of the response can be scaled or graded. An example of a graded response, shown in Figure 5–1, is the relaxant effect of terbutaline in an isolated human bronchial muscle strip (contracted with carbachol), in which the intensity of response varies with the drug concentration. Many other pharmacologic and toxic responses do not occur on a continuous basis, and these are known as *quantal* or *all-or-none* responses. An obvious but extreme example is death. Another is the suppression of an arrhythmia. The arrhythmia either is or is not suppressed. Sometimes, a limit is set on a graded response below which an effect is said not to occur clinically. For example, a potentially toxic effect of antihypertensive therapy is an excessive lowering of blood pressure. The lowering of blood pressure produced by the antihypertensive agents is a graded response, but hypotensive toxicity is said to occur only if the blood pressure falls to too low a value. Here the clinical endpoint is all-or-none, but the pharmacologic response is graded.

Returning to terbutaline, Figure 5–1 is a plot of response as a function of the concentration of drug in the fluid bathing the isolated muscle strip. The plot is characteristic of most graded response curves. A nearly linear relationship between the intensity of response and the concentration at low concentrations, and a tendency to reach a maximal response at high concentrations are apparent.

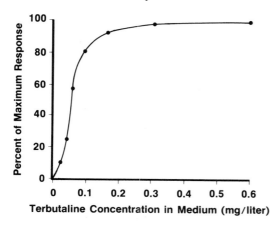

Fig. 5–1. Concentration-response curve for the relaxant effect of terbutaline on an *in vitro* preparation of a human bronchial muscle previously contracted with carbachol. At low terbutaline concentrations, the relaxant effect is essentially proportional to the concentration of terbutaline and approaches a maximum at high concentrations. (One mg/liter = 4.3 micromolar.) (Redrawn from Svedmyr, N., and Thiringer, F.S.: The effects of salbutamol and isoprenaline on beta-receptors in patients with chronic obstructive lung disease. Postgrad. Med. J., 47:44–46, 1971.)

Unlike a graded response, the correlation between a quantal response and concentration is explored by examining the *frequency* of the event with the concentration. The frequency of the suppression of ventricular arrhythmias as a function of the serum procainamide concentration is shown in Figure 5–2. It should be noted that in most patients the arrhythmias are suppressed at concentrations of 2 to 8 milligrams/liter. However, this belies the entire picture.

THERAPEUTIC PLASMA CONCENTRATION RANGE

Figure 5–3 shows the percent of those patients who did not respond to procainamide, those who responded, those who exhibited minor side effects, and those who exhibited serious toxicity. Side effects were considered minor when cessation of the drug was unnecessary and serious when disturbances of cardiovascular function or other adverse effects necessitated discontinuation of the drug. It should be noted in particular that serious toxicity begins to appear above 8 milligrams/liter and occurs with increasing frequency at higher concentrations. Above 16 milligrams/liter, the toxic effects may prove fatal. From these data, it can be concluded that the range of plasma concentrations of procainamide associated with effective therapy and without undue toxicity is 4 to 8 milligrams/liter. This range is commonly known as the *therapeutic concentration range* of the drug.

Clearly, not all patients receiving procainamide for the treatment of ventricular arrhythmias need plasma concentrations between 4 and 8 milligrams/liter. In a few, the arrhythmias are suppressed at concentrations below 4 milligrams/liter; in others, toxicity occurs before efficacy, and for them procainamide is certainly not the drug of choice. Thus, a therapeutic concentration is most appropriately defined in terms of an individual patient's requirements. Usually this infor-

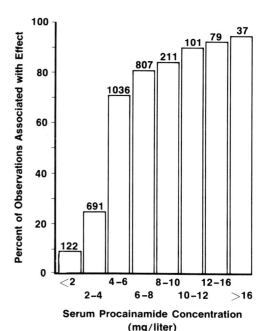

Fig. 5–2. The concentration of procainamide was determined in over 3000 serum samples obtained from 291 patients receiving this drug for the treatment of cardiac arrhythmias. The frequency, expressed as a percent of the number of serum samples with which a serum concentration correlates with effective therapy, increases with each interval of increasing concentration. The value above each bar refers to the number of samples within the respective concentration range. (One mg (base)/liter = 4.3 micromolar.) (From Koch-Weser, J.: *In* Pharmacology and the Future: Problems in Therapy. Edited by G.T. Okita, and G.H. Archeson. Karger, Basel, 1973, Vol. 3, pp. 69–85.)

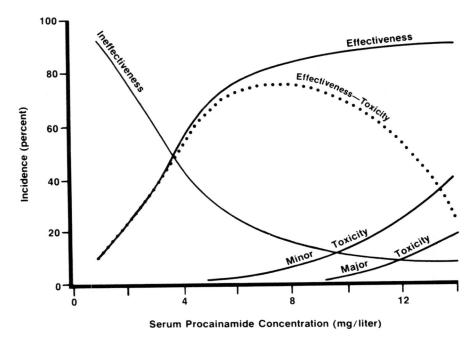

Fig. 5–3. Schematic representation of the frequency of ineffective therapy, effective therapy, minor side effects, serious toxicity, and "therapeutic effectiveness" with serum concentration of procainamide in patients receiving this drug for the treatment of arrhythmias. Therapeutic effectiveness is defined arbitrarily as the difference in the frequency between effective therapy and toxic effects; the therapeutic effectiveness (....) of procainamide reaches a peak at 8 milligrams/liter. (One mg/liter = 4.3 micromolar.) (Adapted from the data of Koch-Weser, J.: In Pharmacology and the Future: Problems in Therapy. Edited by G.T. Okita, and G.H. Archeson, Karger, Basel, 1973, Vol. 3 pp. 69–85.)

mation is unknown, and on initiating therapy, the therapeutic concentration must be estimated from consideration of the probability of therapeutic success within the typical patient population.

The frequency of various effects of procainamide in the patient population is shown schematically in Figure 5–3. A curve is also shown that represents the frequency of therapeutic effectiveness, that is, the frequency of effective therapy minus the frequency of all toxic effects. This may be an inappropriate means of estimating the concentration at which therapeutic success is most probable. Perhaps the minor toxic effects should not be weighted equally against the desired response. Obviously, the major toxic effects should be given more weight. These are considerations of judgment.

Therapeutic Window

Let us expand philosophically on this concept of weighting using the information in Figure 5–3, adding hypersensitivity and assigning values to the responses according to our best judgment. Figure 5–4 shows the probabilities of the responses, plus that of hypersensitivity, each weighted by a judgmental factor versus the logarithm of the plasma concentration. The factor is negative for undesirable effects and the converse. On algebraically adding the weighted probabilities, a *utility curve* is obtained that simply shows the chance of thera-

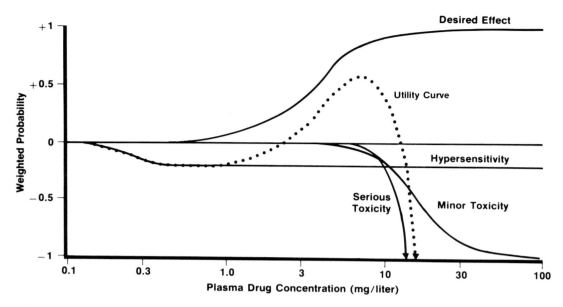

Fig. 5–4. Schematic diagram of the weighted probabilities of responses to procainamide versus the plasma concentration. The probabilities from Figure 5–3 (plus a hypothetical hypersensitivity reaction) are weighted by the following factors: desired effect, 1; hypersensitivity, −5; minor toxicity, −1; serious toxicity, −5. The algebraic sum of the weighted probabilities is the utility curve. According to this scheme, the highest probability of therapeutic success occurs at 7 milligrams/liter and concentrations below 2 milligrams/liter and above 12 milligrams/liter are potentially more harmful than beneficial.

peutic success as a function of the plasma concentration. Both low and high concentrations have a negative utility, that is, at these concentrations the drug is potentially more harmful than helpful. There is an optimum concentration (8 mg/liter) at which therapeutic success is most likely, and there is a range of concentrations (about 4–10 mg/liter) within which the chances of successful therapy are high. This is the *therapeutic window* or *therapeutic concentration range*. Precise limits, of course, are not definable, particularly considering the subjective nature of the utility curve. Each drug produces its own peculiar responses and the values assigned to these responses differ, but both the incidence of the drug effects and the relative importance of each effect must be evaluated to determine the therapeutic concentration range.

There are problems associated with the acquisition of the incidence of the various responses. For example, the procainamide data were obtained in patients who were sometimes titrated with the drug. That is, the dosage was adjusted when the patient had not adequately responded or when toxicity was present. However, patients even on the usual dosage show a wide range of concentrations, leading one to question if selection of patients showing toxicity might have occurred. To avoid this bias, each of the patients should be titrated through all the responses. This is, of course, unacceptable. Our information on toxicity must come from the patient who, for one reason or another, exhibits toxicity because the drug concentration is excessive or who has an unusual response at a low concentration.

For the majority of patients, knowledge of a drug's therapeutic plasma concentration range and pharmacokinetics should lead to a more rapid establishment of a safe and efficacious dosage regimen. However, the narrower this range, the more difficult is the maintenance of values within it. The plasma concentration ranges associated with successful therapy of specific diseases are shown in Table 5–2 for a number of representative drugs.

Several points are worth noting about the data in Table 5–2. First, for most of these drugs, the therapeutic concentration range is narrow; the upper and lower limits differ by a factor of only 2 or 3. Of course, for many other drugs this concentration range is much wider. Second, some drugs are used to treat several diseases, and the therapeutic plasma concentration range may differ with the disease. For example, a much higher plasma concentration of salicylic acid is needed to treat rheumatoid arthritis than is needed to relieve muscle aches. Next, the upper limit of the plasma concentration may be either, like nortriptyline, a result of diminishing effectiveness at higher concentrations without noticeable signs of increasing toxicity or, like digoxin, a result of the possibility of life-threatening toxicity. The upper limit may also be due to limiting effectiveness of the drug, as with the use of salicylic acid to relieve pain. Finally, toxicity may be either an extension of the pharmacologic property of the drug or totally dissociated from its therapeutic effect. The hemorrhagic tendency associated with an excessive plasma concentration of the oral anticoagulant, warfarin, is an example of the former; the ototoxicity caused by the antibiotic, gentamicin, is an example of the latter.

Table 5–2. Representative Drugs and Their Plasma Concentrations Usually Associated with Successful Therapy

Drug	Disease	Therapeutic Window (mg/liter)	(micromolar)
Acetazolamide	Glaucoma	10–30	50–150
Amikacin	Gram-negative infection	12–25[a]	—
Digitoxin	Cardiac dysfunction	0.01–0.02	0.013–0.026
Digoxin	Cardiac dysfunction	0.0006–0.002	0.0008–0.003
Ethosuximide	Epilepsy	25–75	180–540
Gentamicin	Gram-negative infection	4–12[a]	7–21
Kanamycin	Gram-negative infection	12–25[a]	25–50
Lidocaine	Ventricular arrhythmias	1–6	4–25
Lithium	Manic and recurrent depression	—	0.4–1.4[b]
Nortriptyline	Endogenous depression	0.05–0.15	0.2–0.6
Phenobarbital	Epilepsy	10–30	40–120
Phenytoin	Epilepsy	10–20	30–60
	Ventricular arrhythmias	10–20	30–60
Procainamide	Ventricular arrhythmias	4–8	17–34
Propranolol	Angina	0.02–0.2	0.08–0.8
Salicylic Acid	Aches and pains	20–100	150–750
	Rheumatoid arthritis	100–300	750–2200
	Rheumatic fever	250–400	1800–3000
Theophylline	Asthma and chronic obstructive airway diseases	6–20	33–100
Tobramycin	Gram-negative infection	4–12[a]	35–120
Warfarin	Thromboembolic diseases	1–4	3–13
Vancomycin	Penicillin-resistant infection	5–15[c]	3.3–10

[a]Thirty minutes after a 30-minute infusion.
[b]Milliequivalents/liter.
[c]Sample obtained just before next dose.

Therapeutic Correlates

So far, the plasma concentration has been assumed to be a better correlate of a drug's therapeutic response and toxicity, in a population of patients needing a drug, than any other parameter. However, since doses are administered, why not use dose as a therapeutic correlate? Certainly, in most cases, response, plasma concentration, and amount of drug in the body all increase with dose. Still, plasma concentration is expected to be a better correlate than dosage. This must be true following a single dose of drug, since with dose alone no account is taken of time. It is also true for continuous drug administration but for a different reason.

The objective of most drug therapy is to maintain a stable therapeutic response, usually by maintaining an effective plasma concentration. Figure 1–5 (Chap. 1, p. 6) shows the relationship between the steady-state plasma concentration and the rate of administration of phenytoin, expressed as the daily dose per kilogram of body weight. There are large deviations in the plasma concentration at any dosing rate; the plasma concentration ranges from nearly 0 to 50 milligrams/liter when the dosing rate is 6 milligrams/day per kilogram of body weight. Had no correction been made for body weight, the deviations would have been even greater. In contrast, plasma concentration correlates reasonably well with effect. Thus, seizures are usually effectively controlled at concentrations between 10 and 20 milligrams/liter; side effects occur with increasing frequency and severity as the plasma concentration exceeds 20 milligrams/liter, as shown in Figure 5–5. The first sign of toxicity is usually nystagmus, which appears with a concentration of approximately 20 milligrams/liter; gait ataxia usually appears with a concentration approaching 30 milligrams/liter, and prolonged drowsiness and lethargy may be seen with concentrations in excess of 40 milligrams/liter.

It may also be argued that the amount in the body is a better reflection of the pharmacologically active unbound plasma concentration than is the total plasma concentration (Chap. 10, p. 146). Now, instead of a therapeutic plasma concentration range, one may refer to a range of the amount of drug in the body associated with efficacy and with minimal toxicity. While the idea of correlating

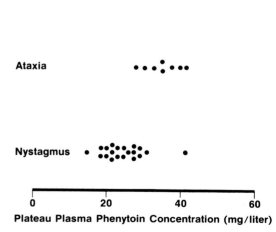

Fig. 5–5. The severity of the untoward effects of phenytoin increases in proportion to its concentration in plasma. (One mg/liter = 4.0 micromolar.) (Modified from Kutt, H., Winters, W., Kokenge, R., and McDowell, F.: Diphenylhydantoin metabolism, blood levels, and toxicity. Arch. Neurol., 11:642–648, 1964. Copyright 1964, American Medical Association.)

response with the amount in the body is attractive, the problem is that in contrast to the plasma concentration the amount in the body is rarely known and cannot easily be measured.

ADDITIONAL CONSIDERATIONS

Measurement of the plasma concentration of a drug, while useful, is not the universal panacea; often it correlates poorly with the measured response. Some examples of poor correlations and their explanations, where known, follow.

Active Metabolites

Unless active metabolites are also measured, poor correlations may exist. For example, based on its plasma concentration, alprenolol is more active as a β-blocker when given as a single oral dose than when administered intravenously. This drug is highly cleared by the liver, and so in terms of the parent drug, the oral dose is poorly available. However, large amounts of metabolites, including an active species, 4-hydroxyalprenolol, are formed during the absorption process, which explains the apparent discrepancy. Other examples of active metabolites and the implications with respect to their pharmacologic response are discussed in Chapter 21.

Tolerance and Acquired Resistance

The effectiveness of a drug can diminish with continual use. Acquired resistance denotes the diminished sensitivity of a population of cells (microorganisms, neoplasms) to a chemotherapeutic agent; tolerance denotes a diminished pharmacologic responsiveness to a drug. The degree of acquired resistance varies; it may be complete, thereby rendering the agent, e.g., an antibiotic, ineffective against a microorganism. The degree of tolerance also varies but is never complete. For example, within days or weeks of its repeated use, subjects develop a profound tolerance but not total unresponsiveness to the pharmacologic effects (euphoria, sedation, respiratory depression) of morphine. Tolerance can develop slowly; for example, tolerance to the central nervous system effects of ethanol takes weeks. Tolerance can also occur acutely (tachyphylaxis). Thus, tolerance, expressed by a diminished cardiovascular responsiveness, develops within minutes following repetitive administration of many β-phenethylamine-type sympathomimetics. At any moment, a correlation might be found between the intensity of response and the plasma concentration of the drug, but the relationship varies with time.

Single-Dose Therapy

One dose of aspirin can often relieve a headache, which does not return even when all the drug has been eliminated. Other examples of effective single-dose therapy include the use of isoproterenol to relieve an acute asthmatic attack, colchicine to treat an acute gouty attack, nitroglycerin to relieve angina, and morphine to relieve acute pain. Although the specific mechanism of action is often poorly understood, the overall effect is known; the drug returns an out-of-balance physiologic system to within normal bounds. Thereafter, feedback control systems within the body maintain homeostasis. The need for the drug has now ended. In these instances of single-dose therapy, a correlation between the effect and the peak plasma concentration of the drug may exist, but beyond the peak, any such correlation is unlikely.

Duration vs. Intensity of Exposure

Some chemotherapeutic agents, e.g., methotrexate, exhibit peculiar relationships between response and dose. The response observed relates more closely to the duration of dosing than to the actual dose used or concentrations produced. This behavior for methotrexate can be explained by its activity as an antimetabolite. It inhibits dihydrofolate reductase, thereby preventing many methylation reactions in the body. These reactions can be inhibited for short periods of time, a few days, without causing permanent biochemical damage. When the exposure is sufficiently prolonged, however, the damage is complete and irreversible.

Time Delays

It often takes some time for a measured response to fully reflect a given plasma concentration of drug. Until then, the continuously changing response makes any correlation between response and plasma concentration extremely difficult to establish. One source of the delay is the time required for equilibration to occur between drug in plasma and that at the site of action, usually in a tissue. This delay may be short if the drug enters the tissue rapidly; when effective, lidocaine suppresses ventricular arrhythmias within a few minutes of giving a

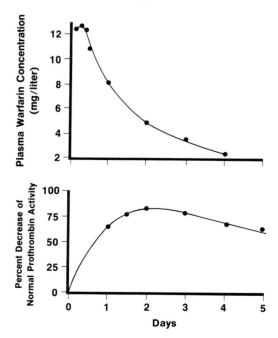

Fig. 5–6. The sluggish response in the plasma prothrombin complex activity to inhibition of its synthesis by warfarin reflects the indirect nature of the measurement and the slow elimination of this complex. For the first two days after giving warfarin, the complex activity steadily decreases. During the first day, the concentration of warfarin is sufficient to almost completely block complex synthesis. As warfarin levels fall, the synthesis rate of the complex increases and by 48 hours equals the rate of degradation of the complex. Thereafter, with the synthesis rate exceeding the rate of degradation, the complex activity rises and eventually, when all the warfarin has been eliminated, it will return to the normal pre-warfarin steady-state level. The data points are the averages following the oral administration of 1.5 milligrams warfarin sodium per kilogram body weight in 5 male volunteers. (One mg/liter = 3.3 micromolar.) (From Nagashima, R., O'Reilly, R.A., and Levy, G.: Kinetics of pharmacologic effects in man: The anticoagulant action of warfarin. Clin. Pharmacol. Ther., *10*:22–35, 1969.)

bolus dose; thiopental induces anesthesia in about the same time. When the target organ resides in a slowly equilibrating tissue, the delay may be many hours. For example, the maximum cardiac effects of digoxin are not seen for an hour or more after administering an intravenous bolus of the drug.

Another source of delay can arise when the response monitored is an indirect measure of drug effect. A change in blood pressure is an indirect measure of either a change in peripheral resistance, in cardiac output, or in both. Plasma uric acid is another example; here, the direct effect is an alteration in uric acid synthesis or elimination. Yet another example of an indirect response is the change in the serum prothrombin complex activity produced by coumarin oral anticoagulants. The more direct effect of these anticoagulants is to inhibit synthesis of the prothrombin complex.

The delay between the attainment of a plasma concentration and the maximal indirect effect varies. Full response in blood pressure to a change in peripheral resistance or in cardiac output occurs within minutes, whereas maximal response of the prothrombin complex activity to warfarin is not seen for one to two days after an oral dose of this anticoagulant (Fig. 5–6).

Uric acid and the prothrombin complex are examples of endogenous materials. Such materials are continuously being renewed, with the pool size reflecting the balance between input and loss. The impact of changes in input and loss on the kinetics of endogenous compounds and the appropriate interpretation of such data are covered in greater detail in Chapter 23, Turnover Concepts.

ACHIEVING THERAPEUTIC GOALS

For those drugs that do not show direct relationships between response and concentration, drug administration must be tailored to the peculiarities of the drug response. Some of these approaches are addressed in Chapter 20 (Pharmacologic Response). The subsequent two chapters present the basic principles for establishing and evaluating dosage regimens for those drugs that show reasonably valid correlations of response with dose and concentration. Chapter 6 examines features of constant-rate input, while Chapter 7 examines the principles underlying the administration of drug in discrete doses to maintain therapy.

Study Problems

(Answers to Study Problems are in Appendix G.)

1. Explain why effect (desired or toxic) is often better correlated with plasma concentration than with dose.

2. List four situations in which poor response-plasma concentration relationships are likely to occur.

3. Define the terms:

   (a) All-or-none response.

   (b) Graded response.

(c) Therapeutic window.

(d) Utility curve.

(e) Tolerance.

4. List the therapeutic plasma concentration ranges of digoxin, gentamicin, lithium, phenobarbital, phenytoin, quinidine, and theophylline, drugs that are commonly monitored.

6

Constant-rate Regimens

Objectives

The reader will be able to:

1. **Define plateau and describe the factors controlling it.**

2. **Describe the relationship between half-life of a drug and time required to approach the plateau following a constant-rate input with or without a bolus dose.**

3. **Estimate the value of half-life, volume of distribution, and clearance of a drug from plasma concentration data obtained during and following constant-rate input.**

4. **Estimate the value of half-life, elimination rate constant, and fraction excreted unchanged from urine data obtained during and following constant-rate input.**

5. **Estimate the value of the renal clearance of a drug from combined plasma and urine data.**

6. **Use pharmacokinetic parameters to predict the plasma drug concentration and the amount of drug in the body with time during and following constant-rate input with or without a bolus dose.**

A single dose of drug may rapidly produce the desired therapeutic concentration of a drug, but this mode of administration is unsuitable when maintenance of plasma or tissue concentrations and effect is desired. To obtain a constant plasma concentration, drug must be administered at a constant rate. This is most reliably accomplished by infusing drug intravenously via either an intravenous drip or a pump, when greater precision is desired. No other mode of administration provides such precise and readily controlled drug administration. It is, however, restricted almost exclusively to hospital settings.

A wider application of constant-rate therapy has become possible with the development and use of constant-rate release devices, which can be ingested or placed at a variety of body sites and which deliver drug for a period of time extending from hours to years. Some examples of these devices and their applications are given in Table 6–1. All such devices are administered extravascularly. When given to produce a systemic effect, absorption is a prerequisite to attain effective plasma concentrations. However, for the purpose of under-

Table 6–1. Representative Constant-Rate Devices and Their Applications

Type of Therapeutic System	Drug	Rate Specification	Application/Comments
Transdermal	Nitroglycerin	2.5, 5, 10, and 15 milligrams over 24 hours	Prophylaxis against attack of angina pectoris. System aims to provide a constant plasma concentration of nitroglycerin. Recommended application site is lateral chest wall.
Transdermal	Clonidine	100, 200, and 300 micrograms/day for one week	Control of blood pressure. System aims to provide constant plasma concentration of clonidine. Recommended application site is upper part of body.
Ocular	Pilocarpine	20 and 40 micrograms/hour for one week	Control of elevated intraocular pressure. System aims to provide a constant rate of input of pilocarpine into the eye.
Oral	Phenylpropanolamine Hydrochloride	25 milligrams immediate release and 3.4 milligrams/hour for 16 hours	Appetite suppressant. System aims to provide a constant and effective plasma concentration of phenylpropanolamine for 16 hours.
Uterine	Progesterone	65 micrograms/day for one year	Contraceptive. System aims to provide a constant and effective uterine concentration of progesterone, an endogenous hormone.

standing the principles in this chapter, drug delivery from these systems is assumed to be equivalent to a constant-rate intravenous infusion.

DRUG LEVEL-TIME RELATIONSHIPS

A drug is said to be given as a constant (rate) infusion when the intent is to maintain a stable plasma concentration or amount in the body. In contrast to the short duration of infusion of a bolus dose, the duration of constant infusion is usually much longer than the half-life of the drug. The essential features of the events following a constant infusion can be appreciated by considering the events depicted in Figure 6–1.

The Plateau Value

At any time during an infusion, the rate of change in the amount of drug in the body (dA/dt) is the difference between the rates of drug infusion and elimination;

$$\frac{dA}{dt} = \underset{\substack{\text{Constant rate} \\ \text{of infusion}}}{R_{\text{o}}} - \underset{\substack{\text{Rate of} \\ \text{elimination}}}{k \cdot A} \qquad\qquad 1$$

or expressing the equation in terms of the concentration of drug in plasma,

$$\frac{V \cdot dC}{dt} = R_{\text{o}} - CL \cdot C \qquad\qquad 2$$

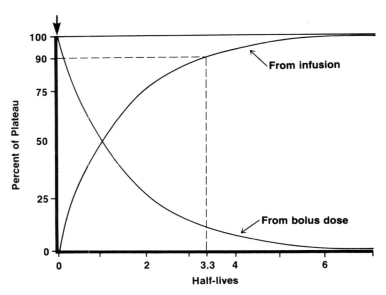

Fig. 6–1.   The approach to plateau is controlled only by the half-life of the drug. Depicted is a situation in which a bolus dose (↓) immediately attains and a constant infusion thereafter maintains a constant amount of drug in the body. As the amount of the bolus dose remaining in the body falls, there is a complementary rise resulting from the infusion. By 3.3 half-lives the amount of drug in the body associated with the infusion has reached 90 percent of the plateau value.

On starting a constant infusion, the amount in the body is zero and hence there is no elimination; therefore the amount in the body rises until the rate of elimination matches the rate of infusion. The amount in the body and the plasma concentration are then said to have reached a *steady state* or *plateau;* these remain stable as long as the same infusion rate is maintained. Since, at plateau, the rate of change of amount of drug in the body is zero, it follows that Equations 1 and 2 simplify to:

★

$$A_{ss} = R_0/k$$

| Amount at steady state | $\dfrac{\text{Infusion rate}}{\text{Elimination rate constant}}$ | 3 |

★

$$C_{ss} = R_0/CL$$

| Concentration at steady state | $\dfrac{\text{Infusion rate}}{\text{Clearance}}$ | 4 |

Clearly the only factors governing the amount of drug at plateau are the rate of infusion and the elimination rate constant. Similarly, only the infusion rate and clearance control the steady-state plasma concentration. Suppose, for illustrative purposes, that a steady-state plasma concentration of procainamide of 4 milligrams/liter is desired. Since the clearance of this drug is 33 liters/hour (Chap. 3), the required infusion rate is 132 milligrams/hour. As the elimination rate constant of procainamide is 0.25 hour^{-1}, the corresponding amount of drug in the body at steady state is 528 milligrams. Alternatively, the amount can be calculated by multiplying the plateau concentration (4 mg/liter) by the volume of distribution of procainamide (133 liters).

To emphasize the factors that control the plateau, consider the following statement: All drugs infused at the same rate and having the same clearance reach the same plateau concentration. This statement is true. The liver and kidneys can clear only what they see. These organs are unaware of differences in tissue distribution among drugs. The rate of elimination depends only on clearance and on the plasma concentration. At plateau, the rate of elimination is equal to the rate of infusion. The plasma concentration must therefore be the same for all drugs with the same clearance if administered at the same rate. However, the amount in the body varies with the volume of distribution. Only drugs for which clearance and volume of distribution are the same will both the plasma concentration and the amount in the body at the plateau be the same when infused at the same rate. Now consider the next statement: When infused at the same rate, the amount of drug in the body at plateau is the same for all drugs with the same half-life. This statement is also true. Drugs with the same half-life have the same elimination rate constant. The elimination rate constant is the fractional rate of drug elimination, that is, the rate of elimination divided by the amount of drug in the body. At plateau the rate of elimination equals the rate of infusion. Hence the amount in the body at plateau must be the same for all drugs with the same half-life. Although the amount in the body is the same, the corresponding plateau concentration of a drug varies inversely with its volume of distribution.

Knowledge of the plateau value at one particular infusion rate helps to predict the infusion rate needed to obtain a different plateau. Thus, provided that clearance is constant, a change in the infusion rate produces a proportional change in the plateau concentration. Returning to the procainamide example, one expects that a rate of 264 milligrams/hour is needed to produce a plateau concentration of 8 milligrams/liter, since an infusion rate of 132 milligrams/hour results in a plateau concentration of 4 milligrams/liter.

Time to Reach Plateau

A delay always exists between the start of an infusion and the establishment of plateau. The sole factor controlling the approach to plateau is the half-life of the drug. To appreciate this point, consider a situation in which a bolus dose is given at the start of a constant infusion to immediately attain the amount at plateau; clearly the size of the bolus dose must be A_{ss}. Thereafter, the amount in the body is maintained at the plateau value by the constant infusion. Imagine that a way exists to monitor separately the drug remaining in the body from the bolus and that accumulating due to the infusion. The events are depicted in Figure 6–1. Drug in the body associated with each mode of administration is eliminated as though the other were not present. The amount associated with the bolus dose declines exponentially and at any time,

$$\text{Amount remaining in the body from bolus dose} = A_{ss} \cdot e^{-kt} \qquad 5$$

However, as long as the infusion is maintained, this decline is always exactly matched by the gain resulting from the infusion. This must be so since the sum always equals the amount at plateau, A_{ss}. It therefore follows that the amount in the body associated with a constant infusion (A_{inf}) is always the difference between the amount at plateau (A_{ss}) and the amount remaining from the bolus dose, namely,

$$A_{inf} = A_{ss} - A_{ss} \cdot e^{-kt} \qquad 6$$

Or, by dividing through by the volume of distribution,

★

$$C_{inf} = C_{ss}[1 - e^{-kt} \qquad 7$$

Thus, both the amount in the body and the plasma concentration (C_{inf}) rise asymptotically toward respective plateau values following constant-rate drug infusion without a bolus dose.

Practically, it may be more useful to discuss accumulation following a constant-rate infusion in terms of the half-life of a drug. Defining n as the number of half-lives elapsed since the start of the infusion ($t/t_{1/2}$), Equations 6 and 7 can be written as,

$$A = A_{ss} [1 - (\tfrac{1}{2})^n] \qquad 8$$

and,

$$C = C_{ss} [1 - (\tfrac{1}{2})^n] \qquad 9$$

The amount of drug in the body, or plasma concentration, expressed as a percent of the plateau value, has been calculated at different times after initiation of an infusion and is shown in Table 6–2. In 1 half-life ($n = 1$), the value in the body is 50 percent of the plateau value. In 2 half-lives ($n = 2$), it is $1 - (\tfrac{1}{2})^2$ or 75 percent of the plateau value. Theoretically, a plateau is only reached when the drug has been infused for an infinite number of half-lives. For practical purposes, however, the plateau may be considered to be reached in 3.3 half-lives (90 percent of the plateau). Thus, the shorter the half-life the sooner is the plateau reached. For example, penicillin G (half-life of 30 minutes) reaches a plateau within minutes (3.3 half-lives is 100 minutes), whereas it takes 2 to 3 weeks of constant phenobarbital administration (half-life of 5 days) before the plateau is reached (3.3 half-lives is 17 days). The important point to remember is that the approach to plateau depends *solely* on the half-life of the drug. For example, because the half-life of procainamide is 2.8 hours, it must be infused

Table 6–2. Percent of the Plateau Level Reached at Various times Following a Constant Infusion of Drug

Time (in half-lives)	Percent of Plateau
0.5	29
1	50
2	75
3	88
3.3	90
4	94
5	97
6	98
7	99

for 9 hours before plateau is reached. This is so whether 132 milligrams/hour is infused to maintain a plateau concentration of 4 milligrams/liter, or the infusion rate is doubled (264 mg/hour) to maintain a plateau concentration of 8 milligrams/ liter. In the latter case, the procainamide plasma concentration at one half-life is one-half the corresponding plateau value of 8 milligrams/liter. So, if one wanted to achieve a plateau concentration of 4 milligrams/liter in 2.7 hours, one could infuse at a rate of 264 milligrams/hour for 1 half-life and then maintain this concentration by halving the infusion rate to 132 milligrams/hour.

Postinfusion

The moment an infusion is stopped, the amount falls by one-half each half-life. Indeed, given only the declining values of a drug, it is impossible to deduce whether a bolus or an infusion had been given. In the example of procainamide, 816 milligrams are in the body at plateau following an infusion rate of 204 milligrams/hour. Approximately 9 hours (3.3 half-lives) after stopping the infusion, only one-tenth of the plateau value or 82 milligrams remains in the body. The same amount of drug would be found in the body 9 hours after an intravenous bolus dose of 816 milligrams of procainamide.

On removal of some transdermal constant-rate release devices, drug continues to be released from binding sites in skin for appreciable periods of time. In these instances, the plasma drug concentration may fall more slowly than after stopping an intravenous infusion.

Changing Infusion Rates

The rate of infusion of a drug is sometimes changed during therapy because of excessive toxicity or an inadequate therapeutic response. If the object of the change is to effect a new plateau, then the time to go from one plateau to another, whether higher or lower, depends *solely* on the half-life of the drug.

Consider, for illustrative purposes, a patient stabilized on a 132 milligram/ hour infusion rate of procainamide, which, according to Figure 6–2, should produce a plateau concentration of 4 milligrams/liter. Suppose the situation now demands a plateau concentration of 8 milligrams/liter. This new plateau value is achieved by doubling the infusion rate to 264 milligrams/hour. Imagine that instead of increasing the drip rate, the additional 132 milligrams/hour was administered at a different site and that a way existed of separately monitoring the procainamide in the body from the two infusions. The events, illustrated in Figure 6–2, show that the procainamide concentration associated with the new infusion will rise to 4 milligrams/liter in exactly the same time as in the first infusion; half the plateau concentration (2 mg/liter) in one elimination half-life (2.7 hours) and so on. Addition of this rising concentration to the pre-existing plateau concentration shows that the half-life is the *sole* determinant of the time required to go from 4 to 8 milligrams/liter. Needless to say, any readjustment in the infusion rate in less than 3.3 half-lives means that a new plateau concentration will not be established.

The decline from a high plateau to a low one is likewise related to the half-life. Consider, for example, the events after stopping the supplementary 132 milligrams/hour infusion rate discussed previously. The procainamide concen-

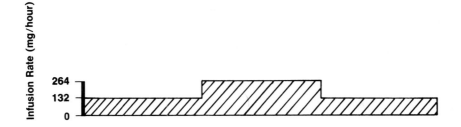

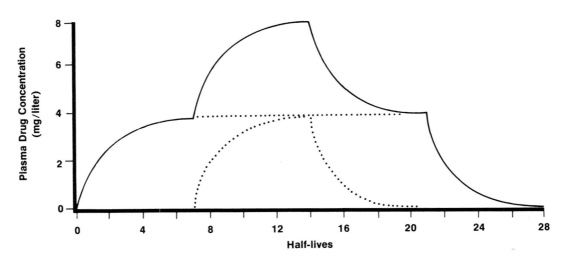

Fig. 6–2. Situation illustrating that the time to reach a new plateau, whether higher or lower than the previous value, depends only on the half-life of a drug. A plateau concentration of 4 milligrams/liter is reached in approximately 3.3 half-lives after starting a constant infusion of 132 milligrams/hour of procainamide. Doubling the infusion rate is like maintaining 132 milligrams/hour and starting another constant infusion of 132 milligrams/hour (....). In approximately 3.3 half-lives the procainamide concentration rises from 4 milligrams/liter to 8 milligrams/liter. Halving an infusion rate of 264 milligrams/hour is analogous to stopping the supplementary 132 milligram/hour infusion. The plasma concentration of procainamide returns to the 4 milligrams/liter plateau in approximately 3.3 half-lives.

tration associated with this supplementary infusion will fall to half the existing value in 1 half-life. In 3.3 half-lives, the total concentration will have almost returned to the preexisting 4 milligrams/liter concentration. Also, it will take another 3.3 half-lives for most of the procainamide to be removed from the body once the original 132 milligrams/hour infusion is stopped.

Bolus and Infusion

It takes approximately 9 hours of constant infusion of procainamide before the plateau concentration is reached. An even longer time is required for drugs with half-lives greater than that of procainamide. Situations sometimes demand that the plateau be reached more rapidly. Figure 6–1 suggests a solution. That is, at the start of an infusion, give a bolus dose, equal to the amount desired in the body at plateau. Usually the bolus dose is a therapeutic dose, and the infusion rate is adjusted to maintain the therapeutic level. When the bolus dose and infusion rate are exactly matched, as in Figure 6–1, the amounts of drug in the body associated with the two modes of administration are complimentary; the gain of one offsets the loss of the other. By 1 half-life, the amounts in the body associated with bolus and with infusion are equal. By 2 half-lives, 75 percent of the plateau results from the infusion. Ultimately, as all the bolus dose is eliminated, the plateau level depends *solely* on the infusion rate.

To emphasize this last point, consider two situations. The first, shown in Figure 6–3, is one in which different bolus doses are given at the start of a constant-rate infusion. In case A, drug is infused alone and the amount rises, reaching a plateau of 200 milligrams in approximately 4 half-lives. In case B, the bolus dose of 200 milligrams immediately attains and the infusion rate thereafter maintains the plateau amount. In case C, the bolus dose of 400 milligrams is excessive. Now, because the rate of loss is initially greater than the rate of infusion, the amount in the body falls. This fall continues until the same plateau as in case B is reached. It should be noticed that the time to reach the plateau depends solely on the half-life of the drug. Thus, in case C at 1 half-life, 300 milligrams, composed of 200 milligrams remaining from the bolus and 100 milligrams from the infusion, lies midway between the bolus dose and the plateau value. By 2 half-lives, the 250 milligrams in the body lies 75 percent of the way toward the plateau. By approximately 4 half-lives, little of the bolus dose remains and the plateau is reached. In case D, the bolus dose of 100 milligrams is below the plateau amount. Because the rate of infusion now exceeds the rate of drug elimination, the amount of drug in the body continuously rises until the same plateau as in the previous cases is reached. Once again the time to approach the plateau is controlled solely by the half-life of the drug.

In the second and more common situation, depicted in Figure 6–4, the same bolus dose and infusion rate are administered to three patients, A, B, and C, with different half-lives and clearance values. The half-lives in these patients are 3, 6, and 9 hours, respectively. All patients start with the same amount of drug in the body. In patient B, this amount is maintained because the rate of infusion is exactly matched by the rate of elimination. Since elimination is slower, the amount in patient C rises until the rate of elimination equals the infusion rate. The time to reach this higher plateau value is governed solely by the half-life of the drug in this patient. Thus, by 1 half-life (9 hours) the amount of drug in patient C is midway between the bolus dose and that at plateau. By the time the plateau is reached all the bolus dose has been eliminated. Also, it follows from Equation 3 that for a given infusion rate, the amount at plateau is proportional to the half-life. This is seen in Figure 6–4, where the amount in patient C at plateau is 50 percent higher than that in patient B. Patient A eliminates the drug more rapidly than does patient B. Accordingly, the amount of drug in patient A falls until a new plateau value, one-half that of patient B, is reached. As always, the approach to plateau is governed solely by the half-life, which in patient A is only 3 hours. Thus, by 3 hours (one half-life) the value has fallen 50 percent of the way toward the plateau, and by 10 hours the plateau is reached.

The approach to plateau during an infusion has been presented so far in terms of the time required to go from the initial concentration (amount) to the plateau. The time to reach any value on approach to plateau can be determined by

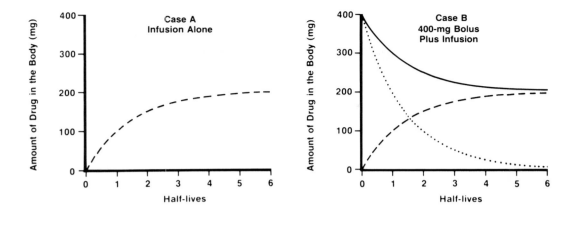

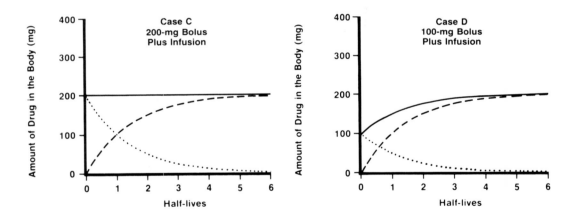

Fig. 6–3. Situations illustrating that the plateau depends upon the infusion rate and not upon the initial bolus dose. Whether a bolus dose is given (Cases B, C, D) or not (Case A) at the start of the infusion, the amount of drug in the body at the plateau is the same. The amount of the bolus dose remaining in the body declines exponentially (....) while the level associated with the infusion in all cases rises asymptotically toward the plateau (——), as portrayed by Case A. In Cases B, C, and D, the observed concentration (○○○○) is the sum of the two. When not initially achieved, it takes approximately 3.3 half-lives to reach plateau (Cases A, B, D). Note in all cases that at 1 half-life the amount in the body lies midway between the initial and plateau amounts.

combining the principles already learned. Recall that the plasma concentration after an intravenous bolus dose is $C = C(0)e^{-kt}$ or $C = C(0)(\frac{1}{2})^n$. The concentration resulting from a constant-rate infusion is given in Equations 7 and 9. As each event is independent of the other, by summing these quantities one obtains the concentration at any time during an infusion when drug is present at the beginning of the infusion.

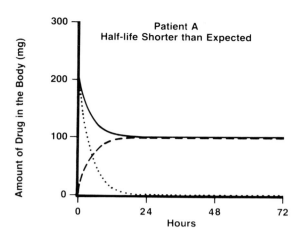

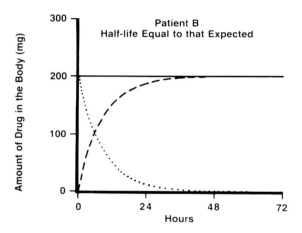

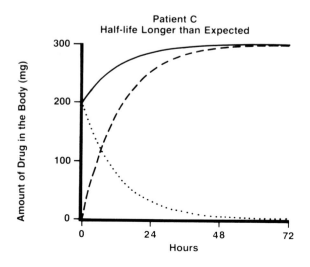

★
10

$$C = C(0)e^{-kt} + C_{ss}(1 - e^{-kt})$$

or

$$C = C(0)(\tfrac{1}{2})^n + C_{ss}[1 - (\tfrac{1}{2})^n]$$

11

For example, if the initial value is 500 micrograms/liter, the plateau value is 100 micrograms/liter, and the concentration to be reached is 110 micrograms/liter, then the time to reach this concentration can be calculated as follows. Rearrangement of Equations 10 and 11 gives

$$e^{-kt} = (\tfrac{1}{2})^n = \frac{C_{ss} - C}{C_{ss} - C(0)}$$

12

Substituting for $C(0)$, C_{ss} and C into Equation 12 yields $(\tfrac{1}{2})^n = 0.025$. Solving for n, a concentration of 110 micrograms/liter is reached in 5.3 half-lives.

Practical Issues

So far, the approach to plateau has been considered in absolute terms. Practically, it is helpful to establish a tolerance, such as ± 10 percent, for the final value. The time required to be within this tolerance varies with the starting and final values. This may be seen by application of Equation 12. For example, if one begins at 80 percent of the final plateau, the time to reach the lower limit of tolerance (90 percent) is only 1 half-life. In contrast, if the starting concentration is 500 percent of the final value, it takes 5.3 half-lives to reach the upper limit of tolerance, 110 percent of the final value. Accepting a tolerance clearly modifies the statement: The time taken to reach plateau is determined solely by the half-life of the drug. Now both the initial and final values must also be considered.

The constant-rate release systems marketed may contain a loading dose to facilitate the more rapid achievement of therapeutic concentrations. Administered extravascularly, however, with the additional absorption step, the attainment of both therapeutic concentrations and plateau will therefore be longer, although perhaps inconsequentially, than that following an equivalent intravenous regimen.

ASSESSMENT OF PHARMACOKINETIC PARAMETERS

Pharmacokinetic parameters are generally determined just as readily from constant-rate data as from intravenous bolus data. Certainly, this is so for an

Fig. 6–4.　Situations illustrating that the plateau depends on the half-life. The same bolus dose and constant infusion are given to patients A, B, and C, with half-lives of 3, 6, and 9 hours, respectively. Although the amount of drug in the initial bolus is the same in all three patients, the amount in the body at the plateau differs in direct proportion to their respective half-lives. The amount of the bolus dose remaining (····) with time depends on the individual's half-life, as does the rise in the amount in the body associated with the constant infusion (----). Only when the rate of loss is immediately matched by the rate of the infusion is the plateau immediately attained and maintained (patient B). Otherwise, the amount in the body (——) changes, until after approximately 3.3 half-lives a plateau is reached (patients A and C).

intravenous infusion. Following the use of constant-rate release devices administered extravascularly, uncertainty exists about availability, which therefore requires reference to intravenous data. Nonetheless, how estimates of pharmacokinetic parameters are made is seen by considering the plasma concentration data in Table 6–3, obtained during and after an intravenous infusion of a drug.

Plasma Data Alone

Consider, for the moment, that measurements only during the infusion were available. What can be estimated?

First, dividing the infusion rate of 40 milligrams/hour by the plateau concentration of 9.5 milligrams/liter gives the clearance, in this case 4.2 liters/hour. Indeed, this is the preferred method for estimating clearance since the plateau concentration can be determined with great precision by averaging those concentrations that clearly lie at the plateau.

Table 6–3. Plasma Concentration of a Drug During and After a Constant Infusion (40 mg/hour) for 12 Hours

	Observation		Treatment of Data
	Time (hours)	Plasma Concentration (C, mg/liter)	$C_{ss}^{a} - C$ (mg/liter)
During infusion			
	1	3.3	6.2
	2	5.4	4.1
	4	7.6	1.9
	6	8.7	0.8
	8	9.3	0.2
	10	9.6	−0.1
	12	9.5	0.0
Postinfusion			
	2	4.1	
	4	1.8	
	6	0.76	
	8	0.33	
	10	0.14	

[a]The concentration at the 12th hour of infusion.

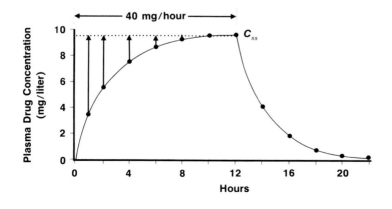

Fig. 6–5. Estimation of pharmacokinetic parameters from plasma data during and after a constant infusion. The vertical arrows represent the differences between the plateau concentration and the concentration observed during the infusion.

Second, the half-life is easily ascertained, being the time taken to reach half the plateau concentration. However, in this example and in most cases, no sample was taken at this time, and so one must interpolate between the observed data. The half-life, estimated in this manner (Fig. 6–5), is approximately 1.5 hours. A more accurate method of estimating the half-life uses all the data obtained during the infusion. Upon rearranging Equation 7, one obtains

$$C_{ss} - C = C_{ss} \cdot e^{-kt} \qquad\qquad 13$$

which upon taking logarithms yields

$$\log (C_{ss} - C) = \log C_{ss} - k \cdot t \qquad\qquad 14$$

Thus, the decline obtained by plotting the difference, between the plateau concentration and that at earlier times, against the corresponding time on semilogarithmic paper should be a straight line. The intercept at time zero is the plateau concentration (C_{ss}) and the slope is $-k$. These differences in concentration, shown by vertical lines in Figure 6–5, are presented in Table 6–3 and have been plotted in Figure 6–6. The data indicate a half-life of 1.7 hours. It should be noted that the longer the period of infusion, the closer the concentration approaches the plateau concentration and the greater is the error in the difference measurement. Generally, difference values calculated from concentrations beyond 90 percent of the plateau are of little value.

Last, the volume of distribution is calculated knowing clearance and half-life; in this case it is 10 liters.

Consider now the concentration data at and after the end of the infusion. Plotting these data on semilogarithmic paper also gives a straight line, from which the half-life can be determined, since after stopping the infusion

$$C = C_{ss} \cdot e^{-kt} \qquad\qquad 15$$

When these data are so plotted, they are observed to superimpose on the previous difference data (Fig. 6–6). In the particular example studied, the half-lives determined from the rising and declining curves are equal. Occasionally they differ, thereby indicating that drug disposition has changed over the period of study.

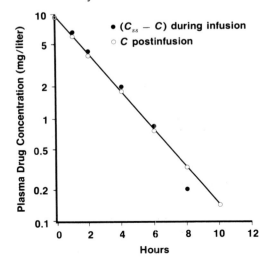

Fig. 6–6. Semilogarithmic plot of the difference (●) between the plateau drug concentration and that observed during the infusion against time. Also plotted are the declining values of the plasma drug concentration (○) against time after stopping the infusion.

Urine Data Alone

If the renal clearance is constant, the rate of excretion is proportional to the plasma concentration. Then excretion rate data can be treated in a manner analogous to that of plasma data, and estimates can be made of elimination half-life and fraction excreted unchanged (*fe*). An estimate of *fe* is obtained at plateau from

$$fe = \frac{\text{Rate of excretion at plateau}}{\text{Rate of infusion}} \qquad 16$$

because the rate of infusion is equal to the rate of elimination. For example, when the infusion rate is 40 milligrams/hour, the observed excretion rate at plateau for the drug is 12 milligrams/hour, so *fe* is 0.3.

Plasma and Urine Data

Without plasma data one cannot estimate a value for volume of distribution or clearance. When both plasma and urine data are available, renal clearance can be estimated in addition to all the other pharmacokinetic parameters. Moreover, a steady-state experiment, achieved with constant infusion is the preferred method for estimating renal clearance. At plateau, accurate measurements can be made of both plasma concentration and urine excretion rate. In the preceding example renal clearance, obtained by dividing excretion rate at plateau by C_{ss}, is 1.26 liters/hour.

Study Problems

(Answers to Study Problems are in Appendix G.)

1. In the text on page 73 the practical view of the approach to plateau was presented. If the tolerance had been 15 percent, instead of 10 percent, what would be the time, in half-lives, to reach this value when the initial concentration is:

   (a) 80 percent of the final value.

   (b) 500 percent of the final value.

2. For prolonged surgical procedures succinylcholine has been given by intravenous drip infusion in order to obtain sustained muscle relaxation. The usual initial dose is 20 milligrams followed by continuous infusion of 0.5 milligram/minute. The infusion must be individualized because of great variation in the kinetics of metabolism of succinylcholine. Estimate the elimination half-lives of succinylcholine in patients requiring 0.5 milligram/minute and 5.0 milligrams/minute, respectively, to maintain 20 milligrams in the body.

3. During an investigational program, the calcium channel blocking agent, nifedipine, was infused at a constant rate (1.5 mg/hour) via a rectal osmotic pump device for 24 hours.

   Table 6–4 lists the plasma nifedipine concentration during and after the infusion. These data indicate that an average plateau concentration of 21 micrograms/liter was attained.

Table 6–4[a]

Time (hours)	Plasma Nifedipine Concentration (micrograms/liter)
0	0
1	4.2
2	14.5
4	21.0
6	23.0
7.5	19.8
10.5	22.0
14	20.0
18	18.0
24	21.0
25	18.0
26	11.6
27	7.1
28	4.2

[a]Abstracted from Kleinbloesem, C.H., van Harten, J., de Leede, L.G.J., van Brummelen, P., and Briemer, D.D. Clin. Pharmacol. Ther., 36:396–401, 1984.

Given that all the infused drug was absorbed and that nifedipine disposition can be characterized by a one-compartmental model:

(a) Calculate the clearance, half-life, and volume of distribution of the drug.

(b) Is the approach of the concentration to plateau in agreement with the half-life of nifedipine observed on removing the infusion pump?

(c) If the infusion rate is increased to 3.0 milligrams/hour, what are the expected concentrations at 1 hour, 2 hours, and at plateau?

(d) If the desire is to instantly achieve the plateau concentration associated with the 3.0 milligrams/hour infusion rate, what is the loading dose required?

4. Estimate the values of volume of distribution, half-life, and clearance from the data in Table 6–5. The drug was administered as an intravenous bolus of 250 milligrams followed immediately by a constant infusion of 10 milligrams/hour for the duration of the study. Assume that the drug instantly distributes throughout the body.

Table 6–5.

Time (hours)	0.3	5.0	20	50
Plasma drug concentration (mg/liter)	9.8	7.6	4.8	4.0

5. Estimate the values of volume of distribution, elimination rate constant, half-life, and clearance from data in Table 6–6, obtained on infusing a drug at the rate of 50 milligrams/hour for 7.5 hours.

Table 6–6.

Time (hours)	0	2	4	6	7.5	9	12	15
Plasma drug concentration (mg/liter)	0	3.4	5.4	6.5	7.0	4.6	2.0	0.9

7

Multiple-dose Regimens

Objectives

The reader will be able to:

1. **Predict the rate and extent of drug accumulation for a given regimen of fixed dose and fixed interval.**

2. **Develop a dosage regimen from knowledge of the pharmacokinetics and therapeutic window of a drug.**

3. **Evaluate a dosage regimen of a drug from a pharmacokinetic point of view.**

4. **Evaluate dosage regimens of controlled-release formulations from a kinetic point of view.**

5. **Derive pharmacokinetic parameters for a drug from plasma concentration (or urine) data following a multiple-dose regimen.**

The previous chapter dealt with constant-rate regimens. Although these regimens possess many desirable features, they are not the most common ones. The more common approach to the maintenance of continuous therapy is to give multiple discrete doses. This chapter covers the pharmacokinetic principles associated with such multiple-dose regimens.

DRUG ACCUMULATION

Drugs are most commonly prescribed to be taken on a fixed dose, fixed time interval basis; e.g., 100 milligrams three times a day. In association with this kind of administration, the plasma concentration and amount in the body fluctuate and, similar to an infusion, rise toward a plateau.

Consider the simplest situation of a dosage regimen composed of equal bolus doses administered intravenously at fixed and equal time intervals. Curve A of Figure 7–1 shows how the amount in the body varies with time when each dose is given successively twice every half-life. Under these conditions the drug accumulates substantially. Accumulation occurs because drug from previous doses has not been completely removed.

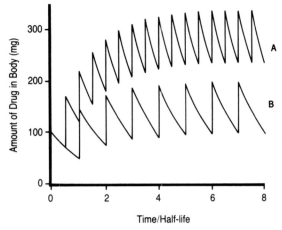

Fig. 7–1. Dosing frequency controls the degree of drug accumulation. Curve A, Intravenous bolus dose (100 mg) administered twice every half-life; curve B, same bolus dose administered once every half-life. Note that time is expressed in half-life units.

Maxima and Minima on Accumulation to the Plateau

To appreciate the phenomenon of accumulation, consider what happens to a drug when given intravenously, as a 100 milligram bolus dose, every elimination half-life. The amounts of drug in the body just after each dose and just before the next dose can readily be calculated; these values correspond to the maximum (A_{max}) and the minimum (A_{min}) amounts obtained within each dosing interval. The corresponding values during the first dosing interval are 100 milligrams ($A_{1,max}$) and 50 milligrams ($A_{1,min}$), respectively. The maximum amount of drug in the second dosing interval ($A_{2,max}$), 150 milligrams, is the dose (100 milligrams) plus the amount remaining from the previous dose (50 milligrams). The amount remaining at the end of the second dosing interval ($A_{2,min}$), 75 milligrams, is the amount remaining from the first dose, 25 milligrams (100 milligrams $\times$ ½ $\times$ ½, because two half-lives have elapsed since administration) plus that remaining from the second dose, 50 milligrams. Alternatively, the value, 75 milligrams, may simply be calculated by recognizing that one-half of the amount just after the second dose, 150 milligrams, remains at the end of that dosing interval. Upon repeating this procedure, it is readily seen (curve B, Fig. 7–1) that drug accumulation, viewed in terms of either the maximum or the minimum amount in the body, continues until a limit is reached. At the limit, the amount lost in each interval equals the amount gained, the dose. For this reason drug in the body is said to be at *steady state* or at *plateau*. In this example, the maximum, denoted by $A_{ss,max}$, and the minimum, denoted by $A_{ss,min}$, amounts in the body at steady state are 200 milligrams and 100 milligrams, respectively. This must be so since at plateau, the difference between the maximum and minimum amounts is the dose, 100 milligrams, and since at the end of the interval, one half-life, the amount must be half that at the beginning.

The foregoing considerations can be expanded for the more general situation in which a drug is given at a dosing interval, τ, which may be different from the half-life. The general equations, derived in Appendix D, for the maximum and minimum amounts in the body after the Nth dose ($A_{N,max}$; $A_{N,min}$) and at plateau ($A_{ss,max}$; $A_{ss,min}$) are

★
Maximum amount in
body after Nth dose, $A_{N,max}$ $= \text{Dose} \cdot \left[\dfrac{1 - e^{-Nk\tau}}{1 - e^{-k\tau}} \right]$
1

★
Minimum amount in
body after Nth dose, $A_{N,min}$ $= A_{N,max} \cdot e^{-k\tau}$
2

★
Maximum amount in
body at plateau, $A_{ss,max}$ $= \dfrac{\text{Dose}}{1 - e^{-k\tau}}$
3

★
Minimum amount in
body at plateau, $A_{ss,min}$ $= A_{ss,max} \, e^{-k\tau} = A_{ss,max} - \text{Dose}$
4

Recall from Chapter 3 that the function $e^{-k\tau}$ is the fraction of the initial amount remaining in the body at time t. Similarly, the amount in the body at the end of a dosing interval τ of a multiple-dose regimen, $A_{N,\tau}$ ($A_{N,min}$), is obtained by multiplying the corresponding maximum amount by $e^{-k\tau}$, that is, $A_{N,\tau} = A_{N,max} \, e^{-k\tau}$ or $A_{ss,\tau} = A_{ss,max} \, e^{-k\tau}$.

For the simple situation in which drug is given every half-life, the fraction remaining at the end of the dosing interval ($e^{-k\tau}$) is 0.5. In this case it can readily be seen from Equations 3 and 4 that the maximum amount at plateau is twice the dose and that the minimum amount at plateau is the dose itself, a conclusion drawn previously.

To further appreciate the phenomenon of accumulation, consider an oral dosage regimen of 0.1 milligram daily of digitoxin, used in the treatment of certain cardiac dysfunctions. Furthermore, assume that absorption is complete and virtually instantaneous, simulating intravenous bolus administration, and that a plateau has been reached.

The average half-life of digitoxin is 6 days; therefore, from Equation 3 the maximum amount at plateau is 0.92 milligram, and from Equation 4 the minimum amount at plateau is 0.82 milligram. Digitoxin clearly undergoes considerable accumulation when given daily.

These calculations of the maximum and minimum values at plateau strictly apply only to intravascular bolus administration. They are reasonable approximations following extravascular administration, when absorption is complete and virtually instantaneous. The following discussion deals with a less restrictive view of accumulation, which applies to all routes of administration.

Average Amount in Body at Plateau

In many respects the accumulation of drugs, administered in multiple doses, is the same as that observed following a constant-rate intravenous infusion. The average amount in the body at steady state, plateau, is readily calculated using the steady-state concept: The average *rate in* must equal the average *rate out*. That is, during each dosing interval, the amount eliminated from the body is equal to the amount absorbed. The average rate in is $F \cdot \text{Dose}/\tau$). The average rate out is $k \cdot A_{ss,av}$, where $A_{ss,av}$ is the average amount of drug in the body over the dosing interval at plateau. Therefore,

$$\frac{F \cdot \text{Dose}}{\tau} = k \cdot A_{ss,av}$$

5

or

$$\frac{F \cdot \text{Dose}}{\tau} = CL \cdot C_{ss,av}$$

6

where $C_{ss,av}$ is the average plasma concentration at the plateau. Since $k = 0.693/t_{1/2}$, it also follows that

$$A_{ss,av} = 1.44 \cdot F \cdot \text{Dose} \cdot t_{1/2}/\tau$$

7

and

$$C_{ss,av} = \frac{F}{CL} \cdot \frac{\text{Dose}}{\tau}$$

8

These are fundamental relationships; they show how the average amount in the body at steady state depends upon rate of administration, Dose/τ, availability, and half-life, and how the corresponding average concentration depends upon the first two factors and clearance.

Drug accumulation is not a phenomenon that depends upon the property of a drug, nor are there drugs that are cumulative and others that are not. Accumulation, in particular the extent of it, is a result of the frequency of administration (half-life of the drug relative to the dosing interval) as shown in Figures 7–1 and 7–2.

From Equations 3 and 4 the maximum and minimum amounts of digitoxin at plateau are 0.92 milligram and 0.82 milligram respectively. Notice that the average amount (0.87 mg), calculated from Equation 7, lies midway between these amounts. Since calculating the average value is the much simpler procedure, under these circumstances the maximum and minimum values can easily be calculated by adding and subtracting one-half the maintenance dose absorbed, respectively, to the average value. With digitoxin, for example, $A_{ss,max}$ is 0.87 + 0.05 = 0.92 milligram; $A_{ss,min}$ is 0.87 − 0.05 = 0.82 milligram. This simple method can be used as long as the dosing interval does not exceed the half-life.

Comparison of Maximum, Average, and Minimum Amounts at Plateau

Fluctuation in the amount of drug in the body, like accumulation, depends on both the frequency of drug administration and the half-life of the drug. Fluctuation also depends upon the rate of absorption; it is greatest for intravenous bolus administration. Figure 7–2A illustrates how the maximum, minimum, and average amounts in the body at plateau depend upon the frequency of intravenous bolus administration. Several observations are pertinent: (1) The average amount increases in direct proportion to the frequency of administration (the inverse of the dosing interval). (2) The maximum amount is not much greater than the dose if the drug is administered less frequently than once every three half-lives, $t_{1/2}/\tau = 0.33$ or less. Then most of the drug from all previous doses has been eliminated before the next dose is administered. (3) Defining fluctuation

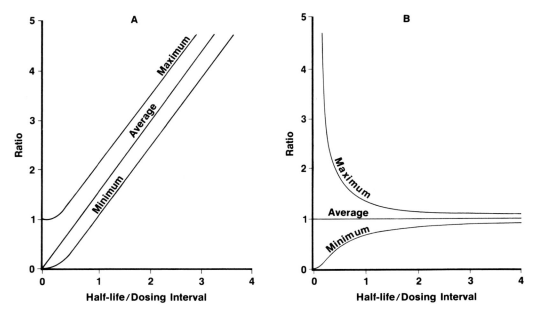

Fig. 7–2. More frequent administration results in a greater degree of drug accumulation and hence smaller relative differences among the maximum ($A_{ss,max}$), average ($A_{ss,av}$) and minimum ($A_{ss,min}$) amounts of drug in the body at plateau. Note that frequency is the reciprocal of the dosing interval expressed here in half-life units. A, Ratios of the maximum, average, and minimum amounts of drug at plateau to the maintenance dose following chronic intravenous bolus administration, as a function of the dosing frequency. B, Ratios of maximum to average, and minimum to average amounts of drug in the body as a function of the dosing frequency.

as the ratio, $A_{ss,max}/A_{ss,min}$, the greater the frequency of administration the smaller is the fluctuation.

Figure 7–2B also demonstrates how the fluctuation at plateau depends on the frequency of administration. The maximum and minimum amounts are each compared with the average amount of drug in the body. Note that the average is arithmetically closer to the minimum than to the maximum value. This is particularly evident for low frequencies of administration.

Rate of Accumulation to Plateau

The amount in the body rises on multiple dosing just as it does following a constant-rate intravenous infusion (Chap. 6). That is, the approach to the plateau depends solely on the drug's half-life. The data for digitoxin, in Table 7–1, which show the ratio of the maximum amount during various dosing intervals to the maximum amount at plateau, illustrate this point. Observe that it takes one half-life (6 days), or 6 doses, to be at 50 percent of the maximum at plateau, two

Table 7–1. Approach to Plateau on Daily Administration of Digitoxin

Time (days)	0	1	2	3	6	12	18	24	30	∞
Number of doses (N)	0	1	2	3	6	12	18	24	30	∞
$\left[\dfrac{\text{Maximum amount}}{\begin{array}{c}\text{Maximum amount}\\\text{at plateau}\end{array}}\right]^{a}$	0	0.11	0.21	0.29	0.5	0.75	0.875	0.94	0.97	1.00

$^{a}A_{N,max}/A_{ss,max} = 1 - e^{-0.116N}$

half-lives (12 days), or 12 doses, to be at 75 percent of the maximum at plateau, and so on.

The accumulation of digitoxin takes a long time because of its long half-life. The degree of accumulation is extensive, because of relatively frequent administration. The frequency of administration also determines the small fluctuation in the amount of drug in the body at plateau; 0.1 milligram is lost in every dosing interval, but there is about 0.9 milligram in the body.

The approach to steady state, observed for the maximum amounts of digitoxin in the body, also holds true for the minimum and average amounts (proof in Appendix D), that is

★

$$\frac{A_{N,max}}{A_{ss,max}} = \frac{A_{N,av}}{A_{ss,av}} = \frac{A_{N,min}}{A_{ss,min}} = 1 - e^{-Nk\tau} \qquad 9$$

where $A_{N,av}$ is the average amount in the body in the dosing interval after the Nth dose.

Accumulation Index

If the amounts at steady state are compared to the corresponding values at time τ after a single dose, then

★

$$\frac{A_{ss,max}}{A_{1,max}} = \frac{A_{ss,av}}{A_{1,av}} = \frac{A_{ss,min}}{A_{1,min}} = \frac{1}{(1 - e^{-k\tau})} \qquad 10$$

The quantity, $1/(1 - e^{-k\tau})$, is a useful index of the extent of accumulation. For digitoxin ($k = 0.116$ day^{-1}, $\tau = 1$ day), the *accumulation index* (R_{ac}) is 9.2. Thus, the maximum, average, and minimum amounts (and for that matter the amount at any time within the dosing interval at plateau) are 9.2 times the values at the corresponding times after a single dose.

Change in Regimen

Suppose that the decision is made to halve the amount of digitoxin in the body at plateau. The need for a twofold reduction in the rate of administration, to 0.05 milligram a day, follows from Equation 7.

As with intravenous infusion, it takes one half-life to go one-half the way from 0.90 to 0.45 milligram, two half-lives to go three-quarters of the way, and so on. For digitoxin it would take about 12 days to go 75 percent of the way to the new plateau. (The same principle applies to an increase in the rate of digitoxin administration.) The fastest way to achieve 0.45 milligram would be to discontinue the drug for one week (approximately one half-life) before initiating the reduced rate of administration.

RELATIONSHIP BETWEEN INITIAL AND MAINTENANCE DOSES

It might be therapeutically desirable to establish the required amount of digitoxin in the body on the first day. When the first or initial dose is intended to be therapeutic it is referred to as the *priming* or *loading dose*. In this case, the patient would require 0.9 milligram initially, followed by 0.1 milligram daily. For digitoxin the initial dose is often administered in divided doses. Several procedures are followed, but the divided dose is commonly given every 6 hours until the desired therapeutic response is obtained. In this way each patient is titrated to the initial therapeutic dose required.

Instead of determining the loading dose when the maintenance dose is given, it is more common to determine the maintenance dose required to sustain a therapeutic amount of drug in the body. The initial dose rapidly achieves the therapeutic response; subsequent doses maintain the response by replacing drug lost during the dosing interval. The maintenance dose, D_M, therefore, is the difference between the loading dose, D_L, and the amount remaining at the end of the dosing interval, $D_L \cdot e^{-k\tau}$. That is,

★

$$\text{Maintenance dose} = \left[\begin{matrix} \text{Loading} \\ \text{dose} \end{matrix} \right] \cdot (1 - e^{-k\tau}) \qquad 11$$

Likewise, if the maintenance dose is known, the initial dose can be estimated:

$$\text{Loading dose} = \frac{\text{Maintenance dose}}{(1 - e^{-k\tau})} \qquad 12$$

Thus, for digitoxin, a daily maintenance dose of 0.1 milligram requires a loading dose of 0.9 milligram.

The similarity between Equations 3 and 11 should be noted. From the viewpoint of accumulation, Equation 3 relates to the maximum amount at plateau on administering a given dose repetitively. If the maximum amount were put into the body initially, then Equation 11 indicates the dose needed to maintain that amount. The relationships are the same, although they were derived using different logic. These equations form the heart of multiple-dose drug administration and might well be called the "dosage regimen equations."

The ratio of loading to maintenance doses depends on the dosing interval and the half-life, and is equal to the accumulation index, R_{ac}. For example, tetracycline has approximately an 8-hour half-life in man, and a dose in the range of 250 to 500 milligrams is considered to provide effective antimicrobial drug concentrations. Therefore, a reasonable schedule is 500 milligrams (two 250-mg capsules) initially, followed by 250 milligrams every half-life, as shown in Figure 7–3. A dosage regimen consisting of a priming dose equal to twice the maintenance dose and a dosing interval of one half-life are convenient for drugs with half-lives between 8 and 24 hours. The frequency of administration for such drugs varies from 3 times a day to once daily, respectively. For drugs with very short to short half-lives, less than 3 hours, or with very long half-lives, greater than 24 hours, this regimen is often impractical.

MAINTENANCE OF DRUG IN THE THERAPEUTIC RANGE

Dosage regimens that achieve therapeutic concentrations are listed in Table 7–2 for drugs with both medium to high and low therapeutic indices and with various half-lives.

Great difficulty is encountered in trying to maintain therapeutic concentrations

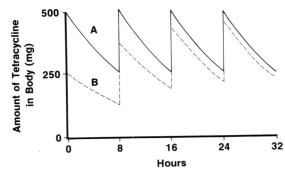

Fig. 7–3. Sketch of the amount of tetracycline in the body with time; simulation of the intravenous administration of 500 milligrams initially and 250 milligrams every 8 hours thereafter, curve A. When the initial and maintenance doses are the same, curve B, it takes approximatley 30 hours (3 to 4 half-lives) before the plateau is practically reached. Thereafter curves A and B are essentially the same.

of a drug with a short to very short half-life (less than 3 hours). This is particularly true for a drug that also has a low therapeutic index, e.g., heparin. Such a drug must be either infused or discarded unless intermittent concentrations are permissible. Drugs with a high therapeutic index may be given less frequently, but the greater the dosing interval the greater is the maintenance dose required to ensure that drug in the body stays above a minimum effective value. Penicillin is a notable example of a drug for which the dosing interval (4–6 hours) is many times longer than its half-life (approximately 0.7 hour). The dose given greatly exceeds that required to yield plasma concentrations of antibiotic equivalent to the minimum inhibitory concentration for most microorganisms.

For a drug of short to intermediate half-life (20 minutes–8 hours) the major considerations are therapeutic index and convenience of dosing. A drug with a high therapeutic index need only be administered once every 1 to 3 half-lives. A drug with a low therapeutic index must be given approximately every half-life, or more frequently, or be given by infusion. Lidocaine, for example has a half-life of only 90 minutes, and the range of plasma drug concentrations associated with the treatment of cardiac arrhythmias is only about threefold. This drug must be given by infusion to ensure prolonged suppression of arrhythmias and minimal toxicity.

For a drug with a long half-life (8–24 hours) the most convenient, common, and desirable regimen is one in which a dose is given every half-life. If immediate achievement of steady state is desired, then, as previously mentioned, the initial dose must be twice the maintenance dose; the minimum and maximum amounts in the body are equivalent to one and two maintenance doses, respectively.

For drugs with very long half-lives (greater than 1 day) administration once daily is convenient and promotes patient compliance. If an immediate therapeutic effect is desired, the therapeutic dose is given initially. Otherwise the initial and maintenance doses are the same, in which case several doses may be necessary before the drug accumulates to therapeutic levels. The decision whether or not to give larger initial doses is often a practical matter. Side effects to large oral doses (gastrointestinal side effects) or to acutely high concentrations of drug in the body may necessitate a slow accumulation.

To summarize the foregoing discussion, consider the antibiotic drug, tetracycline, the nasal congestant, phenylpropanolamine, and the antiepileptic agent, phenobarbital, and their common dosage regimens given in Table 7–3. Listed in Table 7–4 are the corresponding fractions of the initial amount remaining at the end of a dosing interval, the average amounts at steady state, and the

Table 7-2. Dosage Regimens for Continuous Maintenance of Therapeutic Concentrations

Therapeutic Index[a]	Half-life[b]	Ratio of Initial Dose to Maintenance Dose	Ratio of Dosing Interval to Half-life	General Comments	Drug Examples
Medium to High					
	Very short (<20 minutes)	—	—	Candidate for constant-rate administration and/or short-term therapy.	Nitroglycerin
	Short (20 minutes to 3 hours)	1	3–6	To be given any less often than every 3 half-lives, drug must have very high therapeutic index.	Penicillin
	Intermediate (3 to 8 hours)	1–2	1–3	Very common and desirable regimen.	Tetracycline Sulfamethoxazole
	Long (8 to 24 hours)	2	1		
	Very long (>24 hours)	>2	<1	Once daily is practical. Occasionally given once weekly. Initial dose may need to be much greater than maintenance dose.	Chloroquine (suppression of malaria)
Low					
	Very short (<20 minutes)	—	—	Not a candidate except under very closely controlled infusion.	Nitroprusside
	Short (20 minutes to 3 hours)	—	~1	Only by infusion.	Lidocaine
	Intermediate (3 to 8 hours)	1–2		Requires 3–6 doses per day, but less frequently with controlled-release formulation.	Theophylline
	Long (8 to 24 hours)	2–4	0.5–1		
	Very long (>24 hours)	>2	<1	Requires careful control, since once toxicity is produced, drug level and toxicity decline very slowly.	Digitoxin

[a] Usually toxic maintenance dose/usual therapeutic maintenance dose.
[b] Descriptions of half-life are arbitrary.

Table 7–3. Dosage Regimens and Half-lives of Three Drugs

Drug	Loading Dose (mg)	Maintenance Dose (mg)	Dosing Interval (hours)	Half-life (hours)
Tetracycline	500	250	8	8
Phenyl-propanolamine	30	30	8	4
Phenobarbital	30	30	8	120

maximum and minimum values. Instantaneous and complete absorption is assumed.

Dosing intervals for all three drugs are identical. The doses of phenylpropanolamine and phenobarbital are also the same, but the amounts of them in the body with time are certainly not. The explanation is readily visualized with a sketch.

As with any graph, consideration should first be given to scaling the axes. The amount of drug in the body should be scaled to the maximum amount at steady state. The time axis should be scaled to 4 to 5 half-lives, by which time plateau is achieved.

For tetracycline the amount in the body immediately after the first dose is 500 milligrams. At the end of the dosing interval the fraction remaining is 0.5, and the amount therefore is 250 milligrams. A maintenance dose of 250 milligrams returns the level to 500 milligrams and so on. Figure 7–3, curve A, is thus readily drawn. Now consider the sketch had no loading dose been given. The initial amount, 250 milligrams, would then decline to 125 milligrams at the end of the first interval. The amount in the body immediately after the next dose would be 375 milligrams. At the end of the second interval 187 milligrams would remain and so on (curve B of Figure 7–3).

For phenylpropanolamine the maximum and minimum amounts in the body at plateau are 40 milligrams and 10 milligrams, respectively, and a period of 4

Table 7–4. Estimates of Amount of Drug in Body on Regimens Given in Table 7–3

Drug	Fraction Remaining at τ[a]	Average at Steady State $A_{ss,av}$ (mg)[b]	Maximum at Steady State $A_{ss,max}$ (mg)[c]	Minimum at Steady State $A_{ss,min}$ (mg)[d]
Tetracycline	0.5	360	500	250
Phenyl-propanolamine	0.25	22	40	10
Phenobarbital	0.95	650	665	635

[a]Calculated by $e^{-k\tau}$
[b]$1.44 \cdot F \cdot t_{1/2} \cdot D_M/\tau$.
[c]$D_M/(1 - e^{-k\tau})$
[d]$A_{ss,max} - D_M$.

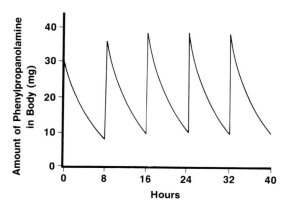

Fig. 7–4. Sketch of the amount of phenylpropanol-amine in the body with time; simulation of 30 milli-grams given intravenously every 8 hours. Because the half-life, 4 hours, is short relative to the dosing interval, the degree of accumulation is small and the fluctuation is large.

half-lives is 16 hours. The fraction remaining at the end of each dosing interval is 0.25; therefore,

Dose	Time (hours)	A (milligrams)
1	0	30
	8	7.5
2	8 +	37.5
	16	9.4
3	16 +	39.4

By the third dose (24 hours) the plateau is virtually achieved. Being given every two half-lives, the accumulation of phenylpropanolamine is minimal. Figure 7–4 is a sketch of the amounts of phenylpropanolamine in the body with time.

The same dosage regimen for phenobarbital produces a dramatically different result. At the end of each dosing interval the fraction remaining is approximately 0.95. Accumulation then occurs until the 5 percent lost in each interval is equal to the dose, and the amount in the body at steady state is therefore about 20 times the dose. From the calculated value of the maximum amount at plateau (650 mg) and the half-life, it is apparent that a sketch must be scaled to 700 milligrams and to 15 to 20 days (Fig. 7–5). The curve is similar to that obtained with constant-rate infusion. The amount of drug in the body at 5 days (120 hours) is one-half of the steady-state amount, and at 10 days (240 hours) the level is 75 percent of the plateau amount and so on. Practically, there is little need to consider the minor fluctuations.

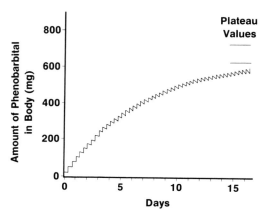

Fig. 7–5. Sketch of the amount of phenobarbital in the body with time; simulation of 30 milligrams given intravenously every 8 hours. Because the half-life, 5 days, is extremely long relative to the dosing interval, the degree of accumulation is large and the fluctuation is low.

The clinical implications of these regimens are manifold. The tetracycline regimen is designed to attain and maintain therapeutic levels. The phenylpropanolamine regimen gives rise to large fluctuations that may be desirable. Tolerance to the drug develops readily; the maintenance of high, effective, decongesting concentrations is questionable. With phenobarbital the appropriate regimen depends on whether the drug is used for sedation or as an antiepilectic. For sedation, the omission of a loading dose is desirable, in that tolerance to the sedative effect develops with time and a large priming dose, 600 milligrams, causes too great a central depressive effect. As an antiepileptic, however, a loading dose may be appropriate. Chronic administration of the drug three times daily is illogical; once daily administration is adequate.

PRACTICAL ASPECTS OF MULTIPLE-DOSE ADMINISTRATION

So far, consideration has been given primarily to the amount of drug in the body following multiple intravenous bolus injections, or their equivalent, at equally spaced time intervals. In practice, chronic administration is usually by the oral route. Furthermore, only drug concentration in plasma or in blood can be measured and not the amount of drug in the body. These aspects are now considered. Problems related to unequal doses and dosing intervals, and to missed doses are covered in Chapter 18, Monitoring.

Extravascular Administration

The oral (also intramuscular, buccal, subcutaneous, and rectal) administration of drugs requires an added step, absorption. Equations 1 to 4 apply to extravascular administration, provided that absorption is essentially completed within a small fraction of a dosing interval, a condition similar to intravenous bolus administration. Even so, a correction must be made if availability is less than 1. When absorption continues throughout a dosing interval, or longer, then the relationships of Equations 7 and 8 still apply. These relationships allow estimation of the average plateau concentration and the average plateau amount in the body, respectively. The slowness of drug absorption affects the degree of fluctuation around, but not the value of, the average level. The exception is when absorption becomes so slow that there is insufficient time to complete absorption, e.g., when limited by the transit time within the gastrointestinal tract.

Fluctuations in the amount in the body within a dosing interval may be very small following oral or other extravascular routes of administration because of continuous absorption. Furthermore, the maximum value at plateau is always close to the average plateau value when the dosing interval is less than one-half of a half-life, irrespective of the route of administration or the rate of absorption. In both instances, the relationshlip between the initial and maintenance doses becomes a simple one, namely

$$\text{Maintenance dose} = k \cdot \tau \cdot \text{Loading dose} \qquad 13$$

This simple relationship is derived from Equation 11. As $k\tau$ approaches zero (less than 0.2), the function $(1 - e^{-k\tau})$ approaches the value of $k\tau$.

Thus, if a drug is administered more frequently than twice every half-life, the error in using Equation 13 is less than 20 percent. This calculation is based on the extreme case of intravenous bolus administration in which fluctuations are the greatest. After extravascular administration the error is even smaller.

The therapeutic impact of differences in absorption kinetics, but not in availability, of extravascularly administered drug products given continuously depends on the frequency of their administration. As illustrated in Figure 7–6, major differences seen following a single dose will only persist and be of potential therapeutic concern at plateau when the drug products are given infrequently, relative to the half-life of the drug. Differences between them will almost disappear at plateau when the products are given frequently. In the latter case, as stated previously, with extensive accumulation of drug, the concentration at plateau is relatively insensitive to variations in absorption rate.

Plasma Concentration Versus Amount in Body

After multiple dosing, the plasma concentration can be calculated at any time by dividing the corresponding equations defining amount by the volume of distribution. Distribution equilibrium between drug in the tissues and that in the plasma takes time. Thus, observed and calculated maximum concentrations may differ appreciably (Chap. 19).

The average plateau concentration may be calculated using Equation 8. This equation is applicable to any route, method of administration, or dosage form, as long as availability and clearance remain constant with both time and dose.

DESIGN OF DOSAGE REGIMENS FROM PLASMA CONCENTRATIONS

Dosage regimens can be designed to maintain concentrations within the therapeutic window. The window is defined by a lower limit (C_{lower}) and an upper

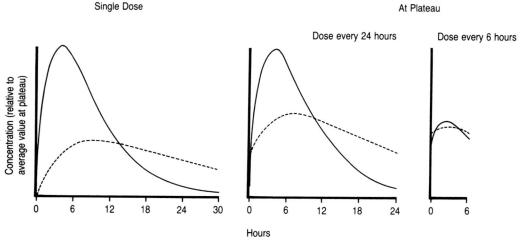

Fig. 7–6. Differences in the absorption rates between two dosage forms, exaggerated here for illustrative purposes, following a single extravascular dose (left panel) can have a major therapeutic impact at plateau during multiple dosing. The relative fluctuation of the plasma concentration when the drug products are given infrequently (middle panel) is much greater than when given frequently (right panel). For comparative purposes, the plateau concentrations during the dosing interval are normalized to the average value within the interval.

limit (C_{upper}). The maximum dosing interval, τ_{max}, and maximum maintenance dose, $D_{M,max}$, can be readily computed from these limits as follows:

$$C_{lower} = C_{upper} \cdot e^{-k\tau max} \qquad 14$$

where τ_{max} is the maximum time interval over which these upper and lower concentrations can occur. By rearrangement of Equation 14, the value of τ_{max} is

$$\tau_{max} = \frac{\log (C_{upper}/C_{lower})}{k} \qquad 15$$

and, from the relationship, $k = 0.693/t_{1/2}$,

$$\tau_{max} = 1.44 \cdot t_{1/2} \cdot \log (C_{upper}/C_{lower}) \qquad 16$$

The corresponding maximum maintenance dose, $D_{M,max}$, that can be given every τ_{max} is then

$$D_{M,max} = \frac{V}{F} (C_{upper} - C_{lower}) \qquad 17$$

When $D_{M,max}$ is administered every τ_{max}, there is an average concentration produced within the dosing interval, defined by

$$\frac{D_{M,max}}{\tau_{max}} = \frac{CL}{F} \cdot C_{ss,av} \qquad 18$$

By dividing Equation 17 by Equation 16 and comparing this ratio to Equation 18, it is apparent that the value of $C_{ss,av}$ is given by

$$C_{ss,av} = \frac{(C_{upper} - C_{lower})}{\log(C_{upper}/C_{lower})} \qquad 19$$

Two approaches are available to design a dosage regimen. One sets the dosing rate to achieve an average concentration. The other uses a peak concentration to set the dosing rate. In both approaches, concentrations are maintained within the therapeutic window throughout the dosing interval.

Maintenance of an Average Concentration

Choosing the average concentration within the dosing interval at plateau to be $C_{ss,av}$ allows the greatest possible dosing interval. This dosing interval (Eq. 16) and the corresponding maintenance dose (Eq. 17) may not be practical, however. Both values may need to be adjusted to make the frequency of administration convenient for patient compliance and to accommodate the dose strengths of the drug products available. The guiding principle is to maintain the same rate of administration and therefore the same chosen average steady-state concentration.

Having chosen a convenient dosing interval, smaller than τ_{max}, the maintenance dose is

$$D_M = (D_{M,max}/\tau_{max}) \cdot \tau \qquad 20$$

and the loading dose, appropriate to attain the steady-state concentration, initially is

$$D_L = D_M/(1 - e^{-k\tau}) \qquad\qquad 21$$

If more (or less) vigorous therapy is desired, resulting in the setting of the average targeted concentration to be higher (or lower) than $C_{ss,av}$, then the dosing rate can be increased (or decreased) proportionately. However, one may wish to adjust the dosing interval to ensure that concentrations remain within the therapeutic window.

Maintenance of a Peak Concentration

The second approach to the design of dosage regimens is based on the desire to maintain a given peak concentration. The peak concentration chosen, C_{peak}, depends on how aggressively one wishes to pursue therapy but usually lies in the upper half of the therapeutic window. The maximum dosing interval is:

$$\text{Maximum dosing interval} = \frac{\log (C_{peak}/C_{lower})}{k} \qquad\qquad 22$$

On choosing a convenient interval, τ, less than the maximum defined in Equation 22, the maintenance dose then becomes

$$D_M = V \cdot C_{peak} (1 - e^{-k\tau}) \qquad\qquad 23$$

and the loading dose, if necessary, is $V \cdot C_{peak}$. Note that C_{peak} is the same as $C_{ss,max}$. This method of regimen design tends to be simpler than the previous one. Figure 7–7 illustrates differences that can occur between these two approaches.

Following extravascular administration, fluctuations in the plasma concentration of drug are less than those after intravascular administration. Depending upon the slowness of the absorption process, it may be possible to administer the drug less frequently than indicated in the regimens designed by either this or the previous method.

When Availability and Volume are Unknown

Oral dosage regimens can also be designed without determining the availability. This is accomplished using the area under the plasma concentration-time curve following a single dose. From the relationship $F \cdot \text{Dose} = CL \cdot AUC$ after a single dose (Eq. 7, Chap. 4) and the relationship $F \cdot \text{Dose}/\tau = CL \cdot C_{ss,av}$ during steady state after multiple doses (Eq. 6), it follows that

★

$$C_{ss,av} = AUC \text{ (single dose)}/\tau \qquad\qquad 24$$

Consequently, either the dosing interval necessary to achieve a desired average steady-state concentration or the average concentration resulting from administering the dose every dosing interval can be calculated.

By definition of $C_{ss,av}$, the value of $\tau \cdot C_{ss,av}$ is the area under the curve within a dosing interval at steady state. Thus, this area is equal to that following a

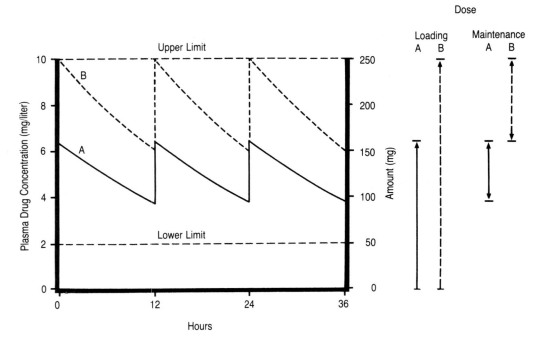

Fig. 7–7. Differences in two methods of dosage regimen design. Regimen A (solid line) is designed to maintain the same average concentration as that obtained when the concentration fluctuates between the upper (10 mg/liter) and lower (2 mg/liter) limits. Regimen B (stippled line) is design to ensure that the peak concentration does not exceed the upper limit. Of course, a lower peak value may have been chosen. The loading doses required to achieve the steady-state concentrations immediately and the maintenance doses for both regimens are indicated.

single dose. This principle is shown in Figure 7–8, and a practical illustration is shown in Figure 7–9.

Given the plasma concentrations with time after a single oral dose, the concentration at any time during repeated administration of the same dose can be readily calculated by adding the concentrations remaining from each of the previous doses. For example, if doses are given at 0, 12, and 24 hours, then the concentration at 30 hours is equal to the sum of the concentration at 30, 18, and 6 hours after a single dose.

Useful relationships have been derived for designing and evaluating a dosage regimen in which the dose and the dosing interval are fixed. Table 7–5 contains some of the more important relationships and their limitations.

Controlled Release

The maintenance of a constant plasma concentration, and usually response, is achieved by constant-rate administration (Chap. 6). While some constant-rate release systems have been developed (see Drug Delivery Systems, Chap. 9), other dosage forms exist from which drug release is much slower than from conventional dosage forms and for which the release kinetics are closer to first-order, than to zero-order. Such controlled-release products do not completely

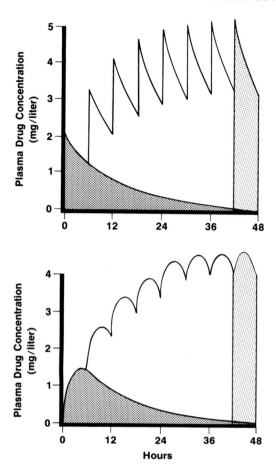

Fig. 7–8.   Plasma concentrations of a drug given intravenously (top) and orally (bottom) on a fixed dose of 50 milligrams and fixed dosing interval of 6 hours. The half-life is 12 hours. Note that the area under the plasma concentration-time curve during a dosing interval at steady state is equal to the total area under the curve following a single dose. The fluctuation of the concentration is diminished when given orally (absorption half-life is 1.4 hours) but the average steady-state concentration is the same as that after intravenous administration, since $F = 1$.

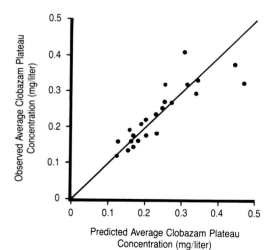

Fig. 7–9.   Twenty-four subjects each received a single 20-milligram oral dose of the benzodiazepine, clobazam, followed one month later by an oral regimen of 10 milligrams of clobazam daily for 22 consecutive days. The observed average plateau clobazam concentration was well predicted by the value calculated from the single dose data, obtained by dividing the *AUC* by the dosing interval and correcting for dose. The solid line is the perfect prediction. (One milligram/liter = 33 micromolar.) (Redrawn from Greenblatt, D.J., Divoll, M., Puri, S.K., Ho, I., Zinny, M.A., and Shader, R.I.: Reduced single-dose clearance of clobazam in elderly men predicts increased multiple-dose accumulation. Clin. Pharmacokin., *8*:83–94, 1983. Reproduced with permission of ADIS Press Australasia Pty Limited.)

Table 7–5. Relationships for Evaluating Dosage Regimens[a]

	Relationship	I.V. Bolus	Extravascular Rapid Absorption $(k_a \gg k)$	Slow Absorption $(k_a > k)$	$(k > k_a)$
Maintenance dose	$D_M = D_L \cdot (1 - e^{-k\tau})$	***[b]	***	**	N
Accumulation index	$R_{AC} = \dfrac{1}{(1 - e^{-k\tau})}$	***	***	**	N
PLATEAU					
Average amount	$A_{ss,av} = 1.44 \cdot F \cdot D \cdot \left(\dfrac{t_{1/2}}{\tau}\right)$	***	***	***	***
Average concentration	$C_{av} = \dfrac{F \cdot D_M}{CL \cdot \tau}$	***	***	***	***
	$C_{ss,av} = \dfrac{AUC \text{ (single dose)}}{\tau}$	***	***	***	***
Maximum concentration	$C_{ss,max} = \dfrac{F \cdot D_M}{V(1 - e^{-k\tau})}$	c	**	*	N
Minimum concentration	$C_{ss,min} = \dfrac{F \cdot D_M \cdot e^{-k\tau}}{V(1 - e^{-k\tau})}$	***	***	*	N

[a]For regimens of equal doses and dosing itervals.
[b]***Generally useful.
**A reasonable approximation.
*Limited usefulness.
cShould not be encouraged because distribution is not instantaneous.
N Not Valid.

obliterate but do reduce considerably the fluctuation in the plasma concentration at plateau, when compared with conventional therapy, and are particularly useful when maintenance of therapeutic concentrations is difficult or inconvenient.

To illustrate the potential value of controlled-release products, consider the events at plateau simulated in Figure 7–10 following oral administration of theophylline in a child with a half-life of 4 hours and a therapeutic window of 6–20 milligrams/liter. With the usual dosage forms, absorption is rapid and, to maintain the plasma concentration within the therapeutic window, the drug must be administered every six hours, an inconvenience. Administering the controlled-release dosage form at the same frequency as the conventional formulation leads to a marked reduction in the fluctuation at plateau. Indeed, the controlled-release formulation can be given at a more convenient dosing interval, 12 hours, and still maintain the plasma concentration within the therapeutic window. To maintain the same average concentration at plateau for the 12-hour interval, the dose of the less frequently administered controlled-release product must be twice that of the conventional product. Obviously, controlled-release products must perform reliably. If all the drug was released immediately an unacceptable fluctuation in the plasma concentration would result.

For oral administration, once or twice daily is desirable. Accordingly, for drugs with half-lives greater than 12 hours, oral controlled-release products may be of little value, not only because the usual regimen is convenient but because protracted release may put drug into the lower intestines, or perhaps out of the

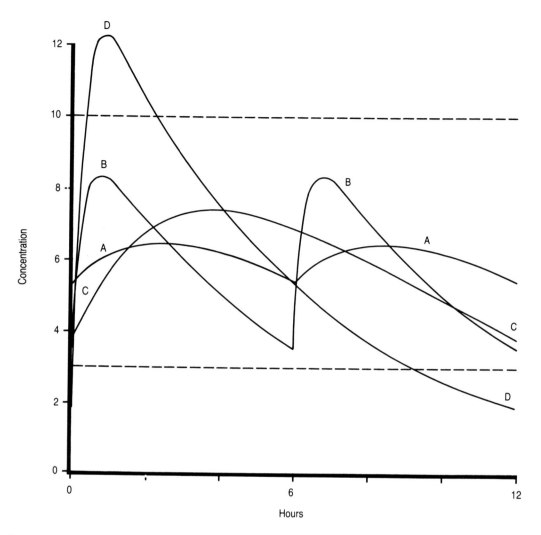

Fig. 7–10. Administering a drug in a controlled-release dosage form may not only decrease the fluctuation in plasma concentration at plateau (Case A) compared to that seen with the usual regimen (Case B), but may also permit the drug to be given less frequently (Case C). Case D shows the concentration-time profile after the usual dosage form. In this example, $t_{1/2} = 4$ hours, $V = 35$ liters, $F = 1$, the half-life of release from the controlled-release product is 3 hours, and the therapeutic window is 3 to 10 milligrams/liter. The dosage regimens are 180 milligrams every 6 hours (Cases A and B) and 360 milligrams every 12 hours (Cases C and D).

body before the release is complete. Decreased availability then becomes a major concern, especially in patients with diseases in which gastrointestinal transit time is shortened.

   For a drug that is usually given intramuscularly or subcutaneously, multiple injections are inconvenient and a controlled-release injectable dosage form may be advantageous. Depending on the total dose required and on the local effects of the injection mixture, it may only be necessary to administer the injection weekly, monthly, or perhaps as a single dose.

Assessment of Pharmacokinetic Parameters

Data obtained on multiple dosing may be used to calculate the pharmacokinetic parameters of a drug. Perhaps the most useful information derived from a multiple oral dosing study is the ratio of clearance to availability. It is obtained from

$$\frac{CL}{F} = \frac{(\text{Dose}/\tau)}{C_{ss,av}} \qquad\qquad 25$$

where $C_{ss,av}$ is determined from the ratio of the area under the plasma concentration curve within a dosing interval at plateau to the dosing interval. Occasionally, the drug is given as a multiple intravenous regimen, then the ratio $(\text{Dose}/\tau)/C_{ss,av}$ is simply clearance, since $F = 1$. The accuracy of the clearance estimate depends on the number of plasma concentrations measured in the dosing interval, that is, on how close the concentration is to the true steady-state value, and on the ratio of $\tau/t_{1/2}$. The estimate, of course, can be improved using several dosing intervals. Equation 25 is also useful for determining the relative availability of a drug administered extravascularly (orally), between two treatments (e.g., dosage forms) A and B. Assuming that clearance remains unchanged, the

$$\text{Relative availability} = \frac{(C_{ss,av})_B}{(C_{ss,av})_A} \cdot \frac{(\text{Dose}/\tau)_A}{(\text{Dose}/\tau)_B} \qquad\qquad 26$$

The renal clearance can be estimated from the amount of drug excreted unchanged in a dosing interval at steady state, $Ae_{\tau,ss}$, the dosing interval and the value of $C_{ss,av}$

$$\text{Renal clearance} = \frac{Ae_{\tau,ss}}{C_{ss,av} \cdot \tau} \qquad\qquad 27$$

Again, the relative availability of an extravascular dose may be determined from urine data

$$\text{Relative availability} = \frac{(Ae_{\tau,ss})_B}{(Ae_{\tau,ss})_A} \cdot \frac{(\text{Dose}/\tau)_A}{(\text{Dose}/\tau)_B} \qquad\qquad 28$$

The half-life is often difficult to assess from multiple-dosing data. In general, the half-life may be determined within a dosing interval at steady state only if the accumulation is minimal, with a large difference between peak and trough concentrations. Half-life is perhaps best determined by observing the decline in concentration after the drug is discontinued.

Study Problems

(Answers to Study Problems are in Appendix G.)

1. Comment on the accuracy of the following statements with regard to drugs given as an oral multiple-dose regimen.

(a) Accumulation always occurs.

(b) The extent of accumulation increases as the drug is given less frequently.

(c) The time to reach plateau following a multiple-dose regimen depends on the frequency of drug administration.

(d) At plateau, the amount of drug lost within a dosing interval equals the maintenance dose.

(e) The larger the volume of distribution, the lower is the average plateau concentration.

(f) The average plateau concentration depends on the absorption kinetics of the drug.

2. The population pharmacokinetics of the oral diuretic agent, chlorthalidone, for a 70-kilogram person are

$$F = 0.64$$

$$V = 280 \text{ liters}$$

$$CL = 4.5 \text{ liters/hour}$$

(a) Assuming that absorption is instantaneous relative to elimination, calculate the following when a 50 milligram dose of chlorthalidone is taken daily at breakfast.

   1. The maximum and minimum amounts of drug in the body at plateau.

   2. The accumulation ratio.

   3. The minimum plasma concentration at plateau.

   4. The time required to achieve 50 percent of plateau.

(b) Complete the table below for the dosage regimen of chlorthalidone given in (a).

Amount of Chlorthalidone in Body (mg)

Dose	1	2	3	4	5	6	7	∞
$A_{N,max}$								
$A_{N,min}$								

(c) Prepare a sketch on regular graph paper of the amount of chlorthalidone in the body with time. Show the salient features of accumulation of this drug during therapy.

(d) If required, what is the loading dose of chlorthalidone needed to immediately attain the condition at plateau?

3. Mr. J.M., a nonsmoking 60-kilogram patient with chronic obstructive pulmonary disease, is to be started on an oral regimen of aminophylline (85 percent of which is theophylline). The pharmacokinetic parameter values for a typical patient population with this disease are:

$$F = 1.0 \text{ (for theophylline)}$$

$$V = 0.5 \text{ liter/kilogram}$$

$$CL = 40 \text{ milliliters/hour per kilogram}$$

Design an oral dosage regimen of *aminophylline* (100- and 200-milligram tablets are available) for this patient to *attain* and *maintain* a plasma concentration within the therapeutic window, 10 to 20 milligrams/liter. Assume complete and rapid absorption of theophylline.

4. Table 7–6 lists a typical plasma concentration-time profile obtained following an oral 50-milligram dose of drug. The *AUC* is 80.6 milligrams-hour/liter, and the terminal half-life is 8 hours.

Table 7–6

Time (hours)	0	1	2	4	8	12	24	36	48
Plasma drug concentration (mg/liter)	0	2.3	4.7	5.2	4.0	2.8	0.6	0.14	0.03

(a) What maintenance oral dosing rate of drug is needed to achieve an average plateau concentration of 10 milligrams/liter?

(b) The decision has been made to give the drug once every 12 hours. What is:

1. The unit dose strength of product needed?

2. The plateau trough concentration expected?

5. The therapeutic dose of a rapidly (compared to elimination) and completely absorbed drug is 50 milligrams. A controlled-release dosage form to be given every 8 hours is designed to release its contents *evenly* and *completely* (no loading dose) over this dosing interval. Given that the half life of the drug is 4 hours:

(a) How much drug should the controlled-release dosage form contain?

(b) To achieve a prompt effect a rapidly absorbed dosage form is administered initially. When should the first controlled-release dosage form be given?

(c) Following the dosage regimen in (b) what is the total dose (i) for day one? (ii) for day two?

(d) In tabular form or on the same graph roughly sketch the relative amounts of drug in the body versus time curves expected when the controlled-release preparation only is given (i) every 4 hours (ii) every 8 hours (iii) every 12 hours.

6. Graffner *et al.* (Clin. Pharmacol. Ther., *17*: 414–423, 1974) compared a rapid-release with a controlled-release formulation of procainamide at steady state. To ensure comparability, the data (presented in Table 7–7) were collected over an 8-hour interval at steady state after administration of 0.5 gram every 4 hours as the rapid-release tablet and 1 gram every 8 hours as the controlled-release formulation.

Table 7–7.

	$AUC_{0\rightarrow\tau}$ (mg-hour/liter)	$Ae_{0\rightarrow\tau}$ (mg)
Rapid-release formulation	22.6	664
Controlled-release formulation	21.1	667

(a) Calculate the relative availability of the controlled-release formulation compared with the rapid-release product.

(b) Calculate the renal clearance of procainamide.

Physiologic Concepts and Kinetics

8

Movement Through Membranes

Objectives

The reader will be able to:

1. **Define passive and facilitated diffusion, active transport, and permeability.**

2. **Distinguish between perfusion rate-limited and permeability rate-limited passage of drugs through membranes.**

3. **Describe the role of pH in the movement of drug through membranes.**

4. **Describe the consequences of the reversible nature of movement of drugs through membranes.**

So far in the book, emphasis has been placed on the kinetic events following drug administration and the application of pharmacokinetic principles to the design and evaluation of dosage regimens. Little has been said about how the underlying physiologic processes control pharmacokinetic parameters, yet such information provides an insight into the interrelationships between drug and body. It also lays a foundation for the individualization of drug therapy, the subject of the next section.

This section explores the physiologic concepts basic to pharmacokinetics. It begins with a chapter dealing with the passage of drugs through membranes, proceeds through the processes of absorption, distribution and elimination, and ends with a chapter on the integration of physiologic kinetics and concepts. Such information helps not only to interpret pharmacokinetic data, obtained under a variety of circumstances, but also to predict the likely outcome when pharmacokinetic parameters change.

Absorption, distribution, and elimination are all processes that require movement through membranes. This movement is known as drug transport. The anatomic and physiologic factors that determine the rapidity of drug transport are the substance of this chapter.

TRANSPORT PROCESSES

Cellular membranes appear to be composed of an inner, predominantly lipoidal, matrix covered on each surface by either a continuous layer or a latticework of protein (Fig. 8–1, upper figure). The hydrophobic portions of the lipid

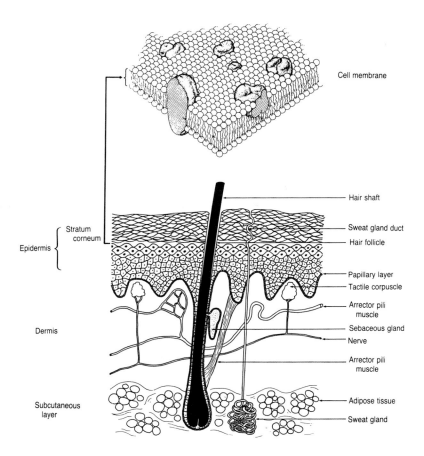

Fig. 8–1.   Functional membranes vary enormously in structure and thickness. They can be as thin as a single-cell membrane, of approximately 1×10^{-6} centimeter thickness (top), to as thick as the multicellular barrier of the skin. This multicellular barrier extends from the stratum corneum to the upper part of the papillary layer of the dermis, adjacent to the capillaries of the microcirculation; a distance of approximately 2×10^{-2} centimeter (bottom). The cell membrane comprises a bimolecular leaflet, with a lipid interior and a polar exterior, dispersed through which are globular proteins, depicted as large solid irregular shaped bodies [Cell membrane—reproduced from Singer, S.J. and Nicolson, G.L.: The fluid mosaic model of the structure of cell membranes. *SCIENCE.*, *175*:720, 1972, copyright 1982 by the AAAS; skin-kindly drawn by Mandy North.]

molecules are oriented toward the center of the membrane and the outer hydrophilic regions face the surrounding aqueous environment. Narrow aqueous-filled channels exist between some cells, and cell membranes contain small aqueous-filled pores.

The transport of drugs is often viewed as movement across a series of membranes and spaces which, in aggregate, serve as a "functional" macroscopic membrane. The cells and interstitial spaces that lie between the gastric lumen and the capillary blood or the structures between the sinusoidal space and the bile canaliculi in the liver are examples. Each of the interposing cellular membranes and spaces impede drug transport to varying degrees, and any one of them can rate-limit the overall process. It is this complexity of structure that makes quantitative prediction of drug transport difficult. A description of the qualitative features of the processes of drug transport across these "functional" membranes follows.

Passive Diffusion

Most drugs pass through membranes by *diffusion*, the natural tendency for molecules to move down a concentration gradient. Movement results from the kinetic energy of the molecules, and since no work is expended by the system, the process is known as *passive diffusion*.

To appreciate the properties of passive diffusion consider a simple system in which a membrane separates two well-stirred aqueous compartments. The driving force for drug transfer is the difference between the concentrations of the diffusing species in the compartments on either side of the membrane:

$$\text{Rate of penetration} = \underset{\substack{\text{Permeability}}}{P} \cdot \underset{\substack{\text{Surface} \\ \text{area}}}{SA} \cdot \underset{\substack{\text{Concentration} \\ \text{difference}}}{(C_1 - C_2)} \qquad 1$$

The importance of the surface area of the membrane is readily apparent. For example, doubling the surface area doubles the probability of collision with the membrane and thereby increases the penetration rate twofold. Some drugs readily pass through a membrane, others do not. This difference in ease of penetration is quantitatively expressed in terms of the *permeability*.

A major source of variation in permeability is the lipophilicity of the molecule, often characterized by its partition between oil and water. Lipid-soluble drugs tend to penetrate lipid membranes with ease and thus have high permeabilities. Polar neutral molecules (e.g., mannitol) and ionized compounds partition poorly into lipids, and they are either unable to pass through membranes or do so with much greater difficulty than do lipophilic molecules. Water-soluble materials may, however, move through the narrow channels between cells. Important functions influencing such paracellular movement are the size, shape and charge of the molecule, water movement through the channels (a convective process), and the nature of the channels themselves. For example, paracellular movement of oxytocin, a cyclic nonopeptide, is quite rapid across the relatively loosely knit nasal membranes but is almost nonexistent across the more tightly knit gastrointestinal membranes. Molecular size and shape are much less important for passive diffusion of lipophilic molecules through cells. Diffusion is related to the square root of the molecular weight, and the molecular weights of most drugs lie within the narrow range of 100 to 400.

Another determinant of permeability is membrane thickness, the distance a molecule has to traverse from the site of interest (e.g., an absorption surface) to a blood capillary. The shorter the distance the higher is the permeability. This distance can vary from about 0.005 to 0.01 microns (for cell membranes) to several millimeters (at some skin sites, Fig. 8–1, lower figure).

Drug transport continues toward equilibrium, a condition in which the concentrations of the diffusing species are the same in the aqueous phases on both sides of the membrane. Movement of drug between regions still continues at equilibrium, but the net flux is zero. Equilibrium is achieved more rapidly with highly permeable drugs, when there is a large surface area of contact with the membrane, and when the volumes of the compartments, to and from which the drug is transported, are small.

Initially, when all the drug is placed on one side of the membrane, it follows from Equation 1 that the rate of drug transport is directly proportional to the concentration (Fig. 8–2). For example, the rate of transport is increased twofold when the concentration of drug is doubled. Stated differently, each molecule diffuses independently of the other and the system cannot be saturated. Unless a drug alters the nature of the membrane, the last statement also applies when the other molecule is a different drug. Both absence of competition between molecules and lack of saturation are characteristics of passive diffusion.

Carrier-mediated Transport

Membranes are not inert barriers; they have a specialized function. Membranes maintain the internal cellular environment by excluding toxic materials and sequestering or selectively retaining vital substances. Many of these compounds are polar, with low lipid solubility. Yet they penetrate membranes much faster than anticipated for passive diffusion through an inert lipoidal barrier. Specialized carrier-mediated transport systems appear to be responsible. The substrates are often endogenous compounds, or close analogs.

The concept of a carrier stems from the observation of a limited rate of transport at increased substrate concentrations (Fig. 8–2). Two types of specialized transport processes have been proposed, passive facilitated diffusion and active transport.

Passive facilitated diffusion is exemplified by the movement of glucose into eryth-

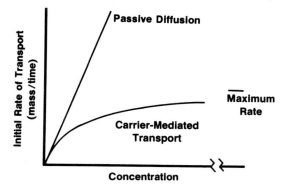

Fig. 8–2. Initial rate of drug transport is plotted against the concentration of drug placed on one side of a membrane. With passive diffusion, the rate of transport increases linearly with concentration. With carrier-mediated transport, the rate of transport approaches a maximum value at high concentrations.

rocytes. It is a passive process; glucose moves down a concentration gradient without expenditure of energy, and at equilibrium, the concentrations in and surrounding the red blood cells are equal. At high plasma glucose concentrations, however, the rate of transport of glucose into the erythrocyte reaches a limiting value or *transport maximum*. Furthermore, in common with other carrier-mediated systems, glucose transport is reasonably specific and is inhibited by other substrates. Few drugs undergo passive facilitated diffusion. An example is the transport of vitamin B_{12} across the gastrointestinal epithelium.

Examples of *active transport* abound and include renal and biliary secretion of many acids and bases, secretion of certain acids out of the central nervous system, and the intestinal absorption of 5-fluorouracil. Characteristics in common with passive facilitated diffusion are saturability, specificity, and competitive inhibition. Active transport is distinguished from passive facilitated diffusion by the net movement of substance against a concentration gradient, which can be large. The maintenance of this gradient requires metabolic energy. Active transport can therefore be impeded by metabolic inhibitors.

BLOOD FLOW

Blood, perfusing tissues, delivers and removes substances. Accordingly, viewing any tissue as a whole, the movement of drug through membranes cannot be divorced from perfusion considerations. Perfusion is usually expressed in units of milliliters per minute per volume (or mass) of tissue.

With highly lipid-soluble drugs, or those that pass freely through the aqueous-filled pores and channels, typical membranes offer virtually no barrier to drug movement. Under these circumstances, the slowest or rate-limiting step controlling the rate of movement through the membrane, and hence into and out of the tissue, is perfusion, not permeability, as shown in Figure 8–3. This perfusion limitation is exemplified in Figure 8–4 for the passage of certain substances across the jejunal membranes of a rat, from lumen to blood. Tritiated water

A. Perfusion-Rate Limitation

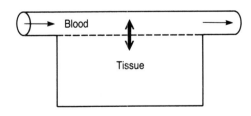

B. Permeability-Rate Limitation

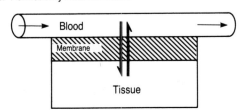

Fig. 8–3. The limiting step controlling the rate of movement of drug across a membrane, from blood to tissue or the converse, varies. A, If the membrane offers no resistance, drug in the blood leaving and in the tissue is in virtual equilibrium; blood and tissue may be viewed as one. Here movement of drug is limited by blood flow. B, A permeability-rate limitation exists if membrane resistance to drug movement becomes high; movement here is both slow and insensitive to changes in perfusion. Also, equilibrium is not achieved by the time the blood leaves the tissue; blood and tissue must now be viewed as separate compartments.

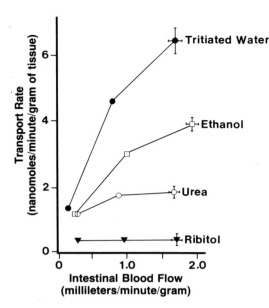

Fig. 8–4.   The rate of passage of a substance across the jejunum of a rat was determined by measuring its rate of appearance in the intestinal venous blood. The passage is blood flow limited when, like tritiated water, the molecule freely permeates the membrane. With poorly permeable substances, like the polar molecule ribitol, the passage is limited by transmembrane penetration, not by blood flow. (Redrawn from Winne, D. and Remischovsky, J.: Intestinal blood flow and absorption of non-dissociable substances. J. Pharm. Pharmacol., 22:640–641, 1970.)

moves freely through the aqueous pores and channels, and its rate of passage increases with increasing perfusion. The passage of ethanol and many lipophilic drugs is similarly perfusion rate-limited.

As membrane resistance to drug increases, the rate limitation moves away from one of perfusion to one of permeability. The problem now lies in penetrating the membrane, not in delivering drug to, or removing it from, the tissue (Fig. 8–3). This increase in resistance may arise for the same drug crossing membranes of increasing thickness; for example, the multiple cell layers of the epidermis are less permeable to a drug than is the single cell layer of the capillary epithelium. For the same membrane, resistance increases with increasing polarity of the molecule. Thus, transport across the jejunum is slower for ribitol and many other polar compounds than for ethanol or water, which results in insensitivity to changes in perfusion (Fig. 8–4).

Some compounds, like urea, have intermediate permeability characteristics across the jejunum. At low blood flow rates, the compound has sufficient time to traverse the membrane so that perfusion becomes rate-limiting. At higher blood flow rates, however, membrane permeability becomes the rate-limiting step, and absorption becomes insensitive to blood flow (Fig. 8–4).

IONIZATION

Most drugs are weak acids or weak bases and exist in solution as an equilibrium between un-ionized and ionized forms. Increased accumulation of drug on the side of a membrane whose pH favors a greater ionization of the drug has led to the *pH partition hypothesis.* According to this hypothesis, only un-ionized nonpolar drug penetrates the membrane, and at equilibrium, the concentration of the un-ionized species is equal on both sides of the membrane.

The majority of evidence supporting the pH partition hypothesis stems from studies of gastrointestinal absorption, renal excretion, and gastric secretion of drugs. The pH of the gastric fluid varies between 1.5 and 7.0; urine pH fluctuates between 4.5 and 7.5. Elsewhere in the body, changes in pH tend to be much smaller and to show less deviation from the pH of blood, 7.4.

The un-ionized form is assumed to be sufficiently lipophilic to traverse membranes. If it is not, theory predicts that there is no transfer, irrespective of pH. The fraction un-ionized is controlled by both the pH and the *pKa* of the drug according to the Henderson-Hasselbalch equation. Thus, for acids,

$$\text{pH} = pKa + \log_{10}\left(\frac{\text{Ionized concentration}}{\text{Un-ionized concentration}}\right) \qquad \text{2a}$$

and for bases

$$\text{pH} = pKa + \log_{10}\left(\frac{\text{Un-ionized concentration}}{\text{Ionized concentration}}\right) \qquad \text{2b}$$

Since $\log_{10}(1) = 0$, the *pKa* of a compound is the pH at which the un-ionized and ionized concentrations are equal. The *pKa* is a characteristic of the drug (Fig. 8–5). Consider, for example, the anticoagulant warfarin. Warfarin is an acid with *pKa* 4.8, that is, equimolar concentrations of un-ionized and ionized drug exist in solution at pH 4.8. Stated differently, 50 percent of the drug is un-ionized at this pH. At one pH unit higher, 5.8, the ratio is 10 to 1 in favor of the ionized drug, i.e., 10 out of 11 total parts or 91 percent of the drug now exists in the ionized form and only 9 percent is un-ionized. At one pH unit lower than the

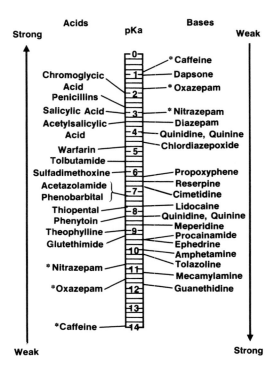

Fig. 8–5. The *pKa* values of acidic and basic drugs vary widely. Some drugs are amphoteric (*).

pKa, 3.8, the percentages in the ionized and un-ionized forms are 9 and 91, the converse of those at pH 5.8.

Figure 8–6 shows changes in the percent of un-ionized drug with pH for acids of different *pKa* values. The pH range 1.0 to 8.0 encompasses the pH values seen in the gastrointestinal tract and the renal tubule. Several considerations are in order and are exemplified by transport across the gastrointestinal barrier. First, very weak acids, such as phenytoin and many barbiturates, whose *pKa* values are greater than 7.5 are essentially un-ionized at all pH values. For these acids drug transport should be rapid and independent of pH, provided the un-ionized form is nonpolar. Second, the fraction un-ionized only changes dramatically for acids with *pKa* values between 3.0 and 7.5, and for these compounds a change in the rate of transport with pH is expected and has been observed. Third, although the transport of still stronger acids, those with *pKa* values less than 2.5, should theoretically also depend upon pH, in practice the fraction un-ionized is so low that transport across the gut membranes may be slow even under the most acidic conditions.

A similar analysis indicates that a base must be very weak, *pKa* less than 5, for transport to be independent of pH. Caffeine (*pKa* 0.8) is an example of a base that is rapidly transported and shows no pH-dependent absorption. Only with stronger bases, those with *pKa* values between 5 and 11, is pH-dependent transport expected. At the usually low pH of the gastric fluid, these bases exist almost exclusively in the ionized form, and for these, gastric transport should be slow. Passage of these bases should be more rapid from a less acidic environment. All evidence supports these expectations.

As originally proposed, the pH partition hypothesis relates to events at equilibrium, yet it has been applied most widely to predict the influence of pH on the rates of absorption and distribution. The likely influence of pH on a rate process depends, however, on where the rate limitation lies. Only if the limitation is in permeability is an effect of pH on rate expected. If the limitation is in perfusion, the problem is not one of movement of drug through membranes and, therefore, any variation in pH is unlikely to have much effect on the rate process. Where the equilibrium lies, however, is independent of what process rate-limits the approach toward equilibrium. Accordingly, pH is predicted to affect the distribution of an ionizable drug across a membrane at equilibrium in all cases in which the membrane is permeable only to un-ionized drug.

Despite its general appeal, the pH partition hypothesis fails to explain certain observations. A variety of quaternary ammonium compounds (e.g., propanthe-

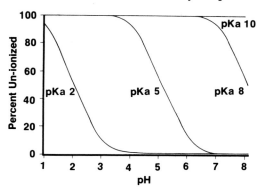

Fig. 8–6. Very weak acids, *pKa* values greater than 8.0, are predominantly un-ionized at all pH values between 1.0 and 8.0. Profound changes in the fraction un-ionized occur with pH for an acid whose *pKa* value lies within the range of 2.0 to 8.0. Although the fraction un-ionized of even stronger acids increases with hydrogen ion concentration, the absolute value remains low at most pH values shown.

line bromide) which are always ionized elicit systemic effects when given orally. Movement of these compounds through the gastrointestinal membranes occurs, although at a slow and erratic rate. Animal studies also indicate penetration of the ionized form of many acids and bases through membranes, though at a slower rate than the un-ionized form. Whether these ionized species traverse the membrane through aqueous pores, through channels between the cells, or by some carrier-mediated transport process is not fully understood. Whatever the mechanism, however, these observations suggest that quantitative predictions of the influence of pH on the movement of drugs across a membrane, the pH partition hypothesis, are unlikely to be accurate.

PROTEIN BINDING

Many drugs bind to plasma proteins and tissue components (discussed in Chap. 10). Such binding is reversible and usually so rapid that an equilibrium is established within milliseconds. Consequently, the associated, bound, and dissociated, unbound, forms of the drug can be assumed to be at equilibrium at all times and under virtually all circumstances.

Only unbound drugs are thought to be capable of passing through membranes, the protein-bound drugs being too large to do so. The influence of protein binding on the rate of movement of drug through a membrane can be viewed in much the same way as that of the influence of pH on the movement of weak acids and bases. Both binding and ionization are virtually instantaneous reactions, with only one species (unbound, un-ionized form) capable of traversing membranes. Thus, only if the limitation is in permeability is an effect of protein binding on rate expected.

If there is a perfusion limitation, dissociation of the bound drug and diffusion of the unbound drug through the membrane occur so rapidly that delivery of drug, rather than protein binding, limits the transport. However, as only unbound drugs diffuse across membranes, protein binding affects distribution of the total concentrations at equilibrium, irrespective of the rate limitation.

REVERSIBLE NATURE
OF TRANSPORT

Except for active transport, it is important to remember that drug transport is bidirectional. One tends, for example, to think of drug absorption in the gastrointestinal tract as being unidirectional. Normally, with very high concentrations of drug placed into the gastrointestinal tract, following oral administration, the net rate of transport is toward blood in the mesenteric capillaries. However, important applications can be made of transport in the opposite direction. For example, the repeated oral administration of charcoal can hasten removal from the body of drugs such as digoxin, phenylbutazone, phenobarbital, and digitoxin in cases of drug overdose. Because of extensive adsorption of drug to charcoal, the lumen of the gastrointestinal tract acts as a sink for removal of drug from the blood. In this case, the site of transfer may be restricted to only a small region of the gastrointestinal tract or may apply to a much larger area. The restriction depends on the distribution of charcoal along the gastrointestinal tract. Even with complete distribution of charcoal, whether the overall transfer from blood to gut lumen is perfusion rate-limited or not depends on the permeability of the various functional membranes along the length of the gut as well as on the blood flow to these various sites.

As previously stated, the concepts of this chapter on the passage of drugs across membranes are important to an understanding of the movement of drugs into, within, and out of the body. In the next three chapters, these concepts are incorporated with other principles dealing with drug absorption, distribution, and elimination.

Study Problems

(Answers to Study Problems are in Appendix G.)

1. Define the terms: passive diffusion, passive facilitated diffusion, and active transport.

2. How accurate are each of the following statements:

   (a) When distribution through a membrane is perfusion-rate limited, the ratio of concentrations across the membrane is virtually one at all times.

   (b) When the surface area of a membrane is doubled so is its permeability.

   (c) Passive diffusion across a membrane stops when the concentrations on both sides are the same.

   (d) Carrier-mediated transport is one in which energy is needed to transfer drug across a membrane.

   (e) Protein binding in the aqueous phases diminishes the permeability of membranes.

3. Briefly discuss the role of ionization in the movement of weak acids and weak bases across membranes.

4. Table 8–1 shows the effect of oral administration of activated charcoal on removal of phenobarbital from the body.

Table 8–1. Effect of Repeated Doses of Activated Charcoal on the Half-life (Hours) of Phenobarbital[a]

During Coadministration of Activated Charcoal[b]	Absence of Charcoal Administration
36 ± 13	93 ± 7

[a]From Pond, S.M. et al.: JAMA, *251*:3101, 1984.
[b]17 grams of charcoal in 70 milliliters of 70% percent sorbitol every 4 hours administered through a nasogastric tube.

Knowing that the volume of distribution of phenobarbital is 0.55 liters/kilogram, calculate the clearance of phenobarbital into the alimentary canal during treatment with charcoal.

Hint: CL (during treatment) $= CL$ (no treatment) $+ CL$ (by charcoal).

9

Absorption

Objectives

The reader will be able to:

1. Describe the steps involved in the absorption of a drug.

2. Distinguish between dissolution and transmembrane rate-limitations in absorption.

3. Anticipate the role of gastric emptying and intestinal transit in the gastrointestinal absorption of a drug, with particular reference to the physicochemical properties of the drug and its dosage form.

4. List the factors influencing the dissolution rate of a drug.

5. Describe the role of pH in drug absorption from solution and solid dosage forms.

Drugs are most frequently administered extravascularly. The majority are intended to act systemically, and for these, absorption is a prerequisite for activity. Delays or losses of drug during absorption may contribute to variability in drug response and, occasionally, may result in failure of drug therapy. It is primarily in this context, as a source of variability in systemic response and as a means of controlling the concentration-time profile of drug in the body, that absorption is considered here and throughout the remainder of the book. It should be kept in mind, however, that even for those drugs intended to act locally (e.g., mydriatics, local anesthetics, nasal decongestants, topical agents, and aerosol bronchodilators), systemic absorption influences the time of onset, the intensity, and the duration of effect.

This chapter deals with the general principles governing the rate and extent of drug absorption. Emphasis is placed on absorption following oral administration. This is not only because the oral mode of administration is the most prevalent for systemically acting drugs, but also because it illustrates essentially all the sources of variability encountered in drug absorption. Where important, distinctions are made between absorption from the gastrointestinal tract and absorption from other sites.

Figure 9–1 depicts the numerous steps involved in the absorption of a drug given orally. Being a complex structure, there are many anatomic and physiologic

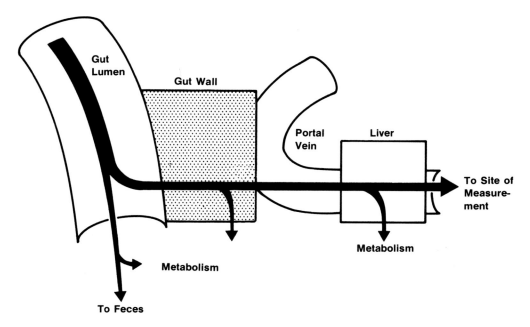

Fig. 9–1. A drug, given as a solid, encounters several barriers and sites of loss in its sequential movement during gastrointestinal absorption. Dissolution, a prerequisite to movement across the gut wall, is the first step. Incomplete dissolution or metabolism in the gut lumen or by enzymes in the gut wall is a cause of poor absorption. Removal of drug as it first passes through the liver further reduces absorption.

factors affecting the overall rate and extent of drug absorption from the gastrointestinal tract, making a precise quantitative prediction difficult. Nonetheless, much can be understood and appreciated.

As elsewhere, passage of drug through the membranes dividing the absorption site from the blood is a prerequisite for absorption to occur from the gastrointestinal tract. To do so, the drug must be in solution. Most drugs are taken orally in solid dosage preparations. Common examples are tablets and capsules. Because solid particles cannot pass through membranes, a drug has to dissolve to be absorbed. Many factors influence the release of drug from a solid pharmaceutical formulation. *Biopharmaceutics* is a comprehensive term denoting the study of the influence of pharmaceutical formulation variables on the performance of a drug *in vivo*.

ABSORPTION FROM SOLUTION

Several physiologic and physical factors that determine the movement of drug through membranes have been discussed generally in Chapter 8. Included among them are the physicochemical properties of the molecule, the nature of the membrane, perfusion, and pH. These factors and others are now considered with respect to drug absorption.

Perfusion and pH

Blood flow assures continuous absorption by removing drug that passes through a membrane. The body into which drug distributes acts as a virtual sink, maintaining a concentration gradient across the intestinal membranes. As was shown in Figure 8–4 (p. 108), absorption from the luminal contents of the jejunum can be perfusion rate-limited for both small and highly lipophilic compounds. This perfusion limitation arises because the small intestine is highly permeable to many substances. For such substances, even if they are weak acids or bases, the effect of changes in pH at this absorption site on the rate of drug absorption is relatively small as long as the perfusion limitation holds. If absorption is permeability rate-limited then a pH effect on absorption is anticipated when the pKa of the molecule is in the range in which substantial changes in the fraction un-ionized occurs with changes in pH. For example, recall from Chapter 8 (p. 110) that this condition is met for acids of pKa 3.0 to 7.5 when placed at the absorption site at which pH varies from 2.0 to 7.0. In practice, changes in small intestinal pH are likely to be small, as the pH is kept reasonably close to neutrality by the buffering action of pancreatic and biliary secretions.

In contrast to the small intestine, and indeed to the gastrointestinal tract as a whole, absorption of drugs in solution from muscle and subcutaneous tissue is invariably perfusion rate-limited; increases in blood flow hasten absorption. This flow dependence can be explained by the nature of the barrier (the capillary wall) between the site of injection (the interstitial fluid) and blood. The capillary wall, a much more loosely knit structure than the epithelial lining of the gastrointestinal tract, offers little impedance to the movement of drugs into blood. For example, gentamicin, a water-soluble, ionized, polar base, has great difficulty penetrating the gastrointestinal mucosa but is rapidly absorbed from the intramuscular site. This lack of impedance by the capillary wall in muscle and subcutaneous tissue applies to drugs, whether ionized or not, of molecular weights below about 5000. Thus, absorption at these sites for almost all drugs is independent of pKa or polarity and is perfusion rate-limited.

Local anesthetics are injected into almost every tissue of the body. Large differences in the absorption rates of these generally highly lipophilic drugs from tissues are observed (Table 9–1), and as expected, many of these differences are associated with tissue perfusion, which varies widely.

Table 9–1. Influence of Site of Injection on the Peak Venous Lidocaine Concentration Following Injection of a 100-milligram Dose[a]

Injection Site	Peak Plasma Lidocaine Concentration (mg/liter)[b]
Intercostal	1.46
Paracervical	1.20
Caudal	1.18
Lumbar epidural	0.97
Brachial plexus	0.53
Subarachnoid	0.44
Subcutaneous	0.35

[a]Taken from Covino, B.G.: Pharmacokinetics of local anaesthetic drugs. In: Pharmacokinetics of Anaesthesia. Edited by C. Prys-Roberts and C.C. Hug. Blackwell Scientific Publications, Oxford, 1984, pp. 270–292.
[b]One milligram/liter = 4.3 micromolar.

Absorption Kinetics

Figure 9–2 is a linear plot of the amount of salicylic acid remaining to be absorbed from a rat stomach and intestine with time. Recall from Chapter 4 that, under these circumstances, absorption of salicylic acid occurs by first-order processes. As a first approximation, absorption of drugs from many other sites is also first-order. An explanation for these observations is now possible. Based on the considerations presented in Chapter 8, the driving force for absorption is the difference between the concentrations of the diffusible form of the drug at the absorption site (C_a) and that unbound in the blood (Cu) perfusing it.

$$\text{Rate of absorption} = W \cdot (C_a - Cu) \qquad\qquad 1$$

where W is a proportionality constant whose value equals either the product of permeability and the effective surface area for absorption ($P \cdot SA$) or blood flow, depending on whether the rate-limiting step is permeability or perfusion. The sheer size of the body, by diluting absorbed drug, tends to maintain sink conditions, in which Cu is much smaller than C_a; therefore

$$\text{Rate of absorption} = W \cdot C_a \qquad\qquad 2$$

Assuming that the volume of fluid at the absorption site (Va) remains relatively constant, then

$$\text{Rate of absorption} = \frac{W}{Va} \cdot Aa \qquad\qquad 3$$

where Aa is the amount of drug at the absorption site. From this last relationship absorption appears to be a first-order process with a rate constant, ka, equal to W/Va. On administering drug in different volumes, because of spreading, there is a tendency for the surface-area-to-fluid-volume ratio (SA/Va) to remain constant. Consequently, the absorption rate constant, ka, is relatively insensitive to volume changes.

Although Equation 3 may be a reasonable approximation of the absorption kinetics at one site, it may not always apply to gastrointestinal absorption as a

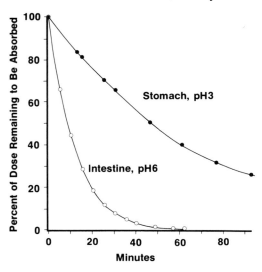

Fig. 9–2. Despite an environment favoring a greater percentage of un-ionized drug, absorption of salicylic acid (*pKa* 3) is slower from the rat stomach at pH 3 (●) than from the rat intestine at pH 6 (○). (Modified from Doluisio, J.T., Billups, N.F., Dittert, L.W., Sugita, E.G., and Swintosky, J.V.: Drug Absorption I. An *in situ* rat gut technique yielding realistic absorption rates. J. Pharm. Sci., *58*: 1196–1199, 1969. Adapted with permission of the copyright owner.)

whole. With exposure of drug to widely different environments along the gastrointestinal tract, gastrointestinal absorption kinetics are sometimes complex and not easily defined by a simple equation.

Gastric Emptying

In accordance with the prediction of the pH partition hypothesis, weak acids are absorbed more rapidly from the stomach at pH 1.0 than at pH 8.0, and the converse holds for weak bases. Absorption of acids, however, is always much faster from the less acidic small intestine (pH 5.0 to 7.0) than from the stomach (Fig. 9–2). These apparently conflicting observations can be reconciled. Surface area, permeability and, for perfusion rate-limited absorption, blood flow are important determinants of the rapidity of absorption. The intestine, especially the small intestine, is favored on all accounts. The total absorptive area of the small intestine, composed largely of microvilli, has been calculated to be about 200 square meters, and an estimated 1 liter of blood passes through the intestinal capillaries each minute. The corresponding estimates for the stomach are only 1 square meter and 150 milliliters/minute. The permeability of the intestinal membranes to drugs is also much greater than that of the stomach. These increases in surface area, permeability, and blood flow more than compensate for the decreased fraction of un-ionized acid in the intestine. Indeed, the absorption of *all* compounds, be they acids, bases, or neutral compounds, is faster from the (small) intestine than from the stomach. The rate of gastric emptying, therefore, is a controlling step in the speed of drug absorption.

Gastric emptying of liquids is approximately a first-order process with a half-life of about 30 minutes. Food, especially fat, slows gastric emptying, which explains why drugs are frequently recommended to be taken on an empty stomach when a rapid onset of action is desired. Drugs that influence gastric emptying also affect the rate of absorption of other drugs (Fig. 9–3).

Retention of drug in the stomach increases the percentage of a dose absorbed through the gastric mucosa, but usually the majority of drug is still absorbed through the intestinal epithelium. In this regard, the stomach may be viewed as a repository organ from which pulses of drug are ejected by peristalsis onto the absorption sites in the small intestine.

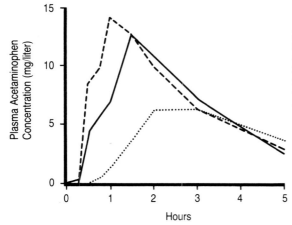

Fig. 9–3. Slowing gastric emptying by propantheline (30 mg intravenously) slows the rate of absorption of acetaminophen (1500 mg), administered orally in a 22-year-old man, as seen by a decrease in the maximum plasma concentration and a longer time to reach this concentration (·······) compared to values when acetaminophen is given alone (——). Metoclopramide (10 mg intravenously), which hastens gastric emptying, hastens the absorption of acetaminophen (– – –). (One mg/liter = 6.6 micromolar.) (Redrawn from Nimmo, J., Heading, R.C., Tothill, P., and Prescott, L.F.: Pharmacological modification of gastric emptying: Effects of propantheline and metoclopramide on paracetamol (acetaminophen) absorption. Br. Med. J., 1:587–588, 1973.)

Causes of Low Availability

When a drug is given in solution and passes readily across membranes, absorption from most sites of administration is complete. This is not always so for drugs placed into the gastrointestinal tract.

A drug must pass sequentially from the gastrointestinal lumen, through the gut wall, and through the liver, before entering the general circulation (Fig. 9–1). This sequence is an anatomic requirement because blood perfusing virtually all the gastrointestinal tissues drains into the liver via the hepatic portal vein. If the only cause of loss is incomplete time for absorption, then the availability would be less than one and the complement, the fraction appearing in the feces unchanged, is a measure of luminal retention. Drug may also be lost by decomposition in the lumen; the fraction entering the tissues, F_F, is then the fraction neither lost in the feces nor decomposed in the lumen. Further loss of drug in the walls of the gastrointestinal tract reduces the fraction of the dose reaching the liver to $F_F \cdot F_G$, where F_G is the fraction of the drug, neither lost in the feces nor decomposed in the lumen, that escapes destruction in the gastrointestinal tract. If drug is also eliminated in the liver, an additional fraction, F_H, of that reaching the liver escapes extraction there. The measured overall availability, F, clearly is then

$$F = F_F \cdot F_G \cdot F_H \qquad\qquad 4$$

For example, if 50 percent of the drug is lost at each step, the availability of the drug, measured systemically, would be $0.5 \times 0.5 \times 0.5$ or 12.5 percent. Note that the drug can be rendered totally unavailable at any one of these steps.

The lungs are excluded from the foregoing considerations of availability even though they may occasionally be an important site of elimination. As discussed in Chapter 4, drug given intravenously is used as a standard to measure availability, with calculation based on measurement of drug at a peripheral venous site. Both intravenously and orally administered drugs must first pass through the lungs to reach this site of measurement. Consequently, the effect of the lungs on the measurement of availability need not be considered.

Insufficient Time for Absorption. Ingested drug is exposed to the entire gastrointestinal mucosa for no more than 1 to 2 days and for only 2 to 4 hours at the main absorption site, the small intestine. If the absorption membranes are poorly permeable to drug, there may be insufficient time for complete absorption. If this occurs, as it does for such polar and relatively large compounds as neomycin and quaternary ammonium drugs, not only is availability low but, with the usual vagaries of intestinal motility and transit time, absorption is often erratic and availability correspondingly variable.

The rectum has a small surface area and a drug given rectally is not always retained for a sufficient length of time to ensure complete absorption. No time limitation exists for a drug injected into muscle, subcutaneous tissue, and most other sites within the body; complete absorption is anticipated unless destruction occurs at the site of administration.

Competing Reactions. Any reaction that competes with absorption may reduce the oral availability of a drug. Table 9–2 lists various reactions that can occur within the gastrointestinal tract. Reactions can be both enzymatic and

Table 9–2. Representative Reactions within the Gastrointestinal Tract that Compete for Drug Absorption from Solution

Reaction	Drug	Comment
Complexation	Tetracycline	Unabsorbed insoluble complexes with polyvalent metal ions, e.g., Ca^{2+}, Al^{3+}
Conjugation		
Sulfoconjugation	Isoproterenol	Loss of activity: product inactive
Glucuronidation	Salicylamide	Loss of activity: product inactive
Decarboxylation	Levodopa	Loss of activity: given with a peripheral dopa decarboxylase inhibitor to reduce gastrointestinal metabolism
Hydrolysis		
Acid	Penicillin G	Loss of activity: product inactive
	Erythromycin	Loss of activity: product inactive
	Digoxin	Product probably inactive
Enzymatic	Aspirin	Salicylic acid formed, active anti-inflammatory compound
	Pivampicillin	Active ampicillin formed: pivampicillin (ester) is inactive
Reduction (micro-flora)	Sulfasalazine	Intended for local (intestinal) anti-inflammatory action; parent drug inactive; product, 5-aminosalicylic acid, active
Adsorption	Digoxin	Adsorption to cholestryamine: adsorbed material not absorbed

nonenzymatic. Acid hydrolysis is a common nonenzymatic reaction. Enzymes in the intestinal epithelium and within the intestinal microflora, which normally reside in the large bowel, metabolize some drugs. The reaction products are often inactive or less potent than the parent molecule. Interactions with constituents of the gastrointestinal fluids also occur; the result may be poor drug availability. For example, one reason why tetracycline is incompletely absorbed when coadministered with milk and with certain antacids is that this antibiotic forms sparingly soluble complexes with the polyvalent cation (e.g., Ca^{2+}, Mg^{2+}, and Al^{3+}) contained in these preparations.

The complexities that occur *in vivo* preclude accurate prediction of the contribution of the competing reaction to a decreased availability. Sometimes the problem of incomplete absorption can be circumvented by physically protecting the drug from destruction in the stomach (see enteric coating p. 36) or by synthesizing a more stable derivative, which is converted to the active molecule within the body. These derivatives are generally referred to as *prodrugs* if they are inactive.

Hepatic Extraction. Aspirin (acetylsalicylic acid) was one of the first prodrugs. It was marketed at the turn of the century to overcome the unpleasant taste and the gastrointestinal irritation associated with the parent drug, salicylic acid. Aspirin was originally thought to be inactive, being designed to be rapidly hydrolyzed within the body to salicylic acid. Only subsequently was aspirin shown to be pharmacologically active. Yet the original design worked; upon ingestion, aspirin, a labile ester, is rapidly hydrolyzed, particularly by esterases in the liver. Indeed, hepatic hydrolysis is so rapid that a sizeable fraction of aspirin is converted to salicylic acid in a single passage through the liver, resulting in a substantial "first-pass effect."

Drugs that show a substantial first-pass effect in man due to hepatic elimination are listed in Table 9–3. Apart from this feature, they have little in common. They are of diverse chemical structure, possess different pharmacologic activities, and are metabolized via a number of pathways. When the metabolite(s) formed during the first pass through the liver is less potent than the parent drug, the oral dose is larger than the intravenous or intramuscular dose required to achieve the same therapeutic effect. This occurs for many of the drugs listed in Table 9–3. In some instances, e.g., isoproterenol, hepatic extraction is so high as to essentially preclude the oral route. Here, no amount of pharmaceutical formulation helps. Either the drug must be given by a parenteral route, or it must be discarded in favor of another drug candidate. A method of estimating the maximum likely decrease in oral availability due to this first-pass effect is discussed in Chapter 11.

Avoiding the first pass through the liver probably explains most of the activity of nitroglycerin administered sublingually. Blood perfusing the buccal cavity bypasses the liver and enters directly into the superior vena cava. This antianginal drug is almost completely metabolized as it passes through the liver, and any drug swallowed is not systemically available. The metabolites seen in blood are only weakly active but under certain circumstances may reach concentrations high enough to contribute to overall activity.

The rectal route has a definite advantage over the oral route for drugs that are destroyed by gastric acidity or by enzymes in the intestinal wall and microflora. Potentially, the rectal route may also partially reduce first-pass hepatic loss. Part of the rectal blood supply, particularly the inferior and middle hemorrhoidal veins, bypasses the hepatic portal circulation and dumps directly into the inferior vena cava. Achieving a reproducible availability, which is important in drug therapy, may be difficult, however, since availability is strongly dependent upon the site of absorption within the rectum.

Table 9–3. Representative Drugs Showing Low Oral Availability Due to Extensive[a] First-Pass Hepatic Elimination

Alprenolol	Methylphenidate
Amitriptyline	Metoprolol
Chlormethiazole	Morphine
Desipramine	Neostigmine
Dextropropoxyphene	Nifedipine
Dihydroergotamine	Nitroglycerin
Diltiazem	Papaverine
5-Fluorouracil	Pentazocine
Hydralazine	Phenacetin
Isoproterenol	Propranolol
Labetolol	Salicylamide
Lidocaine	Testosterone
Mercaptopurine	Verapamil

[a]F = 0.5 or less, on average. Adapted from Pond, S.M. and Tozer, T.N.: First-pass elimination: Basic concepts and clinical consequences. Clin. Pharmacokin. 9:1–25, 1984.

ABSORPTION FROM SOLIDS

Formulation

Solubility and stability limitations, taste, and convenience often argue against administration of solutions; hence the use of solid-medicaments, such as tablets and capsules. Equality of drug content was once assumed to assure equality of efficacy. Evidence now exists that questions this assumption. Therapeutic failures have been reported when one manufacturer's brand of prednisone tablet was substituted by another's. Increased side effects associated with phenytoin have occurred upon switching formulations of this drug. In each case, the amount of drug in the dosage form was the same. The problem arose from differences in absorption of drug from the different formulations. The magnitude of the problem is poorly defined but extends beyond these two drugs. Other drugs that have shown marked differences in absorption from various marketed products of the same dosage form include: chloramphenicol, digoxin, nitrofurantoin, oxytetracycline, tetracycline, and tolbutamide.

Generally, when problems arise in drug therapy because of differences in absorption, availability is the major consideration. Occasionally variations in absorption rate may also be important. Much depends upon whether the drug is taken occasionally or continuously (Chap. 7).

The major cause of differences in absorption of a drug from various formulations is dissolution. Marketed products must meet pharmacopeial standards. These standards, however, have been primarily for content and purity of the active ingredient(s). Few standards exist for the numerous inert ingredients (excipients) used to stabilize the drug; facilitate manufacture of the dosage form; maintain its integrity during handling and storage; and facilitate release of drug following administration of the dosage form. Intended, or otherwise, each ingredient can influence the rate of dissolution of the drug, as can the manufacturing process. The result is a large potential for variability in absorption of a drug between generic products. Sometimes these differences in absorption can be correlated with differences in the dissolution rate of the drug measured in an *in vitro* apparatus. There are dissolution requirements for certain important drug products. However, on occasion, *in vitro* dissolution tests fail to distinguish between products showing inequivalent absorption profiles. At present, evaluation in humans continues to be the best way of discriminating between good and bad formulations.

Dissolution

The reason why dissolution is so important may be gained by realizing that absorption following administration of a solid is a two-step process:

$$\text{Solid drug} \xrightarrow{\text{Dissolution}} \text{Drug in solution} \xrightarrow[\text{the body}]{\text{Entry into}} \text{Absorbed drug}$$

Two situations are now considered. The first, depicted in Figure 9–4A, is one in which dissolution is much faster than the rate of entry of drug into the body. Consequently, most of the drug has dissolved before an appreciable amount has been absorbed. Here, transmembrane passage rather than dissolution rate-

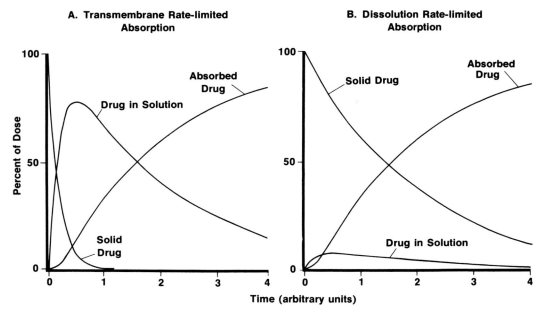

Fig. 9–4.   When absorption is transmembrane rate-limited (case A) most of the drug has dissolved before an appreciable fraction has been absorbed. In contrast, when dissolution rate-limits absorption (case B) very little drug is in solution at the absorption site at any time; drug is absorbed as soon as it dissolves. Notice that the majority of drug not absorbed is always found at the rate-limiting step: in solution in case A and as a solid in case B.

limits absorption. An example is the gastrointestinal absorption of neomycin. This polar antibiotic dissolves rapidly but has difficulty penetrating the gastrointestinal epithelium; little is absorbed. Differences in rates of dissolution of neomycin from different tablets have little or no effect on the speed of absorption of this drug.

In the second and much more common situation, shown in Figure 9–4B, dissolution proceeds relatively slowly, and any dissolved drug readily traverses the gastrointestinal epithelium. Absorption cannot proceed any faster, however, than the rate at which the drug dissolves. That is, absorption is dissolution rate-limited. In this case, changes in dissolution profoundly affect the rate, and sometimes the extent, of drug absorption. Evidence supporting dissolution rate-limited absorption comes from the slower absorption of most drugs from solid dosage forms than from a simple aqueous solution.

Factors Controlling Dissolution

Progress in formulation design, in establishment of useful *in vitro* dissolution tests, and in the ability to anticipate absorption problems with certain drugs comes with an understanding of the factors controlling dissolution. These factors are embodied in the relationship:

$$\text{Rate of dissolution} = K_{dis} \cdot SA \cdot \left[\begin{array}{c} \text{Saturated} \\ \text{solution} \\ \text{at solid} \\ \text{surface} \end{array} - \begin{array}{c} \text{Concentration} \\ \text{in} \\ \text{bulk of} \\ \text{solution} \end{array} \right] \qquad 5$$

where K_{dis} is a constant and SA is the surface area of the dissolving solid. These factors are examined separately.

Surface Area. Expanding the surface exposed to the solvent hastens dissolution. Reducing the size of the solid particles is the most common means of achieving this goal. Yet, for convenience, the opposite is done. For example, fine particles of drugs are compressed or compacted into tablets and capsules. Clearly, this manufacturing process must be reversed if the surface area is to be enlarged sufficiently to ensure adequate dissolution. To this effect, materials (disintegrants) are incorporated into tablets that cause them to swell upon contact with water and then to disintegrate into granules that finally deaggregate into the original fine drug particles.

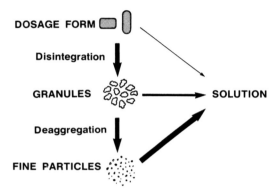

Well-formulated products intended for rapid absorption, disintegrate and deaggregate within minutes of administration. Failure to do so may be the cause of poor absorption.

Solubility. In dissolution rate-limited absorption, the concentration of drug in solution at the absorption site is kept low because dissolved drug rapidly enters the body. The driving force for dissolution is then directly related to the solubility of the drug at the surface of the dissolving solid (Eq. 5). This explains why tablets, capsules, and even suspensions of sparingly soluble drugs are prone to absorption problems. Even if dissolution were not the rate-limiting step and a saturated solution at the absorption site could be maintained, the rate of absorption of these drugs would still be low owing to the low aqueous solubility. Among such drugs are digoxin, griseofulvin, and spironolactone. All have low aqueous solubilities, 10 milligrams/liter or less, as do tolbutamide and warfarin. The last two drugs, however, are weak acids whose dissolution can be markedly increased by using a salt. For example, sodium tolbutamide is absorbed much more rapidly than the free acid. The explanation lies in the different concentration at the surface of the dissolving solid. For tolbutamide this concentration is the low aqueous solubility of the free acid, whereas for sodium tolbutamide the corresponding concentration is the saturated solution of the salt. Since the salt is much more soluble than the free acid, dissolution of the former is much faster. Likewise, the hydrochloride or sulfate salt of a base dissolves more rapidly than does the corresponding free base.

Other means of promoting dissolution have been employed. When a drug exists in more than one crystalline (polymorphic) state, the more rapidly dissolving polymorph or amorphous solid is used.

pH. Any means of increasing the concentration gradient of the dissolving drug that exists between the surface of the solid and the bulk of the solution promotes dissolution. For acids and bases, adjusting the pH of the medium is one way of affecting removal. As an example, consider the dissolution of a base in water and in an acidic solution. In water, as the base dissolves, it produces a saturated solution in the immediate vicinity of the dissolving particle. Further away the concentration falls off as drug diffuses into the body of the solution. Build-up of drug in the water around the solid lowers the concentration gradient and hinders further dissolution. If, however, hydrogen ions are available to consume the dissolved free base by converting it to the solution cation, the gradient of free base is maintained and dissolution is more rapid. Thus, bases dissolve more rapidly in an acid medium, whereas for analogous reasons, acids dissolve more rapidly in an alkaline medium.

Two methods of increasing the dissolution rate of a base have been considered: use of a salt and use of an acidic environment. Of these, using a salt generally results in faster dissolution. The enormous increase in solubility of the salt over that of the free base more than compensates for the continual removal of the base in an acidic solution. This is also true for acids. Thus the sodium salt of an acid generally dissolves more rapidly than does the free acid (Table 9–4).

Stirring. Consider now a common situation, the ingestion of a solid formulation of the sodium salt of a sparingly soluble acid. The salt rapidly dissolves at the surface upon contact with the gastric fluid, forming a saturated solution. However, as the salt diffuses away from the surface it is neutralized by hydrogen ions. The free acid formed is at a concentration in excess of its solubility, so the drug precipitates in a finely divided state. Subsequent events depend largely upon the stirring rate around the dissolving particle. With rapid stirring, the precipitate is swept away into the bulk of the solution, creating fresh surface for neutralization and further dissolution. The result is rapid dissolution of the sodium salt, and the formation of finely divided precipitate of the acid, of large surface area, dispersed in a saturated solution of the acid. These are excellent conditions for rapid absorption. If, on the other hand, stirring is slow, then the less soluble precipitated acid can form a crust around the dissolving particle of the salt. Further dissolution is thereby hindered, especially if the freshly precipitated acid grows to moderately sized crystals, with an associated small surface

Table 9–4. Dissolution of Acids and Their Sodium Salts into Acidic and Neutral Solutions[a]

	Dissolution Rate (mg/100 min/ cm² of dissolving surface)	
	pH 1.5	pH 6.8
Phenobarbital	0.24	1.2
Sodium salt	200	820
Salicylic acid	1.7	27
Sodium salt	1870	2500
Sulfathiazole	<0.1	0.5
Sodium salt	550	810

[a]Taken from the data of Nelson, E.: Comparative dissolution rates of weak acids and their sodium salts. J. Am. Pharm. Assoc., (Sci. Ed.) 47:297–299, 1958.

area. Now, dissolution and absorption may be even slower than from a well-formulated preparation of finely divided free acid. In practice, both situations probably occur.

Peristaltic movements in the stomach are generally feeble but variable. Mixing in the antrum can be quite vigorous. The disintegration rate, deaggregation rate, location of the dosage form in the stomach, food, and the state of the patient each influence the stirring rate around the dissolving particle. Stirring is generally sufficient to ensure complete and rapid drug absorption from solid dosage forms containing the salts of acids and bases.

As mentioned previously, little drug is generally absorbed from the stomach. Nonetheless, dissolution in the gastric fluid is a prerequisite to the absorption of some drugs. This point is well illustrated by tetracycline hydrochloride. Only that which dissolves in the stomach is apparently absorbed. This amphoteric antibiotic, freely soluble in both strongly acidic and alkaline solutions, is minimally soluble at pH 5.8, a typical pH of the intestinal fluid. Perhaps the sparingly soluble tetracycline precipitates onto undissolved particles entering the intestine, thereby limiting further dissolution.

Gastric Emptying and Intestinal Transit

Before discussing the role of gastric emptying on absorption of drugs given as solids, consider the information provided in Figure 9–5. Shown are the mean transit times in the stomach and small intestine of small nondisintegrating pellets (diameters between 0.3 to 1.8 millimeters) and of large single nondisintegrating units (either capsules, 25 millimeters by 9 millimeters or tablets, 8 to 12 millimeters in diameter).

During fasting, gastric emptying of both small and large solids is seen, on average, to be rapid with a mean transit time of around one hour, although there is considerable individual variability. In this state, the stomach displays a complex temporal pattern of motor activity with alternating periods of quiescence and moderate contraction of varying frequency, culminating in an intense contraction, the "housekeeping wave," that propels all gastric contents, including solids almost irrespective of size, into the small intestine. The exact ejection time of a solid particle therefore depends on when the solid is taken during the motor activity cycle, an unpredictable period varying from 20 minutes to a few hours.

The situation is very different after eating. As shown in Figure 9–5, when taken on a fed stomach, the gastric transit time of solids is increased. This increase is greater after a heavy meal than after a light one and is much greater for a large single unit than for small pellets. For example, the mean gastric transit time for large single unit systems is now almost 7 hours, with some of them still in the stomach 11 hours after ingestion. These observations are explained by the sieving action of a fed stomach. The irregular "housekeeping waves" are now replaced by regular and more gentle contractions, which continuously mix and triturate the gastric contents. Furthermore, only solids with diameters less than 2 millimeters are allowed to pass into the small intestine with gastric fluid. Larger food particles are retained until reduced to the requisite size by trituration and partial digestion. With conventional tablets, disintegration and subsequent deaggregation into fine particles achieves the same objective. As long as the

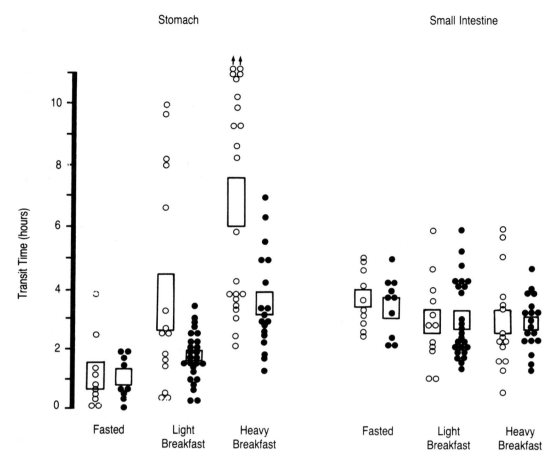

Fig. 9–5. Food, particularly a heavy meal, increases the gastric transit time of small pellets (●) and, even more markedly, of large single units (○). In contrast, neither food nor the physical size of the solid affects the small intestine transit time. The data (individual points, ● or ○, and their mean ± S.E., indicated by the rectangles) were obtained in healthy young adults using drug-free nondisintegrating materials. The points with an arrow indicate that solid was still in the stomach at the time of the last observation, the time indicated. (Adapted from Davis, S.S., Hardy, J.G., and Fara, J.: Transit of pharmaceutical dosage forms through the small intestine. Gut, 27:886–892, 1986.)

stomach remains in a fed state, the conditions above prevail. For those persons who eat three good meals a day, this would be for most of the day.

In contrast to events in the stomach, the transit time of solids within the small intestine varies little among subjects, appears to be independent of either the size of a solid or the presence of food in the stomach, and is remarkably short, approximately 3 hours (Fig. 9–5), a time similar to that found for the transit of liquids. Both solids and liquids appear to move down the small intestine as a plug with relatively little mixing.

As the mouth-to-anus transit time is typically 1 to 2 days, these data on gastric and small intestinal transit times indicate that, for the majority of this time, ingested solids are in either the large bowel or the rectum.

Provided with the physiologic information above, the possible role of gastric emptying and intestinal transit in the absorption of drugs given in solid dosage forms can be understood by considering the following situations.

First, there is the common situation, seen with many conventional tablets and capsules, in which the drug dissolves so rapidly that most is in solution before much has entered the intestine. Here, gastric emptying clearly influences the rate of drug absorption. Hastening gastric emptying, for example, quickens drug absorption from solution.

Next, there is the situation in which a drug does not dissolve in the stomach, whereas in the intestine it both rapidly dissolves and passes across the intestinal wall. Gastric emptying then dramatically affects the time and perhaps the rate of drug absorption. An enteric-coated product is an extreme example of this situation. Erythromycin and penicillin G are rapidly hydrolyzed to inactive products in the acidic environment of the stomach. Salicylic acid is a gastric irritant. A solution to both types of problems has been to coat these drugs with a material resistant to acid but not to the intestinal fluids. Many such enteric-coated products are large single tablets, and the time taken for an intact tablet to pass from the stomach into the intestine will vary unpredictably from 20 minutes to several hours when taken on an empty stomach and up to 12 hours or even more when taken on a fed stomach. Accordingly, such enteric-coated products are not to be used when a rapid and reliable rate of absorption is required. A product composed of enteric-coated granules is an improvement because the rate of delivery of the granules to the intestine is expected to be more reliable, being less dependent on a single event and on food.

Then, there is the situation of a drug, such as griseofulvin, that is sparingly soluble in both gastric and intestinal fluids. There may already be insufficient time for dissolution and absorption when this drug is administered as a solid. With a fixed short time within the small intestine, the slow release of such a drug from the stomach increases the total time it is in the intestine and decreases the concentration at any one site. Both conditions favor increased availability. As mentioned, food, fats in particular, delays gastric emptying, and this delay may be one of the explanations for the observed increase in the availability of griseofulvin when taken with a fatty meal or with fats. Subsequently, as the intestinal fluid and contents move into the large intestine and water is reabsorbed, the resulting compaction of the solid contents may severely limit further dissolution and hence absorption of drug.

The conclusions drawn for sparingly soluble drugs may also apply to certain controlled-release dosage forms. Some of these are coated with a nondisintegrating material through which the release rate of drug is independent of both pH and agitation. In such cases, gastric emptying has little effect on the rate of drug absorption. Even though the solid dosage form may be retained in the stomach, the released drug will be continuously emptied with the gastric fluid into the duodenum and will be available for absorption. Any delay in the gastric emptying of such products will prolong the total period for drug release and absorption. For reasons discussed above, this delay is most likely to be seen with large single units taken on a fed stomach. It would be unwise, however, to depend too much on this delay to achieve a prolonged absorption profile given the well-known unpredictability of patients' eating habits and their general lack of compliance in taking medication. Furthermore, compaction in the large intestine may preclude reliable input of drug beyond 12 hours, which severely limits the design of controlled-release dosage forms of drugs with short half-lives intended for once-a-day administration. Both the absorption rate profile and availability of drug from such products are likely to be poor and highly variable.

Precipitation and Redissolution

Absorption is normally complete within 1 or 2 hours of administering an aqueous solution of a drug intramuscularly or subcutaneously. There are exceptions, however, particularly when injecting a solution of a salt of either a sparingly soluble acid or base. For example, chlordiazepoxide hydrochloride, in solution, is commonly given intramuscularly when rapid sedation is desired. However, large doses sometimes appear to be poorly effective or ineffective. Although it is eventually completely available, absorption of this sedative has been shown to be slow from the intramuscular site. Indeed, it is even slower than from the gastrointestinal tract, when capsules of chlordiazepoxide hydrochloride are administered (Fig. 9–6). The explanation involves consideration of pH, solubility, perfusion, and stirring.

In the study referenced in the figure, the same dose, 50 milligrams chlordiazepoxide hydrochloride, was administered by both routes. The intramuscular dose was dissolved in 1 milliliter of an aqueous vehicle. Chlordiazepoxide is sparingly soluble; its aqueous solubility is approximately 2 milligrams/milliliter. To achieve this high concentration of 50 milligrams chlordiazepoxide hydrochloride/milliliter, the vehicle contains 20 percent propylene glycol and 4 percent polysorbate 80, both water-miscible materials that permit a greater solubility of the drug. Being the salt of a strong acid and a weak base (pKa 4.5), the final pH is low, approximately 3.0. Upon injection, the buffer capacity of both the tissue and the blood perfusing it gradually restores the pH at the injection site to 7.4. This rise in pH and the absorption of the injected water and water-miscible materials cause chlordiazepoxide base to precipitate out of solution. As movement and hence spreading is minimal, a large mass of drug is deposited around the injection site. The rate of absorption now becomes limited by dissolution of the precipitated drug. However, the small surface area, the low solubility, the limited perfusion, and the minimal stirring tend to keep the rate of dissolution down. The result is protracted absorption over many hours or even days. In contrast, absorption following oral administration is relatively rapid. For reasons

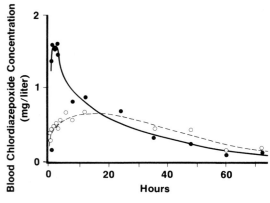

Fig. 9–6. A delayed and lower peak blood concentration of chlordiazepoxide, when given intramuscularly (O---O), as compared to when given orally (●—●), indicates slower absorption from the intramuscular site. On both occasions 50 milligrams of chlordiazepoxide hydrochloride were administered. (One mg/liter = 3.3 micromolar.) (Redrawn from Greenblatt, D.J., Shader, R.I., and Koch-Weser, J.: Slow absorption of intramuscular chlordiazepoxide. N. Engl. J. Med., 291:1116–1118, 1974. Reprinted by permission.)

already discussed, the greater degree of agitation, the larger volume of fluid at the site, and the higher rate of blood flow to the gastrointestinal tract promote more rapid dissolution and absorption following the ingestion of chlordiazepoxide hydrochloride.

Diazepam is sparingly soluble and slowly absorbed when injected intramuscularly. This essentially neutral drug is kept in solution with the aid of propylene glycol. Precipitation at the injection site occurs with the dilution and absorption of this water-miscible solvent.

Drug Delivery Systems

Utilizing the concept that release from a dosage form can rate-limit absorption, various devices have been developed to control the rate of entry of drug into the body. If successful, input becomes more predictable, and differences in membrane permeability at the absorption site, within and between subjects, is less important.

Some of these controlled-release devices, intended for constant-rate drug therapy, are listed in Table 6–1 (p. 64). The techniques for achieving the rate control are almost as numerous as the number of devices developed.

Study Problems

(Answers to Study Problems in Appendix G.)

1. List at least three reasons for reduced oral availability of a drug.

2. How accurate are each of the following statements:

   (a) When transmembrane movement rate limits absorption, the fraction of an orally administered dose in the body at any time is always small.

   (b) Large nondisintegrating controlled-release dosage forms commonly remain in the stomach for 6 hours when taken just after a heavy meal.

   (c) Drugs are more slowly absorbed from muscle than from the gastrointestinal tract.

3. List the factors influencing the dissolution of a drug from a solid dosage form.

4. Listed in Table 9–5 are four drugs together with some of their physical properties.

Table 9–5.

Property or Characteristic	Drug A	Drug B	Drug C	Drug D
Molecular weight	327	273	315	378
pKa	8.4 (Acid)	7.8 (Amine)	Neutral	Quaternary Ammonium Compound
Polarity of un-ionized form	Nonpolar	Nonpolar	Polar	—
Solubility of un-ionized form (milligrams/liter)	1.3	150	—	—

(a) Choose the drug(s) (A,B,C,D) that most appropriately completes each of the following statements:

1. The gastrointestinal absorption of drug _____, when given in solution, is the most sensitive to changes in intestinal pH.

2. The greatest diffusion limitation in crossing the intestinal epithelium is likely to be seen with drug(s) _____.

3. Delayed gastric emptying slows the absorption of drug(s) _____when given orally in solution. (Assume passive diffusion and drug stability in the gastrointestinal tract.)

4. Muscle blood flow is likely to be a major determinant in the absorption of drug(s) _____, when injected intramuscularly as an aqueous solution, pH 7.4.

5. The gastrointestinal absorption of drug(s) _____, when taken as a tablet, is unlikely to be rate-limited by dissolution.

(b) Assuming that the conventional single dose of both drugs A and B is 100 milligrams and that both drugs are stable in the gastrointestinal fluids, circle the most appropriate drug, word, or phrase (in italics) that completes the following statements.

1. The sodium salt of drug A dissolves *much faster, much slower, at essentially the same rate,* in a solution of pH 3.0 than (as) does the free acid in a solution of pH 8.0. (Assume that all other factors, such as surface area and stirring, are the same.)

2. The hydrochloride salt of drug B should dissolve *much faster, much slower, at essentially the same rate,* in the stomach of a patient with achlorhydria (no gastric acid secretion) than (as) in a patient with normal gastric function.

3. Drug A is poorly available when taken orally as the free acid with 100 milliliters of water. The availability of this drug should be significantly increased by taking the drug *with 200 milliliters of water, in divided doses during the day, on an empty stomach.*

4. Absorption problems are likely to be greater with drug A, B, when administered intramuscularly as an aqueous solution of the salt.

10

Distribution

Objectives

The reader will be able to:

1. Define the following terms:
   (a) Apparent volume of distribution
   (b) Plasma protein binding
   (c) Perfusion limitation in distribution
   (d) Permeability limitation in distribution
   (e) Tissue-to-blood equilibrium distribution ratio
   (f) Fraction unbound

2. State the fractions of body volume of an average adult that are assignable to plasma and blood and to extracellular, intracellular, and total body water.

3. Given the volume of distribution and the fraction unbound in plasma, calculate the fraction of drug in the body that is
   (a) In plasma
   (b) Outside plasma
   (c) Unbound, assuming that unbound drug distributes into total body water

4. Determine the plasma concentration, the amount of drug in the body, and the apparent volume of distribution when any two of these values are known.

5. Describe the effects of perfusion limitation, permeability limitation, and the tissue-to-blood equilibrium distribution ratio on the time required for drug distribution to the tissues.

6. Ascertain whether, for a given amount of drug in the body, the unbound plasma concentration is likely to be sensitive to variation in plasma protein binding when the volume of distribution is known.

Distribution refers to the reversible transfer of drug between one location and another within the body. Definitive information on the distribution of a drug requires its measurement in various tissues. This kind of information has been obtained in animals, but is essentially lacking in man. Useful information on both the rate and extent of distribution of drugs in man can be derived, however, solely from observations of blood or plasma drug concentrations. This chapter explores this information and its application to clinical pharmacokinetics. It begins with kinetic considerations and ends with equilibrium concepts.

RATE OF DISTRIBUTION

The distribution of drugs from blood to the body tissues occurs at various rates and to various extents. Several factors determine the distribution pattern of a drug, including the delivery of drug to a tissue, the ability of drug to pass through tissue membranes, and the binding of drug to both plasma proteins and tissue components. Tissue uptake of drug continues toward equilibrium between the diffusible form of the drug in a tissue and in the blood perfusing it.

Perfusion Limitation

The rate of distribution of a drug between blood and a tissue, like the rate of absorption (see Chap. 9), can be limited by either perfusion or permeability. A *perfusion-rate limitation* prevails when the tissue membranes present essentially no barrier to distribution. As expected, this condition is likely to be met by highly lipophilic drugs diffusing across most membranes of the body and, by almost all drugs, diffusing across loosely knit membranes, such as those of muscle and subcutaneous capillary walls (see Chap. 8).

Perfusion is usually expressed in units of milliliters of blood per minute per volume of tissue. As seen in Table 10–1, the perfusion rate of tissues varies from approximately 10 milliliters/minute per milliliter for lungs down to values of only 0.025 milliliter/minute per milliliter for resting muscle or fat. All other factors remaining equal, well-perfused tissues take up a drug much more rapidly than

Table 10–1. Blood Flow, Perfusion Rate, and Relative Size of Different Organs and Tissues Under Basal Conditions in a Standard 70-kg Man[a]

Organ	Percent of Body Volume	Blood Flow (ml/minute)	Percent of Cardiac Output	Perfusion Rate (ml/minute per ml of tissue)
1. Adrenal glands	0.03	25	0.2	1.2
2. Blood	7	(5000)[b]	(100)	—
3. Bone	16	250	5	0.02
4. Brain	2	700	14	0.5
5. Fat	10	200	4	0.03
6. Heart	0.5	200	4	0.6
7. Kidneys	0.4	1100	22	4
8. Liver	2.3	1350	27	0.8
Portal		(1050)	(21)	
Arterial		(300)	(6)	
9. Lungs	0.7	(5000)	(100)	10
10. Muscle (inactive)	42	750	15	0.025
11. Skin (cool weather)	18	300	6	0.024
12. Thyroid gland	0.03	50	1	2.4
Total Body	100	5000	100	0.071

[a]Compiled from data of Guyton, A.C.: Textbook of Medical Physiology, 6th ed., W.B. Saunders, Philadelphia, 1981, p. 232; and Skelton, H.: The storage of water by various tissues of the body. Arch. Intern. Med., *40*:140–152, 1927. Copyright 1927. American Medical Association.
[b]Values in parentheses given for comparison.

do poorly perfused tissues. Moreover, as the subsequent analysis shows, there is a direct correlation between tissue perfusion rate and the time required to distribute a drug to a tissue.

Figure 10–1 shows blood perfusing a tissue in which distribution is perfusion rate-limited and no elimination occurs. The rate of presentation to the tissue is the product of blood flow, Q, and the arterial blood concentration, C_A, that is,

$$\text{Rate of presentation} = Q \cdot C_A \qquad\qquad 1$$

The net rate of uptake into the tissue is the difference between the rate of presentation and the rate of leaving the tissue, $Q \cdot C_V$, where C_V is the emergent venous concentration. Therefore,

$$\text{Net rate of uptake} = Q \cdot (C_A - C_V) \qquad\qquad 2$$

The maximum initial rate of uptake is the rate of presentation, $Q \cdot C_A$. Further, with no effective impedance to movement within the tissue, blood and tissue can be viewed kinetically as one compartment, with the concentration in emergent venous blood concentrtion (C_V) in equilibrium with that in the tissue, C_T.

At any time, therefore,

$$\text{Amount of drug in tissue} = V_T \cdot K_P \cdot C_V \qquad\qquad 3$$

where V_T is the tissue volume and K_P is the equilibrium distribution ratio (C_T/C_V). Since the rate of exit of drug from the tissue is $Q \cdot C_V$, it follows that the fractional rate of exit, k_T, is given by

$$k_T = \frac{\text{Rate of exit}}{\text{Amount in tissue}} = \frac{Q \cdot C_V}{V_T \cdot K_P \cdot C_V}$$

or 4

$$k_T = \frac{(Q/V_T)}{K_P}$$

where Q/V_T is the perfusion rate of the tissue. The parameter k_T, a distribution rate constant with units of reciprocal time, may be regarded as a measure of how rapidly drug would leave the tissue if the arterial concentration were suddenly to drop to zero. It is analogous to the elimination rate constant for loss of drug from the whole body, and like elimination, the kinetics of tissue distribution can be characterized by a tissue distribution half-life for which

$$\text{Half-life} = \frac{0.693}{k_T} = \frac{0.693 \, K_P}{(Q/V_T)} \qquad\qquad 5$$

Fig. 10–1. Drug is presented to a tissue at an arterial blood concentration of C_A and at a rate equal to the product of blood flow, Q, and C_A. The drug leaves the tissue at a venous concentration of C_V and at a rate equal to $Q \cdot C_V$. The tissue concentration, C_T, increases when the rate of presentation exceeds the rate of leaving in the venous blood, and the converse. The amount in the tissue is the product of V_T, the volume of the tissue, and the tissue drug concentration.

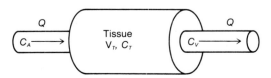

Thus, drug egresses slowly from tissues that have a high affinity (K_P) for it and that are poorly perfused.

Suppose now, that the arterial concentration is maintained constant with time. Then tissue uptake continues, but at a decreasing rate as tissue concentration rises, until equilibrium is achieved, when the net rate of uptake is zero, $C_V = C_A$ and $C_T = K_P \cdot C_A$. This situation is analogous to events occurring during a constant-rate infusion of drug into the body (Chap. 6, p. 65), with the equation defining the rise of tissue concentration to its plateau being given by

$$\text{Tissue concentration} = K_P \cdot C_A \, [1 - e^{-k_T \cdot t}] \qquad\qquad 6$$

Thus, the approach to plateau is determined solely by the tissue distribution half-life. In one half-life, the tissue concentration is 50 percent of its plateau value; in two half-lives, it is 75 percent; and so on.

To appreciate the foregoing, consider the events depicted in Figure 10–2. Shown are plots of concentration in various tissues with time during the maintenance of a constant arterial concentration of 1 milligram/liter. First consider panel A in which the K_P values of a drug in kidneys, brain, and fat are the same and equal to one. Given that the perfusion rates to these tissues are 4, 0.5 and 0.03 milliliter(s)/minute per milliliter of tissue, respectively (Table 10–1), it follows that the corresponding half-lives for distribution are 0.17, 1.4, and 23 minute(s). Thus, by one minute (more than 4 half-lives) drug in the kidneys has reached equilibrium with that in blood while it takes closer to 5 and 75 minutes for 90 percent of equilibrium to be reached in the brain and fat, tissues of lower perfusion. Next consider panel B in which events in fat are shown for drugs with different K_P values, namely 1, 2, and 5. Here the corresponding half-lives are

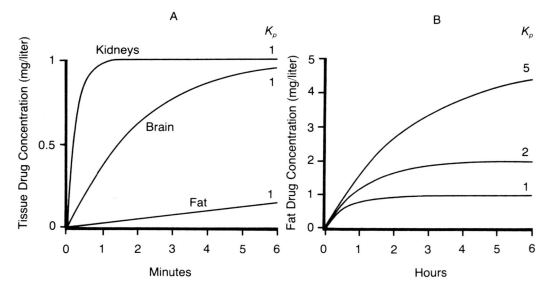

Fig. 10–2. If distribution is perfusion rate-limited, the time to reach equilibrium in tissue, when the arterial concentration is constant (1 mg/liter), depends on perfusion and equilibrum distribution ratio. A, Concentrations with time in kidneys, brain, fat, and tissues with different perfusion rates for $K_P = 1$ for all three tissues. B, Concentrations with time in fat of three drugs with K_P values of 1, 2, and 5, respectively. Note the difference in time scales of A (minutes) and B (hours).

23, 46, and 115 minutes. Now, not only is the time taken for drug in tissue to reach equilibrium different, but so are the equilibrium tissue concentrations.

These simple examples illustrate two basic principles. Namely, both the approach toward equilibrium and the loss of drug from a tissue take longer the poorer the perfusion and the greater the partitioning of drug into a tissue. The latter is contrary to what one might intuitively anticipate. However, the greater the tendency to concentrate in a tissue, the longer it takes to deliver to that tissue the amount needed to reach distribution equilibrium and the longer it takes to redistribute it out of that tissue. Stated differently, the affinity of a drug for a tissue accentuates an existing limitation imposed by perfusion.

Permeability Limitation

A permeability-rate limitation arises for polar drugs diffusing across tightly knit lipoidal membranes, as demonstrated in Figure 10–3 for the passage of compounds into the cerebrospinal fluid. In this study, the concentration of each drug was measured in the cerebrospinal fluid, relative to that in plasma water (unbound), with time following the attainment and maintenance of a constant plasma concentration. Because the vascular perfusion of the central nervous system and the equilibrium distribution ratios of the unbound drug are the same ($K_P = 1$) for each of the drugs studied, the widely differing rates of passage into the cerebrospinal fluid must result from a limitation in the permeation through a lipoidal barrier, a *permeability-rate limitation.* These differences in rate of entry are a function of both the lipid-to-water partition coefficient and the degree of ionization (Table 10–2), suggesting that only the un-ionized drug penetrates the brain. For example, the partition coefficients of salicylic acid and pentobarbital are similar, yet the time required to reach distribution equilibrium is far shorter for pentobarbital than for salicyclic acid because, being the weaker acid, a greater fraction of pentobarbital is un-ionized in plasma, pH 7.4.

With large differences in perfusion and permeability of various tissues it would appear to be impossible to predict tissue distribution of a drug. However, either of these two factors may limit the rate of distribution, thereby simplifying the situation and allowing some conclusion to be drawn. Consider, for example,

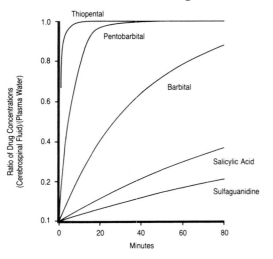

Fig. 10–3. The equilibration of drug in the cerebrospinal fluid with that in plasma is often permeability rate-limited. The ratio of drug concentrations (cerebrospinal fluid/unbound in plasma) is shown for various drugs in a dog. The plasma concentration was kept relatively constant throughout the study. (Redrawn from the data of Brodie, B.B., Kurz, H., and Schanker, L.S.: The importance of dissociation constant and lipid solubility in influencing the passage of drugs into the cerebrospinal fluid. J. Pharmacol. Exp. Ther., *130*:20–25, 1960. Copyright 1960, The Williams and Wilkins Co., Baltimore.)

Table 10–2. Physicochemical Properties and Time for Cerebrospinal Fluid Concentration to Reach 50 Percent of Equilibrium Value for Selected Acidic Drugs[a] of Figure 10–3[b]

Drug	pKa	Fraction Un-ionized at pH 7.4	Partition Coefficient of Un-ionized Form (n-heptane/water)	Effective Partition Coefficient at pH 7.4[c]	Time to Reach 50 Percent of Equilibrium Value (minutes)
Thiopental	7.6	0.6	3.3	2.0	1.4[d]
Pentobarbital	8.1	0.8	0.05	0.042	4
Barbital	7.5	0.6	0.002	0.0012	27
Salicylic acid	3.0	0.004	0.12	0.0005	115
Sulfaguanidine	>10	1.0	0.001	<0.001	231

[a]Similar correlation is observed for basic drugs.
[b]Data from reference in Fig. 10–3 and Hogben, C.A.M., Tocco, D.J., Brodie, B.B., and Schanker, L.S.: On the mechanism of intestinal absorption of drugs. J. Pharmacol. Exp. Ther., *125*:275–286, 1959.
[c]Fraction un-ionized at pH 7.4 times partition coefficient of un-ionized form.
[d]Probably perfusion rate-limited.

the following question: "Why, on measuring total tissue concentration, does the general anesthetic thiopental enter the brain much more rapidly than it does muscle tissue; yet, for penicillin the opposite is true?" The explanation lies in the properties of these drugs and of tissue membranes.

Thiopental is nonpolar, lipophilic and, being a weak acid (pKa 7.6), only partially ionized at the pH of plasma. As such, thiopental readily diffuses into both the brain and muscle; entry into both tissues is perfusion rate-limited. Since perfusion of the brain, particularly gray matter, is one or two orders of magnitude greater than that of muscle (Table 10–1), entry of thiopental into the brain is the more rapid process.

Penicillin, a polar compound, does not readily pass through membranes. The faster rate of entry of penicillin into muscle than into brain is a result of the more porous nature of the muscle capillaries. Recall from Chapter 9 (p. 115) for many tissues, e.g., muscle, the capillary membranes appear to be very porous and have little influence on the entry of drugs of usual molecular weight (100 to 400) into the interstitial fluids, regardless of the drug's physicochemical properties. There may be a permeability limitation at the tissue cell membrane, but in terms of measurement of drug in the *whole* tissue, there would appear to be only a partial impedance to the entry of either ionized or polar compounds, or both. Other tissues, for example, much of the central nervous system, anatomically have a permeability limitation at the level of the capillaries that impedes movement of drug into the tissue as a whole, as observed with penicillin. This observation, especially with a number of polar organic dyes, led to the concept of *blood-to-brain* and *blood-to-cerebrospinal fluid* barriers.

The effect of a high equilibrium distribution ratio on the time to achieve distribution equilibrium, discussed previously for a perfusion-rate limitation, applies equally well to a permeability-rate limitation. A permeability-rate limitation simply decreases the rate of entry to tissue from that of perfusion and hence increases the time to reach distribution equilibrium. Where the equilibrium lies is independent, however, of which process is rate-limiting.

If the concentration of drug in blood is maintained long enough, all drugs should reach distribution equilibrium when the unbound concentrations in tissue

Table 10–3. Representative Proteins to Which Drugs Bind in Plasma

Protein	Molecular Weight	Normal Concentrations	
		grams/liter	micromolar
Albumin	67,000	35–50	500–700
α_1-Acid glycoprotein	42,000	0.4–1.0	9–23
Lipoproteins	200,000–2,400,000	Variable	
Cortisol binding globulin (transcortin)	53,000	0.03–0.07	0.6–1.4

and plasma are equal. Sometimes, however, this equality is not observed. Reasons for lack of equality include maintenance of sink conditions by metabolism, metabolism, active transport out of the tissue, bulk flow of the interstitial fluids through both lymphatic channels and ducts, and pH gradients across cell membranes.

EXTENT OF DISTRIBUTION

Distribution of drug within the tissues of the body involves multiple equilibria. Multiple equilibria also occur within plasma where drug can bind to various proteins, examples of which are listed in Table 10–3. Acidic drugs commonly bind to albumin, the most abundant plasma protein. Basic drugs often bind to α_1-acid glycoprotein and to lipoproteins. Proteins, such as gamma-globulin, transcortin, fibrinogen, and thyroid-binding globulin, bind specific compounds. Tissue distribution can involve both partition into fat and binding to a wide variety of substances (Table 10–4).

Apparent Volume of Distribution

The concentration achieved after distribution is complete is a result of the dose administered and the extent of distribution of drug into the tissues. Recall from Chapter 3 that, at equilibrium, the extent of distribution of a drug is defined by an apparent volume of distribution (V):

★

$$V = \frac{\text{Amount in body at equilibrium}}{\text{Plasma drug concentration}} = \frac{A}{C}$$

7

This parameter is useful in relating amount of drug in the body to plasma concentration, and the converse. Recall, also, that the volumes of distribution

Table 10–4. Representative Tissue Components to Which Drugs Bind

Component	Drug Example
Nucleic acids	Chloroquine
Ligandin	Indocyanine green (diagnostic agent)
Calcified tissues	Tetracycline
Mucopolysaccharides	Propranolol
Na$^+$/K$^+$ ATPase	Digoxin

of drugs vary widely with illustrative values ranging from 7 liters/70 kilograms body weight to 40,000 liters/70 kilograms body weight, a value far in excess of total body size.

Knowing the plasma volume, V_P, and the volume of distribution, V, the fraction of drug in the body in plasma and that outside plasma can be estimated. The amount in plasma is $V_P \cdot C$; the amount in the body is $V \cdot C$. Therefore

$$\text{Fraction of drug in body in plasma } = \frac{V_P}{V} \qquad\qquad 8$$

It is evident that the larger the volume of distribution, the smaller is the fraction in plasma. For example, for a drug with a volume of distribution of 100 liters, only 3 percent resides in plasma.

The remaining fraction, given by

$$\text{Fraction of drug in body outside plasma } = \frac{(V - V_P)}{V} \qquad\qquad 9$$

includes drug in the blood cells. For the example considered above, 97 percent is outside plasma. Although this fraction can be readily determined, the actual distribution of drug outside plasma cannot.

The reason why the volume of distribution is an apparent volume and why its value differs among drugs may be appreciated by considering the simple model shown in Figure 10–4. In this model, drug in the body is entirely accounted for in plasma, of volume V_P, and one tissue compartment, of volume V_T. At distribution equilibrium the tissue-to-plasma ratio of drug concentrations is K_P. The amount of drug in each location can then be expressed in terms of the

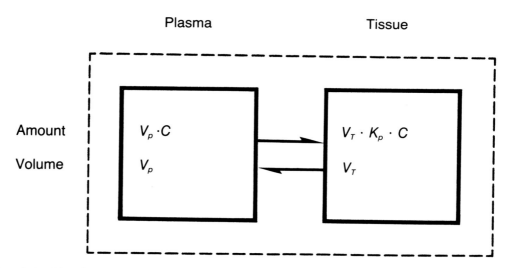

Fig. 10–4. The effect of tissue binding on drug distribution is illustrated by a drug that distributes between plasma and a tissue. The physiologic volumes are V_P and V_T, respectively. At equilibrium the amount of drug in each location depends on the equilibrium distribution (partition) ratio, K_P, the plasma and the tissue volumes, and the plasma concentration.

plasma concentration, C, the volumes of the plasma and the tissue and the distribution ratio, as follows:

$$A = \underset{\substack{\text{Amount} \\ \text{in plasma}}}{V_P \cdot C} + \underset{\substack{\text{Amount} \\ \text{in tissue}}}{V_T \cdot K_P \cdot C} \qquad 10$$

And since $A = V \cdot C$ (Eq. 7), it follows, on dividing the equation above by C, that

★

$$V = V_P + V_T \cdot K_P \qquad 11$$

The product $V_T \cdot K_P$ is the apparent volume of a tissue viewed from measurement of drug in plasma. Thus, by expanding the model to embrace all tissues of the body, it is seen that the volume of distribution of a drug is the volume of plasma plus the sum of the apparent volumes of distribution of each tissue. For some tissues the value of K_P of a drug is large, which explains why the volume of distribution of some drugs can be much greater than the total body size. Fat, for example, occupies approximately 10 percent of body volume. If the K_P value of a drug in fat is 5, then this tissue alone will appear to have an apparent volume of distribution of 50 percent of body volume. Remember, however, that in this case it will take approximately 7 hours for distribution equilibrium in fat to occur (Fig. 10–2B).

The volume of distribution of a drug can vary widely among patients. The reasons for such differences are now explored. Before doing so, however, a general point is considered.

Binding within Blood. Within blood, drug can bind to many components including blood cells and plasma proteins. As a consequence of binding, the concentration of drug in whole blood (C_b), in plasma (C) and unbound in plasma water (Cu) can differ greatly. For ease of chemical analysis, plasma is the most common fluid analyzed. In many respects this choice is unfortunate. One of the primary goals of measuring drug concentration is to relate the measurement to pharmacologic response and toxicity. However, only unbound drug can pass through most cell membranes, the protein-bound drug being too large. Accordingly, the unbound drug concentration is undoubtedly more closely related to the activity of the drug than is the total plasma concentration. Yet unbound concentration is only occasionally measured, primarily because the methods for doing so are often tedious and lack accuracy and precision. Nonetheless, it is helpful to define an unbound volume of distribution, Vu,

★

$$Vu = \frac{\text{Amount in body at equilibrium}}{\text{Unbound plasma concentration}} = \frac{A}{Cu} \qquad 12$$

which permits the amount of drug in the body to be related to the unbound drug concentration.

Sometimes whole blood concentration is measured. Once again an appropriate volume term can be defined. Namely,

★

$$V_b = \frac{\text{Amount in body at equilibrium}}{\text{Concentration in whole blood}} = \frac{A}{C_b} \qquad 13$$

where V_b is the apparent volume of distribution based on concentration in whole blood. As the amount of drug in body is independent of the site of measurement, it follows from Equations 7, 12, and 13 that

$$V \cdot C = Vu \cdot Cu = V_b \cdot C_b$$

★ 14

The values of these volume terms can differ markedly for a given drug. The term most often quoted in the literature is based on measurement of drug in plasma (i.e., V). Examples of drugs with differing values of V are given in Figure 3–2 (p. 22).

Plasma Protein Binding. The principal concern with plasma protein binding is related to its variability within and among patients in various therapeutic settings. The degree of drug binding to plasma proteins is frequently expressed as the ratio of the bound concentration to the total concentration. This ratio has limiting values of 0 and 1.0. Drugs with values greater than 0.9 are said to be highly bound, and those with values less than 0.2 are said to show little or no plasma protein binding.

As stated previously, the unbound concentration, rather than the bound concentration, is frequently more important in therapeutics. Therefore, the value of the fraction of drug in plasma that is unbound to plasma proteins, fu, is of greater utility than is that for bound drug.

$$fu = Cu/C$$

★ 15

Obviously, only if the value of fu is constant will total plasma concentration be a good measure of the changes in unbound drug concentration. Approximate values of fu usually associated with therapy for representative drugs are shown in Figure 10–5.

Binding is a function of the affinity of the protein for the drug. Because of the limited number of binding sites on a protein, binding also depends on the molar concentrations of both drug and protein. Assuming a single binding site on the protein, the association is simply summarized by the following reaction:

$$\text{Drug} + \text{Protein} \rightleftharpoons \text{Drug-protein complex} \qquad 16$$

Equilibrium may lie either to the right or to the left. High affinity, of course, implies that equilibrium lies far to the right. This is a relative statement, however, since the greater the protein concentration for a given drug concentration, the greater the bound drug concentration and the converse. From mass law considerations, the equilibrium is expressed in terms of the concentrations of unbound drug, Cu, unoccupied protein, P, and bound drug, Cbd.

$$K_a = \frac{Cbd}{Cu \cdot P}$$

17

The association constant, K_a, is a direct measure of the affinity of the protein for the drug.

The unoccupied protein concentration depends on the total protein concentration, P_t. These two concentrations are related by $fu_p = P/P_t$, where fu_p is the fraction of the total number of binding sites unoccupied. Furthermore, using the fraction of the total drug concentration that is unbound, fu, the unbound

**Percent
Unbound (100 fu)**

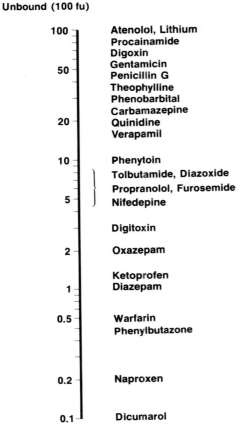

Fig. 10–5.   The fraction of drug in plasma not bound to protein varies widely among drugs.

concentration is $fu \cdot C$ and the bound concentration is $(1 - fu) \cdot C$. Appropriately substituting into Equation 17, it therefore follows that

$$K_a \cdot fu_p \cdot P_t = \frac{1 - fu}{fu} \qquad\qquad 18$$

or

★

$$fu = \frac{1}{1 + K_a \cdot fu_p \cdot P_t} \qquad\qquad 19$$

From this relationship the value of fu is seen to depend on the total protein concentration, as illustrated in Figure 10–6 for the binding of propranolol to α_1-acid glycoprotein. Usually only a small fraction of the available binding sites is occupied ($fu_p \cong 1$) at therapeutic concentrations; the fraction unbound is then relatively constant at a given protein concentration and independent of drug concentration. Occasionally, therapeutic concentrations are sufficantly high

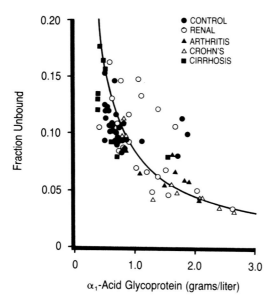

Fig. 10–6. The fraction unbound of propranolol varies with the plasma concentration of α_1-acid glycoprotein in 78 patients with various diseases and in healthy volunteers. The line drawn through the data represents the relationship expected from Equation 19, using a value of 11 liters gram^{-1} (4.84 × 10^5 liters mole^{-1}) for K_a. This relationship appears to account for most of the observed variability in the fraction unbound. In all cases, the protein is not saturated; the molar concentration of propranolol is below that of α_1-acid glycoprotein. (One mg/liter = 22.7 micromolar.) (Redrawn from Tozer, T.N.: Implications of altered plasma protein binding in disease states. *In:* Pharmacokinetic Basis for Drug Treatment. Edited by L.Z. Benet, N. Massoud, J.G. Gambertoglio. Raven Press, New York, 1983, pp. 173–193. Original data from Piafsky, K.M., Borga, O., Odar-Cederlof, I., Johansson, C., and Sjoqvist, F.: Increased plasma protein binding of propranolol and chlorpromazine mediated by disease-induced elevations of plasma α_1-acid glycoprotein. N. Engl. J. Med., 299:1435–1439, 1978. Reproduced with permission of Raven Press.)

that most of the available binding sites are occupied. Then both *fu* and *fu*$_p$ are concentration-dependent (see Chap. 22, Dose and Time Dependencies).

In subsequent chapters, it will be helpful to remember that pharmacologic activity relates to the unbound concentration. Plasma protein binding, then, is often only of interest because the total plasma concentration is measured. The total plasma concentration depends on both the extent of protein binding and the unbound concentration, that is,

$$C = Cu/fu \qquad\qquad 20$$

When conceptualizing dependency and functionality, this equation should not be rearranged.

Tissue Binding. The fraction of drug in body located in plasma depends on a drug's binding to both plasma and tissue components, as shown schematically in Figure 10–7. A drug may have a great affinity for plasma proteins, but may still be located primarily in tissue if the tissue has an affinity for the drug even higher than that of plasma. Unlike plasma binding, tissue binding of a drug cannot be measured directly. The tissue must be disrupted, resulting in the loss of its integrity. Even so, tissue binding is important in drug distribution.

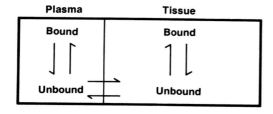

Fig. 10–7. At equilibrium, the distribution of a drug within the body depends upon binding to both plasma proteins and tissue components. In the model, only the unbound drug is capable of entering and leaving the plasma and tissue compartments.

Tissue binding may be inferred from measurement of drug binding in plasma. Consider, for example, the following mass-balance relationship,

$$\underset{\substack{\text{Amount} \\ \text{in body}}}{V \cdot C} = \underset{\substack{\text{Amount} \\ \text{in plasma}}}{V_P \cdot C} + \underset{\substack{\text{Amount} \\ \text{outside plasma}}}{V_{TW} \cdot C_{TW}} \qquad 21$$

in which V_{TW} is the aqueous volume outside the plasma into which the drug distributes and C_{TW} is the corresponding total drug concentration.

Dividing by C,

$$\underset{\substack{\text{Apparent} \\ \text{volume of} \\ \text{distribution}}}{V} = \underset{\substack{\text{Volume} \\ \text{of} \\ \text{plasma}}}{V_P} + \underset{\substack{\text{Apparent} \\ \text{volume of} \\ \text{tissue}}}{V_{TW}} \cdot \frac{C_{TW}}{C} \qquad 22$$

Recall that the fraction of drug in plasma unbound is given by

$$fu = \frac{Cu}{C} \qquad 23$$

Similarly, a fraction unbound to tissue components, fu_T, can be defined by

$$fu_T = \frac{Cu_T}{C_{TW}} \qquad 24$$

Making the reasonable assumption that distribution equilibrium is achieved when the unbound concentrations in plasma, Cu, and in tissues, Cu_T, are equal, then the ratio of Equations 23 and 24 becomes

$$\frac{C_{TW}}{C} = \frac{fu}{fu_T} \qquad 25$$

which on substituting into Equation 22 yields

★

$$V = V_P + V_{TW} \cdot \frac{fu}{fu_T} \qquad 26$$

From this relationship it is seen that the apparent volume of distribution increases when fu is increased and decreases when fu_T is increased.

To appreciate the relationship in Equation 26, consider the data for propranolol shown in Figure 10–8. The linear relationship between volume of distribution and fraction unbound in plasma indicates that V_{TW}/fu_T is constant. Also it is apparent that differences in binding of propranolol in plasma account for most of the variation observed in its volume of distribution.

The relationship expressed in Equation 26 explains why, because of plasma and tissue binding, the volume of distribution, V, rarely corresponds to a real volume, such as plasma volume, extracellular space, or total body water. Even if the volume of distribution of a drug corresponds to the value of a physiologic volume, one cannot conclude unambiguously that the drug distributes only into that volume. The binding of drugs in both plasma and tissues complicates the situation and often prevents making any conclusion about the actual volume into which the drug distributes. An exception is when the drug is restricted to

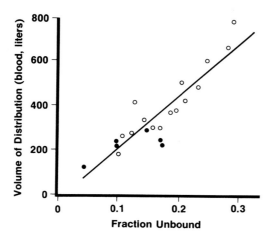

Fig. 10–8.   The volume of distribution of (+)-pro-pranolol varies with the fraction unbound. The observation was made in 6 control subjects (●) and in 15 patients (○) with chronic hepatic disease after an intravenous bolus (40 mg) of (+)-propranolol. (Data from Branch, R.A., Jones, J., and Read, A.E.: A study of factors influencing drug disposition in chronic liver disease, using the model drug (+)-propranolol. Br. J. Clin. Pharmacol., 3:243–249, 1976.)

the plasma; the volumes of distribution, apparent and real, are then the same, about 3 liters in an adult. This last situation occurs only when the drug is highly bound to plasma proteins and is not bound in the tissues. Even here, the apparent volume cannot be an equilibrium value, because plasma proteins equilibrate slowly between plasma and other extracellular fluids. The apparent volume of plasma proteins, about 7 liters for albumin, is perhaps a better estimate of the minimum value for any drug, a point discussed further in Chapter 25.

For drugs that are neither tissue nor plasma protein bound, the volume of distribution varies between the extracellular fluid volume (16 liters) and the total body water (42 liters), depending on the degree to which the drug gains access to the intracellular fluids. For example, the volumes of distribution of aminoglycosides, which are large polar molecules that penetrate cell membranes with great difficulty, are close to 16 liters. Examples of drugs that distribute in total body water are caffeine and alcohol, both small nonpolar molecules that pass freely through membranes.

Since the plasma volume, V_P, is known and the values of fu and V are measurable, the value of V_{TW}/fu_T can be determined.

$$\frac{V_{TW}}{fu_T} = \frac{(V - V_P)}{fu} \qquad\qquad 27$$

Taking warfarin as an example, V is about 10 liters, fu is 0.005, and since V_P is 3 liters, V_{TW}/fu_T is 1400 liters. Clearly this drug must be bound to the tissues somewhere. To say how much is tissue bound requires an assumption about the aqueous volume into which the drug distributes. If a drug does not traverse membranes, drug in the tissues would be restricted to extracellular fluids outside the central nervous system. If it does pass readily through membranes, total body water minus the plasma volume might be a better estimate of V_{TW}. In general, V_{TW} should be between these limits, that is, 12 and 39 liters. Making the reasonable assumption that warfarin, a small lipophilic molecule, passes through membranes, then V_{TW} equals 39 liters, so that the value of fu_T is about 0.03. In other words, 97 percent of warfarin in the tissues is bound despite a small volume of distribution. The small volume of distribution is a consequence of the plasma protein binding being greater than the tissue binding, $fu/fu_T = 0.18$.

A comparison of Equations 11 and 26 shows the following equality

$$K_P = \frac{V_{TW}}{V_T} \cdot \frac{fu}{fu_T}$$

$$28$$

Thus, the distribution ratio is determined by relative binding of drug to plasma and tissue constituents. With the exception of bone and fat, for most tissues, more than 75 percent is water so that V_{TW}/V_T is 0.75 or greater. Accordingly, in most instances, the ratio fu/fu_T may be taken to be approximately equal to K_P.

Percent Unbound in Body. Another view of the effect of binding on drug distribution is gained from the volume of distribution based on the unbound plasma concentration, Vu. For a drug that does not bind to either plasma or tissue, that shows no permeability-rate limitation, and that passes across all cell membranes, the volumes of distribution based on unbound and total drug in plasma are the same and are equal to body water (42 liters). If there is binding, the unbound volume term will be greater than total body water. From Equation 14 it follows that

★

$$\text{Percent unbound in body} = \frac{(\text{Total body water}) \cdot 100}{Vu}$$

$$29$$

The percent unbound in body for three drugs is shown in Table 10–5.

Clearly for caffeine both the unbound and total plasma concentrations reflect drug in the body. For warfarin only 2 percent is unbound, and so the possibility exists of appreciably affecting the unbound concentration, particularly if both plasma and tissue binding are altered simultaneously. This situation can arise because warfarin is predominantly bound to albumin, a protein located in both plasma and tissue. Although it has the same volume of distribution as warfarin, the unbound concentration of salicylic acid is less sensitive to a change in binding since only 58 percent of drug in the body is bound. The consequences of the distribution of plasma proteins in both vascular and extravascular spaces is further explored in Chapter 25, Small Volume of Distribution.

Altered Binding and Loading Dose

Loading doses are given to rapidly achieve a therapeutic response, putatively by rapidly producing a desired unbound concentration. With variations in both plasma and tissue binding, the question arises whether or not the loading dose needs to be adjusted.

Table 10–5. Percent Unbound in Body of Some Drugs

Drug	Volume of Distribution (liters)	Fraction Unbound in Plasma (fu)	Unbound Volume of Distribution (Vu) (liters)	Percent Unbound in Body
Caffeine	37	0.88	42	100
Warfarin	10	0.005	2000	2
Salicylic acid	10[a]	0.1	100	42

[a]At doses of 600 milligrams or less.

For many drugs the volume of distribution is greater than 30 liters, that is, much greater than the plasma volume, implying that only a small fraction of drug in body resides in plasma (Eq. 8). Therefore, ignoring V_P in Equation 26 and realizing that $fu \cdot C = Cu$, it follows that

$$\text{Amount in body} \approx \frac{V_{TW}}{fu_T} \cdot Cu \qquad \qquad 30$$

This equation indicates that Cu is independent of plasma binding and thus no adjustment in loading dose is needed. The total plasma concentration does, of course, change with altered plasma binding, but this is of no therapeutic consequence with respect to loading dose requirements. If, however, tissue binding (fu_T) were to change, so would the initial value(s) of Cu (and C), necessitating a decision to change the loading dose.

Study Problems

(Answers to Study Problems are in Appendix G.)

1. Define the terms: apparent volume of distribution, fraction unbound, tissue-to-blood equilibrium distribution ratio, and perfusion-rate and permeability-rate limitations in drug distribution.

2. Using the information in Table 10–6, calculate the time required for the amounts in each of the tissues listed to reach 50 percent of the equilibrium value for a drug with perfusion rate-limited distribution when the blood concentration is kept constant with time (by giving a bolus and an appropriate infusion). Rank the times and the corresponding tissues.

Table 10–6.

Organ	Equilibrium Distribution Ratio	Perfusion Rate (ml/minute per ml of tissue)
Lungs	1	10
Kidneys	4	4
Heart	3	0.6
Liver	15	0.8
Skin	12	0.024

3. The volume of distribution of quinacrine is about 40,000 liters.
   (a) The plasma concentration when 1 gram of drug is in the body would therefore be _____milligram(s)/liter.
   (b) The amount of drug in the body when the plasma concentration is 0.015 milligram/liter is _____milligram(s).
   (c) The percentage of drug in the body that is outside the plasma is _____.

4. The volume of distribution of a drug in a 70-kilogram man is observed to be 8 liters. Indicate which one (or more) of the following statements is (are) consistent with this observation. The drug is:
   (a) Highly bound to plasma proteins.
   (b) Bound to components outside plasma and is highly bound to proteins in plasma.
   (c) Not bound to plasma proteins.

5. Briefly comment on the validity of each of the following statements.
   (a) The equilibrium distribution ratio for a drug between liver and plasma is 50; therefore, its volume of distribution must be at least 75 liters in a man weighing 70 kilograms.

(b) A drug that reaches distribution equilibrium within 30 minutes, yet whose volume of distribution in a 70-kilogram man is 200 liters, must distribute primarily into highly perfused organs.

6. Digitoxin has a volume of distribution of 38 liters in a 70-kilogram man and is 97 percent bound in plasma. What fraction of drug in the tissues is unbound? Assume that the unbound drug distributes evenly throughout total body water.

7. Digoxin has a volume of distribution of about 550 liters in a 70-kilogram man and is 23 percent bound in plasma. Making the same assumption as in problem 6, is digoxin more or less extensively tissue bound than digitoxin?

11

Elimination

The reader will be able to:

1. Define the following using both words and equations: clearance, blood clearance, unbound clearance, hepatic clearance, biliary clearance, and renal clearance.

2. Calculate the extraction ratio across an eliminating organ given blood clearance and blood flow in that organ.

3. Ascertain from the value of its extraction ratio whether the clearance of a drug by an organ is perfusion rate-limited or is dependent on its binding to plasma proteins.

4. Calculate the maximum oral availability of a drug given either its hepatic extraction ratio or the appropriate information to estimate this value.

5. Determine the biliary clearance of a drug from its bile-to-plasma concentration ratio and the bile flow.

6. Describe the role that biliary secretion can play in drug disposition.

7. Describe where filtration, secretion, and reabsorption of drugs occur within the nephron.

8. State the average value of glomerular filtration rate.

9. Given renal clearance and binding data, determine if a drug is predominantly reabsorbed from or secreted into the renal tubule.

10. Anticipate those drugs for which a change in either urine pH or urine flow may alter the value of their renal clearance.

11. Ascertain the relative contribution of the renal and extrarenal routes to total elimination from their respective clearance values.

12. Explain the statement, "Half-life depends upon clearance and volume of distribution."

This chapter is concerned with the elimination processes and particularly with the concept of clearance. In Chapters 3, 6, and 7 the methods of quantifying clearance were presented. Here its physiologic meaning is given.

Elimination

Elimination occurs by excretion and metabolism. Some drugs are excreted via the bile. Others, particularly volatile substances, are excreted in the breath. For most drugs, however, excretion occurs predominantly via the kidneys.

Metabolism is the major mechanism for elimination of drugs from the body. Some drugs are eliminated almost entirely unchanged by the kidneys, but these drugs are relatively few.

The consequences of drug metabolism are manifold. Biotransformation provides a mechanism for ridding the body of undesirable foreign compounds and drugs; it also provides a means of producing active and toxic compounds. Numerous examples are now recognized in which the administered drug is really an inactive prodrug, which is converted into a pharmacologically active species. Often both the drug and its metabolite(s) are active. The duration and intensity of the pharmacologic and toxic responses vary with the time courses of these substances in the body. The pharmacokinetics of active metabolites, as well as that of the compound administered, is therefore of therapeutic concern. The common pathways of biotransformation and the kinetics of metabolites are presented in Chapter 21, Metabolite Kinetics. The elimination processes are emphasized here.

CONCEPT OF CLEARANCE

Of the concepts in pharmacokinetics, *clearance* has the greatest potential for clinical applications. It is also the most useful parameter for the evaluation of an elimination mechanism.

Loss Across an Organ of Elimination

Recall from Chapter 3 that clearance is defined as the proportionality factor relating rate of drug elimination to the plasma (drug) concentration. That is, rate of elimination = $CL \cdot C$. Clearance may be viewed in another way, namely from the loss of drug across an organ of elimination. This latter physiologic approach has a number of advantages, particularly in predicting and in evaluating the effects of changes in blood flow, plasma protein binding, enzyme activity, or in secretory activity on the elimination of a drug. Figure 11–1 summarizes the various ways of viewing mass balance across an eliminating organ. In this scheme, drug in the eliminating organ is assumed to have reached distribution equilibrium; thus, the sole reason for any difference between the arterial and venous concentrations is elimination. For all but the earliest moments, this assumption is reasonable for the kidneys and the liver, which are among the most highly perfused and hence most rapidly equilibrating organs in the body.

The rate of presentation of a drug to an organ of elimination is the product of blood flow, Q, and the concentration in blood entering the arterial side, C_A, that is, $Q \cdot C_A$. Similarly, the rate at which the drug leaves on the venous side

1. Mass Balance

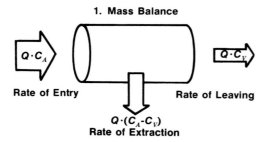

Rate of Entry   Rate of Leaving

$Q \cdot (C_A - C_V)$
Rate of Extraction

2. Mass Balance Normalized to Rate of Entry

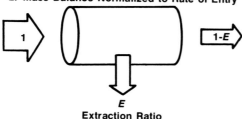

E
Extraction Ratio

3. Mass Balance Normalized to Entering Concentration

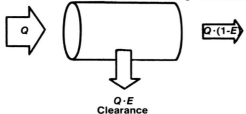

$Q \cdot E$
Clearance

Fig. 11–1. The extraction of a drug by an eliminating organ under steady-state conditions may be considered from the fundamental concepts of mass balance: I, The extraction of drug may be accounted for from its rates in and out of the organ. II, Normalizing to the rate of entry provides a means of determining the fraction extracted, the extraction ratio. III, Normalizing to the entering concentration allows one to account for the drug in terms of clearance and blood flow. The symbols are defined in Equations 1 through 4.

is $Q \cdot C_V$, where C_V is the concentration in the returning venous blood. The difference between these rates is the rate of drug extraction (or elimination) by the organ,

$$\text{Rate of extraction} = Q(C_A - C_V) \qquad \bigstar \quad 1$$

If the rate of drug extraction is related to the rate at which it is presented to the organ, a useful parameter, the *extraction ratio*, E, is derived:

$$E = \frac{\text{Rate of extraction}}{\text{Rate of presentation}} = \frac{(C_A - C_V)}{C_A} \qquad \bigstar \quad 2$$

The value of the extraction ratio can lie anywhere between zero, where no drug is eliminated, and one, where no drug escapes past the organ.

If, instead, the rate of drug extraction is related to the incoming concentration, one obtains, by definition, the value of clearance (Chap. 3),

$$\text{Clearance} = \frac{Q(C_A - C_V)}{C_A} \qquad \bigstar \quad 3$$

in this instance blood clearance, since the concentration in blood is measured.

On substituting Equation 2 into Equation 3, the following important relationship is obtained:

$$\text{Blood clearance} = \text{Blood flow} \cdot \text{Extraction ratio} \qquad \bigstar \\ 4$$

That is, blood clearance may be regarded as the volume of blood from which all the drug would appear to be removed per unit time. For example, if the extraction ratio of a drug across an organ is 0.5 and organ blood flow is 1 liter/minute, then drug in 0.5 liter of the incoming blood is effectively removed each minute as blood passes through the organ. Furthermore, if the arterial concentration is 1 milligram/liter, then the rate of elimination is 0.5 liter/minute times 1 milligram/liter, or 0.5 milligram/minute.

Blood clearance cannot be any value. Examination of Equation 4 shows that if the extraction ratio of the drug across the organ approaches 1.0, then blood clearance approaches its maximum value, organ blood flow. For the kidneys and the liver, the average organ blood flows are 1.1 and 1.35 liters/minute, respectively.

Before considering clearance of drug by specific organs, a number of general comments are in order.

Description of Clearance by Organ, Process, or Site of Measurement

Clearance can be described in terms of the eliminating organ, e.g., hepatic clearance, renal clearance, or pulmonary clearance. It can also be described by the difference between renal excretion and elimination by all other processes, e.g., renal clearance and extrarenal clearance. How an organ clears the blood of drug may also be described by the nature of the elimination process, e.g., metabolic clearance or excretory clearance. Furthermore, the value of the clearance term depends on the reference fluid. Thus, to be specific, the clearance of a drug eliminated, e.g., by metabolism in the liver, using plasma concentration measurements would then be hepatic metabolic plasma clearance. Similarly, "clearance by excretion of drug" in the kidneys would be renal excretory plasma clearance. In practice, the term "plasma" is dropped; it is assumed that plasma is the site of measurement unless stated otherwise. Furthermore, one often drops *metabolic* or *excretory* when describing clearance by the liver and kidneys, respectively, because these processes are generally assumed to occur in these organs. However, metabolism does occur in the kidneys and excretion (into bile) does occur in the liver. Therefore, the assumptions underlying the clearance nomenclature for a specific drug should always be questioned.

Plasma Versus Blood Clearance

For many applications in pharmacokinetics, it matters little whether clearance measurements are based on drug in plasma or in blood. The exception is when a clearance value is used to estimate the extraction ratio. Then the blood clearance value must be used, because it is this parameter that directly relates to organ blood flow and the extraction ratio (see Eq. 4).

Plasma clearance is more frequently reported than blood clearance. Thus, if one wishes to estimate the extraction ratio, one needs to convert this clearance value based on drug concentration in plasma to one based on the concentration in blood. This conversion is accomplished by experimentally determining the blood to plasma concentration ratio. Since, by definition, the products of the respective clearance and concentration terms, based on measurements in blood and plasma, are equal to the rate of elimination, it follows that:

$$\frac{\text{Plasma clearance}}{\text{Blood clearance}} = \frac{\text{Blood concentration}}{\text{Plasma concentration}} \qquad 5$$

The concentration ratio is a function of the hematocrit and of the binding of drug to both plasma proteins and blood cell components. The relationship is derived in Appendix E. Strong binding to plasma proteins produces a ratio less than 1.0. A high affinity for blood cells gives a ratio greater than 1.0.

Clearances of drugs by the liver and the kidneys are now examined. Each organ has special anatomic and physiologic features that require their separate consideration.

HEPATIC CLEARANCE

Although drug metabolism can take place in many organs, the liver frequently has the greatest metabolic capacity and consequently has been the most thoroughly studied. The most direct quantitative measure of the liver's ability to eliminate a drug is hepatic clearance. Hepatic clearance includes biliary excretory clearance, which is subsequently discussed, and hepatic metabolic clearance.

As with other organs of elimination, the removal of drug by the liver may be considered from mass balance relationships. That is

$$\text{Hepatic blood clearance} = \underset{\substack{\text{Hepatic} \\ \text{blood} \\ \text{flow}}}{Q_H} \cdot \underset{\substack{\text{Hepatic} \\ \text{extraction} \\ \text{ratio}}}{E_H} \qquad 6$$

Here Q_H is the sum of hepatic portal and hepatic arterial blood flows, whose average values are 1050 and 300 milliliters/minute, respectively.

Perfusion, Protein Binding, and Enzyme Activity

The following principles, relating changes in clearance and extraction ratio to alterations in perfusion, plasma protein binding, or inherent elimination characteristics, apply in general to all organs of elimination. These principles are exemplified here with hepatic extraction.

Perfusion. There are at least five processes, as shown in Figure 11–2, that may affect the ability of the liver to extract drug from blood. However, when the hepatic extraction ratio approaches 1.0 while in the liver, the drug must have had sufficient time to partition out of the blood cell, dissociate from the plasma protein, pass through the hepatic membranes, and be either metabolized by an enzyme or transported into the bile, or both. At this time blood clearance approaches its maximum value, hepatic blood flow. Under this condition, elimination is limited by perfusion and not by the speed of any of the processes depicted in Figure 11–2; changes in blood flow produce corresponding changes

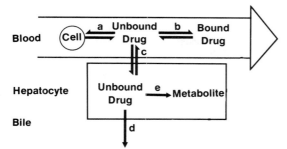

Fig. 11–2. Drug in the blood is bound to blood cells (process *a*) and to plasma proteins (process *b*); however, it is the unbound drug that diffuses (process *c*) into the hepatocyte. Within the hepatocyte, the unbound drug is subject to secretion into the bile (process *d*) or to enzymatic biotransformation (process *e*). The metabolite leaves the hepatocyte via the blood or the bile or it is subjected to further transformation.

in clearance and rate of elimination, but the extraction ratio is virtually unaffected (Table 11–1). Here, clearance is said to be *perfusion rate-limited*. In contrast, elimination of a drug with a low extraction ratio (approaching zero) must be rate-limited somewhere else in the overall scheme. This rate limitation could be a slow enzymatic reaction, process *e*; poor biliary transport, process *d*; poor diffusion into the hepatic cell, process *c*; slow diffusion out of the blood cell, process *a*; or a result of very slow dissociation of drug tightly bound to plasma proteins, process *b*. A combination of these factors could also be involved.

When the extraction ratio of a drug is low, the venous drug concentration is virtually identical with the arterial concentration, by definition. Therefore, changes in blood flow should produce no change in the drug concentration within the organ, the rate of elimination, or clearance. From Equation 6, however, it is seen that the hepatic extraction ratio varies inversely with blood flow when clearance is constant. These expectations regarding perfusion for drugs of high and low extraction ratios are illustrated in Figure 11–3 and are summarized in Table 11–1. Representative drugs and metabolites with low (less than 0.3), intermediate (0.3 to 0.7), and high (greater than 0.7) extraction ratios in both the kidneys and the liver are listed in Table 11–2.

A word of caution is needed here. Although mass-balance principles state that changes in blood flow are not expected to alter the clearance of drugs of low extraction ratio, there are physiologic mechanisms that may secondarily produce such an effect. Examples are the presence of homeostatic control mechanisms and a perfusion-limited supply of cofactors such as oxygen or sulfate.

Plasma Protein Binding. For a drug with a high extraction ratio, the liver is clearly capable of removing all the drug presented to it in spite of binding to blood cells and to plasma proteins. The rate of elimination depends on the total concentration in the blood. Certainly, a decrease in binding aids in removing a

Table 11–1. Changes in Clearance and Extraction Ratio with Changes in Blood Flow[a]

Drug with	Blood Flow	Extraction Ratio	Clearance
High extraction ratio	↑	↔	↑
	↓	↔	↓
Low extraction ratio	↑	↓	↔
	↓	↑	↔

[a]Symbols: ↑ increase; ↔ little or no change; ↓ decrease.

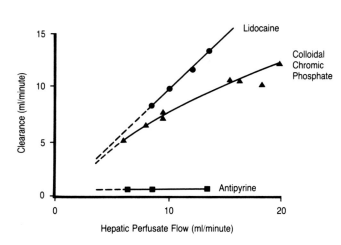

Fig. 11–3. Composite data showing that the sensitivity of the clearance of a compound to changes in blood flow varies. When extraction ratio is low, as occurs with antipyrine (■), clearance is low and independent of blood flow. Clearance varies in direct proportion to flow rate for lidocaine (●), a drug with an extraction ratio close to 1.0. Between these extremes is colloidal chromic phosphate (▲), the clearace of which moves away from a perfusion-rate limitation at higher flows. All data, obtained in an isolated, perfused rat liver, have been normalized to a 10-gram liver. The lines are drawn by eye. (Data abstracted from: Antipyrine and lidocaine—Pang, K.S. and Rowland, M.: Hepatic clearance of drugs I. J. Pharmacokin. Biopharm., 5: 655–680, 1977; Colloidal chromic phosphate—Brauer, R.W., Leong, G.F., McElroy Jr., R.F., and Holloway, R.J.: Circulatory pathways in the rat liver as revealed by ^{32}P chromic phosphate colloid uptake in the isolated, perfused liver preparation. Am. J. Physiol., 184:593–598, 1956.)

Table 11–2. Hepatic and Renal Extraction Ratios of Representative Drugs and Metabolites

	Extraction Ratio		
	Low (<0.3)	Intermediate (0.3–0.7)	High (>0.7)
Hepatic[a] extraction	Carbamazepine Diazepam Digitoxin Indomethacin Phenobarbital Phenytoin Procainamide Salicylic Acid Theophylline Tolbutamide Valproic Acid Warfarin	Aspirin Quinidine Codeine Nortriptyline	Alprenolol Arabinosyl-cytosine Desipramine Doxepin Isoproterenol Lidocaine Meperidine Morphine Nitroglycerin Pentazocine Propoxyphene Propranolol
Renal[a] extraction	Atenolol Cefazolin Chlorpropamide Digoxin Furosemide Gentamicin Lithium Phenobarbital Sulfisoxazole Tetracycline	Cimetidine Cephalothin Procainamide (Some) Penicillins	(Many) Glucuronides Hippurates (Some) Penicillins (Many) Sulfates

[a]At least 30 percent of the drug is eliminated by this route.

drug; but in this case, it is essentially all removed anyway. Therefore, neither the extraction ratio nor the clearance is materially affected by changes in binding.

For a drug with a low extraction ratio, the opposite is observed. This dependency of clearance on plasma protein binding occurs because only unbound drug penetrates membranes and is available for elimination and because the drop in drug concentration across the liver is small. Then the unbound concentration in plasma leaving the liver is almost identical to that in the circulating plasma, Cu. In this case, the rate of drug elimination in the liver is directly related to the concentration of drug unbound in the plasma (except, perhaps, if dissociation of drug from the plasma protein [process b, Fig. 11–2] is rate-limiting). If elimination by metabolism or biliary transport (processes d and e) is slow and distribution into the hepatocyte (process c) is rapid, the concentration in the hepatocyte, available for biliary transport or enzymatic reaction, is that unbound in plasma, Cu. If processes d and e are rapid, but process c is slow, the concentration that determines elimination is still that unbound to plasma proteins, because elimination is rate-limited by diffusion into the hepatic cell, which is dependent on the unbound concentration in plasma. Accordingly, if the extraction ratio of drug is low, the rate of elimination depends on the unbound concentration.

★

$$\text{Rate of elimination} = \underset{\substack{\text{Clearance} \\ \text{based on} \\ \text{unbound} \\ \text{concentration}}}{CLu} \cdot \underset{\substack{\text{Unbound} \\ \text{concentration}}}{Cu} \qquad 7$$

Here the proportionality term, clearance based on the unbound concentration (CLu), is a measure of hepatocellular activity or permeability. Expressing the rate of hepatic elimination relative to the plasma concentration, it is apparent that the hepatic plasma clearance varies proportionally with changes in the fraction unbound.

$$\text{Hepatic clearance} = \underset{\substack{\text{Clearance} \\ \text{based on} \\ \text{unbound} \\ \text{concentration}}}{CLu} \cdot \underset{\substack{\text{Fraction} \\ \text{in plasma} \\ \text{unbound}}}{fu} \qquad 8$$

For example, if the value of fu varies twofold so will the hepatic clearance; the value of the unbound clearance remains unchanged. A similar conclusion is drawn for a drug with a low extraction ratio when relating hepatic blood clearance to the fraction in blood unbound.

The data in Figure 11–4, obtained in the isolated, perfused rat liver, illustrate the points made above. In this preparation, protein binding can be readily altered by changing the concentration of the binding protein, and perfusion can be held constant. Consider first tolbutamide, a drug of low extraction even in the absence of binding ($fu = 1.0$). As expected, the extraction ratio (and clearance) of tolbutamide is directly proportional to fu.

The observations with diazepam are illuminating. The extraction ratio (and clearance) changes from a value close to 1.0 (in the absence of binding, $fu = $

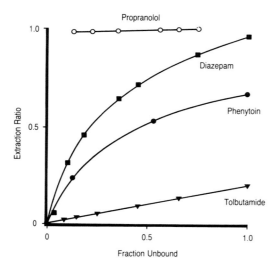

Fig. 11–4. Composite mean data, obtained in an isolated, perfused rat liver, showing that the sensitivity of hepatic extraction ratio to changes in fraction of drug unbound varies. Extraction ratio is proportional to fraction unbound only when the extraction ratio is low, as observed over the entire range of binding for tolbutamide (▼)but only over a limited range for diazepam (■) and phenytoin (●). When the extraction ratio is high, as occurs with phenytoin and diazepam at low binding and with propranolol (○) at all degrees of binding studied, extraction ratio is relatively insensitive to changes in fraction unbound. Notice that in this preparation, in which the fraction unbound is varied over a wide range by modifying the concentration of albumin, the binding protein, a drug such as diazepam can be changed from one of high extraction to one of low extraction. The solid lines are drawn by eye. (Data abstracted from: Phenytoin—Shand, D.G., Cotham, R.H., and Wilkinson, G.R.: Perfusion-limited effects of plasma drug binding on hepatic extraction. Life Sci., *19*: 125–130, 1976; Diazepam—Rowland, M., Leitch, D., Fleming, G., and Smith, B.: Protein binding and hepatic clearance: Discrimination between models of hepatic clearance with diazepam, a drug of high intrinsic clearance, in the isolated, perfused rat liver preparation. J. Pharmacokin. Biopharm., *12*: 129–147, 1984; Tolbutamide—Schary, W.L. and Rowland, M.: Protein binding and hepatic clearance: Studies with tolbutamide, a drug of low intrinsic clearance, in the isolated, perfused rat liver preparation. J. Pharmacokin. Biopharm., *11*: 225–244, 1983; Propranolol—Jones, D.B., Ching, M.S., Smallwood, R.A., and Morgan, D.J.: A carrier-protein receptor is not a prerequisite for avid hepatic elimination of highly bound compounds: A study of propranolol elimination by the isolated, perfused rat liver. Hepatology 5: 590–593, 1985.)

1.0) to one close to zero by decreasing the fraction unbound. Clearly, protein binding can limit extraction if binding is high enough. However, this situation is nonphysiologic in that the fraction unbound is varied between 1.0 and 0.05, a twentyfold change. In practice, a threefold change in *fu* would be considered particularly large. Under these more restricted conditions, the expected relationship between clearance and *fu* holds. Thus, for diazepam, in the region where extraction ratio is low (low *fu*), clearance is directly proportional to *fu*. At the other extreme, in the region where the extraction ratio is high, clearance varies little with a moderate change in *fu*.

Enzyme Activity. As stated above, when clearance is perfusion rate-limited, there is so much hepatocellular activity that modest changes in this activity cause little or no change in clearance. Almost all the drug is extracted anyway. Conversely, if enzyme activity is the rate-limiting step, then clearance is low and directly proportional to activity, e.g., when changed by induction or inhibition by another drug.

A characteristic typical of an enzymatic reaction is a limitation in the capacity of the process. There is only so much enzyme present in the liver, and therefore there is a maximum rate at which metabolism can proceed.

Most of our present knowledge of enzyme kinetics is derived from studies *in vitro* in which substrate, enzyme, and cofactor concentrations are controlled.

Correlation of such studies with those performed *in vivo* has been difficult. Many factors are involved *in vivo* that cannot be isolated. Nevertheless, the basic principles of enzyme kinetics have application in pharmacokinetics.

The upper curve in Figure 11–5 is characteristic of metabolism by a given enzyme both *in vitro* and *in vivo*. The behavior displayed, an apparent statement of the metabolic process, is typical of Michaelis-Menten kinetics if the approach toward the maximum rate, Vm, follows the relationship:

$$\text{Rate of metabolism} = \frac{Vm \cdot Cu}{Km + Cu} \qquad\qquad 9$$

in which Km is a constant, the Michaelis-Menten constant. In enzyme kinetics the value of Vm is directly proportional to the total concentration of enzyme, and Km is an inverse function of the affinity between drug and enzyme. Note in Equation 9 that a value of Cu equal to Km gives a rate that is one-half the maximum; this is a convenient way of defining the constant. An estimate of the true Km requires measurement of the unbound drug concentration at the metabolizing enzyme site. Lacking this capability *in vivo*, the unbound plasma concentration is conventionally used. At unbound plasma concentrations well below Km, which occur for most drugs used therapeutically, the rate and the

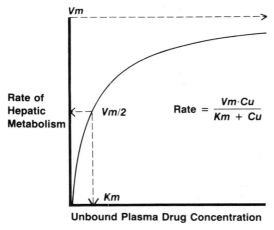

Fig. 11–5. When hepatic metabolism follows Michaelis-Menten kinetics, the rate of metabolism increases (top graph) toward a maximum value, Vm, as the plasma drug concentration is increased. The concentration at which the rate is one-half the maximum is the Km value. The unbound metabolic clearance (bottom graph) falls with increasing drug concentration. The concentration at which the clearance is one-half the maximum is also the Km value. The equations for the relationships are shown.

concentration vary in direct proportion. At concentrations above Km, the rate approaches the value of Vm. Since unbound metabolic clearance is defined as the rate of metabolism relative to the unbound plasma concentration,

$$\text{Unbound metabolic clearance} = \frac{Vm}{Km + Cu} \qquad 10$$

its value decreases at drug concentrations approaching and exceeding the value of Km. This is shown in the lower part of Figure 11–5. Note that the maximum clearance is the ratio Vm/Km, a value often called the *intrinsic metabolic clearance*. *In vivo* the value may be so high that elimination is perfusion rate-limited. In this case the limiting value of blood clearance of drug by the organ is its blood flow. Because of the complexities introduced, the administration of drugs showing saturable metabolism at therapeutic concentrations is difficult. Throughout the rest of the book, except Chapter 22 on Dose and Time Dependencies, drug metabolism is assumed not to show saturability.

A Memory Aid. The general principles just discussed can be difficult to remember. Models of hepatic elimination have been developed to quantify changes in clearance when perfusion, plasma protein binding, and enzyme activity are altered. One of these models, the *well-stirred model*, which assumes instantaneous and complete mixing within the liver, is particularly attractive because it can readily be used to summarize these principles. Even though it may not be quantitative, the model allows one to predict those situations in which either clearance or extraction ratio is affected and their expected direction of change.

The well-stirred model states that

$$CL_{b,H} = \frac{Q_H \cdot CL_{\text{int}} \cdot fu_b}{Q_H + CL_{\text{int}} \cdot fu_b} \qquad 11$$

where Q_H is the hepatic blood flow; CL_{int} is the intrinsic clearance that relates the rate of metabolism at steady state to the unbound concentration at the enzyme site, and fu_b is the fraction unbound in blood. The hepatic extraction ratio, $CL_{b,H}/Q_H$, is then

$$E_H = \frac{fu_b \cdot CL_{\text{int}}}{Q_H + CL_{\text{int}} \cdot fu_b} \qquad 12$$

These two equations have the desired properties at the limits. Thus, when E_H approaches 1.0 (the perfusion rate-limited condition), $CL_{\text{int}} \cdot fu_b$ is much greater than Q_H, and clearance approaches Q_H (Eq. 11). Changes in CL_{int} and fu_b here are not expected to influence $CL_{b,H}$ and E_H much. Conversely, when E_H is small, Q_H must be much greater than $CL_{\text{int}} \cdot fu_b$. Now E_H and $CL_{b,H}$ are approximated by $CL_{\text{int}} \cdot fu_b/Q_H$ and $CL_{\text{int}} \cdot fu_b$, respectively; the value of the extraction ratio depends on all three factors, whereas clearance depends only on CL_{int} and fu_b.

Equation 12 offers an explanation for why the extraction ratios of most drugs appear to be either low ($E < 0.3$) or high ($E > 0.7$). Suppose, for example, that the hepatocellular activity (intrinsic clearance) varied evenly from 0.01 to 100 liters/minute among a large group of compounds, that is, by a factor of 10,000, and that all are unbound in blood ($fu_b = 1.0$). Then substitution of these values into Equation 12 shows that only those drugs with an intrinsic clearance in the narrow range of $0.43 \cdot Q$ to $3.3 \cdot Q$ have an extraction ratio between 0.3 and 0.7.

First-Pass Considerations

To reach the general circulation a drug given orally must pass through the liver via the portal system. The fraction of drug entering the liver that escapes elimination by the organ, F_H, is the upper limit of the oral availability. Its value may be calculated from the hepatic extraction ratio, E_H, since

★

$$\text{Maximum oral availability} = 1 - \text{Hepatic extraction ratio} \qquad 13$$

The hepatic extraction ratio can be estimated if the hepatic (blood) clearance and hepatic blood flow are known or can be approximated.

For illustrative purposes, consider the following data obtained after an intravenous dose (500 mg) of a drug: Cumulative amount excreted unchanged (Ae_∞) = 152 milligrams, AUC = 385 milligram-hours/liter, and C_b/C = 1.2. Extrarenal elimination is assumed to occur only in the liver. The clearance (Dose/AUC) is then 1.3 liters/minute and the blood clearance [$CL/(C_b/C)$] is 1.1 liters/minute since C_b/C is 1.2. The fraction excreted unchanged (Ae_∞/Dose) is 0.304. Accordingly, the renal blood clearance ($fe \cdot CL_b$) is 0.33 liter/minute, and by difference, the hepatic blood clearance [$(1 - fe)CL_b$] is 0.67 liter/minute. Dividing by hepatic blood flow to obtain the hepatic extraction ratio, the maximum oral availability is

$$F \simeq F_H = 1 - (1 - fe)CL_b/Q_H \qquad 14$$

The maximum anticipated availability in this example is 0.50 for a hepatic blood flow of 1.35 liters/minute. Being physiologically determined, no amount of pharmaceutical manipulation can improve on this value for an oral dosage formulation. Any drug with a high hepatic extraction ratio (see Table 11–2) has a low oral availability. There may be other factors that limit the drug reaching the portal vein and so further decrease the availability, as described in Chapter 9.

First-Pass Predictions

The effects of changes in blood flow, intrinsic clearance, and protein binding on first-pass extraction can be predicted using the *well-stirred* model by substituting Equation 12 into the relationship $F_H = 1 - E_H$, that is,

$$F_H = \frac{Q_H}{Q_H + CL_{int} \cdot fu_b} \qquad 15$$

It should be re-emphasized that the prediction here, for changes in $CL_{b,H}$, E_H, and F_H with changes in Q_H, CL_{int}, or fu_b, are based on modest alterations. A low extraction ratio drug can become a high extraction ratio drug if CL_{int} or fu_b is increased or if Q_H is decreased by a sufficiently large factor (Fig. 11–4). The principles here refer to the relative tendencies that modest changes in these factors are likely to produce.

The effect on first-pass extraction can also be visualized by regarding perfusion and protein binding to be in competition with enzymatic activity; perfusion and protein binding help to move drug through the organ, making drug available to the general circulation, whereas enzyme activity removes drug from the perfusing blood.

Consider first the case of a drug with an E_H near zero, that is, Q_H much greater than $CL_{int} \cdot fu_b$. Then F_H is independent of changes in Q, CL_{int}, or fu_b. This is not surprising as the extraction is so small that everything presented gets past the liver anyway. Consider next the condition in which $fu_b \cdot CL_{int}$ is much greater than Q_H, so that E_H approaches 1.0. In this case, $F_H = Q_H/CL_{int} \cdot fu_b$, that is, availability is low and dependent on all three factors. An increase in blood flow increases availability by decreasing the time spent by drug in the liver, where elimination occurs. An increase in either enzymatic activity or in fu_b (which raises the unbound concentration for a given incoming total concentration) decreases availability by increasing the rate of elimination for a given rate of presentation to the liver.

Biliary Secretion

All drugs are excreted into the bile. The ability of the liver to do so is expressed by biliary clearance.

$$\text{Biliary clearance} = \frac{(\text{Bile flow}) \cdot (\text{Concentration in bile})}{\text{Concentration in plasma}} \qquad 16$$

In man, bile flow is a steady 0.5 to 0.8 milliliter/minute. Thus, for a drug with a concentration in the bile equal to or less than that in plasma, the biliary clearance is small. A drug that concentrates in the bile, however, may have a relatively high biliary clearance. Indeed, the bile-to-plasma concentration ratio can approach 1000. Therefore biliary clearances of 500 milliliters/minute or higher can be achieved. Eventually, of course, biliary clearance is limited by hepatic perfusion.

Bile is not a product of filtration, but rather is a product of secretion of bile acids and other solutes. The pH of bile averages about 7.4. The biliary transport of drugs, however, is similar to active secretion in the kidneys (p. 162) in that it may be competitively inhibited.

RENAL CLEARANCE

When the rate of urinary excretion is directly proportional to the plasma drug concentration,

$$\text{Rate of excretion} = CL_R \cdot C \qquad 17$$

renal clearance is constant. This constancy is the basis for the use of urine data to determine the time course of a drug in the body (Chap. 3). Interpretation of urine data with regard to levels of drug in the body is clearly complicated for drugs whose renal clearance varies. Factors that influence renal clearance include plasma drug concentration (see Chap. 22, Dose and Time Dependencies), plasma protein binding, urine flow, and urine pH. How these factors influence renal clearance is seen by considering the physiology of the kidneys.

The Nephron: Anatomy and Function

The basic anatomic unit of renal function is the nephron, shown in Figure 11–6. The basic components of the nephron are the glomerulus, the proximal tubule, the loop of Henle, the distal tubule, and the collecting tubule. The glomerulus receives the blood first and filters about 120 milliliters of plasma water per minute. The filtrate passes down the tubule. Most of the water is

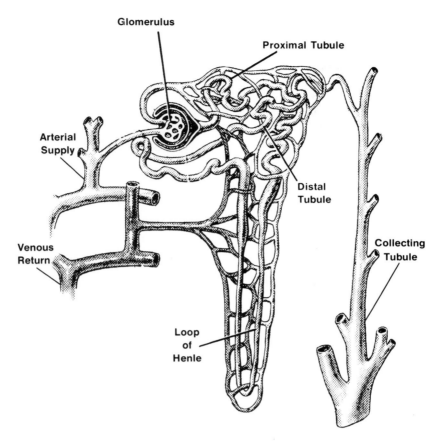

Fig. 11–6.   The functional nephron. (Modified from Smith, H.W.: The Kidney: Structure and Function in Health and Disease. New York, Oxford University Press, 1951.)

reabsorbed; only 1 to 2 milliliters/minute leave the kidneys as urine. On leaving the glomerulus, the same blood perfuses the proximal and distal portions of the tubule through a series of interconnecting channels.

The appearance of drug in the urine is the net result of filtration, secretion, and reabsorption. The first two processes add drug to the lumen of the nephron; the last process involves the movement of drug from the lumen back into the body. The excretion rate of a drug is, therefore,

$$\text{Rate of excretion} = \text{Rate of filtration} + \text{Rate of secretion} - \text{Rate of reabsorption} \qquad 18$$

Let us look at each process in turn.

Glomerular Filtration

Approximately 25 percent of the cardiac output, or 1.1 liters of blood per minute, goes to the kidneys. Of this volume, about 10 percent is filtered at the glomerulus. Only drug unbound in plasma water (concentration Cu) is filtered; drug bound to macromolecules or blood cells is unable to pass across the glomerular membranes.

The rate at which plasma water is filtered, 120 milliliters/minute in a 70-kilogram man, is conventionally called the glomerular filtration rate, *GFR*. It follows that

$$\text{Rate of filtration} = GFR \cdot Cu \qquad ★ \\ 19$$

Recall that the fraction unbound, *fu*, is the ratio of the unbound to total plasma drug concentration; therefore,

$$\text{Rate of filtration} = fu \cdot GFR \cdot C \qquad 20$$

If a drug is only filtered and all filtered drug is excreted into the urine, then the rate of excretion is the rate of filtration. Since renal clearance, CL_R, by definition is

$$CL_R = \frac{\text{Rate of excretion}}{\text{Plasma concentration}} \qquad ★ \\ 21$$

it follows that for such a drug its renal clearance (by filtration) is *fu · GFR*. The extraction ratio of such a drug is low. For example, even if the drug is totally unbound in blood ($Cu = C_b$), the extraction ratio is still only 0.11. This follows since

$$\text{Extraction ratio} = \frac{\text{Rate of extraction } (GFR \cdot Cu)}{\text{Rate of presentation (renal blood flow} \cdot C_b)}$$

$$= \frac{120 \text{ milliliters/minute}}{1100 \text{ milliliters/minute}} = 0.11$$

Creatinine, an endogenous substance, and inulin, an exogenous polysaccharide, are neither bound to plasma proteins nor secreted, and all the filtered load of each substance is excreted into the urine. Accordingly, the renal clearance value of each of these substances is a close measure of *GFR*. Under normal conditions, *GFR* is stable and is relatively insensitive to changes in renal blood flow.

Active Secretion

Filtration always occurs, but as shown above, extraction of a drug by this mechanism alone is low, especially if drug is highly bound within blood. Secretion facilitates extraction.

Secretion is inferred when the rate of excretion exceeds the rate of filtration of a drug (Eq. 18). Stated differently, since substitution of Equation 19 into Equation 18 and division by the plasma drug concentration gives

$$CL_R = fu \cdot GFR + \left[\frac{\text{Rate of} \atop \text{secretion} - \text{Rate of} \atop \text{reabsorption}}{\text{Plasma concentration}} \right] \qquad 22$$

secretion must take place when renal clearance exceeds clearance by filtration. Some reabsorption can occur but it must be less than secretion.

Separate mechanisms exist for secreting acids (anions) and bases (cations), including quaternary ammonium compounds, from the plasma into the tubular lumen. The secretory processes are located predominantly along the proximal tubule. Although active, these acid and base transport systems appear to lack a high degree of specificity, as demonstrated by the wide variety of substances transported by them. As expected, however, substances transported by the same system compete with each other.

Protein Binding and Perfusion

The influence of protein binding on secretion depends on the efficiency of the secretion process and on the contact time of drug at the secretory sites. These conclusions are similar to those drawn for hepatic elimination.

Blood resides at the proximal secretory sites for approximately 30 seconds. When a drug is secreted, but poorly, this contact time is insufficient to transport much drug into the lumen, and accordingly, the drop in drug concentration across the region is small. Then, the unbound concentration at the secretion site is almost identical to the unbound concentration in plasma, Cu. Since the rate of secretion depends on the unbound drug concentration, or $fu \cdot C$, it follows that clearance due to secretion, obtained by dividing rate of secretion by C, is directly proportional to fu. As variation in renal blood flow does not cause any change in the plasma drug concentration, no change in renal clearance with perfusion is expected under these circumstances. Furthermore, the sum of clearances associated with filtration ($fu \cdot GFR$) and secretion, must also be directly proportional to fu. Obviously the extraction ratio of such a drug is low. Figure 11–7 supports these predictions for furosemide in an isolated rat kidney preparation. Furosemide is secreted and is bound to albumin. In this preparation the fraction unbound could be varied over a wide range.

Some drugs are such excellent substrates for the secretory system that they are virtually completely removed from blood within the time they are in contact with the active transport site, even when they are bound to plasma proteins or located in blood cells. In such cases, evidently dissociation of the drug-protein

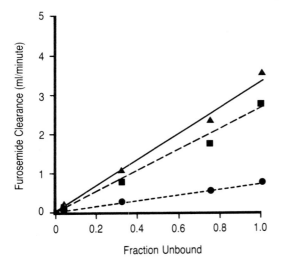

Fig. 11–7. Contribution of glomerular filtration (●) and tubular secretion (■) to the total renal clearance (▲) of furosemide at different values of fraction unbound. Personal communication, S. Hall.

complex and movement of drug out of the blood cells is sufficiently rapid so as to not limit the secretory process. Para-aminohippuric acid (PAH) is handled in this manner and is not reabsorbed. Accordingly, the extraction ratio of PAH is close to 1.0, and hence its renal blood clearance is a measure of renal blood flow. Obviously, under these circumstances, clearance is perfusion rate-limited. Examples of drugs with a variety of renal extraction ratios are listed in Table 11–2.

Reabsorption

Reabsorption is the third factor controlling the renal handling of drugs. Reabsorption must occur if the renal clearance is less than the calculated clearance by filtration (see Eq. 22). Some secretion may still occur but it must be less than reabsorption. Reabsorption varies from being almost absent to being virtually complete. Active reabsorption occurs for many endogenous compounds, including vitamins, electrolytes, glucose, and amino acids. However, for the vast majority of drugs, which are exogenous compounds, reabsorption occurs by a passive process. The degree of reabsorption depends on the properties of the drug, e.g., its polarity, its state of ionization, and its molecular weight. The lipoidal membranes of the cells that form the tubule act as a barrier to water-soluble and ionized substances. Thus, lipophilic molecules tend to be extensively reabsorbed, polar molecules do not. Reabsorption also depends on physiologic variables such as urine flow and urine pH.

Reabsorption occurs all along the nephron, associated with the reabsorption of water filtered at the glomerulus. The majority, 80 to 90 percent, of the filtered water is reabsorbed in the proximal tubule. Most of the remainder is reabsorbed in the distal tubule and collecting tubules. Changes in urine flow are mediated here. If no water is reabsorbed in the distal tubule, urine flow is about 15 to 20 milliliters/minute. Normally, however, water is reabsorbed to the extent that urine flow is 1 to 2 milliliters/minute or lower.

Consequently, with water reabsorption, drugs concentrate in the filtrate. In fact, if a drug is neither reabsorbed (generally polar) nor secreted, the concentration in the urine will be about 100 times as great as that unbound in plasma. This is a result of the rate of excretion being equal to the rate of filtration, that is,

$$GFR \cdot Cu = \text{Urine flow} \cdot \text{Urine concentration}$$

<table>
<tr><td>Rate of
filtration</td><td>Rate of
excretion</td><td>23</td></tr>
</table>

From which it is readily seen that

$$\frac{\text{Urine concentration}}{Cu} = \frac{GFR}{\text{Urine flow}} \qquad 24$$

When the GFR is 100 times the urine flow the urine concentration is 100 times that unbound in plasma. Thus, reabsorption of water favors the reabsorption of a drug that diffuses across tubular membranes.

Urine Flow and Protein Binding. Urine flow can only have a substantial effect on the renal clearance of a drug that is mostly reabsorbed. Certainly, the effect is most dramatic when the reabsorption approaches equilibrium.

As only unbound drug diffuses through membranes, equilibrium is reached when the concentration in urine and that unbound in plasma, Cu, are identical. Consequently, since

★

$$CL_R = \frac{\text{Urine flow} \cdot \text{Urine concentration}}{\text{Plasma concentration}} \qquad 25$$

and since $Cu = fu \cdot C$, it follows that

$$\text{Renal clearance} = fu \cdot \text{Urine flow} \qquad 26$$

This last relationship is a simple test of how close reabsorption is to equilibrium. A nonpolar drug may have a renal clearance below this value only if it is actively reabsorbed. Moreover, if drug is highly bound to plasma proteins, renal clearance (and extraction ratio) would be extremely small since the urine flow is normally only 1 to 2 milliliters/minute. Note also that at constant urine flow, its renal clearance is directly proportional to the fraction unbound.

Ethyl alcohol and methyl alcohol are examples of compounds that are reabsorbed to the extent that the concentration in the urine is virtually the same as that in the plasma regardless of urine flow. Consequently, from Equations 25 and 26, the renal clearance is approximately equal to urine flow and is, therefore, urine-flow dependent.

Urine pH. For weak acids and weak bases the pH of the urine is an additional factor that can determine reabsorption. Although there is some change in the pH of the filtrate as it passes down the proximal tubule, the major adjustment is at the end of the distal tubule and in the collecting tubule. The extremes of urine pH are 4.5 and 7.5 under forced acidification and alkalinization, respectively; on the average, urine pH is 6.3. These extremes contrast with the narrow range of plasma pH, 7.3 to 7.5. Thus, a large pH gradient may exist between plasma and urine.

Urine pH is altered by diet, by drugs, and by the clinical state of a patient. The pH of the urine also varies during the day. Respiratory and metabolic acidosis produces acidification, and respiratory and metabolic alkalosis produces alkalinization. An exception to this is when the metabolic acidosis is of renal origin, for example, renal tubular acidosis, in which case the urine is alkaline. Drugs such as the carbonic anhydrase inhibitor, acetazolamide, produce an alkaline urine.

The influence of pH on reabsorption can be thought of in equilibrium terms or in terms of the rate of reabsorption.

Equilibrium Considerations. The renal clearances of several weak acids and bases, listed in Table 11–3, were calculated using Equation 25. The urine-to-plasma concentration ratio was calculated using the Henderson-Hasselbalch equation (Chap. 8), assuming that these acids and bases do not bind to plasma proteins, that equilibrium is achieved between un-ionized drug in urine and plasma, and that the ionized form is not diffusible. From the values in the table it appears that the renal clearance of acids, pKa less than 6.0, can be much less than urine flow, whereas that of bases can be only slightly less than urine flow, because urine pH is never much higher than plasma pH.

An interesting observation may be made with regard to the renal clearance of weak bases. At low urine pH the renal clearance, by calculation, approaches renal blood flow. Such a high clearance value usually suggests active secretion. It is unlikely, however, that such a high clearance value can be obtained by passive diffusion—for three reasons. First, the fraction of renal blood flow that reaches the end of the distal tubule and the collecting tubule, where the major change in pH occurs, is small. Second, the calculation of renal clearance in Table 11–3 is based on the ratio of urine concentration to plasma concentration leaving, rather than entering, the kidneys. The venous concentration here is less than that entering the kidneys, particularly when the extraction ratio of the drug is high—a perfusion rate-limited condition. Third, the high values of calculated clearance apply to bases, which at blood pH values tend to be almost completely ionized; thus the rate of movement through the membranes, which depends on the concentration of un-ionized drug, is reduced. A similar argument applies to weak acids. Accordingly, an unbound renal clearance value greater than the *GFR* for either acids or bases at normal urine pH probably suggests active secretion.

A Rate Process in Reality. The foregoing discussion was based on equilibrium concepts, but passive reabsorption seldom approaches equilibrium. The primary consideration is how rapidly equilibrium is approached. In reality, then, reabsorption must be considered from a kinetic rather than from an equilibrium point of view, as was true for absorption of drugs from the gastrointestinal tract (Chap. 9).

The rate at which reabsorption occurs depends on the ability of the un-ionized drug to diffuse across membranes, its polarity, and the fraction of drug in the lumen that is un-ionized. The percentages un-ionized for the same drugs listed in Table 11–3 are given in Table 11–4. The calculation is based on the Henderson-Hasselbalch equation (Chap. 8).

Weak Bases. The effect of urine pH on the cumulative amount of unchanged methamphetamine (pKa 10) that is excreted in the urine is shown in Figure 11–8. After 16 hours about 16 percent of the dose is excreted unchanged when the urine pH is not controlled. On alkalinizing the urine by ingesting sodium bicarbonate, only 1 to 2 percent of the dose is in the urine, while acidification by ingesting ammonium chloride results in 70 to 80 percent recovery in the urine. Clearly, for this drug, urine pH is important in determining the contribution of the renal route to total elimination.

Under conditions of no pH control, urine pH varies throughout the day and

Table 11–3. Calculated Renal Clearances (ml/minute) of Selected Nonpolar Weak Acids and Weak Bases at Various Values of Urine pH Under Equilibrium Conditions[a]

Drug	Nature	pKa	Urine pH		
			4.4	6.4	7.9
A		2.4	0.001	0.1	3
B	Acid	6.4	0.1	0.2	3
C		10.4	1.0	1.0	1.0
D		2.4	1.0	1.0	1.0
E	Base	6.4	90	2	0.9
F		10.4	1000	10	0.3
G		12.4	1000	10	0.3

[a]Conditions: no binding of drug to plasma proteins; *fu* = 1.0; urine flow of one milliliter/minute; pH of plasma is constant at 7.4.

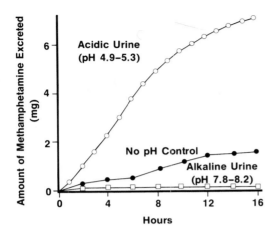

Fig. 11–8. The cumulative urinary excretion of methamphetamine (11 mg orally) in man varies with the urine pH. (Adapted from Beckett, A.H. and Rowland, M.: Urinary excretion kinetics of methylamphetamine in man. Nature, *206*: 1260–1261, 1965.)

Table 11–4. Percent Un-Ionized of Selected Weak Acids and Weak Bases at Various Values of Urine pH[a]

Drug	Nature	pKa	Urine pH 4.4	Urine pH 6.4	Urine pH 7.9
A		2.4	1.0	0.01	0.0003
B	Acid	6.4	99	50	3
C		10.4	100	100	99.7
D		2.4	99	100	100
E	Base	6.4	1.0	50	97
F		10.4	0.0001	0.01	0.3
G		12.4	10^{-6}	0.0001	0.003

[a]Same drugs as in Table 11–3.

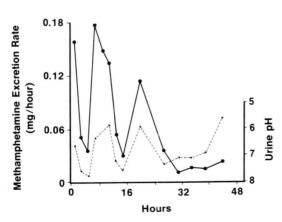

Fig. 11–9. The urinary excretion rate (—) of methamphetamine (11 mg orally) is dramatically influenced by the urine pH (– – –). The urine pH is clearly not controlled. (Adapted from Beckett, A.H. and Rowland, M.: Urinary excretion kinetics of methylamphetamine in man. Nature, *206*: 1260–1261, 1965.)

the excretion of methamphetamine fluctuates accordingly. The excretion rate after a single dose increases during periods of lower pH and decreases during periods of higher pH (Fig. 11–9). The explanation for these observations is contained in Tables 11–3 and 11–4. At low urine pH both equilibrium and kinetic considerations favor high renal clearance of a drug of pKa 10. In particular, the percent un-ionized, and hence the un-ionized concentration in the renal tubule is so small that there is little opportunity for reabsorption within the time that the drug resides in the nephron. At high urine pH with a greater percent of drug un-ionized in the tubule, both equilibrium and rate considerations favor reabsorption. Drugs that show these substantial changes in renal clearance are said to be pH sensitive.

The effect of urine pH on the reabsorption of basic drugs, in general, can be summarized as follows:

1. A basic drug that is polar in its un-ionized form is not reabsorbed, regardless of its degree of ionization in the urine, unless actively transported. The aminoglycoside gentamicin is an example; its renal clearance is independent of urine pH.

2. A very weakly basic nonpolar drug, whose *pKa* is around 6.0 or below, such as propoxyphene, is extensively reabsorbed at all values of urine pH because the percent of drug in the diffusible un-ionized form is sufficient to have no limiting effect on the rate of reabsorption, regardless of urine pH. Furthermore, equilibrium favors reabsorption. The renal clearance of such a drug may vary with urine pH but its value is low, especially if the drug is highly bound to plasma proteins.

3. For a strong base with a *pKa* value approaching 12 or greater, such as guanethidine, little or no reabsorption is expected throughout the range of urine pH because ionization is so extensive that it limits the rate of reabsorption. Accordingly, its renal clearance is independent of urine pH and is generally high.

4. For a basic nonpolar drug with a *pKa value between 6.0 and 12* the extent of reabsorption varies from negligible to almost complete (equilibration) with changes in urine pH. The renal clearance of such a drug varies markedly with urine pH.

Weak Acids. The principles developed for weak bases also apply to weak acids. However, for acids, an increase in pH causes more ionization, not less. Consequently acids are reabsorbed less and have larger renal clearance values at higher values of urine pH.

Again, the effect of *pKa* in reabsorption is seen by inspecting Tables 11–3 and 11–4. An acid with a *pKa* value of 2.0 or less, e.g., chromoglycic acid, is so completely ionized at all urine pH values that it is simply not reabsorbed; its renal clearance is generally high and insensitive to pH. At the other extreme, a very weak acid with a *pKa* value above 8.0, such as phenytoin, is mostly un-ionized throughout the range of urine pH; its renal clearance is always low and insensitive to pH. Only for an acid whose *pKa lies between 3.0 and 7.5* is renal clearance pH sensitive. Note in Table 11–3 that for all nonpolar acids equilibrium favors reabsorption.

The effect of pH on the renal clearance of basic and acidic drugs of various *pKa* values is summarized in the schematic diagram of Figure 11–10. Curves are shown for extremes of both acidic (pH 5.0) and alkaline (pH 7.5) urine. The

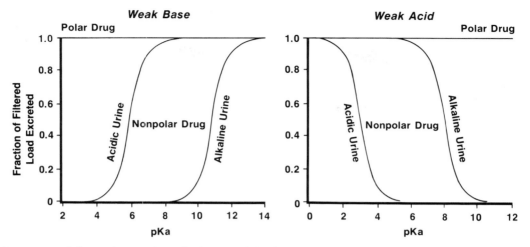

Fig. 11–10. Scheme showing how the fraction of the filtered load excreted (renal clearance relative to the clearance by filtration [*fu* · *GFR*]) of nonpolar weak bases (left) and weak acids (right) depends on both *pKa* and urine pH: the drugs are assumed to be equally nonpolar. Also shown is how the value for polar compounds (top horizontal lines) is high and independent of ionization. All drugs are assumed not to be secreted.

scheme is not intended to be accurate. Variations in urine flow and polarity of the un-ionized form of a drug, as well as active secretion and active reabsorption, preclude it from being so.

Weak acids and bases that show pH-sensitive reabsorption also generally show flow-rate dependence. Again, however, the degree to which the renal clearance is changed by flow depends on the extent of reabsorption. If 50 percent of that filtered and secreted is reabsorbed at normal urine flow, 50 percent is excreted. Increased urine flow decreases reabsorption toward zero, but renal clearance cannot be increased by more than a factor of two. Figure 11–11 shows how the renal clearance of phenobarbital (*pKa* 7.2) varies with urine flow. As expected the renal clearance of this drug is pH sensitive as well as urine flow-rate dependent.

For polar substances that are not reabsorbed, e.g., gentamicin, penicillin, and para-aminohippuric acid, the rate of excretion is the rate of filtration plus the

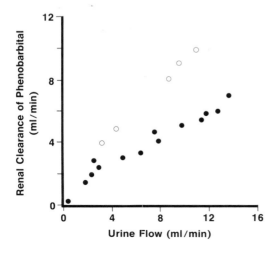

Fig. 11–11. The renal clearance of phenobarbital varies with urine flow in man. It is also a function of urine pH: without alkalinization (●), with alkalinization (○). (Redrawn from Linton, A.L., Luke, R.G., and Briggs, M.D.: Methods of forced diuresis and its application in barbiturate poisoning. Lancet, 2:377–380, 1967.)

rate of secretion. For a given plasma drug concentration the rate of excretion is constant. An increase in the urine flow only produces a more dilute urine.

Forced Diuresis and Urine pH Control. Increased urine flow by forced intake of fluids and, in some cases, the coadministration of mannitol or another diuretic, can increase the excretion of some drugs. More rapid elimination is, of course, desirable for the purpose of detoxifying a patient who is overdosed. There are several criteria that must be met for forced diuresis to be of value:

1. Renal excretion under conditions of forced diuresis must become the major route of drug elimination. Increasing the renal clearance of a drug tenfold, for example, does little to hasten drug elimination from the body if renal clearance normally is only 1 percent of total clearance.

2. The compound must normally be extensively reabsorbed in the renal tubule.

3. If the reabsorption is pH sensitive, both forced diuresis and pH control may be of value. This applies if forced diuresis or pH control alone only partially prevents reabsorption.

The last point bears further discussion. Suppose that, on alkalinizing the urine, the reabsorption of a weak acid is decreased from 90 to 10 percent of that filtered and secreted. The addition of forced diuresis will be of little additional value; the excretion rate can only be increased by a further 10 percent. The converse applies to the use of pH control when forced diuresis almost completely prevents reabsorption.

Additivity of Clearance

The anatomy of the human body dictates that the clearance of a drug by one organ adds to the clearance of another. This is a consequence of the circulation. Consider, for example, a drug that is eliminated by both renal excretion and hepatic metabolism. Then

$$\frac{\text{Rate of}}{\text{elimination}} = \frac{\text{Rate of}}{\text{renal excretion}} + \frac{\text{Rate of}}{\text{hepatic metabolism}} \qquad 27$$

Dividing the rate of removal associated with each process by the incoming drug concentration (blood or plasma), which for both organs is the same (C), gives the clearance associated with that process:

$$\frac{\dfrac{\text{Rate of}}{\text{elimination}}}{C} = \frac{\dfrac{\text{Rate of}}{\text{renal excretion}}}{C} + \frac{\dfrac{\text{Rate of}}{\text{hepatic metabolism}}}{C} \qquad \bigstar$$

or   28

$$\frac{\text{Total}}{\text{clearance}} = \frac{\text{Renal}}{\text{clearance}} + \frac{\text{Hepatic}}{\text{clearance}}$$

Thus, total clearance is the sum of the clearances by each of the eliminating organs.

Because of the additivity of clearance, the relative contribution of any organ to drug elimination is readily calculated. For example, the fraction of drug excreted unchanged (designated *fe*, see Chap. 3), being the fraction of total elimination that occurs via renal excretion, is just renal clearance divided by total clearance.

One exception to the additivity of clearance is pulmonary clearance. This is due in part to the blood supply to the lungs being in series, rather than in parallel, with other organs of elimination and in part to the total cardiac output passing through the lungs before reaching the site of measurement, usually blood in a peripheral vein. The concentration measured is that leaving, rather than entering, the lungs. The use of this concentration to calculate clearance is inconsistent with its definition (see Eq. 3). Indeed, if the pulmonary extraction ratio is high, clearance values calculated in the usual manner may even exceed cardiac output, making interpretation difficult.

The physiology of the body dictates that several pharmacokinetic parameters are related to and dependent on one another. Perhaps the most fundamental dependency in clinical pharmacokinetics is that of half-life on clearance and volume of distribution. This dependency is derived as follows.

DEPENDENCE OF ELIMINATION KINETICS ON CLEARANCE AND DISTRIBUTION

Half-life in Plasma

Recall from Chapter 3 that the elimination rate constant (i.e., fractional rate of drug elimination), k, is related to total clearance, CL, and volume of distribution, V, by the expression

★

$$k = \frac{\text{Rate of elimination}}{\text{Amount in body}} = \frac{CL}{V} \qquad 29$$

Because clearance is the volume of plasma that is cleared of drug per unit of time and V is the volume that drug appears to occupy at a concentration equal to that in plasma, it is apparent from Equation 29 that the fractional rate of drug elimination can be thought of as the fraction of the volume of distribution from which drug is removed per unit time.

Furthermore, recall that the half-life, $t_{1/2}$, is related to k, or to V and CL through the expressions

★

$$t_{1/2} = \frac{0.693}{k} = \frac{0.693\,V}{CL} \qquad 30$$

To appreciate the dependence of half-life on clearance and volume of distribution, consider a drug that undergoes complete enterohepatic cycling, yet distributes to bile and subsequently to the intestines in significant amounts as a result of slow intestinal reabsorption. The consequence of biliary obstruction would be a decreased volume of distribution, but no change in total clearance, and therefore a shorter half-life. On the other hand, if there is no enterohepatic cycling, the bile and the intestines are not part of the volume of distribution. Biliary obstruction, by decreasing clearance without affecting distribution, would then cause the half-life to increase.

Figure 11–12 illustrates half-lives of drugs with various combinations of clearance and volume of distribution. When clearance is low and volume of distribution is large, the half-life can be weeks or months. There is a paucity of drug

1. Penicillin V
2. Aspirin
3. Penicillin G
4. Oxacillin
5. Furosemide
6. Morphine
7. Meperidine
8. Propranolol
9. Procainamide
10. Quinidine
11. Chloramphenicol

12. Tetracycline
13. Gentamicin
14. Amikacin
15. Theophylline
16. Acetazolamide
17. Sulfisoxazole
18. Tolbutamide
19. Desmethylimipramine
20. Doxepin
21. Chlorpromazine
22. Nortriptyline

23. Digoxin
24. Clonazepam
25. Diazepam
26. Carbamazepine
27. Sulfamerazine
28. Valproic Acid
29. Warfarin
30. Phenylbutazone
31. Amphotericin B
32. Phenobarbital
33. Digitoxin

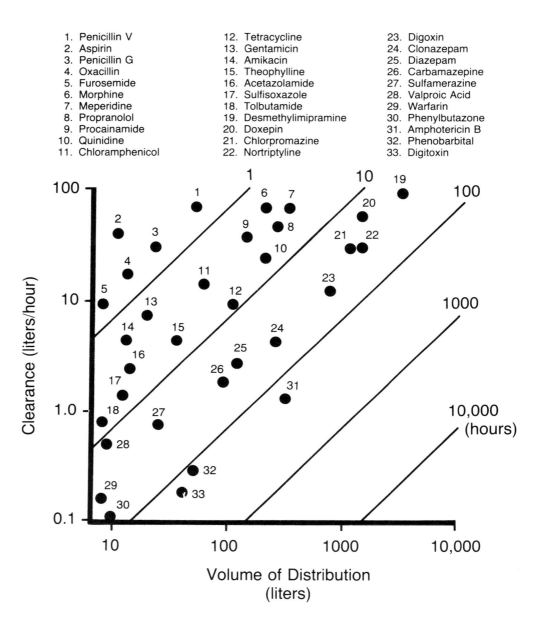

Fig. 11–12. Clearance (ordinate) and volume of distribution (abscissa) of selected drugs vary widely. The diagonal lines show the combinations of clearance and volume with the same half-life (hours). Note that drugs with low clearances and large volumes (right lower quadrant of graph) are difficult to find: their half-lives are too long for these drugs to be used practically in drug therapy. (Adapted from Tozer, T.N.: Concepts basic to pharmacokinetics. Pharmacol. Ther., 12, 109–131, 1981. Reproduced with permission of author and publisher.)

examples with these characteristics. This is not surprising as drug accumulation would be extenisve and very slow on daily multiple dosing. Furthermore, detoxification of a patient who exhibits toxicity on such a drug would be slow.

Half-life in Blood and Plasma Water

The interrelationships expressed in Equations 29 and 30 are just as readily derived from clearance and volume parameters based on measurements of drug in blood (CL_b, V_b) or in plasma water (CLu, Vu). Thus, by definition,

$$\text{Rate of elimination} = CL \cdot C$$
$$= CL_b \cdot C_b = CLu \cdot Cu$$

★ 31

and

$$\text{Amount in body} = V \cdot C$$
$$= V_b \cdot C_b = Vu \cdot Cu$$

★ 32

Note that each clearance or volume term can be related to the other using the definitions $fu = Cu/C$ and $fu_b = Cu/C_b$. For example, $CL = fu \cdot CLu$. Dividing each term in Equation 31 by the respective term in Equation 32 gives

$$k = \frac{CL}{V} = \frac{CL_b}{V_b} = \frac{CLu}{Vu}$$

★ 33

and on substituting Equation 33 into Equation 30, it follows that

$$t_{1/2} = \frac{0.693\ V}{CL} = \frac{0.693\ V_b}{CL_b} = \frac{0.693\ Vu}{CLu}$$

★ 34

Thus, the value of the elimination rate constant, k, or the half-life, $t_{1/2}$, is independent of the site of measurement in blood.

The clearance parameter based on measurement of drug in blood is useful in considerations of drug extraction in the eliminating organs. Volume and clearance parameters based on the unbound drug concentration are particularly useful in therapeutics, because it is the unbound drug that is thought to relate most closely to the effects of a drug. Both sets of parameters are of value in anticipating and evaluating the pharmacokinetic and therapeutic consequences of alterations in protein binding, blood flow, and other physiologic variables. For convenience of chemical analysis, plasma drug concentrations are usually measured, but the application of the volume and clearance parameters so obtained are limited.

Study Problems

(Answers to Study Problems are in Appendix G.)

1. The renal clearances and the fractions unbound to plasma proteins of three drugs in a 70-kilogram man are listed as follows:

	Renal Clearance (ml/minute)	Fraction Unbound
Theophylline	10	0.50
Phenytoin	0.15	0.10
Cefonicid	20	0.02

State the likely contribution of filtration, secretion, and reabsorption to the renal handling of each of these drugs. Assume a *GFR* of 120 milliliters/minute and a urine flow of 1.5 milliliters/minute.

2. For each of the following multiple choice questions indicate the letters of all (one or more) of the correct answers.

(a) The conditions that indicate the possibility of renal clearance of a weakly acidic drug being sensitive to urine pH are

1. It is secreted and not reabsorbed.

2. It has a pKa value of 5.0.

3. It has a small volume of distribution.

4. All of the drug is renally excreted unchanged, *fe* = 1.0.

(b) Forced diuresis is likely to enhance significantly the elimination kinetics of a drug

1. Which is both polar and slowly removed from the body.

2. For which most of the filtered and secreted drug is reabsorbed and *fe* is greater than 0.5.

3. Which is neutral, polar, and has a value of *fe* greater than 0.9.

4. Which is not secreted and for which the ratio of its unbound renal clearance to creatinine clearance is 1.0.

(c) A renal blood clearance of 567 milliliters/minute for oxacillin indicates that:

1. It is secreted into the luminal contents of the nephron.

2. Its renal extraction ratio is 0.1.

3. The majority of drug entering the body is excreted in the urine unchanged.

4. It is not bound to plasma proteins.

(d) The renal clearance of a drug is constant with time if

1. Its value exceeds 300 milliliters/minute.

2. The concentration in urine is independent of urine flow.

3. A constant fraction of filtered and secreted drug is reabsorbed.

3. Payne *et al.* (Br. Med. J., 3:819, 1967) were interested, for legal reasons, in determining if the concentration of alcohol in urine could be related to its blood concentration. Table 11–5 summarizes their findings.

(a) Knowing that alcohol is not bound to components in blood, what explanation(s) can you offer for the very close correlation between concentrations of alcohol in blood and in urine?

(b) Would you expect the excretion rate of alcohol to correlate with the blood alcohol concentration? Discuss briefly.

Table 11-5. Frequency Distribution of the Ratio of Alcohol Concentrations, Urine/Blood

Percent of Observations	9	51	32	8
$\dfrac{\text{Urine Concentration}}{\text{Blood Concentration}}$	<1.2	1.2–1.4	1.4–1.6	>1.6

4. Three different drugs are listed in Table 11–6 together with some of their physical properties and disposition characteristics in a 70-kilogram man.

Table 11-6.

Property or Characteristic	Nafcillin	Tocainide	Cyclosporine A
Polarity of un-ionized form	Polar	Non-polar	Non-polar
pKa	3.0 (weak acid)	9.0 (amine)	Not an acid or a base
Usual dose (mg)	250	400–600	350
Volume of distribution (liters)	25	210	245
Fraction unbound (fu)	0.1	0.9	*
Half-life (hours)	1	14	8
Fraction excreted unchanged	0.27	0.14	<0.01

*Information not given.

(a) Indicate the drug(s) for which each of the following statements is probably most applicable:

1. The renal clearance of this drug is the most sensitive to changes in urine pH.

2. This drug has the highest renal clearance of the three listed.

3. This drug most likely shows the greatest diffusion limitation in crossing the placenta to the fetus.

4. Forced diuresis is most likely to be of value for this drug in a case of drug overdose.

5. For 100 milligrams in the body, the plasma concentration is highest for this drug after distribution equilibrium is achieved.

6. This drug has the lowest total clearance.

(b) Write in the space provided the most appropriate word, term, or value for the following statements:

1. The renal clearance of nafcillin will _____

   increase, decrease, show little change

   if the drug is significantly displaced from plasma protein binding sites.

2. For the drug with a renal clearance that is most sensitive to changes in urine pH, _____of the urine should decrease the renal

   alkalinization, acidification

   clearance.

3. Nafcillin _____ distributed evenly throughout and accounted for within the
                is, is not
   extracellular fluids.

4. Cyclosporine A is primarily eliminated by _____ .
                                            metabolism, renal excretion

5. Cyclosporine A _____ be highly bound (fu less than 0.1) to plasma pro-
                  can, cannot
   teins since it has such a large apparent volume of distribution.

6. _____ percent of tocainide in the body is located outside the plasma.
   51,97,99,99.9

12

Integration with Kinetics

Objectives

The reader will be able to:

1. **List examples of physiologic variables that may alter the primary pharmacokinetic parameters: absorption rate constant, availability, hepatic clearance, renal clearance, and volume of distribution.**

2. **Given plasma (or blood) concentration versus time data in normal and altered states, determine the changes that have occurred in the primary and secondary pharmacokinetic parameters and list the possible physiologic mechanism(s) involved.**

3. **Predict and graphically demonstrate the effects of an alteration in plasma protein or tissue binding, perfusion or metabolic activity on the time course of drug in blood when the appropriate primary pharmacokinetic parameters are known.**

4. **Predict the pharmacologic consequences of each of the alterations given in objective 3.**

Reference is frequently made to the value of *the* half-life of a drug or *the* value of its clearance. The pharmacokinetic parameters of a drug may, however, change—with disease, with concomitant drug therapy, and even within the same individual with time. An ability to assign likely physiologic and pathologic mechanisms to these observed changes in the kinetics of a drug is important, as is the prediction of the kinetic consequences of an alteration in a physiologic variable. Both approaches are taken in this chapter in order to integrate and practice the physiologic and pharmacokinetic concepts learned to this point. No attempt is made to examine situations involving all possible changes of physiologic variables as the theoretical possibilities are too numerous. In subsequent chapters, especially Chapters 17 (Drug Interactions) and 22 (Dose and Time Dependencies), additional examples that demonstrate and require an integration of physiologic and kinetic concepts are given.

Frequently, conditions that produce a change in one physiologic parameter cause changes in others as well. For example, renal disease appears not only to decrease the renal clearance of digoxin, but to decrease its tissue binding and extrarenal clearance as well (see Chap. 16). The interaction of quinidine and digoxin is another example. Similar to renal disease, quinidine decreases tissue binding and both renal and extrarenal clearances of digoxin. Thus, neither of these situations is a good example of the kinetic consequences of any *one* of the alterations that occur. Yet, these kinds of observations occur frequently. The first step in analyzing them is to examine the expectations for an alteration in each physiologic variable involved. The overall picture is then gained by integrating these expectations.

INTERRELATIONSHIPS AMONG PHARMACOKINETIC PARAMETERS AND PHYSIOLOGIC VARIABLES

A summary of the interrelationships among pharmacokinetic parameters and physiologic variables is appropriate here.

Dependence of Primary Parameters on Physiologic Variables

The processes of absorption and disposition depend on many physiologic variables. Gastrointestinal absorption may be affected by blood flow at the absorption site, gastric emptying, and gastrointestinal motility. Distribution is influenced by binding to both plasma proteins and tissue components, and by body composition. Renal excretion may depend on secretion (active transport), urine pH, and urine flow. Each of these physiologic variables is affected by numerous factors. Thus, rubbing increases subcutaneous and muscle blood flow, food slows gastric emptying, and diseases and drugs produce many effects.

The pharmacokinetics of a drug often can be described by relatively few parameters. Recall that: absorption can be characterized by availability and by an absorption rate constant, when absorption is first order; distribution can be characterized by the volume of distribution; and elimination can be characterized by hepatic and renal clearance. As discussed in Chapters 8 through 11, each of these parameters may be directly affected by changes in physiologic variables. Because of this direct relationship, these parameters may be referred to as *primary pharmacokinetic parameters*. The dependence of the primary pharmacokinetic parameters on selected physiologic variables is summarized in Table 12–1.

Table 12–1. Dependence of Primary Pharmacokinetic Parameters on Physiologic Variables

Primary Pharmacokinetic Parameters	Physiologic Variables
Absorption rate constant	Blood flow at absorption site, gastric emptying (oral), intestinal motility (oral)
Hepatic clearance; availability[a]	Hepatic blood flow, binding in blood, intrinsic hepatocellular activity
Renal clearance	Renal blood flow, binding in blood, active secretion, active reabsorption, urine pH, urine flow, glomerular filtration rate
Volume of distribution	Binding in blood, binding in tissues, partition into fat, body composition, body size

[a]Hepatic elimination is assumed to be the only cause of a decrease in the oral availability.

Secondary Pharmacokinetic Parameters and Derived Values

Half-life, elimination rate constant, and fraction excreted unchanged in urine are examples of *secondary pharmacokinetic parameters*, in that their values depend on those of the primary pharmacokinetic parameters. Furthermore, there are several derived values, such as plateau plasma concentration, that depend not only on the primary pharmacokinetic parameters, but also on either dose or rate of administration. These dependencies are summarized briefly in Table 12–2.

The equations in Table 12–2 plus three other previously given equations provide the basic relationships for interpreting and predicting alterations in kinetic behavior. One of the three additional equations is a modification of Equation 22 in Chapter 10. Expressing the volume of distribution in terms of the concentration of drug in blood, this equation becomes

$$V_B = V_B + V_T \cdot \frac{fu_b}{fu_T} \qquad 1$$

where V_B, the blood volume, is about 5 liters and fu_b is the fraction unbound in blood. The two other equations derive from the memory aids given as Equations 9 and 13 in Chapter 11, namely,

$$CL_{b,H} = \frac{Q_H \cdot CL_{int} \cdot fu_b}{Q_H + CL_{int} \cdot fu_b} \qquad 2$$

and

$$F_H = \frac{Q_H}{Q_H + CL_{int} \cdot fu_b} \qquad 3$$

The subsequent examples are analyzed using these relationships. They exemplify alterations in intrinsic hepatocellular activity (induction and inhibition), hepatic blood flow, active tubular secretion, and plasma protein binding.

Table 12–2. Dependence of Secondary Pharmacokinetic Parameters and Other Derived Values on Primary Pharmacokinetic Parameters

	Equations
Secondary Pharmacokinetic Parameters	
Elimination half-life	$0.693 \cdot \dfrac{\text{Volume of distribution}}{\text{Clearance}}$
Elimination rate constant	Clearance/(Volume of distribution)
Fraction excreted unchanged	(Renal clearance)/(Total clearance)
Other Derived Values	
Area under curve (i.v.)	Dose/Clearance
Steady-state concentration (i.v.)	(Infusion rate)/Clearance
Area under curve (oral)	$\dfrac{\text{Dose} \cdot (\text{Oral availability})}{\text{Clearance}}$
Average plateau concentration (oral)	$\dfrac{\text{Dose} \cdot (\text{Oral availability})}{\text{Clearance} \cdot (\text{Dosing interval})}$

Induction of Metabolism

Some drugs can induce the metabolism of others by increasing the rate of synthesis of the enzyme(s) involved. The kinetic and therapeutic consequences depend on whether the affected drug initially has a low or a high extraction ratio in the eliminating organ in which induction occurs and on the route of administration.

Low Extraction Ratio. Figure 12–1 demonstrates the kinetic effect of induction of warfarin metabolism by the antitubercular agent, rifampin. Warfarin is predominantly metabolized in the liver; little is excreted in urine unchanged. Warfarin is also well and rapidly absorbed when given orally.

The data in Figure 12–1 support warfarin having a low hepatic extraction ratio. This conclusion is based on a rough calculation of clearance. Thus, during the control phase clearance, obtained by dividing dose (1.5 mg/kg) by AUC [1356 mg-hours/liter, calculated from $C(0)/k$], is 0.0011 liter/hour per kilogram. Making the reasonable assumption of a blood/plasma concentration ratio of 0.6, since warfarin is restricted in blood to plasma (see Appendix E, hematocrit of 0.4 is assumed), the corresponding blood clearance is therefore 0.0018 liter/hour per kilogram. This value is low compared to the hepatic blood flow of 81 liters/hour per 70 kilograms or 1.2 liters/hour per kilogram. In the presence of rifampin the AUC of warfarin is decreased compared to that of the control value, reflecting a higher clearance. This observation is consistent with induction of hepatic enzymes; the clearance of a drug of low hepatic extraction ratio is expected to be sensitive to changes in hepatocellular enzymatic activity. There are no data to suggest an effect of rifampin on warfarin distribution. The estimated volumes of distribution, obtained from CL/k, are 0.079 and 0.068 liter/kilogram during the control and rifampin phases, respectively. These values are probably not significantly different.

The therapeutic consequence of induction can be appreciated from the difference in the response-time curves, shown in the bottom graph of Figure 12–1. Response here is defined as the elevation in prothrombin time above a baseline value of 14 seconds. The overall response, given by the area under the response-

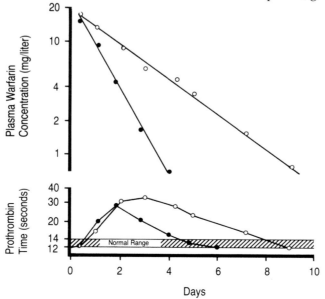

Fig. 12–1. The half-life of warfarin, a drug with a low extraction ratio, is shortened and clearance is increased when it is given in a single dose (1.5 mg/kg) before (○) and while (●) the inducer, rifampin, is being administered in a 600-milligram dose daily for 3 days prior to warfarin administration. The peak and duration of the elevation in the prothrombin time (response) are decreased when rifampin is coadministered (lower graph). (One mg/liter = 3.3 micromolar.) (Reproduced, with permission, from: O'Reilly, R.A.: Interaction of sodium warfarin and rifampin. Ann. Intern. Med., 81:337–340, 1974.)

time curve after the single oral dose, is substantially reduced in the presence of rifampin. Consequently, one would expect under steady-state conditions that the dosage of warfarin must be increased in the presence of rifampin to maintain the same prothrombin time. The reason for the apparently poor correlation between response and plasma warfarin concentration during the first 48 hours after warfarin administration, when response is increasing and concentration is falling, is discussed in Chapter 23, Turnover Concepts.

High Extraction Ratio. Induction of metabolism of a drug with a high hepatic extraction ratio has kinetic consequences very different from those of a drug with a low hepatic extraction ratio, as illustrated in Figure 12–2. Pretreatment with the inducer pentobarbital appears to have little effect on the pharmacokinetics of alprenolol after its intravenous administration. Following oral administration, however, both the peak concentration and the area under the curve are dramatically reduced, although there is little apparent change in the half-life. These observations, at first glance, appear to be inconsistent. Knowing that this drug is metabolized only in the liver and on calculating (from dose and AUC following intravenous administration) a clearance of 1.2 liters/minute in this individual, an explanation can be offered. Pentobarbital induces alprenolol metabolism, which manifests itself as a decrease in alprenolol availability. The argument for this conclusion follows.

The hepatic extraction ratio of alprenolol is high; its clearance approaches hepatic blood flow, approximately 1.35 liters/minute, and its oral availability (F), calculated by comparing the dose-corrected AUC after oral and intravenous administrations, is 0.22. Assuming that the low availability is due solely to hepatic extraction, the hepatic extraction ratio ($1 - F$) is 0.78. Availability reflects the balance between perfusion, which forces drug through the organ, and enzymatic activity, which removes drug. After induction, which increases enzyme

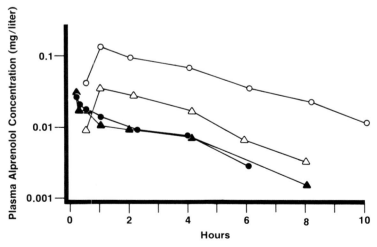

Fig. 12–2. Induction of alprenolol metabolism by pentobarbital treatment produces marked differences in the plasma concentration when the drug is given orally (200 mg), but not when given intravenously (5 mg). Alprenolol was administered before (●, i.v.; ○, oral) and 10 days into (▲, i.v.; △, oral) a pentobarbital regimen of 100 milligrams at bedtime. (One mg/liter = 4.0 micromolar.) (From Alvan, G., Piafsky, K., Lind, M., and von Bahr, C.: Effect of pentobarbital on the disposition of alprenolol. Clin. Pharmacol. Ther., 22:316–321, 1977.)

activity, oral availability (based on comparison of *AUC* values) decreases to 0.06, almost a fourfold change, and hence the hepatic extraction ratio increases to 0.94. Because clearance is perfusion rate-limited and because there is no evidence in man that pentobarbital alters hepatic blood flow, there is only a small increase in clearance. The increase in hepatic extraction ratio, and hence clearance, is only 20 percent (from 0.78 to 0.94). The lack of change in terminal half-life after induction also indicates that pentobarbital has no effect on the volume of distribution of alprenolol. Thus, induction of the metabolism of this drug, or any other drug with a high hepatic extraction ratio, has therapeutic implications when administered orally, but not when given intravenously. A larger oral dose is needed in the presence of the inducer to produce the same effect, assuming all activity resides with the drug.

Decreased Hepatocellular Activity

Examples of drugs that inhibit the metabolism of other drugs are given in Chapter 17, Interacting Drugs. Reduced metabolism can also be a consequence of hepatic disease (Chap. 16), dietary deficiencies, and other conditions. Whatever the cause of decreased metabolic activity, the kinetic consequences depend on the hepatic extraction ratio of the drug.

Low Extraction Ratio. The effect of decreasing hepatocellular activity for a drug of low hepatic extraction ratio is shown in Figure 12–3. The half-life of chlordiazepoxide is increased and its clearance is decreased in patients with hepatic cirrhosis. The availability and volume of distribution (not shown) are unaffected.

That chlordiazepoxide has a low hepatic extraction ratio even in healthy subjects can be deduced from the data in the figure if one also knows that: the drug is eliminated primarily by hepatic metabolism, the blood-plasma concentration ratio is close to 1.0, and an average hepatic blood flow is 19 milliliters/minute per kilogram. In subjects with normal hepatic function the hepatic extraction ratio $[CL_b/Q_H = (0.55 \text{ ml/minute per kg})/(19 \text{ ml/minute per kg})]$ is then expected to be only about 0.03 or less.

Typical of many studies of hepatic metabolism, the variation in pharmacokinetic parameters in cirrhotic patients is much greater than in patients with

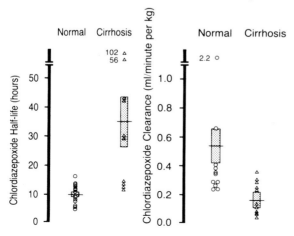

Fig. 12–3. Chlordiazepoxide's half-life is increased and total clearance is decreased in patients with hepatic cirrhosis compared to normal subjects. Mean ($\pm$ SEM) and individual values are shown. (Redrawn from Sellers, E.M., Greenblatt, D.J., Giles, H.G., Naranjo, C.A., Kaplan, H., and MacLeod, S.M.: Chlordiazepoxide and oxazepam disposition in cirrhotics. Clin. Pharmacol. Ther., 26:240–246, 1979. Reproduced with permission of C.V. Mosby.)

normal hepatic function. Furthermore, in some patients diagnosed with the disease the drug shows normal kinetics. In others, clearance is greatly (5 to 10 times) reduced. Such observations for many drugs undergoing extensive metabolism have led to the conclusion that drug therapy must be monitored more closely in cirrhotic patients than in patients with normal hepatic function.

High Extraction Ratio. The kinetic consequences of inhibition of metabolism of a drug with a high hepatic extraction ratio are illustrated by the coadministration of cimetidine and labetolol (Fig. 12–4). That labetolol is a drug of high hepatic extraction ratio is deduced from its clearance, 1.06 liters/hour (estimated by dividing the intravenous dose by the corresponding *AUC* given in the article), approaching hepatic blood flow and from the knowledge that labetolol is eliminated almost exclusively by hepatic metabolism. The intravenous dose of labetolol is much smaller than the oral dose because the drug is highly extracted in the liver, and hence subject to extensive first-pass hepatic loss, and because the pharmacologic activity primarily resides with the drug, rather than with its metabolites.

There is a large increase in the area under the curve for labetolol when administered orally, but not when given intravenously, in the presence of cimetidine therapy. This observation is expected following inhibition of the elimination of a drug with a high hepatic extraction ratio. The lack of change in area following intravenous administration reflects the minor decrease caused by cimetidine in the hepatic extraction ratio, and hence in clearance. Evidently blood flow continues to limit the hepatic elimination of labetolol even when inhibition occurs. This would not be so if the degree of inhibition were such as to reduce labetolol to a drug of low hepatic extraction ratio. The large increase in area following oral administration is a consequence of increased availability; here the increment is about 56 percent, while only a minor decrease (20 percent) was seen in the hepatic extraction ratio. The therapeutic corollary of the kinetic changes in the presence of cimetidine is heightened activity of labetolol when given orally, but not when given intravenously.

Altered Blood Flow

As presented in Chapter 11, changes in organ blood flow only affect clearance when the extraction ratio is high. This conclusion is based on the concept of a perfusion-rate limitation. It should be borne in mind, however, that effects

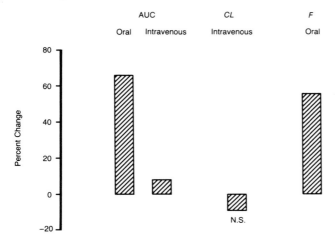

Fig. 12–4. Availability increased, but clearance showed no significant (N.S.) change, when 6 healthy volunteers were given labetolol either in a 200-milligram dose orally or in a 0.5-milligram/kilogram dose intravenously before and on the fourth day of cimetidine treatment (400 mg every 6 hours). This conclusion is based on a significant change in the area under the curve after oral, but not after intravenous, administration. (Adapted from Daneshmend, T.K. and Roberts, C.J.C.: The effects of enzyme induction and enzyme inhibition on labetolol pharmacokinetics. Br. J. Clin. Pharmacol., *18*:393–400, 1984.)

secondary to an altered blood flow, particularly when decreased, may supersede perfusion considerations alone. For example, a decreased blood flow may produce anoxia, which in turn may affect hepatocellular activity and hence the extraction ratio. The extraction ratio may also be altered by a decreased blood flow because every blood vessel in the organ may not provide the same exposure of the drug to hepatic parenchymal cells, and the pattern of distribution of blood flow within the eliminating organ may change. This alteration in the degree of shunting or bypassing of the parenchymal cells may occur in certain hepatic diseases and under a variety of conditions.

Good examples of the kinetic consequences of altered blood flow are hard to find. This is not because they are uncommon, but because a number of additional complications always seem to occur concurrently. For example, conditions such as congestive cardiac failure, in which cardiac output is decreased, are often associated with: increased third-spacing, that is, build-up of fluid in intestinal spaces and body cavities; diminished hepatic and renal functions; and slowed distribution to the tissues. A decrease in hepatic blood flow, brought about by cirrhosis, chronically leads to portal hypertension and extrahepatic shunting of portal blood. Thus, the kinetic consequences of altered blood flow are subsequently examined alone, with the realization that in therapeutic scenarios the effects of changes in more than one physiologic variable need to be considered.

For this theoretical presentation, consider the three drugs given in Table 12–3. Drug L is eliminated in both the liver and the kidneys; its major property is low extraction in both organs. Drug K has a high renal extraction ratio, while Drug H has a high hepatic extraction ratio and is almost exclusively eliminated by the liver.

Low Hepatic Extraction Ratio. Figure 12–5 shows the effect of a doubling of the blood flow to each of the organs of elimination for the poorly cleared drug, Drug L, and for the one highly cleared by the kidneys, Drug K. Because Drug L has a low hepatic extraction ratio, altered blood flow has little or no effect on the pharmacokinetics of this drug.

High Renal Extraction Ratio. For Drug K, with elimination being perfusion rate-limited, the increased blood flow increases renal clearance, which in turn shortens the half-life and decreases the area under the curve after both oral and intravenous administrations.

High Hepatic Extraction Ratio. The events following intravenous administration of a drug with a high hepatic extraction ratio, Drug H, when hepatic blood flow is increased, are readily apparent. Being well-extracted, clearance is increased, and hence half-life is shortened, as occurred with Drug K. Not so apparent are the likely events that follow when Drug H is given orally. Recall

Table 12–3. Pharmacokinetic Parameters of Three Hypothetical Drugs

Drug	Availability[a]	Volume of Distribution (liters)	Clearance[b] (liters/hour)	Fraction Excreted Unchanged	Extraction Ratio	
					Hepatic	Renal
L	0.97	26	6	0.60	0.03	0.05
K	1.00	330	77	1.00	0	0.95
H	0.05	430	100	0.05	0.95	0.08

[a]Availability is fully accounted for by first-pass metabolism in the liver.
[b]Clearance is based on measurement of drug in blood.

INCREASED BLOOD FLOW

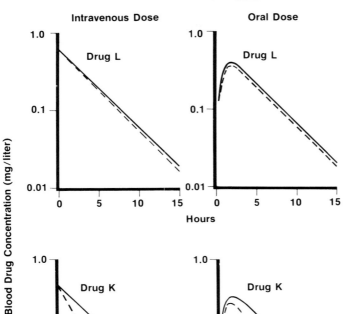

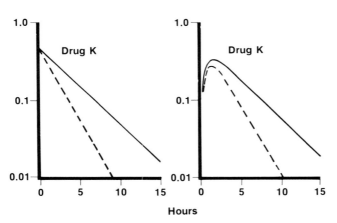

Blood Drug Concentration (mg/liter)

Hours

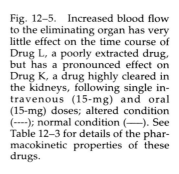

Fig. 12–5. Increased blood flow to the eliminating organ has very little effect on the time course of Drug L, a poorly extracted drug, but has a pronounced effect on Drug K, a drug highly cleared in the kidneys, following single intravenous (15-mg) and oral (15-mg) doses; altered condition (----); normal condition (——). See Table 12–3 for details of the pharmacokinetic properties of these drugs.

that $F \cdot Dose = CL \cdot AUC$ or $AUC = F \cdot Dose/CL$. Although the half-life is shortened, clearance and availability are increased simultaneously; availability is elevated because drug in blood remains in the hepatic sinusoids for a shorter period of time with an increased blood flow, and therefore there is less chance of drug being eliminated. Accordingly, the result may be little or no change in area under the curve (Fig. 12–6). The outcome depends on whether or not the increase in availability is exactly matched by that of clearance when the blood flow is increased. The memory aids of Equations 2 and 3 predict equal effects, in that the ratio of these equations ($CL_{b,H}/F_H = CL_{int} \cdot fu_b$) is independent of blood flow. Unfortunately, there is a lack of good quantitative information to generalize here.

The effect of an increased blood flow is further exemplified by comparing data for propranolol in subjects during fasting and high protein meal intake conditions (Table 12–4). The high protein meal causes the oral availability of the drug to increase 70 percent. This is accompanied by a 38 percent increase in the clearance and an insignificant change in AUC after an oral dose. The explanation given by the authors of the kinetic changes is an increase in the hepatic blood flow

INCREASED BLOOD FLOW

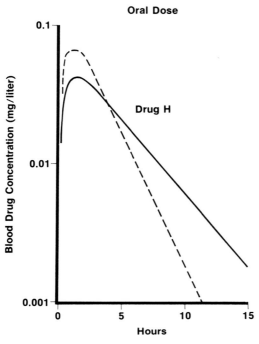

Fig. 12–6. Increased hepatic blood flow alters the blood drug concentration-time profile after an oral dose (500 mg) of Drug H, a drug of high hepatic extraction ratio; altered condition (----); normal condition (——). Note that the corresponding (linear plot) area under the curve is not altered; a consequence of clearance and availability being increased to an equal extent. (The change in availability was calculated using Equation 3.)

produced by the high protein meal. The consistency of this explanation with kinetic theory is now evaluated.

First, it must be recognized that this drug is of high extraction ratio (clearance, 1.0 liter/minute). Recall that an increase in hepatic blood flow produces an increase in availability. Similarly, one expects clearance to increase as, under high extraction conditions, clearance is perfusion rate-limited. The observation of different extents of increase in availability (70 percent) and clearance (38 percent) can be explained by the increased blood flow being restricted to early

Table 12–4. Effect of Food and Consequent Increased Hepatic Blood Flow on the Availability, Systemic Clearance, and Oral *AUC* of Propranolol[a]

	State of Subject	
Parameters	Fasting	Food
Availability (percent)	27 ± 2[b]	46 ± 4[c]
Clearance[d] (liters/minute)	1.00 ± 0.06	1.38 ± 0.12[c]
Oral AUC[e] (mg-hour/liter)	21.8 ± 2.6	27.8 ± 10.0[f]

[a]Data from Olanoff, L.S., Walle, T., Cowart, T.D., Walle, U.K, Oexmann, M.J., and Conradi, E.C.: Food effects on propranolol systemic and oral clearances: Support for a blood flow hypothesis. Clin. Pharmacol. Ther., *40*:408–414, 1986.

[b]Mean ± SEM; N = 6.

[c]Significantly different; P<0.05.

[d]Dose$_{i.v.}$/AUC$_{i.v.}$ (blood).

[e]AUC$_{p.o.}$ (blood) of deuterated propranolol given concurrently with the intravenous dose.

[f]Not significant; P>0.05.

times when the food is digested and absorbed. It is during this period that absorption of drug occurs, while elimination of absorbed drug (half-life of about 3.6 hours) occurs predominantly thereafter. The small change in *AUC* is now explained.

Altered Active Tubular Secretion

Figure 12–7 shows the effect of inhibiting the renal tubular secretion of amoxicillin by probenecid. An increased sojourn (area) of amoxicillin in the body is obvious; it reflects a decrease in clearance. The prolongation of elimination half-life is also due primarily to the reduced clearance; the volume of distribution (CL/k) is changed relatively little, indicating that probenecid does not affect the distribution of amoxycillin. The inhibition of renal excretion of this penicillin by probenecid becomes apparent when this pathway is isolated. Renal clearance, that is, the excretion rate relative to the plasma concentration of amoxicillin, is clearly reduced by probenecid. The substantial renal excretion of amoxicillin explains why a reduced renal clearance has such a pronounced affect on total clearance.

The decrease in renal clearance occurs by inhibition of the tubular secretory mechanism for amoxicillin. The degree of inhibition of this process is masked by the contribution of filtration at the glomerulus. If secretion is completely blocked, renal clearance of this polar antibiotic is expected to have a lower limit of $fu \cdot GFR$, because it is not reabsorbed in the tubule.

Altered Plasma Protein Binding

Conditions in which the binding to plasma proteins is altered are critical to plasma drug concentration monitoring (Chap. 18). Under the assumption that activities, desired and undesired, relate to the unbound concentration, changes in binding directly affect the interpretation of total concentration data. This problem applies to drugs of both low and high extraction. Whether or not the altered binding affects the unbound concentration, and therefore the effect, is therapeutically important. These aspects are now addressed in turn.

Low Extraction Ratio. Changes in the therapeutic window of phenytoin as a function of the serum creatinine concentration, an index of renal function, is shown in Figure 12–8. The higher the creatinine concentration, the lower the

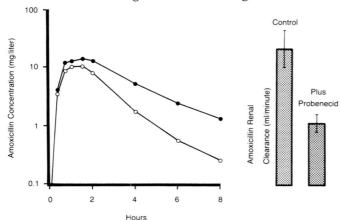

Fig. 12–7. The plasma concentration (on left), and hence the area under the curve, for amoxicillin is increased when 500 milligrams are administered orally in solution to fasting subjects in the absence (O) and presence (●) of probenecid (1 gram, 12 hours and then 1 hour before the antibiotic). The effect is due to probenecid decreasing the renal clearance of amoxicillin (on right), its primary route of elimination. (One mg/liter = 2.7 micromolar.) (Data from Staniforth, D.H., Jackson, D., Clarke, H.L., and Horton, R.: Amoxicillin/clavulanic acid: The effect of probenecid. J. Antimicrob. Chemother., *12*: 273–275, 1983.)

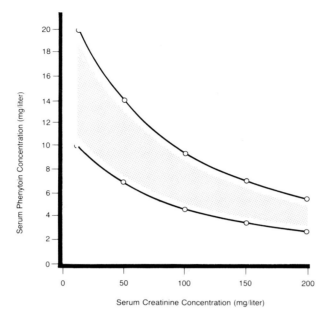

Fig. 12–8. The therapeutic range of phenytoin decreases with the degree of renal function impairment, as measured by serum creatinine, from the usual value of 10 to 20 milligrams/liter. This decrease is a consequence of reduced binding, which is related to the severity of the renal disease. (One mg/liter = 4.0 micromolar.) (Redrawn from Reidenberg, M.M. and Affrime, M.: Influence of disease on binding of drugs to plasma proteins. Ann. N.Y. Acad. Sci., 226:115–126, 1973.)

renal function. The window falls because the fraction unbound, normally about 0.1, increases to about 0.25 to 0.3 in patients with severe renal function impairment.

For example, on the assumption that the unbound concentration required to produce a given response in the presence of renal disease is the same as that in the absence, it follows that

$$fu \cdot C = fu' \cdot C' \qquad\qquad 4$$

where fu' and C' are the unbound fraction and total drug concentration in the presence of the disease, respectively. On rearrangement

$$C' = \frac{fu}{fu'} \cdot C \qquad\qquad 5$$

Concentrations of 10 and 20 milligrams/liter in normal conditions thus become equivalent to 4 and 8 milligrams/liter when fu and fu' are 0.1 and 0.25, respectively.

Phenytoin is a low extraction drug eliminated by hepatic metabolism. Consequently, its elimination is related to its unbound concentration (Chap. 11). Total clearance ($fu \cdot CLu$) increases in renal disease, but there is no requirement for dosing rate adjustment because the unbound clearance, the proportionality constant between rate of input and unbound concentration at steady state, is not affected by the binding change.

High Extraction Ratio. Figure 12–9 shows how clearance, volume of distribution, and half-life of propranolol vary with the fraction unbound in 6 healthy male volunteers. The value of clearance (based on concentration in blood) appears to be independent of protein binding. The volume of distribution (blood) and half-life are both observed to increase with an increase in the fraction unbound in blood. This is the behavior expected for a drug whose elimination is

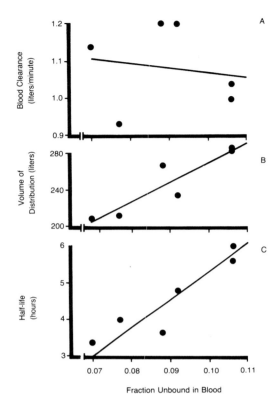

Fig. 12–9. The clearance of propranolol (Graph A), based on its concentration in blood, does not appear to correlate with the fraction unbound in blood of six healthy male volunteers after intravenous administration of 20 milligrams. On the other hand, the volume of distribution (Graph B) and the half-life (Graph C) are observed to increase with an increase in the fraction unbound. This kinetic behavior is anticipated for a drug, such as propranolol, that is highly extracted in the liver. Clearance here is perfusion-limited. Binding to plasma proteins does not influence clearance, but does affect the volume of distribution and, therefore, the half-life. The lines are the best fits by linear regression. (Data from Evans, G.H. and Shand, D.G.: Disposition of propranolol. VI: Independent variation in steady-state circulating drug concentrations and half-life as a result of plasma drug binding in man. Clin. Pharmacol. Ther., 14:494–500, 1973. Reproduced with permission of C.V. Mosby.)

perfusion rate-limited and which has a large volume of distribution. The drug is primarily eliminated by hepatic metabolism, and the metabolic (blood) clearance approaches hepatic blood flow (1.35 liters/minute on average). The increase in the volume of distribution with the fraction unbound is anticipated, as is the correlation of half-life with fraction unbound.

With the increase in fraction unbound and no change in clearance, there must be a corresponding decrease in unbound clearance, since $CL_b = fu_b \cdot CLu$. This means that the unbound concentration under constant-rate intravenous infusion conditions is increased when binding is decreased and the converse; an effect with potentially important therapeutic consequences.

An alternative view of this situation is to remember that when the clearance approaches blood flow in the eliminating organ, the total steady-state concentration is not expected to change with altered plasma binding. An increase in the fraction unbound thereby raises the unbound concentration and the drug's effects. Although there are many drugs with a high hepatic extraction ratio, they are fortunately seldom given chronically by the parenteral route under conditions in which binding is altered.

The availability of a drug with a high extraction ratio is expected to decrease with an increase in fraction unbound, as seen from Equation 15 of Chapter 11, when CLu is much greater than Q/fu. Here $CLu/F = CL_{int}$. The memory aid model of Chapter 11 predicts little or no change in the steady-state unbound concentration or the therapeutic response after oral administration, because CL_{int} is unchanged. Whereas, after intravenous administration, the decrease in CLu

Table 12–5. Anticipated Effects of Alterations in Selected Physiologic Variables on Various Parameters and Observations for a Drug Eliminated Solely by the Liver

Administration	Parameters or Observations	Increased Enzyme Activity[a]	Inhibition of Metabolism	Decreased Blood Flow	Increased Fraction Unbound in Blood
		Low Hepatic Extraction Ratio Drug			
Intravenous	Half-life	↓ [b]	↑	↔	↔
	Area under curve (blood)	↓	↑	↔	↓
Oral	Availability	↔	↔	↔	↔
	Area under curve (blood)	↓	↑	↔	↓
		High Hepatic Extraction Ratio Drug			
Intravenous	Half-life	↔	↔	↑	↑
	Area under curve (blood)	↔	↔	↑	↔
Oral	Availability	↓	↑	↓	↓
	Area under curve (blood)	↓	↑	↔[c]	↓

[a]Enzyme activity is increased by one of several mechanisms, such as enzyme activation, induction, or increased availability of cofactors, if rate-limiting.
[b] ↑ Increased; ↓ decreased; ↔ little or no change.
[c]The decrease in availability is assumed to be equally matched by a decrease in clearance.

is not compensated for by a decrease in availability. A decrease in the intensity of response is then expected with chronic administration when the fraction unbound is increased, and the converse.

The combinations of conditions and scenarios in drug therapy are multitudinous. This chapter has presented approaches and examples toward integrating kinetic principles and physiologic concepts. To complete this integration, Table 12–5 summarizes the effects expected from increased enzyme activity, inhibition of metabolism, decreased blood flow, and increased fraction unbound in blood for a drug eliminated exclusively in the liver. Conditions involving drugs of both low and high extraction ratios are considered. The expectations are similar for a drug eliminated only by the kidneys; however, increased active tubular secretion rather than increased enzyme activity applies. Also, oral availability of a drug highly extracted in the kidneys is unaffected by changes in the physiologic variables considered here.

Study Problems

(Answers to Study Problems are in Appendix G.)

1. List ten examples of physiologic variables that alter pharmacokinetic parameter values.

2. Complete Table 12–6 below by marking: ↑ for increase, ↓ for decrease, and ↔ for little or no change in the empty spaces. The drug is only eliminated in the liver and its volume of distribution is greater than 100 liters.

Table 12–6.

Hepatic Extraction Ratio	Hepatic Blood Flow	Fraction in Blood Unbound	Fraction in Tissue Unbound	Total Clearance[a]	Volume of Distribution[a]	Half-life	Oral Availability
High	↑	↔	↔				
High	↔	↓	↔				
High	↔	↔	↑				
Low	↑	↔	↔				
Low	↔	↔	↑				
Low	↔			↑	↔		

[a]Based on drug concentration in blood.

3. Although recognized for many years, the interaction between allopurinol, used in the treatment of gout, and 6-mercaptopurine, an antineoplastic agent, was not well understood until the kinetics of the interaction was elucidated. The *AUC* values of 6-mercaptopurine before and after pretreatment with allopurinol (100 mg orally three times a day for 2 days) following oral and intravenous administrations of 0.8 millimole of 6-mercaptopurine are given in Table 12–7. Both drugs are mostly eliminated by metabolism in the liver.

Table 12–7. Average Areas under the Plasma 6-Mercaptopurine Concentration-Time Curves (micromoles—minute) Before and After Allopurinol Pretreatment[a]

	Before	After
Oral	142	716
Intravenous	1207	1405

[a]Adapted from data in Zimm, S., Collins, J.M., O'Neill, D., Chabner, B.A., and Poplack, D.G.: Clin. Pharmacol. Ther., *34*:810–817, 1983.

The half-life of 6-mercaptopurine was not significantly changed by allopurinol treatment. For the purpose of this problem use a blood/plasma concentration ratio of 0.6.

(a) Calculate the clearance and availability of 6-mercaptopurine before and after allopurinol.

(b) Provide a logical kinetic explanation for the enhanced efficacy of 6-mercaptopurine in the presence of allopurinol.

4. A drug highly bound to plasma proteins ($fu = 0.01$) has a volume of distribution of 240 liters/70 kilograms. The liver is the only organ of elimination. The hepatic extraction ratio is 0.95 despite the fact that the fraction in blood that is unbound, fu_b, is only 0.005. Use a hepatic blood flow of 81 liters/hour.

(a) Estimate the values of the following parameters for this drug: blood clearance (CL_b), clearance (CL), volumes of distribution based on drug concentrations in plasma water (Vu) and in blood (V_b), and half-life.

(b) In uremic patients the volume of distribution and the fraction unbound in plasma, fu, average 140 liters and 0.03, respectively. Is there any evidence that the uremic state affects the tissue binding? If so, in what direction and by what factor is the tissue binding altered?

(c) When this drug is infused intravenously at the same constant rate to a patient who is and has been receiving another drug, the value of fu_b is now found to be 0.03. Under steady-state conditions for both drugs, predict the ratio of the unbound concentrations of the drug in the presence and absence of the other drug.

Altered Binding to Plasma Proteins

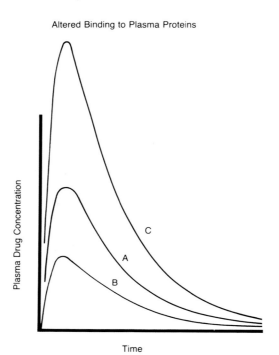

Altered Tissue Binding

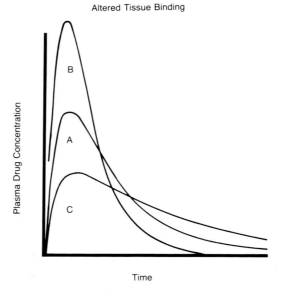

Fig. 12–10.

5. Figure 12–10 shows plasma drug concentration-time profiles following oral administration of two drugs under the following conditions:

   Top Graph. Low extraction ratio. Plasma protein binding is: normal (Case A); halved
   (Case B, twofold increase in *fu*); and doubled (Case C, twofold decrease in *fu*).

   Bottom Graph. Low extraction ratio. Tissue binding is: normal (Case A); halved
   (Case B, twofold increase in *fu*); and doubled (Case C, twofold decrease in *fu*).

   Draw the corresponding time profiles of the unbound concentrations for the three
   situations given for each of the two drugs. Be sure that each graph shows the salient
   features including: relative areas under the curve, peak times, and half-lives. The
   volumes of distribution of both drugs are greater than 100 liters.

6. Ampicillin has the following average pharmacokinetic parameter values in a 70-
   kilogram man:

$$F \text{ (oral)} = 0.6 \qquad\qquad V = 20 \text{ liters}$$
$$CL = 160 \text{ milliliters/minute} \qquad\qquad fe = 0.8$$

   Determine the minimum oral maintenance dose of ampicillin, to be given every 6
   hours, that will keep the urinary drug concentration (in ureters) above 50 milligrams/
   liter. This value is the minimum inhibitory concentration against an antibiotic-resis-
   tant organism believed to be producing the patient's urinary tract infection. Use an
   average urine flow of 1 milliliter/minute. Instantaneous absorption and distribution
   of ampicillin, and steady-state conditions are assumed.

SECTION FOUR

Individualization

13

Variability

Objectives

The reader will be able to:

1. **List major sources of variability in drug response.**

2. **Evaluate whether the variability in drug response is caused by a variability in pharmacokinetics, in pharmacodynamics, or in both, given pharmacokinetic data.**

3. **State why the variability around the mean value and the shape of the frequency distribution histogram of a parameter are as important as the mean itself.**

4. **Explain how variability in hepatic enzyme activity manifests itself in variability in both pharmacokinetic parameters and plateau plasma drug concentrations for drugs of high and low hepatic extraction ratios.**

5. **Suggest an approach to the establishment of a dosage regimen for an individual patient, given patient population pharmacokinetic data.**

Thus far, the assumption has been made that all people are alike. True, as a species, man is reasonably homogeneous, but differences among people do exist including their responsiveness to drugs. Accordingly, there is a frequent need to tailor drug administration to the individual patient. A failure to do so can lead to ineffective therapy in some patients and toxicity in others.

This section of the book is devoted to individual drug therapy. A broad overview of the subject is presented in this chapter. Evidence for and causes of variation in drug response, and approaches to individualized drug therapy are examined. Subsequent chapters deal in much greater detail with genetics (Chap. 14), age (Chap. 15), disease (Chap. 16), interactions between drugs within the body (Chap. 17), and monitoring of plasma concentration of a drug as a guide to individualizing drug therapy (Chap. 18).

Before proceeding, a distinction must be made between the individual and the population. Consider, for example, the results of a study designed to examine the contribution of an acute disease to variability in drug response. Suppose, of thirty patients studied during and after recovery, only two showed a substantial difference in response; in the remainder the difference was insignificant. Viewed as a whole, the disease would not be considered as a significant source of variability, but to the two affected patients it would. Moreover, to avoid toxicity, the dosage regimen of the drug may need to be reduced in these two patients during the disease. The lesson is clear: Average data are useful as a guide; but ultimately, information pertaining to the individual patient is all-important.

EXPRESSIONS OF INDIVIDUAL DIFFERENCES

Evidence for interindividual differences in drug response comes from several sources. Variability in the dosage required to produce a given response was illustrated in Figure 1–4 (Chap. 1), which showed the wide range in the daily dose of warfarin needed to produce a similar degree of anticoagulant control. Variability in the intensity of response to a set dose is illustrated in Figure 13–1, which shows a frequency distribution histogram of the blood glucose-lowering effects of intravenous tolbutamide. As illustrated in Figures 13–2 and 13–3, which show frequency distribution histograms of the plateau plasma concentration of nortriptyline to a defined daily dose of the drug and the plateau plasma concentration of warfarin required to produce the same degree of anticoagulant control, variability exists in both the pharmacokinetics and the pharmacodynamics of a drug. Variability in the pharmacokinetics of a drug was also illustrated by the wide scatter in the plateau plasma concentration of phenytoin seen following various daily doses of this drug (see Fig. 1–5, Chap. 1).

DESCRIBING VARIABILITY

Knowing how a particular parameter varies within the patient population is important in therapy. To illustrate this statement consider the frequency distributions in clearance of the three hypothetical drugs shown in Figure 13–4. The mean, or central tendency, for all three drugs is the same, but the variability about the mean is very different. For Drugs A and B, the distribution is unimodal and normal; here the mean represents the typical value of clearance expected

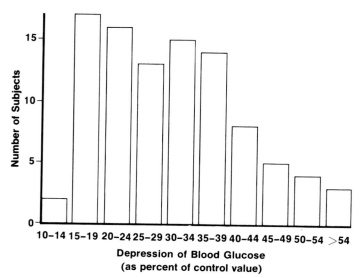

Fig. 13–1. The depression of blood glucose at 30 minutes, after a test dose of 1 gram tolbutamide intravenously in 97 subjects, varies widely. (Adapted from the data of Swerdloff, R.S., Pozefsky, T., Tobin, J.D., and Andres, R.: Influence of age on the intravenous tolbutamide response test. Diabetes, 16:161–170, 1967. With permission from the American Diabetes Association, Inc.)

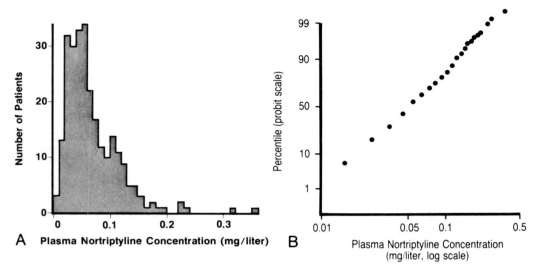

Fig. 13-2. A, The plateau plasma concentration of nortriptyline varies widely in 263 patients receiving a regimen of 25 milligrams nortriptyline orally three times daily. B, The concentrations are log-normal distributed, as seen from the straight line, when the percentiles on probit scale are plotted against the logarithm of the concentration. (One mg/liter = 3.8 micromolar.) (Redrawn and calculated from Sjoqvist, F., Borga, O., and Orme, M.L.E.: Fundamentals of clinical pharmacology. In: Drug Treatment. Edited by G.S. Avery. Churchill Livingstone, Edinburgh, 1976, pp. 1–42.)

in the population. As the variability about the mean is much greater for Drug B than for Drug A, one has much less confidence that the mean value of Drug B applies to an individual patient. For Drug C, the distribution in clearance is bimodal, signifying that there are two major groups within the population: those with a high clearance and those with a low clearance. Obviously, in this case, the mean is one of the most unlikely values to be found in this population.

Generally distributions of pharmacokinetic parameters are unimodal rather than polymodal, and they are often skewed rather than normal, as seen, for example, in the frequency distribution of plateau plasma concentrations of nor-triptyline (Fig. 13–2A). A more symmetrical distribution is often obtained with the logarithm of the parameter; such distributions are said to be log-normal. A common method of examining for log-normal distribution is to plot the cumu-

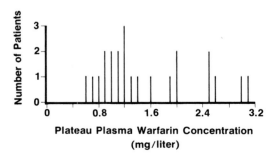

Fig. 13–3. The plateau plasma concentration of war-farin (expressed to the nearest 0.1 mg/liter), required to produce the same degree of anticoagulant control in 23 patients, varies widely. (One mg/liter = 3.3 mi-cromolar.) (Redrawn from Breckenridge, A. and Orme, M.L.E.: Measurement of plasma warfarin concentrations in clinical practice. In: Biological Effect of Drugs in Relation to Their Plasma Concentrations. Edited by D.S. Davies and B.N.C. Prichard. Macmillan, London and Basingstoke, 1973, pp. 145–154.)

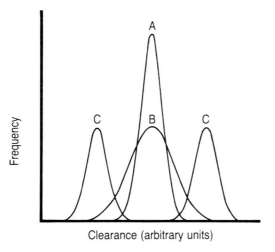

Fig. 13–4. As the frequency distributions for the clearance of three hypothetical drugs (A, B, C) show, it is as important to define the variability around the mean value and the shape of the frequency distribution as it is to define the mean value itself.

lative frequency, or percentile, on a probit scale against the logarithm of the variable. The distribution is log-normal if all the points lie on a straight line. As can be seen in Figure 13–2B, this is the case for the plateau plasma concentration of nortriptyline. In such cases the median, or value above and below which there are equal numbers, differs from the mean. For nortriptyline, examination of Figure 13–2B indicates that the median concentration is 0.05 milligram/liter, which is less than the average value of 0.069 milligram/liter.

When describing variability a distinction should be made between variation within an individual and variation among individuals. Substantial interindividual variability in pharmacokinetics and pharmacodynamics exists for most drugs and is reflected for many by the variety of dose strengths available. Because intraindividual variability is generally much smaller than interindividual variability, once well-established, there is often little need to subsequently readjust an individual's dosage regimen. Clearly if intraindividual variability were large and unpredictable, trying to titrate dosage for an individual would be an almost impossible task.

WHY PEOPLE DIFFER

The reasons why people differ in their responsiveness to drugs are manifold and include, in general order of importance, genetics, disease, age, pharmaceutical formulation and route of administration of drug, drugs given concomitantly, and a variety of environmental factors. Although inheritance accounts for a substantial part of the differences in response between individuals, this source of variability is largely unpredictable.

Disease can be an added source of variation in drug response. Usual dosage regimens may need to be modified substantially in patients with renal function impairment, hepatic disorders, congestive cardiac failure, thyroid disorders, gastrointestinal disorders, and other diseases. The modification in the dosage may apply to the drug used to treat the specific disease, but may apply equally well to other drugs the patient receives. For example, to prevent excessive accumulation and so reduce the risk of toxicity, the dosage of the antibiotic, gentamicin, used to treat a pleural infection of a patient, must be reduced if the patient also has compromised renal function. Similarly, hyperthyroidic patients require higher doses of digoxin, a drug used to improve cardiac efficiency. Moreover, a modification in dosage may arise not only from the direct impairment of a diseased organ, but also from secondary events that accompany the disease. Drug metabolism, for example, may be modified in patients with renal disease; plasma and tissue binding of drugs may be altered in patients with uremia and with hepatic disorders.

Table 13–1 lists examples of other factors known to contribute to variability in drug response. Perhaps the most important factor is noncompliance. Noncompliance includes the taking of the drug at the wrong time, the omission or supplementation of the prescribed dose, and the stopping of therapy, either because the patient begins to feel better or because of the development of side-effects that the patient considers unacceptable. Whatever the reason, these problems lie in the area of patient counselling and education, backed occasionally by plasma concentration data as an objective measure of noncompliance.

Pharmaceutical formulation and the process used to manufacture the product can be important as both can affect the rate of release, and hence entry, of drug into the body (Chap. 9). A well-designed formulation diminishes the degree of variability in the release characteristics of a drug *in vivo*. Good manufacturing practice, with careful control of the process variables, ensures the manufacture of a reliable product. Drugs are given enterally, topically, parenterally, and by inhalation. The route of administration can not only affect the drug concentration locally and systemically, but can also alter the systemic concentration of metabolite compared with that of drug (Chap. 21). All these factors can profoundly affect the response to a given dose or regimen of drug.

Table 13–1. Examples of Certain Factors Known to Contribute to Variability in Drug Response

Factors	Observations and Remarks
Noncompliance	A major problem in clinical practice; solution lies in patient education.
Pharmaceutical formulation	Formulation and manufacturing process can affect both rate and extent of drug absorption.
Route of administration	Patient response can vary on changing the route of administration. Not only pharmacokinetics of drug, but also metabolite concentrations can change.
Age	Pharmacokinetics and pharmacodynamics of many drugs vary with age.
Drugs	Pharmacokinetics and pharmacodynamics of many drugs vary with concurrent drug therapy.
Food	Rate and occasionally extent of absorption are affected by eating. Effects depend on composition of food. Severe protein restriction may reduce the rate of drug metabolism.
Pollutants	Drug effects appear to be lessened in smokers and workers occupationally exposed to pesticides; enhanced drug metabolism is hypothesized.
Time of day and season	Diurnal variations are seen in pharmacokinetics and in drug response. These effects have been sufficiently important to lead to the development of a new subject, chronopharmacology.
Location	Dose requirements of some drugs differ between patients living in town and in the country.
Gender	Intramuscular absorption of some drugs is slower in females than in males; this observation is explained by differences in blood flow.

Age and concomitantly administered drugs are important because they are sources of variability that can be accounted for. Gender-linked differences in hormonal balance, body composition, and activity of certain enzymes manifest themselves in differences in both pharmacokinetics and responsiveness; but the effect of gender tends to be generally small.

Food, particularly fat, slows gastric emptying and so decreases the rate of drug absorption. Oral drug availability is not usually affected by food, but there are many exceptions to this statement. Food is a complex mixture of chemicals, each potentially capable of interacting with drugs. Recall from Chapter 9, for example, that the availability of tetracycline is reduced when taken with milk, because of the formation of an insoluble complex with calcium. Recall also that a slowing of gastric emptying may increase the oral availability of a sparingly soluble drug, such as griseofulvin, and of some of the actively transported water-soluble vitamins. Diet may also affect drug metabolism. Enzyme synthesis is ultimately dependent on protein intake. When protein intake is severely reduced for prolonged periods, particularly because of an imbalanced diet, drug metabolism may be impaired. Conversely, a high protein intake may cause enzyme induction.

Chronopharmacology is the study of the influence of time on drug response. Many endogenous substances, for example hormones, are known to undergo cyclic changes in concentration in plasma and tissue with time. The amplitude of the change in concentration varies among the substances. The period of the cycle is often diurnal, approximately 24 hours, although there may be both shorter and longer cycles upon which the daily one is superimposed. The menstrual cycle and seasonal variations in the concentrations of some endogenous substances are examples of cycles with a long period. Drug responses may therefore change with the time of day, with the day of the month, or with the season of the year.

Cigarette smoking tends to reduce the clinical and toxic effects of some drugs, including chlordiazepoxide, chlorpromazine, diazepam, propoxyphene, and theophylline. The drugs affected are extensively metabolized by hepatic oxidation, and induction of the drug-metabolizing enzymes appears likely. Patients living in rural areas tend to be more sensitive to the analgesic effects of pentazocine than those living in towns. Enzyme induction may explain this effect of location. Many compounds that are environmental pollutants and that exist in higher concentrations in the city than in the country can stimulate the synthesis of hepatic metabolic enzymes.

In practice, all these factors contribute to observed variability, and great care must be taken in experimental design to ensure that an appropriate conclusion is reached when trying to assign variability to a given factor. Consider, for example, the data displayed in Figure 13–5, which show the half-lives of phenylbutazone in normal subjects and in patients with hepatic disease (primarily cirrhosis). Initially, no difference was revealed between the two groups, except for a greater variability in the half-life among the patients with hepatic disease (Fig. 13–5A). When, however, both groups were further subdivided on the basis of whether they received other drugs, a clearer picture emerged (Fig. 13–5B). Of those receiving no other drugs, patients with hepatic disease handled phenylbutazone more slowly than did normal subjects. Evidently some of the drugs received can hasten phenylbutazone elimination.

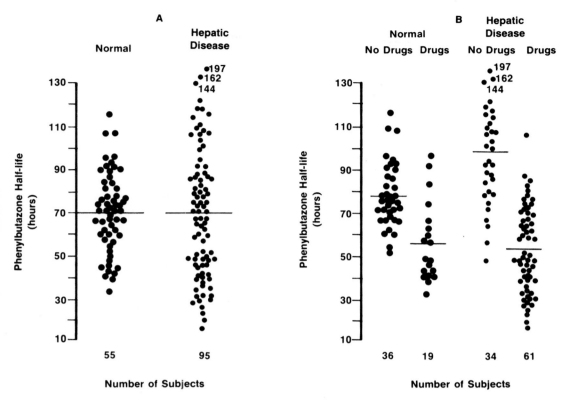

Fig. 13–5. A, No difference is seen between the average half-life of phenylbutazone (horizontal line) in normal subjects (●) and that in patients with hepatic disease (●). B, After separating drug takers from nondrug takers, the prolonged elimination of phenylbutazone in patients with hepatic disease becomes evident. (Redrawn from Levi, A.J., Sherlock, S., and Walker, D.: Phenylbutazone and isoniazid metabolism in patients with liver disease in relation to previous drug therapy. Lancet, 1:1275–1279, 1968.)

Genetic factors can also obscure the picture. Many metabolic pathways are under genetic control and when, as with phenylbutazone, metabolism is a major route of elimination, interindividual variability in the pharmacokinetics of a drug in the normal population can be wide. With such wide interindividual variability, a change in the pharmacokinetics of a drug associated, for example, with a disease is difficult to detect. This is particularly so when studying the effect of chronic disease on pharmacokinetics; assessment is usually made by comparing average drug handling in the patient population with the disease to that in an otherwise comparable population without the disease. Had, for example, the sample size in the phenylbutazone study been smaller and the effect of the disease less consistent, a difference between normal subjects and cirrhotic patients may not have been detected.

Pharmacokinetics of a drug may also change with age (Chap. 15), and care should be taken in population studies to age match the control group. In reversible conditions, such as acute viral hepatitis, genetic and other factors may be removed from consideration with a longitudinal study in which the kinetics of a drug is studied in the individual during and after the condition. Since each person now acts as his or her own control, the influence of the condition can be assessed on an individual basis. It is also important to divide total clearance into hepatic and renal clearances. For example, if a drug is primarily renally excreted, a depressed formation of an important metabolite in hepatic disease may go undetected by measuring only the total clearance of the drug. Similarly, a lack of change in total clearance does not exclude the possibility of compensating changes in renal and hepatic clearances.

KINETIC MANIFESTATIONS

There is considerable variability in enzymatic activity and, to a lesser extent, in plasma and tissue binding even among healthy individuals. How such variability manifests itself, in pharmacokinetic parameters and in such measurements as plateau plasma concentration, depends on the extraction ratio of the drug and the route of administration. For example, the large interindividual variability in the half-life of theophylline (Fig. 13–6) can be explained primarily by variations in hepatic enzyme activity, probably associated with variations in the amounts of the enzymes responsible for the metabolism of this compound. This conclusion is based on theophylline being predominantly metabolized in the liver, having a low hepatic extraction ratio, and being only moderately bound to plasma and tissue components. In contrast, such a high degree of variability in enzymatic activity is expected to be masked in the clearance of a drug having a high hepatic extraction ratio, because clearance tends to be perfusion rate-

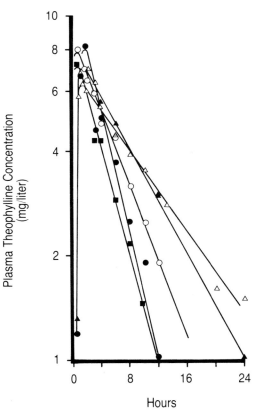

Fig. 13–6. Five healthy subjects each received 350 milligrams theophylline orally, in solution as an elixir. Large differences in *AUC* are seen, but in contrast to propranolol (Fig. 13–7), the peak concentrations are almost identical. These observations are as expected for theophylline, a drug of low hepatic extraction that is extensively metabolized in the liver. Variability in hepatic enzyme activity is manifested primarily in variability in clearance, and hence half-life; the weight corrected volume of distribution of theophylline is relatively constant. The oral availability is close to 100 percent in all subjects, and because absorption occurred much faster than elimination, the peak concentrations are similar. Each symbol refers to a different subject. (Data provided by S. Toon, personal observations.)

limited and hepatic blood flow is relatively constant among healthy individuals. Moreover, unless plasma and tissue binding are highly variable, the volume of distribution, and hence the disposition kinetics, of such a drug will be much the same for all healthy individuals. This is the case for propranolol (Fig. 13–7), a drug of high hepatic clearance.

As described in Chapter 11, when considering induction and inhibition, changes in hepatic enzyme activity result in variations in availability for a drug with a high hepatic extraction ratio. Accordingly, with subsequent disposition being controlled by hepatic perfusion, a series of similarly shaped plasma drug concentration-time profiles, but reaching different peak concentrations, should be seen among individuals with varying enzyme activity receiving the same oral dose of drug. This is indeed seen with propranolol (Fig. 13–7). In contrast, for a drug with a low hepatic extraction ratio, such as theophylline, variation in enzymatic activity is reflected by variation in clearance (and half-life) rather than in availability (and maximum plasma concentration), which is always high (Fig. 13–6).

The impact of variability in availability, because of a high first-pass effect, depends on the intended use of the drug. It may result in subjects needing different single oral doses of drug to produce the same effect, as might be the case if the drug is to be used as a sedative hypnotic. However, if the drug is

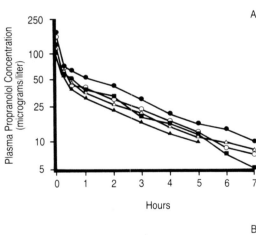

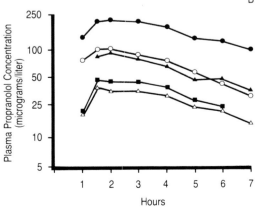

Fig. 13–7. Five healthy subjects each received propranolol intravenously (10 mg over 10 minutes) and orally (80 mg) on separate occasions. The plasma concentration-time profiles were very similar following intravenous administration (A), but showed large differences, particularly in peak concentration and *AUC*, following oral administration (B). Such differences in variability with the two routes of administration are expected for propranolol, a drug of high hepatic extraction. Variability in hepatic enzyme activity among the group is manifested primarily in variability in oral availability (16–60 percent), rather than in differences in clearance, which is perfusion rate-limited, and hence half-life. (One mg/liter = 3.9 micromolar.) (Redrawn from Shand, D.G., Nuckolls, E.M., and Oates, J.A.: Plasma propranolol levels in adults, with observations in four children. Clin. Pharmacol. Ther., *11*: 112–120, 1970. Reproduced with permission of C.V. Mosby.)

intended for chronic use, the degree of variability in the average plateau concentration should not be inherently different from that which exists for a drug of low hepatic clearance and having the same degree of variability in enzymatic activity (Fig. 13–8). This statement is based on the following reasoning. At plateau, the average concentration ($C_{ss,av}$) is given by

$$C_{ss,av} = \frac{F \cdot Dose}{CL \cdot \tau} \qquad\qquad 1$$

where τ is the dosing interval. For a drug of high hepatic clearance, the variability in $C_{ss,av}$ reflects variability in enzyme activity through F; whereas, for a drug of low hepatic clearance, the variability in $C_{ss,av}$ reflects variability in enzyme activity through CL (with $F \simeq 1$). In both cases the dosing rate (Dose/τ) would need to be adjusted by the same degree to maintain a common $C_{ss,av}$ within subjects. This is achieved by simply adjusting the dose for the high-clearance drug (as half-life is relatively constant) and perhaps by a mixture of adjusting the dose and the dosing interval (given that half-life varies) for the low-clearance drug. Of major importance is the underlying variation in enzyme activity, which differs from one enzyme system to another. Obviously, to minimize variation in pharmacokinetics, molecules should be selected that, if metabolized, are substrates of enzyme systems that show the least variability among subjects. Unfortunately, current information is insufficient to make this selection.

It follows from the foregoing that there is no inherent reason to believe that a set variation in enzyme activity (caused by a variation in concentration of enzymes, inhibitors, or inducers) should cause a greater *intra*individual variation in pharmacokinetic parameters, or in $C_{ss,av}$, for a drug of high hepatic extraction than for one of low hepatic extraction. Certainly there is no greater *intra*individual variation in the plasma concentration of propranolol than is seen with theophylline.

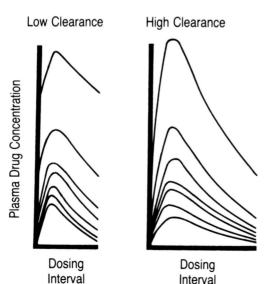

Low Clearance   High Clearance

Plasma Drug Concentration

Dosing Interval   Dosing Interval

Fig. 13–8. Expected plasma drug concentration-time profiles during a dosing interval at steady state and following chronic oral administration of a drug; changes in hepatic enzyme activity for a drug of low extraction ratio (left) and high extraction ratio (right). In this simulation both drugs are substrates for the same enzyme, the concentration (and intrinsic clearance) of which varies ninefold. The result is a corresponding ninefold variation in the average concentration. Prediction is based on the well-stirred model of hepatic elimination.

DOSE STRENGTHS

Products are frequently marketed as unit doses of defined strength, such as 50 or 100 milligrams. The number of dose strengths required depends on various factors, including the therapeutic index of the drug and the degree of interindividual variability in pharmacokinetics and pharmacodynamics. Obviously, if the therapeutic index is sufficiently wide, all patients can receive the same dose strength almost irrespective of any differences in pharmacokinetics among the patient population. A narrow therapeutic index necessitates the manufacture of several dose strengths, however. Although, in practice, the final number of strengths chosen depends on many practical issues, a rough estimate of the numbers can be calculated in the following manner for drugs intended for chronic maintenance therapy.

Assume that the maximum and minimum clearance values that encompass 95 percent of the patient population, designated CL_{max} and CL_{min}, respectively, differ by a factor of six. That is, $CL_{max} = 6 \cdot CL_{min}$. It would then follow from the familiar relationship

$$\frac{F \cdot \text{Dose}}{\tau} = CL \cdot C_{ss,av} \qquad\qquad 2$$

that the range of dosing rates needed would be six-fold if the object was to obtain the same $C_{av,ss}$ in all patients. In practice, the therapeutic index is sufficiently wide to allow some tolerance, and so let us suppose that an average plateau concentration within 20 percent of the optimal value is acceptable. Accordingly, the highest dosing rate that could be given to a patient with a clearance value of CL_{min} is one that produces an average plateau concentration that is 1.2 times the optimal population value; the lowest dosing rate that could be given to a patient with a clearance value of CL_{max} is one that produces an average plateau concentration that is 0.8 times the optimal value. It then follows that the range of associated dosing rates (and hence amounts, if the dosing interval is kept constant) is fourfold. Now, usually, adjacent dose strengths differ by a factor of two. Therefore, in the current example, if the smallest dose strength is 50 milligrams, it would be reasonable to market three dose strengths, 50-milligram, 100-milligram, and 200-milligram products, which would suffice for 95 percent of the population. Of the outstanding 5 percent, those with a particularly high clearance value may be accommodated with a larger-than-usual maintenance dose, comprising a combination of the available unit dose strengths, or they may receive an available dose strength more frequently. Those with a particularly low clearance value may be accommodated by taking the lowest available dose strength less frequently than usual, because the half-life in this group is likely to be the longest in the population.

ACCOUNTING FOR VARIABILITY

It remains to be seen how information on variability can be used to devise an optimal dosage regimen of a drug for the treatment of a disease in an individual patient. Obviously, the desired objective would be most efficiently achieved if the individual's dosage requirements could be calculated *prior to administering the drug*. While this ideal cannot be totally met in practice, some success may be achieved by adopting the following type of approach, which assumes that all patients require the same (unbound) plasma concentration range.

The approach is to move from the population pharmacokinetic parameter estimates to the individual patient's values. This may be accomplished by first assessing the variability of each parameter within the patient population and then determining how much of the variability can be accounted for in terms of characteristics, such as weight, age, renal function, and so forth, that are known or can be measured readily. The greater the variability that can be accounted for, the greater the likelihood of achieving the objective.

The variability in the various pharmacokinetic parameters within the patient population differs widely among drugs, as shown in Table 13–2 for a number of representative drugs. For some drugs, such as digoxin and propranolol, there is substantial variability in absorption, but for different reasons. With digoxin the variability is caused primarily by differences in pharmaceutical formulation, but with propranolol it is caused by differences in the extent of first-pass loss, as mentioned previously (Fig. 13–7). For other drugs, such as theophylline, almost all the variability in their pharmacokinetic parameters resides in the substantial variability in clearance. With others, phenytoin and propranolol included, significant variability exists in all pharmacokinetic parameters, and finally, for some considerable variability exists in either the degree of plasma binding or the time taken for equilibration of drug between plasma and the active site.

The next step is to try to accommodate as much of the variability as possible in terms of measurable characteristics. If the characteristic is discrete, this can be achieved by partitioning the population into subpopulations. For example, as illustrated in Figure 13–9, if the discrete characteristics are hepatic disease and smoking, then the population would be divided into four categories: those that smoked and had no hepatic disease; those that smoked and had hepatic disease; those that had hepatic disease but did not smoke; and those that neither

Table 13–2. Degree of Variability in the Absorption, Disposition, and Specific Distribution of Representative Drugs Within the Patient Population[a]

| Drug | Absorption–Disposition | | | Specific Distribution | |
	F	V	CL	Plasma Protein Binding	Delayed Equilibrium with Active Site
Digitoxin	−	+	+	+	+ +
Digoxin	+ +	+	+ +	−	+ +
Lidocaine	NA	+	+ +	−	−
Lithium	−	−	+	−	+ +
Phenobarbital	−	−	+	−	−
Phenytoin	+	+ +	+ +	+ +	−
Procainamide	+	+	+ +	−	−
Propranolol	+ +	+	+	+ +	−
Quinidine	+	+	+	+	−
Salicylic Acid	−	+	+ +	+ +	−
Theophylline	−	−	+ +	−	−

[a]Symbols: − = little variability; + = moderate variability; + + = substantial variability; NA = not applicable.
Modified from Sheiner, L.B. and Tozer, T.N.: Clinical Pharmacokinetics: The use of plasma concentrations of drugs. *In:* Clinical Pharmacology. Edited by K.L. Melmon and H.F. Morrelli. 2nd Ed., Macmillan Publishing Co., New York, 1978, pp. 71–109.

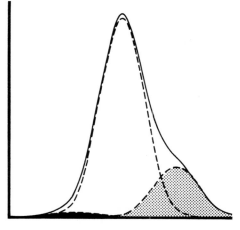

Frequency

Clearance (arbitrary scale)

Fig. 13–9. The frequency distribution of a parameter within the total patient population (——) is a function of the frequency distribution of the parameter within the various subpopulations that comprise the population and the relative sizes of each of these subpopulations. In this simulation the variables are smoking and hepatic disease, and the subpopulations are: (----)–those who neither have hepatic disease nor smoke (78.4 percent), the majority; (shaded gray)–those who smoke but have no hepatic disease (19.6 percent); (shaded black)–those who have hepatic disease but do not smoke (1.6 percent); and those that both smoke and have hepatic disease. The size of the last subpopulation is too small (0.4 percent) to be seen in this figure. The average values for clearance in the four subpopulations were set at 1, 1.5, 0.5, and 0.75 units, respectively, assuming that smoking increases clearance by induction and that clearance is reduced in hepatic disease.

had hepatic disease nor smoked. For each subpopulation, the pharmacokinetic parameter is characterized by its mean and associated variability. And, it is the relative size of each subpopulation that determines the shape of the overall frequency distribution histogram of a pharmacokinetic parameter for the entire population. If, on the other hand, the measurable characteristic is continuous, such as age, weight, or degree of renal function, it may be possible to find a functional relationship with one or more pharmacokinetic parameters, as seen, for example, between the renal clearance of the cephalosporin, ceftazidime (and many other drugs), and creatinine clearance, a graded measure of renal function (Fig. 13–10).

To envisage how the entire strategy would work, consider the data in Figure 13–11 for a drug, partly metabolized in the liver and partly excreted unchanged, whose population pharmacokinetics are availability, 0.82; volume of distribution, 10.3 liters; renal clearance, 6.7 liters/hour; and metabolic clearance, 16.2 liters/

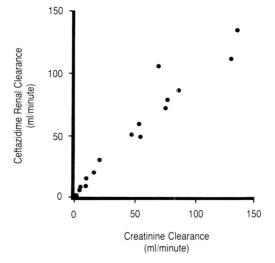

Ceftazidime Renal Clearance (ml/minute)

Creatinine Clearance (ml/minute)

Fig. 13–10. The renal clearance of the cephalosporin, ceftazidime, varies in direct proportion to creatinine clearance in a group of 19 patients with varying degrees of renal function. (Drawn from the data of van Dalen, R., Vree, T.B., Baars, A.M., and Termond, E.: Dosage adjustment for ceftazidime in patients with impaired renal function. Europ. J. Clin. Pharmacol., 30:597–605, 1986.)

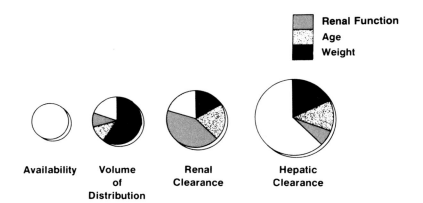

Fig. 13–11. Schematic representation of variability in various pharmacokinetic parameters within a population. The size of each tablet is related to the degree of variability in the parameter. The portion of the tablet labeled weight, age, and renal function reflects the fraction of the variability in a parameter that is accounted for by each of these factors.

hour. Depicted are four tablets, representing availability, volume of distribution, renal, and metabolic clearances. The size of each tablet is a measure of the variability of that parameter within the patient population. For this drug, availability is the least variable and hepatic clearance is the most variable parameter. Stated differently, the greatest confidence exists in assuming that the availability of the drug in the patient is the population value; the least confidence exists in assuming that the hepatic clearance in the patient is the corresponding population value. Moreover, since the population value for hepatic clearance is much greater than that for renal clearance, the variability in the value of the total clearance within the population is also high.

It should also be noted that, not unexpectedly, weight accounts for most of the variability in volume of distribution and for some of the variability in renal and hepatic clearances. Age, separated from its influence on body weight, accounts for some of the variability in renal and hepatic clearances and, to a much lesser extent, for some of the variability in the volume of distribution. Renal function also accounts for much of the variability in renal clearance. Indeed, together with age and weight, renal function helps explain almost all the variability in this parameter. Surprisingly perhaps, renal function helps to explain some of the variability in metabolic clearance and volume of distribution, but drug distribution and metabolism can be altered in patients with renal function impairment (see Chap. 16). None of the variability in availability is accounted for but, as mentioned, this variability is small and is acceptable.

Finally, the inability to account for most of the variability in metabolic clearance should be noted. None of the characteristics included, or indeed any other known characteristic, could adequately account for the influence of genetics, disease, and other drugs on this parameter.

Returning to the individual patient, correcting the population pharmacokinetics for the patient's weight, age, and renal function should give reasonable individual estimates of F, V, and CL_R, but poor estimates of CL_H and hence total clearance. Since the ratio F/V strongly influences the peak plasma drug concentration after a single dose, assuming absorption is rapid relative to elimination, reasonable confidence can be expected in estimating the patient's loading dose, if required. However, since the ratio F/CL controls the average plateau drug concentration, less confidence can be expected in estimating the patient's maintenance dose requirements. If the therapeutic index of the drug is sufficiently narrow, there may be a case for monitoring the plasma drug concentration and adjusting the maintenance dosing rate through feedback, as will be described in Chapter 18 (Monitoring). Nonetheless, the estimate of the maintenance dose based on the information provided in Figure 13–11 should be better than using the population values. Clearly, if the drug had just been excreted unchanged, the probability of being able to estimate the correct dosage regimen for the patient would have been much higher.

Study Problems

(Answers to Study Problems are in Appendix G.)

1. (a) List three major sources of variability in response to drugs.

   (b) What pharmacokinetic parameters vary the most in the patient population for digoxin, phenytoin, and theophylline.

2. Discuss briefly why the mean pharmacokinetic parameters alone are not sufficient to characterize how a drug is handled in the patient population.

3. Suggest which pharmacokinetic parameter is most likely to explain the variation in the plateau concentration of nortriptyline shown in Figure 13–2. The drug is lipophilic, stable in the gastrointestinal tract, and little is excreted unchanged.

4. Explain the following observation: By coincidence, the weight, age, and renal function of the patient, discussed under the section, "Accounting for Variability," corresponded to the patient population values. Yet, when the pharmacokinetics of the drug was studied in the patient, the values of F, 0.42, and V, 22 liters, were considerably different (outside the 99 percent confidence intervals) from the population values of F, 0.82, and V, 10.3 liters.

5. In a group of healthy subjects the average pharmacokinetic parameters of the β-adrenergic blocking agent, alprenolol, which is eliminated almost exclusively by hepatic metabolism, were found to be: volume of distribution, 230 liters; clearance, 1.05 liters/minute; and half-life, 2.5 hours. After intravenous administration, values of these parameters differed little within this group; yet, when the drug was ingested orally, both the peak plasma concentration and the AUC were observed to vary over a fivefold range. Suggest why the variability in the observed plasma concentration-time curve is much greater after oral than after intravenous administration.

6. The following data (Table 13–3) were obtained in a study of the pharmacokinetic variability of a renally eliminated drug, $fe = 0.98$. The drug was intravenously infused in five subjects at a constant rate of 20 milligrams/hour for 48 hours. The value of the fraction unbound was found to be independent of drug concentration, but did vary among the subjects.

Table 13–3.

Subject	1	2	3	4	5
Steady-state plasma concentration (mg/liter)	5.0	3.2	5.9	3.0	4.5
Postinfusion Half-life (hours)	14.4	5.9	4.7	9.9	8.2
Fraction unbound	0.1	0.15	0.09	0.16	0.11

(a) Analyze the data to identify the most and the least variable (use the *range/mean value* as your index of variability) of the following parameters: Clearance based on unbound drug (CLu), fraction unbound in plasma (fu), and fraction unbound in tissue (fu_T). Assume V_{TW} to be 39 liters.

(b) Discuss briefly the therapeutic implications of these data with regard to the rate of attainment and maintenance of a "therapeutic" concentration in the various subjects.

14

Genetics

Objectives

The reader will be able to:

1. **Give examples of inherited variability in pharmacokinetics and pharmacodynamics.**

2. **Define the terms: pharmacogenetics, polymorphism, idiosyncrasy, phenotype, allele, homozygous, and heterozygous.**

3. **Demonstrate how population studies and studies in twins can be used to indicate the existence of genetic polymorphism.**

4. **State under what circumstances phenotype status is of therapeutic value.**

Inheritance accounts for a large part of the differences among individuals, including much of the variation in the response to an administered drug. *Pharmacogenetics* is the study of hereditary variations in drug response.

When a distinguishable difference in a given characteristic exists and is under genetic control, it is called genetic polymorphism. The mode of inheritance is either monogenic or polygenic depending on whether it is transmitted by a gene at a single locus or by genes at multiple loci on the chromosomes. Table 14–1 lists genetic conditions that affect the pharmacokinetics and the pharmacodynamics of some drugs. Many of these conditions are probably transmitted monogenically, and some are rare events. Indeed, monogenically controlled conditions are often detected as an abnormal drug response, that is, a *drug idiosyncrasy*. They may also be detected in population studies by a polymodal frequency distribution of the characteristic or some measure of it. Polygenically controlled variations give rise to a unimodal frequency distribution and are usually detected in studies of twins.

An *allele* is one of two or more different genes containing specific inheritable characteristics that occupy corresponding positions (loci) on paired chromosomes. An allele is dominant if it expresses itself and recessive if it does not. An individual possessing a pair of identical alleles, either dominant or recessive, is *homozygous* for the gene. A union of a dominant gene with its recessive allele produces a *heterozygous* individual for that characteristic. A *phenotype* is a characteristic expressive of an individual. Both homozygous individuals with dominant alleles and heterozygous individuals may show the same phenotype, and

Table 14–1. Some Genetically Determined Drug Responses[a]

Inherited Variation in Pharmacokinetics

Condition	Response	Abnormal Enzyme and Location	Frequency	Drugs That Produce the Response
Slow and fast acetylation	Slow acetylators may show toxicity	N-Acetyltransferase in liver	40 percent of USA population are fast acetylators; much higher percentage among Orientals and Eskimos	Isoniazid, procainamide, hydralazine, sulfasalazine, phenelzine; dapsone, aminoglutethimide, and many sulfonamides
Poor and extensive hydroxylation of debrisoquine	Poor metabolizers may show toxicity	Deficiency of one (or more) hepatic P-450 cytochrome(s)	6–10 percent of Caucasians have deficiency; much lower percentage among Arabs, and much higher percentage among Orientals	Many drugs are found to cosegregate with debrisoquine, including nortriptyline, metoprolol, mephenytoin, phenformin, dextromethorphan, sparteine, and perhexiline
Slow succinylcholine hydrolysis	Prolonged apnea	Cholinesterase in plasma	Several abnormal genes; most common disorder occurs 1 in 2500	Succinylcholine

Inherited Variation in Pharmacodynamics

Condition	Response	Abnormal Enzyme and Location	Frequency	Drugs That Produce the Response
Warfarin resistance	Resistance to anticoagulation	Altered receptor or enzyme in liver with increased affinity for vitamin K	2 large pedigrees	Warfarin
Favism or drug-induced hemolytic anemia	Hemolysis in response to certain drugs	Glucose-6-phosphate dehydrogenase (G6PD) deficiency	Approximately 100 million affected in world; occurs in high frequency where malaria is endemic; 80 biochemically distinct mutations	Variety of drugs, e.g., acetanilide, primaquine, nitrofurantoin, and chloramphenicol
Phenylthiourea taste insensitivity	Inability to taste certain drugs	Unknown	Approximately 30 percent of Caucasians	Drugs containing N-C-S group, e.g., phenylthiourea, methyl and propylthiouracil
Glaucoma	Abnormal response of intraocular pressure to steroid eye drops	Unknown	Approximately 5 percent of USA population	Corticosteroids
Malignant hyperthermia	Uncontrolled rise in body temperature with muscular rigidity	Unknown	Approximately 1 in 20,000 anesthetized patients	Various anesthetics, especially halothane
Methemoglobin reductase deficiency	Methemoglobinemia	Methemoglobin reductase deficiency	Approximately 1 in 100 are heterozygous carriers	Same drugs as listed above for G6PD deficiency

[a]Adapted, with expansion, from Vesell, E.S. TRIANGLE, Sandoz Journal of Medical Science, 14:125, 1975.

homozygous individuals with recessive alleles may show another. More than one inheritable characteristic may be present on the same pair of alleles. For example, the genes for blood types A, B, and O are in the same position on alleles.

INHERITED VARIATION IN PHARMACOKINETICS

Isoniazid

Individuals vary widely in their elimination kinetics of the antitubercular drug, isoniazid. The bimodality of the frequency distribution histogram of the 6-hour plasma isoniazid concentration following a single oral dose (Fig. 14–1) was taken as evidence of polymorphism under monogenic control. Although subsequent evidence confirmed that polymorphic isoniazid elimination exists, the use of a single time-point measurement could have been misleading. One does not know, a priori, whether a low concentration reflects poor availability, slow absorption, with perhaps the concentration still rising, or rapid elimination, with the concentration falling. Moreover, if the measurements had been taken at 2 hours, when the concentration primarily reflects absorption rather than elimination, one might have obtained a unimodal frequency distribution and excluded monogenic control. Isoniazid is primarily acetylated in the liver to N-acetylisoniazid, a precursor of a hepatotoxic compound; the differences in the elimination kinetics of isoniazid reflect polymorphism of the N-acetyltransferase enzyme involved. As shown in Table 14–2, there are large genetically controlled ethnic differences in the distribution of acetylator status. Both Caucasians and Negroes have approximately equal numbers of slow and fast acetylators, but in Oriental and Eskimo populations the percent of slow acetylators is much smaller. Slow acetylators are genetically homozygous with a recessive allele pair, and since acetylator status is under monogenic control, it is possible to calculate the frequency of heterozygous and homozygous fast acetylators from gene frequencies. The results displayed in Table 14–2 for each ethnic group are calculated in the following manner: if p and q are the frequency of two alleles, so that $p + q = 1$, then the frequency of the genotype (consisting of a combination of the alleles) is $p^2 + 2pq + q^2 = 1$. For example, in the data in Table 14–2 for Caucasians, p^2 (for the homozygous slow acetylators) is 0.586, so that $p = 0.766$, that is, 76.6

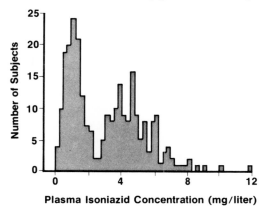

Fig. 14–1. The bimodal distribution of the 6-hour plasma isoniazid concentration in 483 subjects after 9.8 milligrams/kilogram isoniazid orally results from acetylation polymorphism. (One mg/liter = 7.3 micromolar.) (Redrawn from Evans, D.A.P., Manley, K.A., and McKusick, V.A.: Genetic control of isoniazid metabolism in man. Br. Med. J., 2:485–491, 1960.)

Table 14–2.   Distribution of Acetylators of Isoniazid in Different Populations

Population	Number	Slow acetylators (percent)	Fast acetylators (percent)	
			heterozygotes	homozygotes
South Indians (Madras)	1477	59	35.6	5.4
Caucasians	1958	58.6 (52–68)	35.9	5.5
Negroes	531	54.6 (49–65)	38.6	6.8
Eskimos	485	10.5 (5–21)	43.8	45.7
Japanese	2141	12.0 (10–15)	45.3	42.7
Chinese	682	22	49.8	28.2

From Kalow, W.: Ethnic differences in drug metabolism. Clin. Pharmacokinet., 7:373–400, 1982. Reproduced with permission of ADIS Press Australasia Pty Limited.

percent of Caucasians have one slow acetylator allele. Hence, the frequency for the fast acetylator allele is 0.234, which leads to distributions for heterozygous and homozygous fast acetylators of 0.359 ($2pq$) or 35.9 percent and 0.055 (q^2) or 5.5 percent, respectively.

Isoniazid is an exception. In most cases the frequency of occurrence of an allele is linked with other factors, such as gender. Also, often there are several subpopulations within the general population of a given ethnic group. These effects make it difficult to calculate the genotype frequency. However, notwithstanding the difficulties in making precise calculations, knowledge of the existence of large ethnic differences in pharmacokinetics, such as seen with isoniazid and some other drugs including debrisoquine (see below), is clearly important for the optimal use of drugs. This is particularly true for drugs prescribed worldwide or used in a multiracial society.

Interest in acetylation polymorphism is not just academic. Peripheral neuropathy, associated with elevated concentrations of isoniazid, occurs more prevalently in slow acetylators unless an adjustment is made in the dosage of isoniazid or vitamin B_6 is concomitantly administered. The awareness of the prevalence of homozygous and heterozygous rapid acetylators may also be clinically relevant, as they appear to differ in their susceptibility to adverse reactions, such as isoniazid-induced hepatic damage. Acetylation polymorphism also occurs and is important for several other drugs besides isoniazid, such as procainamide and hydralazine (Table 14–1). For both drugs the N-acetyl derivative is the major metabolite. A systemic lupus erythematous syndrome, a generalized inflammatory response, often limits procainamide use; it occurs more frequently in long-term than in short-term therapy and in slow rather than rapid acetylators. The mechanism remains obscure, but does appear to be associated with an elevated plasma procainamide concentration. Rapid acetylators require higher doses of hydralazine to control hypertension.

Debrisoquine

In common with many drugs, debrisoquine, an antihypertensive agent, is metabolized by a cytochrome P-450 mixed function oxidase system within the liver. What is distinctive about debrisoquine is that oxidation of this compound was the first shown to exhibit genetic polymorphism. There is a deficiency in the metabolism of this drug in 6 to 10 percent of Caucasians, with wide differences in other ethnic groups (Table 14–1). It is a recessive trait, caused perhaps by a defect on a single chromosome, that affects a particular oxidative enzyme. Since its discovery, the oxidation of other drugs, including metoprolol (Fig. 14–2), nortriptyline, and mephenytoin (Table 14–1), have been found to cosegregate with that of debrisoquine. In general, unless the dose is reduced, these drugs accumulate excessively in subjects with the deficiency, producing a more pronounced effect and potentially more frequent occurrence of adverse reactions.

Many drugs are metabolized with widely differing efficiencies by the different forms of cytochrome P-450 now known to exist in addition to the one responsible for debrisoquine oxidation. Although definitive data are currently lacking, many of the other cytochromes are also likely to be under genetic control, and at least for some, the clearance values associated with the oxidation of certain drugs cosegregate (Fig. 14–3). Further evidence, favoring genetic control of many of these processes, is gained from studies with twins. Figure 14–4 illustrates such an investigation with the antidepressant drug, nortriptyline. Variability in the plateau plasma nortriptyline concentration after oral administration among identical twins is much less than among fraternal twins or, indeed, among any randomly selected, age-matched group. Similar data exist for phenylbutazone, bishydroxycoumarin, and antipyrine, a model compound frequently used in drug metabolism studies. Although the evidence presented in Figures 14–2 and 14–4 is striking, analysis based solely on the unchanged drug in plasma may be misleading. Consider, for example, a drug that is eliminated by several metabolic

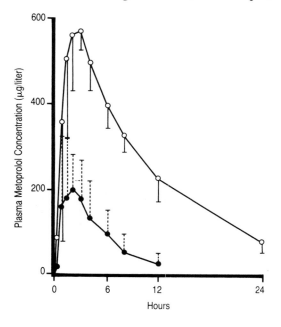

Fig. 14–2. The plasma metoprolol concentrations after a single oral dose of 200 milligrams metoprolol tartrate were much higher in poor (○) than in extensive (●) hydroxylators of debrisoquine. Because metoprolol is a drug of high hepatic clearance, the difference between poor and extensive metabolizers is expressed in the large difference in availability, due to differences in first-pass hepatic loss. The vertical lines indicate the standard deviation. (One mg/liter = 3.7 micromolar.) (Redrawn from Lennard, M.S., Silas, J.H., Freestone, S., Ramsay, L.E., Tucker, G.T., and Woods, H.F.: Oxidative phenotype—a major determinant of metoprolol metabolism and response. Reprinted by permission of The New England Journal of Medicine, *307*:1558–1560, 1982.)

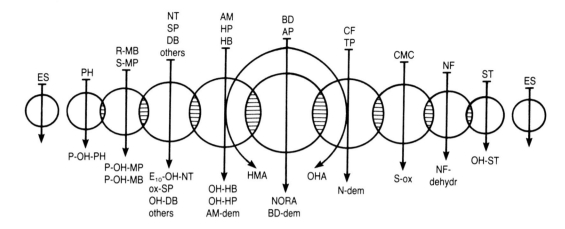

Fig. 14–3. Graphic representation of the different forms of cytochrome P-450 (circles) in man with different, but probably overlapping, substrate and product specificities. The arrows indicate single metabolic pathways. ES = endogenous substrate; PH = phenytoin; MP = mephenytoin; MB = methylphenobarbital; DB = debrisoquine; SP = sparteine; NT = nortriptyline; HB = hexobarbital; HP = heptabarbital; AM = amino-pyrine; AP = antipyrine; BD = benzodiazepine; TP = theophylline; CF = caffeine; CMC = carboxyme-thylcysteine; NF = nifedipine; ST = steroid; P-OH = para-hydroxy; ox = oxy; OH = hydroxy; dem = demethylation; HMA = hydromethylation; NORA = norantipyrine; OHA = hydroxyantipyrine; S-ox = sulfoxidation; dehydr = dehydrogenation. (Redrawn and updated from Breimer, D.D.: Interindividual dif-ferences in drug disposition: Clinical implications and methods of investigation. Clin. Pharmacokinet., 8:371–462, 1983. Reproduced with permission of ADIS Press Australasia Pty Limited.)

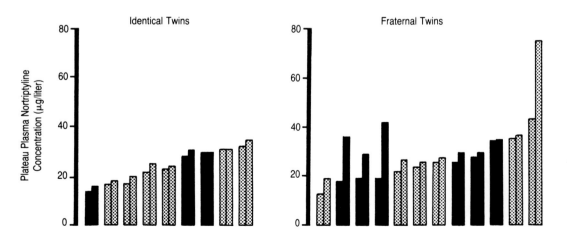

Fig. 14–4. The much smaller intrapair variability in plateau plasma concentration of nortriptyline between (nine) identical twins than between (twelve) fraternal twins indicates that genetics plays a major role in nortriptyline pharmacokinetics. Female ■; male ▨. (From Alexanderson, B., Price-Evans, D.A., and Sjöqvist, F.: Steady-state plasma levels of nortriptyline in twins: Influence of genetic factors and drug therapy. Br. Med. J., 4:764–768, 1969.)

pathways of which only a minor one is under genetic control. Looking solely at the elimination half-life or at the total clearance of the drug may fail to detect this genetically controlled source of variability. Yet, if the affected metabolite is very potent or toxic, identifying this source of variation may be therapeutically important. The need to measure both drug and metabolites under these circumstances and to calculate the clearance associated with the formation of each metabolite is self-evident.

Succinylcholine

Typically, muscle paralysis wears off within minutes of discontinuing the neuromuscular blocking agent succinylcholine, because it is rapidly hydrolyzed to inactive products, choline and monosuccinylcholine, by plasma and hepatic pseudocholinesterases. In the occasional patient, however, the neuromuscular blockade lasts up to several hours after stopping the infusion, because hydrolysis is much slower than usual. The reason is the existence of an atypical enzyme rather than a lower concentration of the typical cholinesterase; the atypical cholinesterase has only $\frac{1}{100}$ the usual affinity for succinylcholine, and it behaves differently from the typical cholinesterase to various enzyme inhibitors. Many aberrant forms of the enzyme are now known to exist, each determined by a different gene.

One drug can hasten the elimination of another by inducing the synthesis of metabolizing enzymes. Conversely, one drug can retard the elimination of another by competing for the same metabolizing enzymes. Large interindividual variations exist in the degree of induction or inhibition produced by concurrent drug therapy; part of the variability is undoubtedly under genetic control.

In contrast to many metabolic pathways, the renal handling of drugs does not appear to show genetic polymorphism. Thus, the renal clearance value for any drug tends to be the same in age- and weight-matched, healthy subjects. This last observation suggests that much of the interindividual variability in pharmacokinetics might be avoided if drugs were entirely excreted unchanged. Whether any of the variations in drug absorption and distribution are also under genetic control is poorly defined. Slow and fast gastrointestinal absorption of several drugs has been traced to differences in gastric emptying rate, but extensive twin studies and family studies to further define this aspect are lacking.

INHERITED VARIATION IN PHARMACODYNAMICS

As previously noted, patients vary in the dosage requirements of warfarin needed to produce adequate anticoagulant control. At most, the variation in dosage requirements is fivefold. In several members of two families, however, massive doses of warfarin were needed to achieve a therapeutic response. Figure 14–5 illustrates the findings in two families. In common with other genetic traits, warfarin resistance is not found in all kindred. Analysis of the frequency of the resistance in several generations indicates that the resistance is a dominant characteristic transmitted as a single gene effect. A normal pharmacokinetic profile of warfarin in the resistant subjects points to a pharmacodynamically based resistance. A probable mechanism is either a reduced affinity of warfarin

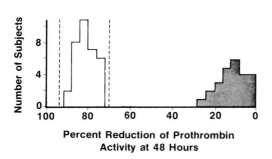

**Percent Reduction of Prothrombin
Activity at 48 Hours**

Fig. 14–5. Reduction of the one-stage prothrombin activity (an index of anticoagulability) from 0 to 48 hours, after an oral dose of 1.5 milligrams/kilogram sodium warfarin, for 59 members of two warfarin-resistant kindreds. The dotted lines represent the 99 percent confidence limits for the response in 50 normal subjects given the same dose. The 34 members of both kindreds with a normal response are indicated by the lightly shaded bars, and 25 of the 26 members with a resistant response are indicated by the darkly shaded bars. (Redrawn from O'Reilly, R.A.: Symposium on pharmacogenetics. Genetic factors in the response to the oral anticoagulant drugs in human genetics. Proceedings of the Fourth International Congress of Human Genetics, International Congress Series 250. Excerpta Medica, Amsterdam, 1972, pp. 428–438.)

at the site of action, or an increased affinity of the receptor for vitamin K, with which warfarin competes to produce its anticoagulant effect.

Other examples of genetically determined variation in pharmacodynamics are given in Table 14–1. Undoubtedly others will emerge as more concentration-response relationships are investigated in the patient population.

PHENOTYPING

Phenotyping patients for a particular metabolic pathway, such as acetylation or oxidation, prior to drug administration has been proposed. This approach aims to better anticipate the dosage regimen of a drug required in an individual. Its appeal is greatest in those situations in which the therapeutic index of the drug is low; the analyses of the drug and its metabolites in plasma are difficult; and the marker is relatively safe, easy to measure, and its phenotypic characteristic is highly correlated with that of the drug. The value of this approach has not been fully evaluated, and although the indications may be few, it does appear promising in certain cases. For example, slow acetylators receiving isoniazid have an increased susceptibility to phenytoin toxicity and phenotyping them for acetylator status with dapsone as the marker (see Table 14–1) may be advisable.

Study Problems

(Answers to Study Problems are in Appendix G.)

1. Give two examples each of inherited variation in pharmacokinetics and pharmacodynamics.

2. Define the terms: drug idiosyncrasy, polymorphism, and phenotype.

3. Discuss briefly how an inherited source of variation in pharmacokinetics can be identified within the patient population.

4. Subjects phenotyped according to their debrisoquine oxidation status (poor or extensive metabolizers) ingested one of the following four β-adrenergic blocking drugs: atenolol, metoprolol, propranolol, and timolol. Table 14–3 lists the mean values of

various pharmacokinetic parameters for each drug and whether the correlation with debrisoquine status was weak or strong. Discuss briefly possible reasons for the observed correlations.

Table 14–3.

| Drug | Pharmacokinetic Parameters (mean value) | | | Correlation with Debrisoquine Oxidation Phenotype |
	CL (liters/hour)	V (liters)	CL_R (liters/hour)	
Atenolol	5.0	38	4.3	weak
Metoprolol	63.0	290	6.0	strong
Propranolol	50.0	280	<0.3	weak
Timolol	31.0	150	4.7	strong

5. The frequency within the population of an allele associated with slow oxidation of a drug is 0.15. If slow oxidizors are homozygous with a recessive allele pair, what are the expected frequencies of slow and fast oxidizors in the population? Assume that oxidation status is under monogenic control and that all the variability within the population is of genetic origin.

15

Age and Weight

Objectives

The reader will be able to:

1. **Determine those drugs for which the loading dose, normalized for body weight, is likely to be independent of age, given the values of the volume of distribution and the fraction of drug in plasma unbound.**

2. **Describe the likely changes with age in the pharmacokinetics of a drug that is predominantly excreted unchanged in urine, from the neonate to the elderly patient.**

3. **Adjust, based on age and weight, the usual adult dosage regimen for an individual older than one year of age.**

Aging, characterized by periods of growth, development, and senescence, is an additional source of variability in drug response and, as a result, the usual adult dosage regimen may need to be modified, particularly in both the young and the old, if optimal therapy is to be achieved. Unfortunately, the pharmacokinetic and therapeutic information required to make these necessary modifications in dosage is only now becoming available. It is the very young and the aged who often are in most critical need of drugs. It is against this background of limited data that this chapter, in which an attempt is made to develop a framework for making dosage adjustments for age, must be viewed.

The life of a human is commonly divided into various stages: that of the newborn, the infant, and so forth. For the purposes of this book the various stages are defined as follows: *neonate*, up to two months *post utero; infant*, between the ages of two months and one year; *child*, between one year and 12 years of age; *adolescent*, between the ages of 12 and 20 years; *adult*, between 20 and 70 years; and *elder*, older than 70 years of age. It is recognized, however, that this stratification of human life is arbitrary. Life is a continuous process with the distinction between one period and the next often ill-defined. It is also recognized that chronologic age does not necessarily define functional age, and accordingly, statements made in this chapter pertain to the average person within the age bracket rather than to the individual.

Expediency and practicality dictate against the use of longitudinal studies in individuals to examine the influence of age on pharmacokinetics. Rather, single observations are made in individuals of differing ages. The information obtained therefore pertains to the population and does not necessarily reflect how an individual may change with age.

A POINT OF REFERENCE

Throughout this chapter reference is made to the "(usual) adult dosage regimen" of a drug. Before proceeding it is necessary to define this phrase more precisely. The word "adult" refers here to the average adult patient with the disease or condition requiring the drug. The "(usual) adult dosage regimen" is defined as that regimen which when given to this population, on the average, achieves therapeutic success. Clearly, the characteristics of the adult patient population vary with the disease. This is certainly true of age.

The data in Figure 15–1 show different age trends for the use of two drugs. Thus, patients taking digoxin, used to treat congestive cardiac failure, are generally older than those taking nitrofurantoin, used to treat urinary tract infections, a condition more evenly affecting people of all ages. Patients with incontinence are generally even older, 70 to 80 years, than those with congestive cardiac failure. However, there are few drugs for which pharmacokinetic data are obtained at the mean age of the adult patient population. Since most patients taking drugs tend to be middle-aged, for the purposes of subsequent calculations, an adult age of 55 years is assumed.

The data in Table 15–1 illustrate a point about age and disease. Listed are estimates of the population pharmacokinetics of digoxin in a group of young healthy adults and in a group of inpatients receiving digoxin for the treatment of severe congestive cardiac failure. Notice the differences in the values of the estimates, particularly for renal clearance, between the two groups. Evidently the estimates in the young healthy group are of little therapeutic value. Yet, much pharmacokinetic data on drugs are obtained in this selected group. Of greater clinical value are estimates of the pharmacokinetic parameters in the patient population requiring the drug.

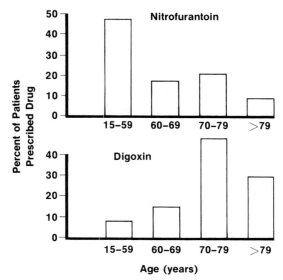

Fig. 15–1. Age distribution of drug consumption. Outpatients in the county of Jämtland, Sweden, taking digoxin are generally older than those taking nitrofurantoin. (Abstracted from Boethius, G. and Sjöqvist, F.: Doses and dosage intervals of drugs— clinical practice and pharmacokinetic principles. Clin. Pharmacol. Ther., 24:255–263, 1978.)

Table 15–1. Estimates of the Population Pharmacokinetics of Digoxin in Young Healthy Subjects and in Inpatients with Severe Congestive Cardiac Failure

	Age (years)	Weight (kilograms)	Availability (percent)	Volume of Distribution (liters)	Renal Clearance (liters/hour)	Extrarenal Clearance (liters/hour)
Young healthy subjects[a]	28	71	40–70	760	8.52	3.48
Inpatients, severe congestive cardiac failure[b]	54	68	60	476	3.50	1.37

[a]Abstracted from the data of Koup, J.R., Greenblatt, D.J., Jusko, W.J., Smith, T.W., and Koch-Weser, J.: Pharmacokinetics of digoxin in normal subjects after intravenous bolus and infusion dose. J. Pharmacokinet. Biopharm., 3:181–192, 1975.

[b]Abstracted from the data of Sheiner, L.B., Rosenberg, B., and Marthe, V.V.: Estimation of population characteristics of pharmacokinetic parameters from routine clinical data. J. Pharmacokinet. Biopharm., 5:445–479, 1977.

Part of the difference in renal clearance of digoxin between the two groups is accounted for by the disease. Part, however, is accounted for by age. One objective of this chapter is to suggest means of correcting the values of pharmacokinetic parameters for age. The intent thereby is to permit a better estimate to be initially made of the dosage required to treat a disease in an individual patient or in a patient population whose age differs substantially from the mean age of the patient population in which the usual adult dosage regimen was established. It is assumed that the influence of all other factors on the pharmacokinetics of a drug, such as the disease being treated, concurrent diseases, and other drugs, is independent of age or that the age-related effects are known and can be accounted for independently.

PHARMACODYNAMICS

Throughout this chapter, the range of unbound plasma drug concentrations associated with successful therapy is assumed to be independent of the age of the patient. This assumption may well be substantiated for most drugs in the future, but at present, data are very limited. At least for those antiepileptic drugs studied and for digoxin, effective plasma drug concentrations appear to be the same in both children and adults, although children appear to tolerate a higher concentration of these drugs before any toxic manifestations become apparent. It is likely, however, that differences in response with age do exist for certain drugs. For example, the observed increased sensitivity of elderly patients to the central nervous effects of the benzodiazepines cannot be explained on the basis of differences in the pharmacokinetics of this group of drugs.

ABSORPTION

Drug absorption does not appear to change dramatically with age. Nonetheless, all the factors discussed in Chapter 9 that affect drug absorption, including gastric pH, gastric emptying, intestinal motility, and blood flow, do change with age. Thus, in the neonate, a condition of relative achlorhydria persists for the first week of life, and it is not until after three years of age that gastric acid secretion approaches the adult value. Gastric emptying is also prolonged and peristalsis is irregular during the early months of life. Skeletal muscle mass is also much reduced, and muscle contractions, which tend to promote both blood flow and spreading of an intramuscularly administered drug, are relatively feeble. An elevated gastric pH, a delay in gastric emptying, and both diminished intestinal motility and blood flow are also seen in old people. A difference in drug absorption between the adult and both the very young and the old is therefore expected. Generally, changes in rate (usually slower) rather than in extent of absorption are found. These changes tend to be less apparent in the elderly than in the very young. Children often appear to absorb drugs as completely and, if anything, more rapidly than adults. Accordingly, in subsequent calculations of dosage, absorption is assumed not to vary with age.

BODY WEIGHT

One aspect of aging is body weight. Weight, three kilograms at birth, increases rapidly in childhood and in adolescence and then declines slowly during later years (Fig. 15–2). Because body water spaces, muscle mass, organ blood flow, and organ function are related to body weight, so too should be volume of distribution, clearance, and hence the dosage regimen of drugs. Owing to large variability in drug response, however, a weight adjustment is generally thought necessary only if the weight of an individual differs by more than 30 percent from the average adult weight (70 kg). In practice, then, adjustments for weight

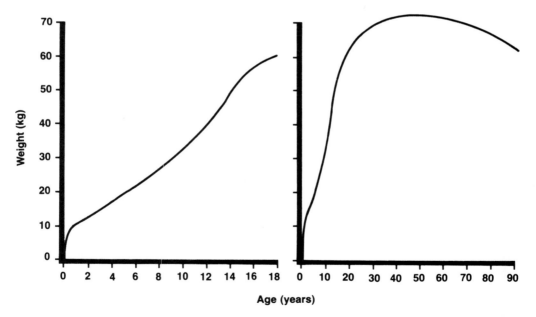

Fig. 15–2.   Variation in average weight with age, from the neonate to the elder. Weight increases rapidly in the young, particularly during the first year of life, and during puberty. It declines slowly after 50 years of age. (Data from: 0–20 years, Documenta Geigy. 5th Ed., Basle, Karger, 1959, pp. 255–256; 20–75 years, 2nd National Health and Nutrition Examination Survey, 1976–80. Maryland, U.S. National Center for Health Statistics; 75–94 years, CRC Handbook of Nutrition in the Aged. Edited by R.R. Watson. Florida, CRC Press, 1985, p. 18.)

are made only for the child and for the adult who is petite, emaciated, big, or obese.

LOADING DOSE

Clinically, correcting the adult loading dose proportionately for body weight appears reasonable. The volume of distribution based on unbound drug, Vu, is frequently both directly proportional to body weight and independent of age, but not always so. Much depends on the physicochemical properties of the drug and on the reason for the difference in weight.

Shown in Table 15–2 are values for the degree of plasma protein binding, the volume of distribution (V), the unbound volume of distribution (Vu), and the percent of drug in the body unbound, for a number of drugs in neonates and in adults. The last two parameters were calculated from the fraction unbound in plasma and the volume of distribution (see Chap. 10). As commonly found, plasma drug binding is lower in the neonate than in adults. Yet, for the first three drugs, phenobarbital and the two sulfonamides, the value of Vu, corrected for body weight, is the same because most of the drug is unbound in the body. Clearly, for these drugs a weight-normalized dose produces the same unbound drug concentration in both neonates and adults or in any other age group. In contrast, little of either digoxin or phenytoin is unbound in the body. Even so, a difference in binding only occurs in plasma (Vu is the same) and so a weight-corrected loading dose, if required, should suffice.

During adulthood the value of fu remains unchanged or tends to rise for those drugs bound to albumin, the concentration of which falls slightly with advancing years. The change in binding is generally too small, however, to warrant any consideration of dose adjustment.

Body composition is important. A dose correction must be considered for emaciated and obese patients. However, the difference in the required loading dose may not be as great as anticipated from body weight alone. As with age-related changes in drug distribution, much depends upon the physicochemical properties of the drug. Digoxin and polar drugs, for example, do not partition well into fat. Accordingly, for these drugs the volume of distribution correlates

Table 15–2. Plasma Protein Binding and Distribution Data for Some Drugs in Neonates and Adults[a]

Drug	Fraction Unbound in Plasma (fu)		Volume of Distribution (V, liters/kg)		Unbound Volume of Distribution (Vu, liters/kg)		Percent of Drug in Body Unbound[b]	
	Neonate	Adult	Neonate	Adult	Neonate	Adult	Neonate	Adult
Phenobarbital	0.68	0.53	1.0	0.55	1.4	1.0	56	58
Sulfisoxazole	0.32	0.16	0.38	0.16	1.2	1.0	65	58
Sulfamethoxypyrazine	0.43	0.38	0.47	0.24	1.1	0.63	72	92
Digoxin	0.80	0.70	5–10	7.0	6–12	10	6–12	6
Phenytoin	0.2	0.1	1.3	0.63	6.5	6.3	12	9

[a]Adapted from the data collected by Morselli, P.L.: Clinical pharmacokinetics in neonates. Clin. Pharmacokinet., 1:81–98, 1976.

[b]Calculated from Equation 29, Chapter 10, assuming that the unbound drug distributes evenly throughout total body water.

better with lean body mass, which is similar between obese and average persons of the same height and frame, than with total body weight.

DISPOSITION KINETICS

Figure 15–3 shows the changes with age in the half-life of creatinine and the clearance of creatinine expressed per kilogram of body weight. Creatinine distributes into total body water spaces, is negligibly bound to tissue or plasma constituents, is eliminated almost entirely by renal excretion, and has a clearance equal to the glomerular filtration rate. The example of creatinine was chosen because changes in total body water and glomerular filtration rate with age are understood reasonably well. To the extent that creatinine mimics other drugs, the data displayed in Figure 15–3 further our understanding of age-related changes in the pharmacokinetics of drugs and suggest a means of individualizing dosage regimens for age. Let us consider the various parts of Figure 15–3 in some detail.

Clearance, if normalized for body weight, is depressed in the neonate, but rapidly increases to reach a maximum value at 6 months, when it is almost twice that in the adult. Thereafter, weight-normalized clearance falls but still remains, throughout childhood, considerably above the adult value. Also, an often forgotten point is that throughout adulthood many functions decrease (Fig. 15–4). This is certainly so for creatinine clearance (glomerular filtration rate), which diminishes at a rate of about 1 percent per year; therefore, as an approximation, beyond 20 years of age,

★

$$\text{Creatinine clearance (milliliters/minute)} = [140 - \text{Age}] \cdot \frac{\text{Weight}}{70} \qquad 1$$

where age is expressed in years and weight in kilograms. Thus, in the average 95-year-old adult, who weighs 55 kilograms, the creatinine clearance is only one-third (35 ml/minute) of that in the average young adult (120 ml/minute). More exact relationships between creatinine clearance and age, for males and females, are given in Chapter 16.

Because total body water as a percent of body weight, and hence distribution, changes relatively little during life, the change in the half-life of creatinine inversely reflects the change in clearance. That is, the half-life is shortest around one year of age; it is longest in both newborn and elderly patients. Although extensive data are lacking, similar age-related changes in disposition of drugs seem to occur.

First, consider the data on diazepam, a drug metabolized primarily in the liver. As seen in Figure 15–5, the elimination half-life of diazepam is longest in the neonate, particularly within the first few days, and in adults greater than 55 years of age. Infants eliminate the drug most rapidly. With creatinine, the long half-life in the neonate is caused by depressed renal function, which takes several months to mature. With diazepam the long half-life in the neonate reflects an undeveloped drug-metabolizing activity. Metabolic activity may take months to mature; the time required for full maturation varies with the enzyme system. That the premature neonate has the longest half-life of diazepam is not surprising

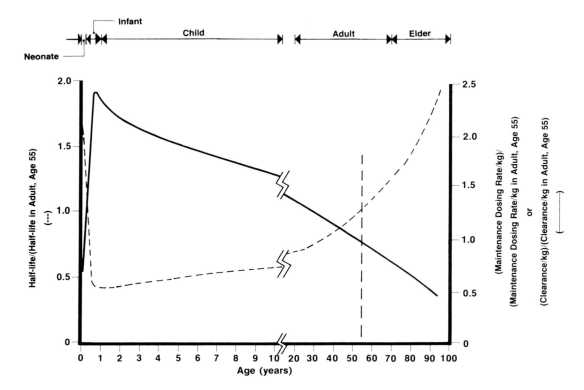

Fig. 15–3. How half-life (---) and both the clearance and the maintenance dosing rates (—) of a drug might vary with age. The values were calculated from data on creatinine. The drug, like creatinine, distributes into total body water, is eliminated entirely by renal excretion, and has a clearance equal to the glomerular filtration rate. The half-life is expressed as a fraction of the average value for a typical adult patient, 55 years old; the dosage regimen is calculated on the assumption that the desired average plateau concentration of drug remains constant throughout life. Notice that, because of poor renal function, elimination is slow in the neonate, but function rapidly improves such that, by 1 year, the elimination half-life is about one-half of the adult value. During childhood and adolescence the half-life becomes longer because, with growth, clearance, a function of surface area, increases more slowly than does volume of distribution, a function of body weight. Although body weight and therefore volume of distribution change only slightly beyond 30 years, because renal function and therefore clearance progressively diminish, the half-life is longer in the aged. By 95 years the half-life is twice the adult value. These changes in clearance and weight with age explain why the maintenance dose per kilogram of body weight is higher in the child and lower in both the neonate and the aged than in the adult.

The data used in the calculations were obtained as follows: Half-life–Calculated from volume of distribution and clearance. The half-life in an average adult, 55 years, is 5.9 hours. Volume of distribution–Taken as 78 percent of body weight at birth, 67 percent of body weight at 6 months, and 60 percent of body weight thereafter (Friis-Hansen, B.: Changes in body water compartments during growth. Acta Paediatr., (Supp.) 110:1–68, 1956). Clearance–at birth, taken as the inulin clearance, 3 milliliters/minute (Weill, W.B.: The evaluation of renal function in infancy and childhood. Am. J. Med. Sci., 229:678–694, 1955); between 6 months and 20 years, calculated by multiplying the creatinine clearance, 120 milliliters/minute per 1.8 square meters, in an average, healthy, young adult; 21–29 years, by body surface area; between 30 and 99 years, taken from the data of Siersbaek-Nielsen (Siersbaek-Nielsen, K., Hansen, J.M., Kampmann, J., and Kristensen, M.: Rapid evaluation of creatinine clearance. Lancet, 1:1133–1134, 1971). Surface Area–Calculated from body weight using the relationship: Surface area = 1.8 square meters · [Weight (kg)/70]$^{0.7}$.

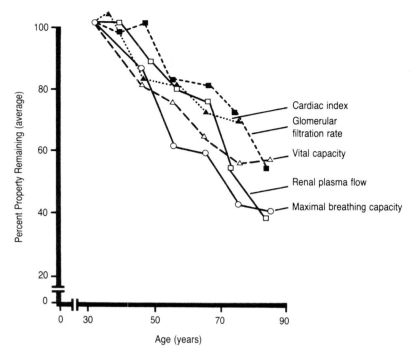

Fig. 15–4.   Many physiologic functions diminish with increasing age during adulthood. (Adapted from Shock, N.W.: Age changes in physiological functions in the total animal: The role of tissue loss. Edited by B.L. Strehler. The biology of aging. Washington, D.C., American Institute of Biological Sciences, 1960, pp. 250–264.)

and stresses a point made earlier: chronologic and functional age must be distinguished, especially in neonates.

The shorter half-life of diazepam in the infant than in the 20 to 55 year-old adult reflects differences in clearance, because the volume of distribution of this drug is approximately the same (1.2 liters/kg) in both groups. The further prolongation in half-life in the most elderly group, clearly shown to be age-related (Fig. 15–6), requires some discussion. Clearance remains essentially constant, and volume of distribution is increased with age from 20 to 80 years, but only because of the tendency for lower plasma binding of drug. Diazepam is a drug

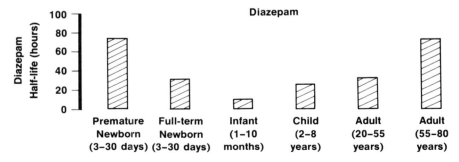

Fig. 15–5.   The elimination half-life of diazepam is shortest in the infant and longest in the newborn and the aged. (Adapted from the data of Morselli, P.L.: Drug Disposition During Development. New York, Spectrum Publications, 1977, pp. 311–360 and p. 456; and from the data of Klotz, U., Avant, G.R., Hoyumpa, A., Schenker, S., and Wilkinson, G.R.: The effect of age and liver disease on the disposition and elimination of diazepam in adult man. J. Clin. Invest., 55:347–359, 1975.)

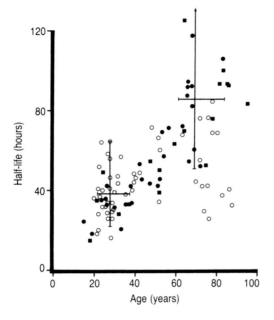

Fig. 15–6. The half-life of diazepam increases with age, from 20 to 80 years. (Composite data from (●)–Klotz, U., Avant, G.R., Hoyumpa, A., Schenker, S., and Wilkinson, G.R.: The effects of age and liver disease on the disposition and elimination of diazepam in adult man. J. Clin. Invest., 55:347–359, 1975; (+, mean and range)–Greenblatt, D.J., Allen, M.D., Harmatz, J.S., and Shader, R.I.: Diazepam disposition determinants. Clin. Pharmacol. Ther., 23:301–312, 1979; (○)–Macleod, S.M., Giles, H.G., Bengert, B., Lui, F.F., and Sellers, E.M.: Age and gender-related differences in diazepam pharmacokinetics. J. Clin. Pharmacol., 19:15–19, 1979; (■)–Macklow, A.F., Barton, M., James, O., and Rawlins, M.D.: The effect of age on the pharmacokinetics of diazepam. Clin. Sci., 59:479–483, 1980.)

of low extraction and large volume of distribution, and both its clearance and volume of distribution are dependent on protein binding. The unbound volume of distribution changes relatively little with age. However, the all important unbound clearance is reduced (Fig. 15–7), probably reflecting diminished capacity for hepatic metabolism, which occurs primarily by oxidation.

A decrease in unbound metabolic clearance in the elderly patient has been demonstrated for an increasing number of drugs, especially those eliminated principally by oxidation. For example, the clearance (predominantly metabolic) of antipyrine, a model compound used to assess hepatic oxidative metabolic status, decreases by approximately 1 percent per year (Fig. 15–8). However, the overall variability in oxidative clearance of drugs is usually large, and as with antipyrine, age may capture only a small percent of the total variance in clearance. Conjugative capacity also decreases but by a lesser extent than oxidative capacity. These changes may be associated, in part, with the decrease in the size of the liver, as a proportion of body weight, from 2.5 percent in the young adult to 1.6 percent at 90 years of age. As a rough approximation, the decline for unbound metabolic clearance with age is the same as that for renal clearance, 1 percent per annum.

Next consider the increasing ratio of the plateau plasma drug concentration to the dosing rate/kilogram, determined after chronic oral dosing of several antiepileptic drugs with increasing age in children (Fig. 15–8). All these drugs are completely available and since

$$\frac{C_{ss,av}}{(\text{Dose/kilogram})/\tau} = \frac{1}{\text{Clearance/kilogram}} \qquad 2$$

it follows that the weight-corrected clearance must be higher in the younger and smaller child. All these antiepileptic drugs are extensively metabolized, and in none studied does the protein binding appear to change substantially between

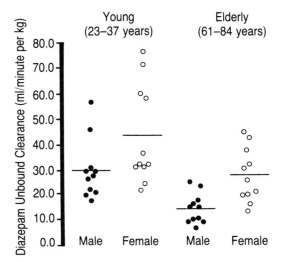

Fig. 15–7. The unbound clearance of diazepam is reduced in elderly patients compared with young adults. Differences also exist between males and females. The reduced unbound clearance is the primary reason for a prolonged half-life of diazepam in the elderly patient. (Redrawn from Greenblatt, D.J., Allen, M.D., Harmatz, J.S., and Shader, R.I.: Diazepam disposition determinants. Clin. Pharmacol. Ther., 27:301–312, 1980. Reproduced with permission of C.V. Mosby.)

the different age groups. Greater hepatic metabolic capacity per unit body weight is therefore implicated in the younger group.

MAINTENANCE DOSE THERAPY

The Neonate

The lack of maturation of renal and hepatic function necessitates that the rate of administration of drugs to both the neonate and the young infant be reduced, even on a body weight basis, if toxicity is to be avoided. Unfortunately, events occur so rapidly in these stages of life that it is impossible to predict clearance and hence the required dosage regimen. Caution must clearly be exercised in administering drugs to this patient population. Besides carefully noting the effects, monitoring of the plasma concentration of drugs with a narrow therapeutic index should be helpful.

In passing, noteworthy here is the incidental exposure of the fetus and the suckling infant to drugs. For those drugs that can pass the placenta, the unbound plateau concentration in the fetus is likely to equal that in the pregnant mother if she ingests the drug chronically. With eliminating capacity generally poorly developed, the fetus acts for the most part as an additional "tissue" of distribution, with the half-life in the fetus being the same as that in the mother. A drastic change occurs, however, on delivery. Deprived of access to the fully developed eliminating organs of the mother, elimination of drug from the newborn child can be very slow indeed.

The suckling infant is exposed to those drugs taken by the mother. As suckling occurs regularly, of concern are the events at plateau. The risks are greatest for drugs, particularly lipophilic ones, that concentrate in breast milk, that are poorly cleared by the infant, and that have a narrow therapeutic index.

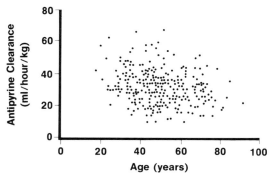

Fig. 15–8. The clearance of antipyrine, an extensively metabolized drug, declines but marginally with age when studied in 307 healthy subjects, each of whom received 1 gram antipyrine intravenously. Age accounts for little of the variability in clearance within this population. (Adapted from Vestal, R.E., Norris, A.H., Tobin, J.D., Cohen, B.H., Shock, N.W., and Andres, R.: Antipyrine metabolism in man: Influence of age, alcohol, caffeine, and smoking. Clin. Pharmacol. Ther., *18*:425–432, 1975.)

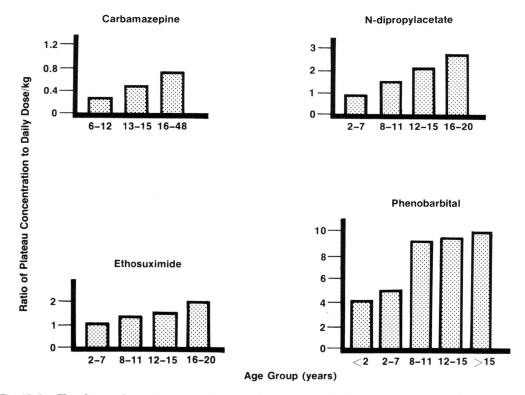

Fig. 15–9. The plateau plasma drug concentrations of several antiepileptic drugs were measured after chronic oral medication in children. An increased clearance per kilogram of body weight explains the lower ratio of concentration to daily dose per kilogram in the youngest children. (Adapted from the data of Morselli, P.L.: Antiepileptic drugs. *In* Drug Disposition During Development. Edited by P.L. Morselli. Spectrum Publications, New York, 1977, Chap. 11, p. 311–360.)

The Child

The evidence in Figures 15–3 and 15–9 suggests that a maintenance regimen, calculated by correcting the adult dosage for body weight, would prove inadequate for children, especially for the very young. *Body surface area* has been found to be a much better correlate of dosage requirements, cardiac output, hepatic and renal blood flow, and glomerular filtration rate in children and in adults of varying sizes than body weight. Because clearance relates dosing rate to the plateau plasma concentration of a drug and because renal clearance is proportional to the glomerular filtration rate (see Fig. 13–10), the choice of surface area over weight as the method of calculating maintenance therapy has some justification. According to this concept a child's maintenance dosage is calculated from the formula:

$$\text{Child's maintenance dosage} = \left[\frac{\text{Surface area of child (square meters)}}{\text{1.8 square meters}}\right] \cdot \text{Adult maintenance dosage} \qquad 3$$

where 1.8 square meters is the surface area of an average 70-kilogram adult. The surface area of a child can be determined from its body weight using the observation that surface area is proportional to body weight to the 0.7 power (weight$^{0.7}$). Using this last relationship, Equation 3 may be rewritten as

★

$$\text{Child's maintenance dosage} = \left[\frac{\text{Weight of child (kilograms)}}{\text{70 kilograms}}\right]^{0.7} \cdot \text{Adult maintenance dosage} \qquad 4$$

To illustrate the use of the relationship expressed in Equation 4, consider the example of phenobarbital; the usual adult antiepileptic maintenance dose is 100 milligrams daily. Question: What is the phenobarbital dosage needed in a 15-kilogram child? Answer: 34 milligrams daily. This answer can be estimated from the ratio of surface areas (estimated from body weight) using Equation 4.

$$\text{Child's dosage of phenobarbital} = \left(\frac{15}{70}\right)^{0.7} \cdot 100 \text{ milligrams/day}$$

$$= 34 \text{ milligrams/day}$$

Notice that the weight-normalized dosage of phenobarbital in the child, 2.3 milligrams/kilogram, is much higher than that in the adult, 1.43 milligrams/kilogram. The reason is that clearance is proportional to surface area, and surface area per kilogram *increases* disproportionately with decreasing weight. To appreciate this point, consider a cube of length L. The area of each face is L^2 and having 6 sides the total surface area is therefore $6 L^2$. The weight is proportional to volume, that is L^3. Thus, since the ratio of surface area to volume is $6/L$, diminishing the size by decreasing L increases the surface-area-to-volume ratio. The need for a higher maintenance dose per kilogram body weight, the smaller and hence usually the younger the child, is seen in Figure 15–3 for children between the ages of 6 months and 12 years. Note the complementary decrease in the half-life with decreasing size and age. Thus, not only may a child of one year of age require a larger maintenance dose per kilogram body weight than an adult, but also, because of a shorter half-life, the drug may need to be given more frequently, especially if the drug has a low therapeutic index and large fluctuations around the plateau concentration are to be avoided.

The Adult

Within the age range of 35 to 75 years, there is generally no need to adjust dosage for age when the typical patient is 55 years old. A need may exist, however, when the difference between the individual and the typical patient exceeds 20 years. This situation might arise, for example, if the age of the typical patient is close to 70 years and the patient is a young adult.

The Elder

As a broad generalization, drug dosage should be reduced in elderly patients, reflecting the general decline in body function with age (Fig. 15–4). A reduction in dosage is needed particularly in the weak and infirm elderly patient, who often suffers from several diseases, who receives multiple drug therapy, and whose body functions decrease very sharply with advancing years.

Certainly, the marked and progressive decrease in renal function implies that the dosage regimens of drugs that are predominantly excreted unchanged should be reduced in the elderly population. For example, an 80-year-old patient requires, on the average, only 70 percent of the usual adult dosage expressed on a body weight basis; the actual dose required would be even less because the elderly patient is lighter. Despite the obvious need for dosage adjustment, little appears to be made in practice. Perhaps it is a therapeutic oversight; a depressed clearance without dose adjustment probably explains, in part, the increased frequency and degree of adverse drug effects often noted in elderly patients.

General Equation

To return to the example of creatinine and similarly handled drugs, from 1 year to 20 years of age the relationship between renal clearance and age is expressed in Equation 4; beyond 20 years, this relationship is expressed in Equation 1. These equations can now be combined to give the general equation:

★

$$\text{Maintenance dosage} = \frac{[140 - \text{Age (years)}] \cdot [\text{Weight (kilograms)}]^{0.7}}{1660} \cdot \text{Usual adult maintenance dosage}$$

5

that permits the calculation of a maintenance dosage for a patient of any age, except the infant and the neonate, when maintenance of the same average plateau plasma concentration is needed. The value of the denominator, 1660, in Equation 5 is the product of the age-related decline in renal clearance for a 55-year-old: 85 (140 − 55) and $70^{0.7}$ or 19.5.

These relationships are shown graphically in Figure 15–10. The maintenance dosing rate is observed to increase almost linearly between 1 and 12 years of age. These predictions are based on changes in body surface area with age, which are estimated from average weights, and the general correlation observed between clearance and body surface area in children. Because clearance increases up to 20 years of age and then declines, note that there are pairs of age values in which the same rate of administration is required. For example, on the average, a 4-year-old child (16 kg) requires the same rate of drug administration as a 90-year-old person (60 kg).

Hopefully these equations will serve to facilitate and to improve the initial estimate of the dosage regimen needed for a patient of any age beyond 1 year. In general, a correction in the usual adult dosage is worthwhile when administering drugs to the very young, to the child, and to the aged. A correction is also worthwhile in emaciated and obese patients.

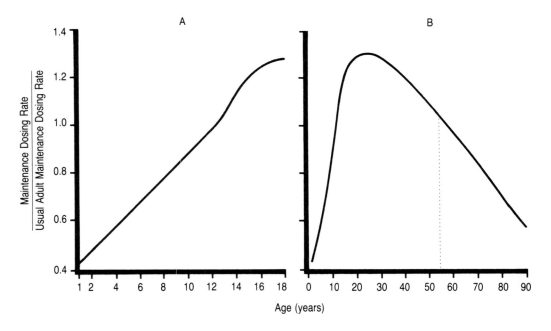

Fig. 15–10. Variation in the maintenance dosing rate expressed as a fraction of the maintenance dosing rate in a 55-year-old adult (dotted vertical line) as a function of age, from 1 year to 90 years. Note the almost linear increase in maintenance dosing rate with age from 1 to 12 years (A), associated primarily with an increase in body size, and the almost linear decline between 30 and 90 years (B), associated primarily with diminished organ function with advancing years. Also note that the total range of dosing rates as a function of age differs by no more than about twofold from the usual adult dosing rate. Values are calculated using Equation 5 and the weight-for-age relationships given in Figure 15–2.

Study Problems

(Answers to Study Problems are in Appendix G.)

1. Calculate a dosage regimen of gentamicin to treat a severe infection caused by *Pseudomonas aeruginosa* with the objective of maintaining the same average concentration in:

   (a) A child, age 4 years, weight 15 kilograms, with normal renal function.

   (b) An elderly patient, age 87 years, weight 63 kilograms, with normal renal function.

   The adult dose of gentamicin usually recommended (for a typical 55-year-old, 70-kg patient) is 1 milligram/kilogram administered intramuscularly every 8 hours. This antibiotic is almost completely renally excreted unchanged.

2. Figure 15–11 shows the variation in clearance per square meter (M^2) of body surface area of the cephalosporin antibiotic ceftriaxone in individuals from 1 day to 92 years of age. Renal and biliary excretion are about equally involved in the elimination of this drug in normal adults.

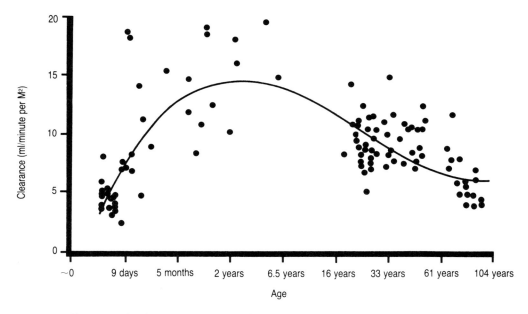

Fig. 15–11.   Clearance of ceftriaxone in subjects from 1 day to 92 years of age. Each symbol represents a single value. Note the scale for age, which is age raised to the power of 0.25 (age $^{0.25}$). (Redrawn from Hayton, W.L. and Stoeckel, K.: Age-associated changes in ceftriaxone pharmacokinetics. Clin. Pharmacokin., 11:76–86, 1986. Reproduced with permission of ADIS Press Australasia Pty Limited.)

   (a) Discuss briefly the changes observed.

   (b) Given that no change in drug distribution with age is observed, superimpose on the figure the expected trend of half-life with age.

   (c) What are the general implications of the finding for the administration of ceftriaxone?

3. When administering drugs to obese patients, a concern exists whether or not dose should be weight-corrected. Table 15–3 lists information on the volume of distribution of three drugs in control and obese patients; an individual was classified as obese if their weight for height was in excess of 150 percent of ideal body weight. Neither theophylline nor digoxin, relatively polar drugs, showed a difference in the volume of distribution between normal and obese individuals; the weight-corrected values were lower in the obese individuals. In contrast, the volume of distribution of diazepam, a nonpolar drug, was much greater in the obese group, even after correcting for differences in body weight. No significant difference in plasma binding of these three drugs has been found between obese and normal weight subjects.

Table 15–3[a].

Drug	Volume of Distribution (liters)		Weight-Corrected Volume of Distribution (liters/kilogram)		Average Ratio of Weight to Ideal Body Weight (percent)	
	Obese	Control	Obese	Control	Obese	Control
Theophylline	29	27	0.32	0.47	165	91
Digoxin	981	937	10.7	14.3	162	98
Diazepam	292	91	2.81	1.53	164	95

[a]Abstracted from Abernethy, D.R. and Greenblatt, D.: Clin. Pharmacokin., *11*:199–213, 1986.

(a) What explains the difference in the effect of obesity on the volume of distribution for each of the drugs?

(b) What impact do such findings have on the dosage regimens of these drugs?

16

Disease

Objectives

The reader will be able to:

1. **List at least six diseases in which the pharmacokinetics of drugs is known to be altered.**

2. **List and briefly discuss the pharmacokinetic parameters that are often altered in patients with hepatic and renal diseases.**

3. **Judge, using pharmacokinetic principles, on when alteration of drug administration should be considered for patients with hepatic or renal diseases.**

4. **Estimate the creatinine clearance of a patient from the patient's age, weight, gender, and serum creatinine.**

5. **Estimate how much the clearance of a drug of known fraction excreted unchanged is decreased in a patient with known renal function.**

6. **Establish, from pharmacokinetic principles, a dosage regimen for the patient in Objective 5.**

7. **Sketch the amount in the body with time following the dosage regimen recommended in Objective 6.**

8. **List the assumptions that underlie the application of renal function tests in dosage regimen adjustment for patients with renal insufficiency.**

Disease is a major source of variability in drug response. For many diseases this variability is due primarily to differences in pharmacokinetics, the area of principal focus in this chapter. The chapter begins with a general discussion of the diseases known to affect drug kinetics and concludes with extensive details on adjusting drug administration in patients with renal insufficiency.

DISEASE STATES

The pharmacokinetics, as well as the pharmacodynamics, of many drugs has been shown to be influenced by the concurrent presence of diseases other than the one for which a drug is used. Examples of concurrent diseases that increase the variability in drug response are listed in Table 16–1. The subsequent discussion centers on the first three groups of disease listed, namely hepatic, cardiovascular, and renal diseases.

Hepatic Disorders

Because the liver is the major site for drug metabolism, an impression prevails that special care should be taken in administering drugs to patients with disease states modifying hepatic function. Objective data, while generally supporting this impression, are occasionally in conflict.

One reason for the conflict arises from an attempt to classify hepatic disorders as a single entity. However, disorders of the liver, local or diffuse, are caused by many diseases; each disease affects various levels of hepatic organization to a different extent. On grouping clearance data together for numerous drugs, there appears to be no consistent relationship between hepatic disease and drug handling. Many drugs show a decreased clearance, some drugs show no change. When, however, hepatic disease is divided into chronic (especially cirrhosis) and acute and reversible situations, e.g., acute viral hepatitis, a much clearer picture emerges. With few exceptions, the clearance of drugs is decreased in cirrhosis. In contrast, in acute viral hepatitis, there appears to be a fairly even division between those drugs for which clearance is decreased, or half-life prolonged, and those for which no change is detected. The meager existing data suggest that drug elimination is diminished in chronic active hepatitis and obstructive jaundice.

Another potential pitfall is to equate prolongation of half-life with diminution of hepatic drug-metabolizing activity. Half-life is controlled by both total clearance and volume of distribution, two independent parameters (Chap. 11). To assess clearance and volume of distribution, the drug should be given intravenously to ensure complete availability. When so studied, the volumes of distribution of some drugs remain unaltered in hepatic disease, but those of others are increased. An increase in volume of distribution is found particularly with drugs bound to albumin in patients with cirrhosis. The explanation lies in the depressed synthesis of albumin and many proteins, including various enzymes and clotting factors, in these patients. The resultant fall in albumin is responsible for a decreased plasma binding of drug, an associated increase in volume of distribution, and an associated increase in clearance for a drug of low extraction. The fall in hepatic enzymes is responsible, in large part, for a diminished hepatic unbound clearance of many drugs, although oxidized drugs appear to be more affected than those eliminated by conjugation. Care must therefore be taken in interpreting a change in half-life.

The influence of hepatic disease on drug absorption is poorly understood. The problem is complicated by the need to separate disposition from absorption when analyzing plasma drug concentration-time data. It is likely, though, that the oral availability of drugs highly extracted by the liver is increased in cirrhosis (Fig. 16–1). There are two reasons for this increase. One is a diminished first-pass hepatic loss due to depressed hepatocellular activity. The other is because many cirrhotic patients develop portal bypass, a condition in which a significant fraction of the portal blood bypasses the liver and enters directly into the superior

Table 16–1.   Examples of Increased Variability in Drug Response Associated with Concurrent Disease States

Condition	Drug	Class	Observation	Variation in Pharmaco-kinetics	Variation in Pharmaco-dynamics	Comments
Hepatic Diseases						
Cirrhosis	Theophylline	Bronchodilator	Slower fall in plasma concentration	+	−	Clearance reduced; reduce dosage to avoid toxicity
Acute viral hepatitis	Warfarin	Anticoagulant	Excessive anticoagulant response	−	+	Reduce dosage to lessen risk of hemorrhage
Cardiovascular Disease						
Congestive cardiac failure	Lidocaine	Antiarrhythmic agent	Elevated plasma concentration after usual dosage	+	−	Clearance and volume of distribution diminished; reduce dosage to lessen risk of toxicity
Renal Disease						
Uremia	Gentamicin	Gram-negative antibiotic	Increased toxicity with usual dosage	+	−	Renal clearance diminished; reduce dosage to lessen risk of toxicity
Uremia	Thiopental	Anesthetic	Prolonged anesthesia	NS	NS	Reduce dose to avoid excessive sleeping time
Gastrointestinal Diseases						
Celiac Disease	Fusidic acid	Antibacterial agent	Elevated plasma concentration after usual oral dose	+	−	Availability increased and/or clearance diminished
Crohn's Disease	Propranolol	β-Blocker	Elevated plasma concentration after an oral dose	+	NS	Increased plasma binding, elevated α₁-acid glycoprotein suspected cause; observed only in active phase
Respiratory Diseases						
Asthma	Tolbutamide	Hypoglycemic agent	More rapid fall in plasma concentration	+	−	Therapeutic consequences uncertain
Emphysema	Morphine	Analgesic	Increased sensitivity to respiratory depressant effect	NS	NS	Reduce dose to diminish risk of respiratory complications
Cystic Fibrosis	Dicloxacillin	Antibiotic	Reduced area under plasma drug concentration-time curve	+	−	Renal clearance increased
Pneumonia	Theophylline	Bronchodilator	Elevated plasma concentration	+	−	Metabolic clearance decreased; reduce dose to lessen risk of toxicity
Endocrine Disease						
Thyroid Disease	Digoxin	Cardioactive agent	Diminished response in hyperthyroidism; increased response in myxedema	−	+	Adjust dosage according to thyroid activity
Down's Syndrome	Atropine	Spasmolytic	Heart rate increase to standard dose is greater than usual	NS	NS	Therapeutic consequences are uncertain
Fever	Quinine	Antimalarial agent	Plasma concentration of drug elevated, of metabolite depressed, after usual dosage	+	NS	Impaired metabolism suspected; may need to reduce doses in severe febrile states

+, established source of variability.
−, no evidence that variability is increased due to disease.
NS, not studied.

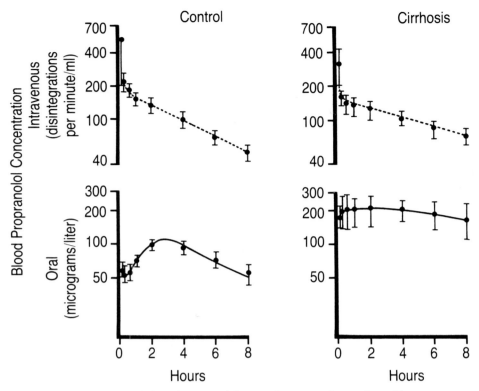

Fig. 16–1. In cirrhosis, the availability of propranolol is greatly increased as evidenced by comparison of the concentration of unlabeled drug in whole blood after oral administration (——) with the concentration of tritiated drug after intravenous administration (-----), following simultaneous determination of the kinetics of propranolol during the seventh dosing interval of an oral 8-hour dosing regimen in 9 normal subjects and 7 patients with cirrhosis (mean ± SE). (One mg/liter = 3.9 micromolar.) (Redrawn from Wood, A.J.J., Kornhauser, D.M., Wilkinson, G.R., Shand, D.G., and Branch, R.A.: The influence of cirrhosis on steady-state blood concentrations of unbound propranolol after oral administration. Clin. Pharmacokin., 3:478–487, 1978. Reproduced by permission of ADIS Press Australasia Pty Limited.)

vena cava via esophageal varices. These portacaval shunts can greatly increase availability; an increase of greater than 200 percent has been reported for some drugs with extensive first-pass metabolism.

From the foregoing discussion, it is apparent that drug dosage may need to be reduced in patients with hepatic function impairment as a result of both decreased clearance and increased availability. An adjustment in dosage is particularly warranted when the usual regimen results in the unbound drug concentration at plateau approaching or exceeding the upper limit of the therapeutic concentration window. This condition arises when the clearance based on unbound drug is substantially depressed, since it is this clearance that controls the unbound drug concentration at plateau (see Chaps. 11 and 12).

Hepatic dysfunction is a graded phenomenon, and theoretically a correlation should exist between changes in the pharmacokinetics of drugs, especially hepatic clearance, and an appropriate measure of hepatic function. Attempts to establish such relationships, although occasionally encouraging, have been generally unsuccessful. This failure probably arises because, unlike drug excretion, there are numerous pathways of drug metabolism, each with a different set of cofactor requirements and each affected to a different degree in hepatic disorders. The contribution of each pathway to total drug elimination also varies with the drug. Nonetheless in severe cirrhosis, signified by the combination of a low albumin (less than 3 grams/deciliter) and an elevated clotting time (prothrombin time in excess of 15 seconds), drug metabolism is likely to be sufficiently depressed to warrant reducing the dose and monitoring the patient carefully for adverse reactions. Consideration should also be given to whether the drug is truly needed or if alternative drugs might be preferred.

Circulatory Disorders

Circulatory disorders, which include shock, malignant hypertension, and congestive cardiac failure, are generally characterized by diminished vascular perfusion to one or more parts of the body. Since blood flow may influence drug absorption, distribution, and elimination, it is not surprising that the pharmacokinetics of drugs may be altered in circulatory disorders.

A diminished perfusion of absorption sites, e.g., gastrointestinal tract and muscle, with an associated protracted and erratic drug absorption, tends to be seen in patients with depressed cardiovascular states; it may be necessary to give the drug intravenously if a prompt response is desired. However, in these conditions the distribution kinetics of the drug is also affected, with perfusion to many organs diminished. Exceptions are the brain and the myocardium, which consequently receive an increased fraction of an intravenous bolus dose, particularly in the earlier moments of administration. For centrally acting and cardioactive agents, the rate of administration of a bolus dose to patients with circulatory depression must be tempered if the risks of toxicity are to be reduced. In these depressed circulatory states, cardiac output and therefore hepatic blood flow and, to a much lesser extent, renal blood flow are also reduced. Thus, the same response should be observed in the clearance of highly extracted drugs. Evidence supporting this concept is illustrated in Figure 16–2 by a strong positive correlation between the clearances of lidocaine and indocyanine green in patients both without and with varying degrees of congestive cardiac failure. Both indocyanine green, used as a dynamic test of hepatic function, and lidocaine are high hepatic extraction ratio drugs whose clearances should therefore reflect a diminished hepatic blood flow. Notice in Figure 16–2 the almost sixteenfold

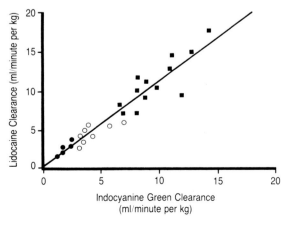

Fig. 16–2. A strong positive correlation exists between the clearance of lidocaine and indocyanine green in patients without (■) and with both mild (○) and severe (●) congestive cardiac failure. (From Zito, R.A. and Reid, P.R.: Lidocaine kinetics predicted by indocyanine green clearance. Reprinted, by permission of The New England Journal of Medicine, *298*: 1160–1163, 1978.)

variation in clearance of both lidocaine and indocyanine green. This range is almost certainly greater than the range of hepatic blood flows in these patients. The hepatic flow, usually about 18 milliliters/minute per kilogram, is unlikely to fall to a value as low as 2 milliliters/minute per kilogram because severe anoxia is expected to result at even higher flow rates. Hepatocellular enzyme activity is most probably also depressed when perfusion is severely diminished; this would further depress the clearances of both lidocaine and indocyanine green. As lidocaine has a narrow therapeutic window (see Table 5–2), dosage should be reduced in patients with congestive cardiac failure if the risk of toxicity is to be kept low.

RENAL DYSFUNCTION

When the usual intramuscular regimen of amikacin is administered to a patient with severe renal function impairment, the drug accumulates excessively as shown in Curve B of Figure 16–3. The figure reminds us that the extent of accumulation depends on both the frequency of administration and the half-life, and that the time required to approach the plateau is a function of the half-life only (Chap. 7). Having a much longer half-life than usual, the time to reach steady state is much longer in this patient than in a patient with normal renal function. Obviously, to avoid excessive accumulation, the dosage regimen of the drug must be reduced in the patient with renal dysfunction.

The clinician needs information on which drugs accumulate excessively in renal dysfunction and, more importantly, how to adjust drug administration to achieve an optimal therapeutic response. The basic principles that permit this calculation follow.

Decrease in Clearance

The elements of the problem of renal dysfunction are shown in Figure 16–4. Ceftazidime clearance, unbound clearance here because the drug is not bound to plasma proteins, is low when renal function, measured by creatinine clearance, is low and increases linearly with renal function. Note that some clearance remains (y-intercept) even when there is no renal function. This represents clearance by nonrenal pathways. The magnitude of the change in unbound clearance depends on the renal function remaining and on the fraction that renal clearance is of total clearance.

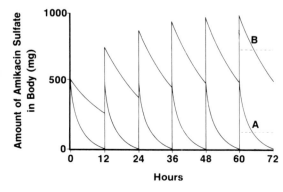

Fig. 16–3. Sketch of the amount of amikacin sulfate in the body with time following a regimen of 500 milligrams every 12 hours in a patient whose renal function is normal, Curve A, and in a patient whose age and weight are the same but whose renal function is 17 percent of normal, Curve B. Intravenous bolus administration is simulated. The normal half-life is assumed to be 2 hours. The dashed lines are the average plateau values.

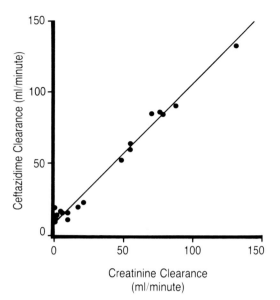

Fig. 16–4. The total clearance of the cephalosporin, ceftazidime, varies linearly with creatinine renal clearance in a group of 19 patients with varying degrees of renal function. Note that some clearance remains (y-intercept) when there is no renal function. (Drawn from the data of van Dalen, R., Vree, T.B., Baars, A.M., and Termond, E.: Dosage adjustment for ceftazidime in patients with impaired renal function. Europ. J. Clin. Pharmacol., *30*:597–605, 1986.)

Defining renal function, *RF*, as the ratio of the renal clearance of a drug in an individual patient $CLu_R(d)$, to that in the typical 55-year-old, 70-kilogram patient with normal renal function, $CLu_R(n)$, then

$$CLu_R(d) = RF \cdot CLu_R(n) \qquad 1$$

Renal function, as defined here, is a relative value and takes into account changes with age, weight, and the presence of renal disease. In the typical patient with normal renal function, renal clearance is a fraction, *fe(n)*, of the total clearance, that is,

$$CLu_R(n) = fe(n) \cdot CLu(n) \qquad 2$$

The typical unbound clearance by extrarenal routes is therefore,

$$\text{Extrarenal unbound clearance} = (1 - fe(n)) \cdot CLu(n) \qquad 3$$

Estimation of its value in the individual patient requires adjustment for age and weight. Using the approximation $\dfrac{(140 - \text{Age}) \cdot wt(d)^{0.7}}{1660}$ for the factor by which nonrenal clearance deviates from that in the typical patient (Chap. 15), its value in the individual patient becomes

$$\begin{matrix}\text{Extrarenal} \\ \text{unbound} \\ \text{clearance}\end{matrix} = (1 - fe(n)) \cdot CLu(n) \cdot \frac{(140 - \text{Age}) \cdot wt(d)^{0.7}}{1660} \qquad 4$$

where age and weight are in years and kilograms, respectively. Now, under any condition,

$$\begin{matrix}\text{Total} \\ \text{unbound} \\ \text{clearance}\end{matrix} = \begin{matrix}\text{Renal} \\ \text{unbound} \\ \text{clearance}\end{matrix} + \begin{matrix}\text{Extrarenal} \\ \text{unbound} \\ \text{clearance}\end{matrix} \qquad 5$$

Given that extrarenal, usually metabolic, clearance based on unbound drug does not change in renal insufficiency, but does change with age and weight, then on substituting Equations 1 to 4 into Equation 5 the following useful relationship is derived for R_d, the ratio of the unbound drug clearance in the individual patient with renal insufficiency and that in the typical patient requiring the drug.

★

$$R_d = \frac{CLu(d)}{CLu(n)} = RF \cdot fe(n) + (1 - fe(n)) \cdot \frac{(140 - \text{Age}) \cdot wt(d)^{0.7}}{1660} \qquad 6$$

Figure 16–5A illustrates the relationship between unbound clearance ratio, R_d, and renal function for various values of $fe(n)$ in a 55-year-old, 70-kilogram patient. It is apparent that R_d changes the most when $fe(n) = 1$ and is unchanged when $fe(n) = 0$. The value of $fe(n)$ is, by definition,

$$fe(n) = \frac{CLu_R(n)}{CLu(n)} = \frac{CL_R(n)}{CL(n)} \qquad 7$$

where $CL_R(n)$ and $CL(n)$ are the renal and total clearances of the drug in the typical patient for whom the usual regimen is intended. Experimentally, the value of $fe(n)$ is given by the fraction of an intravenous dose that is recovered unchanged in urine in a typical patient with normal renal function.

Recall that $t_{1/2} = 0.693\, Vu/CLu$. The value of the half-life of a drug in a patient with renal insufficiency, $t_{1/2}(d)$, compared to that in a patient with fully functioning kidneys, $t_{1/2}(n)$, is then

$$\frac{t_{1/2}(d)}{t_{1/2}(n)} = \frac{Vu(d)}{Vu(n)} \cdot \frac{1}{R_d} \qquad 8$$

where $Vu(d)$ and $Vu(n)$ are the unbound volumes of distribution in the patient with renal insufficiency and in the typical patient, respectively.

Also, recall that volume of distribution tends to vary in direct proportion to body weight. If renal function does not affect the unbound volume of distribution, then

$$\frac{t_{1/2}(d)}{t_{1/2}(n)} = \frac{wt(d)}{wt(n)} \cdot \frac{1}{R_d} \qquad 9$$

Figure 16–5B illustrates the dependence of half-life on both renal function and fraction excreted unchanged. Notice that half-life changes the most for a drug that is excreted entirely unchanged when renal function approaches zero.

An additional point needs to be made with respect to the data acquired in the different individuals in Figure 16–4. The x-axis, creatinine clearance, is a function of age, weight, and renal disease. One might expect that nonrenal clearance may also be related to age and weight. Higher values of nonrenal clearance occur in younger and larger patients, who have higher creatinine clearances, and smaller values are expected in older and smaller patients. This positive correlation of nonrenal clearance with creatinine clearance may distort the regression so that the y-intercept is lower and the slope is greater than expected. Ideally, the renal clearance of a drug should be correlated with creatinine clearance, and the nonrenal clearance should be examined separately for its dependence on age, weight, and perhaps renal disease.

Estimation of Renal Function

The commonly employed measures of renal function are based on creatinine, an endogenous substance that is derived from muscle catabolism and almost entirely excreted unchanged. The usefulness of creatinine lies in its clearance varying in direct proportion to the renal clearance of many drugs (e.g., Fig. 13–10).

In clinical practice, creatinine clearance is usually estimated from serum creatinine alone rather than from measurements of creatinine in both plasma and urine. Apart from the extra analysis involved, incomplete urine collection is a major problem resulting in the underestimation of creatinine clearance. The utility of serum creatinine, which can be used alone to estimate creatinine clearance, depends on the fact that under normal circumstances the daily production of creatinine is matched by its elimination. Consequently, serum creatinine is related to creatinine clearance by

$$\text{Serum creatinine} = \frac{\text{Rate of creatinine production}}{\text{Creatinine clearance}} \qquad \bigstar \atop 10$$

Table 16–2 summarizes some of the relationships currently found to approximate creatinine clearance from serum creatinine values. These relationships include corrections of creatinine production for age, weight, and gender. It should be emphasized that they are most accurate for individuals with an average muscle mass (source of creatinine) for their age, weight, and height. For emaciated, highly muscular, or obese adult patients, poor estimates are obtained. For these patients a creatinine clearance measurement may be more accurate than an estimate of its value from serum creatinine alone. This also applies to patients in whom there is an acute change in renal function, as discussed further

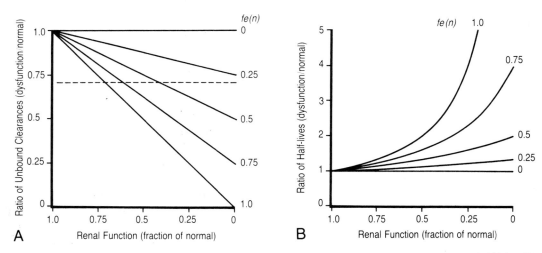

Fig. 16–5. The extent of decrease in unbound clearance, (A), and corresponding increase in half-life, (B), caused by renal dysfunction also depend on the fraction of available drug excreted in urine unchanged, *fe(n)*. Note that generally dose adjustment would not be considered unless the unbound clearance in the patient fell below 70 percent of the value for a typical patient with normal renal function for his/her age, that is, below the horizontal dotted line. The calculations have been made for a 70-kilogram patient of comparable age to a typical patient. The unbound volume of distribution of the drug is kept constant.

Table 16–2. Estimation of Creatinine Clearance in Adults[a] and Children[b]

| Population | Creatinine Clearance (ml/minute) | |
	Serum Creatinine in milligrams/deciliter	Serum Creatinine in micromolar units
Adults (20–100 years of age)[c]		
Males	$\dfrac{(140 - \text{Age}) \times \text{Weight}}{72 \times \text{Serum creatinine}}$	$\dfrac{1.23 \times (140 - \text{Age}) \times \text{Weight}}{\text{Serum creatinine}}$
Females	$\dfrac{(140 - \text{Age}) \times \text{Weight}}{85 \times \text{Serum creatinine}}$	$\dfrac{1.04 \times (140 - \text{Age}) \times \text{Weight}}{\text{Serum creatinine}}$
Children (1–20 years of age)[d]		
	$\dfrac{0.48 \times \text{Height}}{\text{Serum creatinine}} \times \left(\dfrac{\text{Weight}}{70}\right)^{0.7}$	$\dfrac{42.5 \times \text{Height}}{\text{Serum creatinine}} \times \left(\dfrac{\text{Weight}}{70}\right)^{0.7}$

[a]Adults 20 years of age and older. Poor estimates are obtained for obese and emaciated patients. Adapted from the review by Lott, R.S. and Hayton, W.L.: Estimation of creatinine clearance from serum creatinine concentration. Drug Intel. Clin. Pharm., *12*: 140–150, 1978.

[b]Children 1 to 20 years of age. Adapted from Traub, S.L. and Johnson, C.E.: Comparison of methods of estimating creatinine clearance in children. Am. J. Hosp. Pharm., *37*: 195–201, 1980.

[c]Age in years; body weight in kilograms.

[d]Height in centimeters; body weight in kilograms. The equation given by the authors has been modified to adjust for body surface area. A child of normal weight for height is assumed.

in Chapter 23, Turnover Concepts. Finally, on passing, it should be noted that both the rate of production of creatinine and creatinine clearance tend to decline in parallel with age. Consequently, serum creatinine remains relatively constant (about 1 mg/deciliter) from age 20 onward for patients with normal renal function for their age.

It remains to calculate the renal function in the individual patient. This value is given by

$$RF = CL_{cr}(d)/CL_{cr}(n)$$

★ 11

where $CL_{cr}(d)$ and $CL_{cr}(n)$ are the creatinine clearances in this patient and in the typical patient with normal renal function, respectively. The use of both renal function and fraction of drug excreted unchanged in dosage regimen adjustment for patients with renal disease is now presented.

Adjustment of Dosage Regimens

The alternatives for adjustment of maintenance and loading doses in patients with renal function impairment apply, in principle, to all disease conditions in which drug elimination is altered. For no other condition, however, is the adjustment required as readily predicted and assessed as for renal dysfunction.

Maintenance Rate. The simplest way of conceiving the adjustment of a maintenance regimen for a patient with renal insufficiency is to maintain the same average unbound concentration, $Cu_{ss,av}$, at steady state:

$$F \cdot \frac{D_M}{\tau} = CLu \cdot Cu_{ss,av}$$

12

The rate of administration of a drug in renal insufficiency, $(D_M/\tau)(d)$, compared to the normal rate of administration, $(D_M/\tau)(n)$, is then

$$\frac{(D_M/\tau)(d)}{(D_M/\tau)(n)} = \frac{CLu(d)}{CLu(n)} \cdot \frac{F(n)}{F(d)} \qquad\qquad 13$$

where $F(d)$ and $F(n)$ are the availabilities of drug in the patient with renal insufficiency and in the typical patient with normal renal function, respectively. When availability does not change, the rate of administration in a patient with renal dysfunction is

$$(D_M(\tau)/(d) = R_d \cdot (D_M/\tau)(n) \qquad\qquad \bigstar \quad 14$$

The reduction in dosing rate is therefore seen to depend only on the unbound clearance ratio, R_d. Associated with the reduction in renal function is a prolongation in half-life, which means that the time taken to achieve the desired plateau takes longer the more severe the dysfunction (Eq. 9). This last feature is illustrated in Figure 16–6 for constant-rate administration. In practice, administration is by discrete doses and an adjustment of a maintenance regimen may be made in one of several ways: decrease the frequency of administration, decrease the maintenance dose, or a combination of both. The outcome of these approaches is different. To appreciate the differences consider the adjustment of the usual regimen of amikacin sulfate, 7.5 milligrams/kilogram intramuscularly every 12 hours, to a 23-year-old, 68-kilogram patient with an estimated creatinine clearance of 14 milliliters/minute.

With the expected creatinine clearance in a typical 55-year-old, 70-kilogram patient with normal renal function being 85 milliliters/minute (Chap. 15), the value of RF in this patient is 0.165. Using Equation 14, it is apparent that the maintenance dosing rate of amikacin sulfate should be decreased by a factor of 6. Thus, the maintenance regimen might be one of the following: (1) The dosing interval may be increased sixfold, regimen: 500 milligrams (7.5 mg/kg · 68 kg)

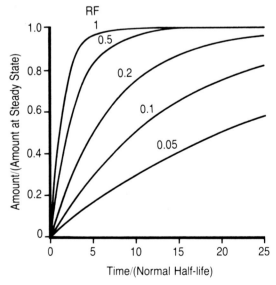

Fig. 16–6. It takes longer to reach plateau following constant-rate administration of a drug as renal function (RF) is reduced because half-life is correspondingly increased. The effect of renal insufficiency is particularly marked in this simulation in which $fe(n) = 1$. No effect is expected if $fe(n) = 0$. Note that time is expressed in units of half-life for a typical patient with normal renal function.

every 72 hours; (2) The maintenance dose may be reduced by a factor of 6, regimen: 83 milligrams every 12 hours; (3) Both the dosing interval and the maintenance dose may be adjusted to reduce the average dosing rate by sixfold, regimen: e.g., 167 milligrams every 24 hours.

The normal half-life of amikacin sulfate is 2 hours, so for the patient under consideration the half-life is prolonged sixfold to 12 hours (Eq. 9). Figure 16–7A is a sketch of the amount of drug in the body with time for the three maintenance regimens considered, assuming absorption from the intramuscular site is complete and instantaneous. Although both the time taken to reach plateau and the average amount of drug in body at plateau are the same for all three regimens, the picture is very different for each one. Clearly, changing the interval only (stippled curve) results in the greatest fluctuation, with many hours at both high and low levels. The desirability of this is difficult to support except in terms of convenience to the patient since the intramuscular dose need only be given every three days. Changing the maintenance dose only (solid curve) reduces fluctuation but suffers from the inconvenience of frequent intramuscular injections. Changing both the maintenance dose and the dosing interval (dotted curve) reduces both fluctuation and inconvenience to the patient and as such may be preferred for this drug and for many others.

In this example with amikacin, the administration of the usual dosage regimen to the patient with renal dysfunction resulted in a twofold increase in the maximum amount in the body and a sixfold increase in the average amount at plateau (Fig. 16–3). It is important, however, to consider whether the maximum amount (or concentration) or the average amount is more closely related to the efficacy and toxicity of the drug. Only a twofold reduction in the maintenance dosing rate would be required (Chap. 7) if the former were true. An argument can be made for wanting to attain high concentrations of this antimicrobial drug intermittently in order to optimize efficacy. However, chronic toxicity of the aminoglycosides has been shown to be related to the total exposure to the drug. Thus, elevation of the average level by a factor of three, when the maintenance

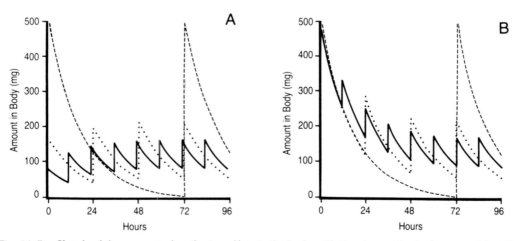

Fig. 16–7. Sketch of the amount of amikacin sulfate in the body with time in a patient whose renal function is 16.5 percent of normal. Shown are regimens without (A) and with (B) a 500-milligram loading dose. The maintenance regimens are: (---)–500 milligrams every 72 hours; (—)–83 milligrams every 12 hours; (···)–167 milligrams every 24 hours. Note: intravenous bolus administration is simulated.

dose is decreased by only one-half, may be undesirable. Which adjustment is the most appropriate for amikacin, as well as for other aminoglycosides, is debatable.

Loading Dose. Particularly large differences in the amount of amikacin in the body exist following the first dose of the three regimens just considered (Fig. 16–7A). With the regimen of 500 milligrams given every 72 hours to a patient with renal dysfunction, as with the regimen of 500 milligrams given every 12 hours to a patient with normal renal function, there is little accumulation because the dosing interval is much longer than the half-life. Accordingly, effective levels are reached after the first dose of drug. In contrast, in the patients with renal dysfunction appreciable accumulation occurs with the relatively frequent regimens of once every 12 or 24 hours. The initial dose is now much less than the average amount in the body at plateau. Under these circumstances, a case for a loading dose may be made. The size of the loading dose is open to debate, however. Making it the usual dose of 500 milligrams can lead to high levels in the body for an extended period after initiating therapy (Fig. 16–5B), which might increase the chance of an adverse effect. A smaller loading dose might be prudent. In the particular case of amikacin, based on experience, the manufacturer recommends not changing the usual loading dose.

General Guidelines and Limitations

Except for drugs with very low therapeutic indices, a reduction of less than 30 percent in the dosing rate, based on a change in renal function alone, is probably unwarranted. Variability in the absorption, distribution, and extrarenal elimination of drugs for a variety of reasons is usually at least of this magnitude, and the therapeutic range is often sufficiently large to make adjustment here unnecessary. Consequently, as long as the fraction excreted unchanged, $fe(n)$, is 0.30 or less and the metabolites are inactive, no change in a regimen is called for, based on renal function, regardless of the function. Similarly, regardless of the contribution of the renal route, if renal function is 0.70 of normal or greater, no change is needed (see Eq. 14). These recommendations are summarized in Figure 16–5A. The exception is the condition in which nonrenal clearance is changed by 0.30 or more and $fe(n)$ is less than 0.70.

As renal function approaches zero, the importance of nonrenal clearance increases. However, nonrenal clearance usually varies widely within the population, making calculation of the optimal dosage difficult for an individual with minimal renal function. When the fraction excreted unchanged approaches one and the renal function approaches zero, there is little elimination, and the dosing rate must be drastically reduced. Two particularly difficult problems are encountered here. One is the large change in the chronic requirements for a drug with only a small change in renal function, e.g., a change of 0.05 to 0.20 in renal function gives a quadrupling in the required rate of administration. The second problem is associated with the accuracy of measurements of renal function and the stability of the function itself. Administration of drugs with an $fe(n)$ approaching one to a patient with severe renal function impairment requires great caution. The plasma concentration and the therapeutic and toxic effects should be closely monitored in this situation.

A further complication in patients with severe renal function impairment is the concurrent and regular use of a dialysis technique to remove unwanted endogenous toxic substances, which would otherwise accumulate and cause problems. Unfortunately, dialysis sometimes also hastens the elimination of drugs from the body. This complication exacerbates drug therapy in these patients, a topic covered in Chapter 24 (Dialysis).

There are, of course, a number of assumptions on which the preceding adjustments are made. The method falters if: availability changes in renal dysfunction, which is relatively uncommon; metabolites are either therapeutically active, toxic, or both, or are converted back to drug, complications that are further discussed in Chapter 21 (Metabolite Kinetics); compromised renal function alters the ability to metabolize the drug, which occurs when the kidney is an organ of metabolism as well as excretion; or metabolism or renal excretion exhibits concentration-dependent kinetics, as the relationship between total clearance and renal function then becomes extremely complex. Also, the renal function is assumed to be constant with time, and the renal clearance of the drug is assumed to be directly proportional to the renal clearance of the compound used to determine renal function.

A note of caution should be emphasized on the last qualification. It is assumed that, regardless of whether the compound is eliminated primarily by glomerular filtration or by active secretion, the renal clearance of the compound decreases in proportion to the clearance of the compound used to determine renal function. This assumption appears to be valid to a first approximation. Para-aminohippuric acid, procainamide, carbenicillin, and penicillin are examples of actively secreted compounds whose renal clearances are apparently proportional to endogenous creatinine clearance and inulin clearance, regardless of the cause of renal function impairment.

Furthermore, no consideration has been given to intersubject differences in: absorption, distribution and metabolism, the response to a given plasma concentration, or disease state and physiologic functions. Renal function is only one of several sources of variability. Adjustment of drug administration based on renal function alone must be put into perspective.

Further Considerations

Renal disease often affects more than just renal clearance. Furthermore, other diseases that may alter dosage requirements are sometimes concurrently present. Digoxin, as previously mentioned, binds much less to tissues in uremia, resulting in a smaller volume of distribution and a shorter half-life than that predicted from the loss of renal function. This decreased tissue binding reduces the loading dose required, but has little or no effect on the maintenance dose of the drug. However, the presence of severe congestive cardiac failure, the condition for which the drug is most often used, is associated with decreased metabolic clearance and with a daily maintenance dosage requirement reduced beyond that expected for renal function impairment alone. The changes in digoxin clearance and volume of distribution with renal function and congestive cardiac failure, obtained from population pharmacokinetic studies, are summarized in Table 16–3.

Phenytoin and many other acidic drugs are two to three times less well-bound to plasma proteins in uremia than normal (Chap. 12). Part of this change is due

Table 16–3. Estimation of Clearance and Volume of Distribution of Digoxin in Patients with Mild and Severe Congestive Cardiac Failure[a]

Congestive Cardiac Failure	Clearance (liters/hour per kg)	Volume of Distribution (liters/kg)
Mild	CL_{cr}[b] $+ 0.048$[c]	$3.8 + 52 \cdot CL_{cr}$
Severe	$0.9 \cdot CL_{cr} + 0.02$	$3.8 + 52 \cdot CL_{cr}$

[a]Adapted from Sheiner, L.B., Rosenberg, B., and Marathe, V.V.: Estimation of population characteristics of pharmacokinetic parameters from routine clinical data. J. Pharmacokin. Biopharm., 5: 445–479, 1977.
[b]CL_{cr} = Creatinine clearance in liters/hour per kilogram.
[c]Approximation of nonrenal (metabolic) clearance.

to a decreased concentration of plasma albumin. The mechanism accounting for the rest of the change is uncertain, although displacement by an endogenous compound(s) that accumulates in renal impairment has been suggested. The unbound values of both clearance and volume of distribution of these principally metabolized drugs remain essentially unchanged, and no change in dosage regimen is anticipated in renal function impairment. The total plasma clearance, however, increases two- to threefold, giving rise to a corresponding drop in the steady-state plasma concentration. This change must be carefully considered when interpreting plasma concentrations of these drugs in patients with renal disease.

Perhaps, the *most* commonly invalid assumption is that metabolites are pharmacologically and toxicologically inactive. For example, the metabolite of procainamide, N-acetylprocainamide, is also active. Prediction of the total activity of the drug and of the dosage adjustment needed in renal failure can be much more complex. Nonetheless, there are ways of treating such situations, as given in Chapter 21, Metabolite Kinetics.

In this chapter, approaches have been presented for predicting changes in the clearance of drugs in various disease states. Rules for estimating the renal clearance of a drug from creatinine clearance or serum creatinine values have been given. This kind of information is useful for initiating drug therapy in an individual patient, but the variability remaining is often sufficiently large that plasma drug concentration monitoring, the topic of Chapter 18, is still prudent. In fact, the measurement of the drug concentration may allow estimation of the clearance of the drug in the individual patient, which is the information specifically sought.

Study Problems

(Answers to Study Problems are in Appendix G.)

1. List and briefly discuss six diseases in which the pharmacokinetics of drugs is known to be altered.

2. (a) Rank the situations in Table 16–4, from most important to least important, for considering a change in a dosage regimen of the cephalosporins listed in adult patients with varying degrees of renal function. Assume comparable therapeutic indices for all compounds. Use anticipated change in clearance as the basis of your ranking.

(b) Name the situations in Table 16–4 for which you would recommend a change in the usual dosage regimen.

Table 16–4.

Situation	Drug	Percent of Dose Normally Excreted Unchanged (fe(n))	Renal Function (percent of typical patient)
A	Ceftizoxime	28	10
B	Cefonicid	98	5
C	Cefamandole	96	40
D	Ceforanide	80	20
E	Ceftazidime	84	60

3. Table 16–5 summarizes pharmacokinetic observations of two different opioid analgesics in patients with and without hepatic cirrhosis.

Table 16–5[a].

	Pentazocine		Meperidine	
	Control	Cirrhotic	Control	Cirrhotic
Availability[b]	0.18	0.68	0.48	0.87
Blood Clearance[c] (liters/minute)	1.25	0.68	0.90	0.57

[a]Average of data from Neal, E.A., Meffin, P.J., Gregory, P.B., and Blaschke, T.F.: Gastroenterology, 77:96–102, 1979.
[b]From ratio of areas after oral and intravenous administrations on separate occasions.
[c]From Dose/AUC_b after an intravenous dose.

(a) Knowing that pentazocine and meperidine are eliminated primarily by hepatic metabolism, suggest a mechanism to explain the altered kinetics in hepatic cirrhosis.

(b) Explain why the availability of pentazocine is affected much more than that of meperidine.

4. In Table 16–6, various data on four patients with varying degrees of renal function are listed. None of them is undergoing a dialysis procedure.

Table 16–6.

Patient:	S.W.	B.J.	D.A.	B.T.
Gender	M	F	F	M
Age (years)	25	82	3	15
Weight (kilograms)	84	60	15	68
Height (centimeters)	182	160	96	169
Serum Creatinine (milligrams/deciliter)	1.0	2.5	1.6	3.0

(a) Estimate the creatinine clearance in each of these individuals.

(b) Calculate the renal function in each of these patients. Express renal function as a ratio of creatinine clearances in the patient to the value expected in a typical 55-year-old, 70-kilogram patient.

5. Vancomycin is chosen for the therapy of a 17-kilogram, 4-year-old, 108-centimeter tall boy with staphylococcal pneumonia, which is refractory to other antibiotics. The child has moderately impaired renal function as indicated by a serum creatinine of 2.7 milligrams/deciliter. Approximately 95 percent of a dose of vancomycin is normally excreted unchanged. Its half-life and volume of distribution are 6 hours and 0.4 liter/kilogram, respectively, in a typical 55-year-old patient.

   (a) Estimate the maximum and minimum steady-state concentrations associated with therapy in a typical 55-year-old patient who receives a 1,000-milligram bolus dose intravenously every 12 hours.

   (b) Determine a dosage regimen for the 4-year-old to attain and maintain the amount (or concentration) within the limits you derived in (a) above to minimize the likelihood of the child developing ototoxicity and a further decrease in renal function, both toxic manifestations of excessively high concentrations of vancomycin.

   (c) Prepare sketches of the anticipated amount of vancomycin in the body with time had the usual maintenance dose been adjusted for:

      1. The child's age and weight only (no adjustment for renal disease).

      2. The child's age, weight, and renal function.

      No loading dose is given in either situation.

17

Interacting Drugs

Objectives

The reader will be able to:

1. Explain why drug interactions are graded phenomena.

2. Ascertain whether the pharmacokinetics or the pharmacodynamics of a drug, or both, are altered by another drug, given unbound plasma drug concentration-time data.

3. Show graphically the consequence of a pharmacokinetic drug interaction when the mechanism of the interaction and the circumstances of its occurrence are given.

4. Anticipate the likely changes in the plasma and unbound concentrations of a drug with time when its pharmacokinetics is altered by concurrent drug therapy.

5. Suggest an approach to the modification in the dosage regimen of a drug when its pharmacokinetics is altered by concurrent drug administration.

Patients commonly receive two or more drugs concurrently; indeed, an in-patient on the average receives five drugs during a hospitalization. The reasons for multiple drug therapy are many. One reason is that combination drug therapy has been found to be beneficial in the treatment of some conditions, including a variety of cardiovascular diseases, infections, and cancer. Another reason is that patients frequently suffer from several diseases or conditions, and each may require the use of one or more drugs. Furthermore, drugs are prescribed by different clinicians, and each clinician may be unaware of the others' therapeutic maneuvers.

Multiple drug therapy can give rise to a *drug interaction*. A drug interaction occurs when either the pharmacokinetics or the pharmacodynamics of one drug is altered by another. Drug interactions are of concern because, occasionally, the outcome of concurrent drug administration is diminished therapeutic efficacy or increased toxicity of one or more of the administered drugs. A *therapeutic drug interaction* has then occurred. The undesirable consequences of a drug interaction may arise from a lack of understanding of, or a failure to recall, the mode of action and the pharmacokinetics of each drug; many undesirable interactions are therefore potentially avoidable.

255

The possibilities for interactions among drugs within the body are almost limitless. Yet few of these interactions are of a type or of a sufficient magnitude to be clinically important. Many interactions between drugs within the body take place without affecting either the unbound drug concentration or the therapeutic activity of the drugs involved. Also, the dosage of many drugs needed to demonstrate a clinically significant drug interaction can exceed the median lethal dose. Moreover, many affected processes and pathways of drug elimination are too minor to be of concern.

Implicit in the definition of drug interactions is the concept that, like essentially all responses of the body, they are graded. The degree of interaction depends on the concentration of the interacting species and hence on dose and time. Thus, drug interactions are a source of variability in drug response; they are a cause of additional variability within a patient population receiving the interacting drugs. This last point is well illustrated by the data in Table 17–1. Chloral hydrate, a sedative hypnotic, is thought to potentiate transiently the anticoagulant effects of warfarin. Yet in only 22 of 237 patients, who were studied prospectively and who received chloral hydrate during warfarin therapy, was potentiation of warfarin's effect unambiguously demonstrated. The reasons for these differences in response are many. Included are individual differences in the dosage regimen and duration of administration of each drug, in the sequence of drug administration, and in patient compliance. Pharmacodynamic and pharmacokinetic differences due to genetics, to concurrent disease states, and to many other factors also contribute. Thus, the circumstances associated with a clinically significant interaction in an individual should always be carefully documented.

A final general comment needs to be made before considering specific mechanisms of drug interactions. It deals with the sequence of drug administration. A drug interaction is likely to be detected only when the interacting drug is initiated or withdrawn. For example, given the usual large degree of variability in patients' response to drugs, it is unlikely that a drug interaction would be detected if the drug is administered to a patient stabilized on the interacting drug. Certainly the dosage regimen of the affected drug would be different than otherwise in *that* patient, but the resulting regimen is unlikely to be outside of

Table 17–1. Prospective Study of 237 Warfarin-Treated Patients for Detection of Interaction Between Warfarin and Chloral Hydrate[a]

Received chloral hydrate during warfarin therapy	237
During warfarin therapy received chloral hydrate for at least 3 consecutive days and did not receive chloral hydrate for at least 3 consecutive days before or after this period	69
Impossible to evaluate interaction (clinically unstable or multiple drug changes)	28
Potentiation of hypoprothrombinemic action of warfarin	22
No demonstrable interaction	19

[a]Abstracted from Koch-Weser, J.: Hemorrhagic reactions and drug interactions in 500 warfarin-treated patients. Clin. Pharmacol. Ther., *14*:139–146, 1973.

the normal range. In this case, only if the offending drug is withdrawn first, when the patient is stabilized on the drug combination, can the interaction be seen. Obviously the interaction would also have been detected if the interacting drug had been administered to the patient already stabilized on the original drug.

CLASSIFICATION

One system of classifying drug interactions is to note whether drug response is increased or decreased. While perhaps clinically useful, this classification does not help to define the mechanism of the interaction. In this book, interactions are classified on the basis of whether the pharmacokinetics or pharmacodynamics of a drug is altered; occasionally, both are changed. Distinction between the two is best made by relating response to the unbound concentration of the pharmacologically active species. No change in the unbound concentration-response curve implies a pharmacokinetic drug interaction, which can arise either through a physical interaction, such as competition for protein binding sites, or through altered physiology, such as altered blood flow at an absorption site. The result is a change in one or more of the primary pharmacokinetic parameters, ka, F, V, CL_R, CL_H, which in turn alter the secondary pharmacokinetic parameters, such as half-life and fe.

Before proceeding, a discussion of what is meant by the word *interaction* is worthwhile. Strictly speaking, this word implies a *mutual effect*. The interaction between two drugs, A and B, might thus be denoted by A ↔ B. An example is the competition between two drugs for a common binding site on albumin: One drug displaces but is also displaced by the other. Generally, however, the term interaction is interpreted more broadly to indicate any situation in which one drug affects another. For example, phenobarbital appears to reduce the absorption of the diuretic, furosemide, but the renal clearance of phenobarbital is increased by the diuresis produced by furosemide. This might be regarded as a *bidirectional interaction* and may be denoted by A ⇌ B. Clearly in the case of mutual and bidirectional interactions, the measured response of one drug cannot be considered without also defining the level of the other.

When given in sufficient quantities, two drugs almost always affect each other; this may not be the case, however, at concentrations achieved in therapy. For example, the H_2 antagonist, cimetidine, inhibits the metabolism of warfarin, but warfarin, at doses normally given, does not affect the response or the pharmacokinetics of cimetidine. This interaction is *unidirectional* and may be denoted by A → B. In a unidirectional interaction, the unaffected Drug, A, can be considered independently, but the change in response of the affected Drug, B, cannot be adequately defined without also considering the concentration-response curve of the effect of Drug A on Drug B.

The material in Chapters 8 to 12 forms the basis for discussing many aspects of pharmacokinetic drug interactions. For convenience, in this chapter, the effect of one drug on another is examined under the separate headings of altered absorption, displacement, and altered clearance. However, it should be borne in mind that several pharmacokinetic parameters can be altered simultaneously. Examples of drug interactions are listed in Table 17–2.

Table 17–2. Classification and Examples of Drug Interactions

	Pharmacodynamic Interactions		
	Response	Example	Comment
	↑	Digoxin ←[a] Chlorothiazide	By inducing hypokalemia chlorothiazide enhances digoxin cardiotoxicity.
		Chlorpheniramine ↔[b] Alcohol	Mutual sedative effects.
	↓	Guanethidine ← Chlorpromazine	Chlorpromazine blocks uptake of guanethidine at postganglionic adrenergic neuron.
		Warfarin ↔ Vitamin K₁	Each lowers the effectiveness of the other.

		Pharmacokinetic Interactions	
Parameter	Response	Example	Comment
Absorption rate	↑	Acetaminophen ← Metoclopramide	Metoclopramide hastens gastric emptying.
	↓	Lidocaine ← Epinephrine	Epinephrine decreases blood flow to subcutaneous and intramuscular sites of administration.
Availability	↑	Metoprolol ← Cimetidine	Cimetidine inhibits metoprolol metabolism, expressed as diminished first-pass effect.
	↓	Tetracycline ← Calcium	Calcium forms an insoluble complex with tetracycline.
Volume of distribution	↑	Salicylic acid ↔ Phenylbutazone	Competitive displacement from plasma (and tissue) binding sites.
	↓	Digoxin ← Quinidine	Quinidine displaces digoxin from tissue binding sites
Hepatic clearance	↑	Warfarin ← Phenobarbital	Phenobarbital induces microsomal enzymes.
	↓	Theophylline ← Erythromycin	Erythromycin inhibits theophylline metabolism.
Renal clearance	↑	Salicylic acid ← Bicarbonate	Elevated urine pH by bicarbonate diminishes tubular reabsorption of salicylate.
	↓	Benzylpenicillin ← Probenecid	Probenecid inhibits the secretion of penicillin.

[a]Denotes a unidirectional interaction; the arrow points to affected drug.
[b]Denotes a mutual interaction.

ALTERED ABSORPTION

It was stated in Chapters 4 and 7 that the more rapid the absorption process the higher and earlier is the peak plasma drug concentration and that neither the total area under the concentration-time curve after a single dose nor the area within a dosing interval at the plateau after chronic dosing changes unless the availability of the drug is altered. Therapeutic consequences of a change in either the rate or the extent of drug absorption were discussed in Chapter 7.

Considered now are situations in which availability is altered, with emphasis on the changes in average plasma concentration with time; an altered rate of absorption changes the degree of fluctuation around the average value. The situation considered pertains to the common ones of chronic drug therapy. These events are illustrated in Figure 17–1.

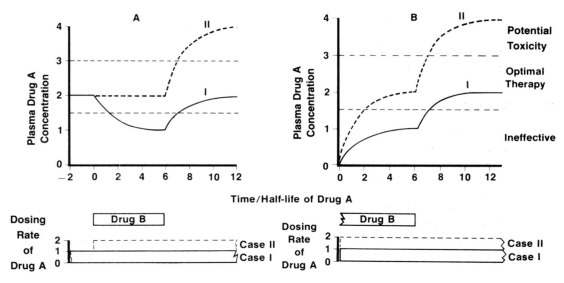

Fig. 17–1. Altered absorption. As long as Drug B is administered, the availability of Drug A is reduced by one-half. For simplicity, Drug A is assumed to be given at a constant rate; intermittent administration will produce fluctuations, but the general shape of the curve will not be altered. The therapeutic concentration range is assumed to lie between 1.5 and 3 units/liter for Drug A.

A, Patient stabilized on Drug A. The plasma concentration of Drug A will fall by one-half (case I), unless the dosing rate is doubled (case II), when Drug B is concurrently administered. A problem potentially arises if administration of Drug A is not reduced to its preexisting rate when Drug B is removed (case II).

B, Patient stabilized on Drug B. An adequate concentration of Drug A will not be achieved (case I) unless the usual dosing rate of this drug is doubled (case II). When Drug B is withdrawn, there is a potential problem similar to that considered in A.

Figure 17–1A depicts the situation in which a patient is stabilized on Drug A and receives Drug B, which reduces the availability of Drug A. It is apparent that if no steps are taken to change the dosing rate of Drug A, its concentration will fall to a lower plateau, the time being determined by the elimination half-life of this drug. Suppose that it was then noticed that the patient was no longer being treated effectively with Drug A, and that, having recognized the problem, the offending drug was withdrawn. The concentration of Drug A would then return, in 3.3 of its elimination half-lives, to the previous plateau value. Therapeutic control would again be restored. Alternatively, on another occasion, in anticipation of the problem but desiring to give the two drugs together, the dosing rate of Drug A is increased appropriately at the time that Drug B is introduced. As long as Drug B continues to be administered, therapeutic control is satisfactory. A problem arises, however, if Drug B is subsequently withdrawn, but the dosing rate of Drug A is not correspondingly reduced. Then, in 3.3 of its elimination half-lives, the concentration of Drug A in the body reaches a higher plateau and toxicity may result.

Another possible situation is one in which Drug A is added to the regimen of a patient stabilized on Drug B (Fig. 17–1B). Here, as before, optimal therapy with Drug A in the presence of Drug B is achieved only if the usual dosing rate is appropriately increased. However, the danger of the concentration of Drug A rising too high, if the dosing rate of Drug A is not readjusted when Drug B is withdrawn, must always be kept in mind.

The previous considerations emphasize the dependence of the time scale of events on the half-life of the affected drug. Thus, for drugs with very long half-lives, such as phenobarbital ($t_{1/2}$ of 5 days), changes in response of the affected drug will be insidious and the clinician may not associate the interaction with the causative drug, which was either initiated or stopped sometime previously.

DISPLACEMENT

The most common explanation for altered distribution in a drug interaction is displacement. Displacement is the reduction in the binding of a drug to a macromolecule, usually a protein, caused by competition of another drug, the *displacer*, for the common binding site(s). The result is a rise in the fraction of drug unbound in plasma or tissue, or both. Sometimes, drug binding is diminished through an allosteric effect. The second drug, binding at another site, induces a conformational change in the protein, thereby reducing the affinity of the first drug for the protein. Occasionally, an allosteric effect causes an enhanced affinity between drug and protein; drug binding is then increased.

Conditions Favoring Displacement

Two conditions must be met before substantial displacement occurs. First, in the absence of a displacer, most of the drug must be bound to a protein, that is, its value of *fu* must be low. Obviously, if the drug is not bound it cannot be displaced. Second, the displacer must occupy most of the binding sites, thereby substantially lowering the number of sites available to bind the drug. This second condition is most likely to be met when the displacer has a high affinity for the binding site and its concentration approaches or exceeds the molar concentration of the protein binding sites.

Table 17–3 lists two groups of acidic drugs that bind to albumin, a protein that exists abundantly in plasma (120 grams/3 liters; 0.6 millimolar) and in the interstitial fluids (150 grams). Not all of the drugs bind to and hence compete for the same primary binding site on albumin. Albumin and some other proteins have many binding sites, each exhibiting some degree of specificity; possessing an acidic function is not a sufficient criterion for predicting the ability of one

Table 17–3. Binding of Selected Acidic Drugs to Albumin[a]

Drugs That Bind to and Compete for One of Two Sites, Designated A and B, on Albumin

Site A	Site B
Chlorothiazide	Benzodiazepines
Furosemide	Cloxacillin
Indomethacin[b]	Dicloxacillin
Naproxen[b]	Glibenclamide
Phenylbutazone	Ibuprofen
Phenytoin	Indomethacin
Sulfadimethoxine	Naproxen
Tolbutamide[b]	Probenecid
Valproate	Tolazamide
Warfarin	Tolbutamide

[a] Abstracted from Sjöholm, J., Ekman, B., Kober, A., Ljungstedt-Pohlman, I., Seiving, B., and Sjödin, T.: Binding of drugs to human serum albumin: XI. Mol. Pharmacol., *16*:767–777, 1979.
[b] These drugs bind to both sites.

acidic drug to displace another. Moreover, even though almost all those drugs that compete for the same site have a high affinity for albumin, only a few are generally listed as displacers, such as salicylic acid, phenylbutazone, and some sulfonamides. This list is limited because the plasma concentration achieved during therapy must approach or exceed 0.6 millimolar, the concentration of plasma albumin. For a substance with a molecular weight of 250, this concentration corresponds to 150 milligrams/liter. This concentration is achieved during salicylate and sulfonamide therapy, because these drugs are commonly given in doses approaching 1 gram and because they possess relatively small volumes of distribution, 10 to 20 liters. With phenylbutazone the plasma concentration achieved with the usual dose, 100 milligrams (V = 10 liters), is only 10 milligrams/liter, but because its clearance is low and half-life is long (3 days), the plateau concentration ultimately achieved is high when the usual maintenance regimen of 100 to 300 milligrams daily is administered.

Displacers share an expected common property, that is, their value of *fu* changes with plasma concentration. With most sites occupied by the displacer, the fraction unoccupied is sensitive to a change in the concentration of displacer. Therefore, displacers must show concentration-dependent disposition kinetics (Chap. 22, Dose and Time Dependencies).

So far, distinction has been made between displacers and the displaced drug, but it should be apparent that this classification is arbitrary. Phenylbutazone is said to displace warfarin from albumin, but only because the plasma concentration of phenylbutazone (100 mg/liter) approaches the molar concentration of albumin, whereas that of warfarin (1 to 4 mg/liter) does not. Both drugs have approximately the same affinity for the same site on albumin, and if the concentrations were reversed, warfarin would be called the displacer.

The conclusions drawn from the interactions between acidic drugs and albumin are generally applicable to all drug-protein interactions, bearing in mind the widely differing molar concentrations of the various binding proteins in plasma (Chap. 10, p. 137). For example, the molar concentrations of the specialized transport proteins, which avidly bind many hormones, are very low, and therefore displacement interactions between synthetic and endogenous steroids can occur at low plasma concentrations of these substances.

Therapeutic Implications

Displacement interactions in plasma have been studied primarily *in vitro*. The drug of interest is added to a sample of plasma and any changes in its binding are measured. Substantial displacement from plasma proteins can frequently be demonstrated *in vitro*; yet this may be of little therapeutic consequence. It depends on whether one considers acute events or events at plateau.

Acute Events. Two situations can be envisaged. One involves the administration of a loading dose of drug to a patient already stabilized on the displacer. The other involves the administration of a dose of displacer to a patient already stabilized on the drug. In both situations, the question of altering the usual dose of drug would arise only if, in the presence of the displacer, the unbound drug concentration was to be much higher than usual, or stated differently, the unbound volume of distribution (Vu) was to decrease significantly. This decrease in Vu would occur only if, in the absence of the displacer, the drug was substantially bound in the body and the displacer caused significant displacement of drug from the major binding sites. That is, the unbound concentration would rise if displacement occurred from plasma binding sites for a drug with a small volume of distribution, around 10 liters/70 kilograms, or if displacement occurred from tissue binding sites for a drug with a large volume of distribution. An example of the former situation is the displacement of warfarin from albumin binding sites by phenylbutazone. An example of the latter situation is the displacement of digoxin from tissue binding sites by quinidine. These situations are relatively uncommon, however. More common is displacement from plasma binding sites for a drug with a large volume of distribution. Then, because so little drug resides in plasma, there would be only a minimal change in the unbound drug concentration even if all the drug in plasma is displaced, as discussed in Chapter 10. For example, if the volume of distribution of a drug is 100 liters and 99 percent of the drug in plasma is bound ($fu = 0.01$), then only 3 percent (($1 - fu$) · (plasma volume)/V) of drug in the body would reside bound in plasma. Even if completely displaced, the small amount affected would redistribute throughout the rest of the body and so would only marginally increase the unbound body pool, and hence unbound concentrations in plasma and tissue. Conceivably, if the displacer was injected rapidly the unbound drug concentrations in plasma would rise appreciably, but only momentarily, because displaced drug would move rapidly down the newly created unbound concentration gradient into the large tissue water space. In practice, this last situation is unlikely to occur because of the problems experienced with a drug injected rapidly. An exception is the rapid injection of some drugs used in an emergency setting, but even then many do not have the required properties of a displacer.

Returning to the two examples above: With digoxin, quinidine causes a sufficiently large increase in Vu to warrant considering a reduction in the loading dose of digoxin in the presence of quinidine. With warfarin, because the clinical response (prothrombin time) is so insensitive to acute changes in warfarin concentration (Fig. 5–6, Chap. 5), no adjustment in dosage of this oral anticoagulant would be contemplated in the event of acute displacement. A more important consideration for both these drugs and for most others is the effect of displacement on events at plateau, as most drugs, including displacers, are given chronically.

Events at Plateau. The influence of displacement on the unbound concentration at steady state (Cu_{ss}) depends on the extraction ratio of the drug and perhaps on the route of drug administration.

Consider a drug with a low extraction ratio. Recall the following facts: Clearance depends on fu, but unbound clearance (CLu) does not; the rate of drug elimination is directly proportional to the unbound concentration, Cu. Recall also the equality (Eq. 3, Chap. 11)

$$\text{Rate of elimination} = CLu \cdot Cu = CL \cdot C \qquad 1$$

When drug is infused at a constant rate, R_0, and steady state is achieved,

$$R_0 = CLu \cdot Cu_{ss} = CL \cdot C_{ss} \qquad 2$$

However, since unbound clearance, e.g., that of a glomerularly filtered drug, is unaffected by displacement, the same is true of the value of Cu_{ss}. Thus, although displacement by increasing fu increases clearance (and hence causes the total plasma concentration to fall), no change in response and therefore in dosing rate is anticipated at steady state. Neither is any change anticipated, following displacement, in the average unbound concentration at plateau, $Cu_{ss,av}$, upon chronic oral dosing.

Now consider a drug with a high extraction ratio. Since clearance is unaffected by displacement, the steady-state blood concentration is also unaffected following a constant-rate intravenous infusion. However, as binding is diminished, the value of Cu_{ss} and therefore the response to the drug must be increased. The maintenance dose of the drug may need to be reduced.

Prediction of the outcome when a drug with a high extraction ratio is given orally and when elimination occurs predominantly in the liver is difficult. In the presence of the displacer, both unbound drug clearance and availability decrease (see Chap. 12); the effect of displacement on the unbound drug concentration at plateau is therefore likely to be relatively small. Irrespective of any effect of displacement, however, the unbound concentration at plateau is always lower than that achieved following an equivalent intravenous dosing rate.

The events predicted at plateau before and after displacement for drugs of low and high extraction are shown in Figure 17–2. Shown in Figure 17–3 are the total and unbound plateau plasma concentrations of the antiepileptic drug, phenytoin, in patients before and after receiving valproate, another antiepileptic drug, which displaces phenytoin from albumin binding sites. As predicted for phenytoin, a drug of low extraction, although the total plasma concentration is decreased, the unbound concentration is unaltered. Accordingly, there is no need to alter the dosing rate of phenytoin in patients receiving valproate. Corresponding data for a drug of high extraction is currently unavailable. It is likely, however, that the predictions made for such a drug will hold.

Kinetic Features. Both acute events and events at plateau have been discussed. It remains to discuss the kinetic consequences of displacement on approach to plateau under the usual condition in which both drug and displacer are given chronically. To do this, the expected changes in the disposition kinetics of a drug, with displacement, need to be considered.

Disposition Kinetics. The points made here summarize those made in Chapters 10 to 12. Because clearance of a drug with a high extraction ratio is unaffected

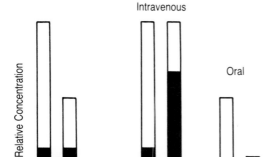

Low Extraction   High Extraction

Intravenous

Oral

Relative Concentration

C D   C D   C D

Fig. 17–2. The influence of displacement (D) on the control values (C) of the total (▣) and unbound (■) concentrations at plateau depends on the extraction ratio for the drug and the route of drug administration. For a drug of low extraction ratio, diminished binding (fu ↑) reduces the total, but not the unbound, concentration regardless of the route of administration. For a drug of high hepatic extraction ratio, clearance, and so total concentration, is unaffected by diminished binding when the drug is given intravenously. The unbound concentration, however, is elevated. Because diminished binding decreases availability of the highly cleared drug, the likely outcome of displacement is a decrease in the total concentration and little or no change in the unbound concentration, depending on whether the effect on availability or clearance predominates.

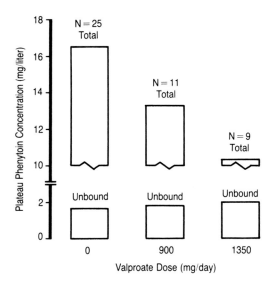

Fig. 17–3. The valproate-phenytoin interaction involves displacement only. Although plasma protein binding of phenytoin is decreased when sodium valproate is administered chronically to a group of patients stabilized on phenytoin, with a resultant fall in the steady-state plasma phenytoin concentration, there was no substantial change in the unbound phenytoin concentration. These observations are consistent with a displacement interaction of phenytoin by valproic acid. Note that the degree of phenytoin displacement depends on the dose of sodium valproate. Of the 25 patients stabilized on phenytoin, 11 received 900 milligrams sodium valproate per day; 9 received a 1350-milligram daily dose; and some received both. (One mg/liter = 4.0 micromolar.) (Taken from Mattson, R.H., Cramer, J.A., Williamson, P.D., Novelly, R.A.: Valproic acid in epilepsy: Clinical and pharmacological effects. Ann. Neurol., 3: 20–25, 1978.)

by displacement, the half-life changes with volume of distribution, which generally increases. In contrast, for a drug of low extraction, because unbound clearance, CLu, does not change, half-life either does not change (when Vu does not change) or shortens (if Vu decreases) with displacement.

Plasma Concentration-Time Profile. Although there are many possible combinations of events, only one situation, the most common, is considered. In this case (Fig. 17–4), the displacer is added to the regimen of a patient stabilized on a low extraction ratio drug. To simplify matters, both drug and displacer are

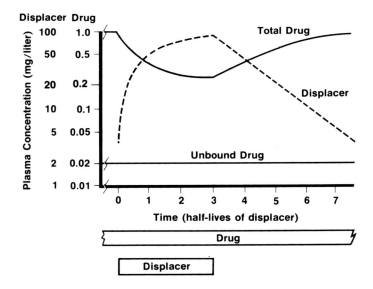

Fig. 17–4. When constantly infused, the unbound concentration of a drug with a low extraction ratio remains virtually unchanged if a displacer with a long half-life, relative to the drug, is either infused or withdrawn. The change in plasma drug concentration reflects the displacement.

administered by constant-rate infusion and both are assumed to always be at distribution equilibrium. While these conditions are somewhat restrictive, the situation chosen does illustrate the importance of both kinetics and the manner of drug administration on the likely therapeutic outcome.

Considered next is the chronic administration, without a loading dose, of a displacer, which has a half-life longer than that of the drug. This is a relatively common situation in practice, for two reasons. First, because of the previously mentioned potential risks, administration of a loading dose of the displacer is uncommon. Second, because the high concentration required for significant displacement is, in general, more likely to be achieved with a drug that has a long half-life, one with a short half-life would have to be given either in a large dose or frequently, both unlikely events.

Notice in Figure 17–4 that slow accumulation and correspondingly slow elimination of the displacer results in insignificant changes in the unbound drug concentration and therefore response. This is a consequence of the kinetics of the displacer being the rate-limiting step. The concentration of the displacer is changing so slowly relative to that of the drug that at all times the drug is at a virtual steady state, with rate of elimination ($CLu \cdot Cu_{ss}$) matching the rate of administration. That is, although there is a tendency for the unbound drug concentration to rise above the concentration at steady-state during accumulation of the displacer, it is compensated for by the opposing tendency for the unbound concentration to fall because the rate of elimination ($CLu \cdot Cu$) would then exceed the rate of administration ($CLu \cdot Cu_{ss}$). The reverse tendencies occur on stopping the displacer, but once again they balance each other out. Accordingly, although the unbound concentration remains essentially unaltered, the total plasma drug concentration changes with that of the displacer, reflecting the changing degree of displacement. A transient change in unbound concentration might occur if the kinetics of the drug, rather than that of the displacer, had been the slower or rate-limiting step, but as mentioned previously, this is an unlikely situation.

In the case just discussed no change in the effect and hence in the dosage regimen of the drug is anticipated even though displacement had occurred. Indeed, if only response were monitored, displacement would not have been suspected.

DIMINISHED UNBOUND CLEARANCE

A reduction of the unbound clearance of a drug is potentially the most dangerous type of drug interaction. The unbound drug concentration can rise to a toxic level, unless an adjustment in dosage is made. Consequently, it is extremely important to be able to identify, to characterize, and where possible, to avoid this type of interaction. Inhibition of drug metabolism is the major cause of reduced unbound clearance.

An Equilibrium Consideration

The phenylbutazone→warfarin interaction, whereby phenylbutazone produces a sustained enhancement in the anticoagulant effect of warfarin and sometimes causes serious bleeding episodes, is well documented. Warfarin is highly bound in plasma to albumin. Phenylbutazone, devoid of inherent anticoagulant activity, displaces warfarin. Consequently, displacement has been advocated as the primary mechanism for this interaction.

Figure 17–5 shows the temporal effects of phenylbutazone administration on the plasma and unbound concentrations of warfarin in a subject who ingested 10 milligrams warfarin daily. The half-life of warfarin is approximately 2 days, and therefore, as anticipated, a steady state for this drug was reached within the first 12 days, when warfarin alone was administered. At that time the warfarin plasma concentration was approximately 4 milligrams/liter and only 0.5 percent (0.02 mg/liter) is unbound, that is, $fu = 0.005$. Warfarin is completely absorbed, and therefore its clearance, estimated by dividing the daily dosing rate by the steady-state plasma concentration, is 0.1 liter/hour. Thus, warfarin is a highly bound drug with a low extraction ratio.

Phenylbutazone is also poorly extracted, is highly bound ($fu = 0.004 - 0.010$), and has a half-life (approximately 3 days) even longer than that of warfarin. Accordingly, when on day 13 the subject commenced the usually recommended dosage regimen of phenylbutazone, 100 milligrams 3 times a day, the plasma concentration of this drug rose and eventually reached a plateau of approximately 100 milligrams/liter, after approximately 8 days. During this period, the plasma warfarin fell steadily in half, to 2 milligrams/liter, and the value of fu for warfarin rose approximately threefold.

At this point, the situation and the events appear remarkably similar to those depicted in Figure 17–4: A pure displacement interaction. However, there is one important difference: The unbound warfarin concentration rose and remained

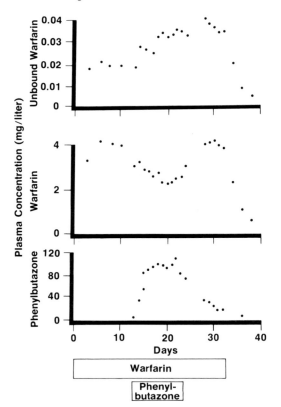

Fig. 17–5. Warfarin-phenylbutazone interaction. A subject received 10 milligrams warfarin orally each day and 100 milligrams phenylbutazone three times a day on days 13 to 22. As the phenylbutazone concentration rose, bound warfarin was displaced and the plasma warfarin concentration fell. The sustained elevation in the unbound warfarin during phenylbutazone administration implies inhibition of warfarin elimination. (Phenylbutazone: One mg/liter = 3.2 micromolar; warfarin: One mg/liter = 3.3 micromolar.) (Modified from Schary, W.L., Lewis, R.J., and Rowland, M.: Warfarin-Phenylbutazone interaction in man: A long term multiple-dose study. Res. Commun. Chem. Pathol. Pharmacol., 10:663–672, 1975.)

elevated during phenylbutazone administration. Because the effect of warfarin is related to its unbound concentration, this sustained elevation is in accord with the observed sustained augmentation of the effect as long as phenylbutazone is coadministered. Examination of Equation 2 indicates that to account for the elevated values of unbound drug, either the rate of entry of drug into the body is increased or the value of CLu is decreased. Since the dosage regimen of warfarin was unaltered and warfarin is fully available, CLu must have decreased.

Warfarin is almost exclusively metabolized in the liver to either weakly active or inactive metabolites. Thus, a lower value for CLu implies a decrease in the ability of the liver to metabolize warfarin. Analysis of several metabolites of warfarin in both plasma and urine subsequently confirmed that, indeed, phenylbutazone inhibits warfarin elimination, and it is this inhibition and not displacement that accounts for the clinical picture.

The interaction between phenylbutazone and warfarin is even more complex than portrayed above. Commercial warfarin is a racemate, that is, a 50:50 mixture of $R(+)-$ and $S(-)-$ warfarin, and the $S(-)$ isomer is five times more active than the $R(+)$ isomer. Phenylbutazone primarily inhibits the formation of 7-(S)-hydroxywarfarin, the major metabolite of the more active isomer. The lesson is clear: Drug interactions can be complex; careful observations are required to unravel the facts.

A Graded Response

The pharmacokinetics of warfarin is independent of dose because the unbound plasma concentration, Cu, is below the value for the Michaelis-Menten constant, Km. Thus, for each metabolic pathway

$$\text{Rate of metabolite formation} = \frac{Vm}{Km} \cdot Cu \qquad 3$$

or expressed in terms of the unbound clearance associated with the metabolite formation, CLu_f,

$$\text{Rate of metabolite formation} = CLu_f \cdot Cu = fm \cdot CL \cdot Cu \qquad 4$$

where fm is the fraction of the dose of drug that is converted to the metabolite. In the presence of an inhibitor the rate of metabolite formation is slowed; the value of the new rate being given by the expression

★

$$\text{Rate of metabolite formation} = \frac{CLu_f \cdot Cu}{1 + Cu_I/K_I} \qquad 5$$

where Cu_I is the unbound concentration of the inhibitor and K_I is the inhibition constant, given by the unbound concentration of inhibitor that decreases the clearance associated with the metabolite formation twofold. According to this relationship, the degree of inhibition of warfarin 7-hydroxylation should vary with the plasma concentration of phenylbutazone. Unfortunately, such data are not presently available, but they are for the interaction between the sulfonamide, sulfaphenazole, and the oral hypoglycemic agent, tolbutamide.

Sulfaphenazole is no longer prescribed. One reason is that it inhibits the metabolism of a number of drugs and thereby causes excessive drug accumulation and toxicity. For example, hypoglycemic crises have been reported when patients, stabilized on tolbutamide, have had sulfaphenazole added to their drug therapy; the half-life of tolbutamide, usually 4 to 8 hours, was prolonged to values ranging from 24 to 70 hours. Moreover, oxidation to hydroxytolbutamide is the obligatory pathway of tolbutamide elimination, that is, $CLu_f = CLu$ and $fm = 1$. If it is assumed that sulfaphenazole does not substantially affect the volume of distribution of tolbutamide and its volume of distribution is constant, then Equation 5 can be written for tolbutamide in the simple form:

$$\text{Rate of tolbutamide elimination} = \frac{k \cdot A}{1 + A_I/K_I} \qquad 6$$

where A and A_I are the amounts of tolbutamide and sulfaphenazole in the body, and K_I may now be defined as the amount of inhibitor that diminishes the apparent elimination rate constant, $k/(1 + A_I/K_I)$, of tolbutamide by one-half, or doubles the half-life of tolbutamide. For sulfaphenazole, the K_I value is 200 milligrams. This value is small compared to the 1- to 2-gram daily dose of the sulfonamide that was usually recommended.

Given the preceding information it is now possible to appreciate why a hypoglycemic crisis did not usually occur until many days after sulfaphenazole had been added to the patient's regimen and why treatment of the crisis often had to be continued for several days, even though the administration of both drugs was stopped.

The likely events following oral administration of 0.5 gram tolbutamide and 1.0 gram sulfaphenazole twice daily are portrayed in Figure 17–6. Initially, when only tolbutamide is given the expected plateau is reached within 3 to 4 half-lives or by 30 hours. When sulfaphenazole is also given, it accumulates and blocks tolbutamide oxidation, ultimately causing a rise in the amount of the sulfonylurea to approximately seven times its usual value. Also a period of 2 to 3 days is required before this elevated amount of tolbutamide falls to the level observed in the absence of sulfaphenazole or falls to zero if both drugs are stopped.

A more exact quantitative picture of the events may be gained from two equations. One, previously examined (Eq. 7, Chap. 7), defines the average amount of drug at plateau

$$A_{ss,av} = \frac{1.44 \cdot \text{Dose} \cdot \text{Half-life}}{\text{Dosing interval}} \qquad 7$$

The other follows from Equation 6. The term $k/(1 + A_I/K_I)$ can be considered as the new (and smaller) elimination rate constant of tolbutamide in the presence of the inhibitor. It follows therefore that the new half-life of tolbutamide ($t_{1/2,\text{inhibited}}$) is related to the normal half-life ($t_{1/2,\text{normal}}$) by

★

$$t_{1/2,\text{inhibited}} = t_{1/2,\text{normal}} \cdot [1 + (A_I/K_I)] \qquad 8$$

Obviously, the value of the half-life changes continuously with changes in the amount of inhibitor in the body, but once sulfaphenazole reaches a plateau, the half-life of tolbutamide becomes constant. For example, when 1 gram of sulfaphenazole ($t_{1/2} = 12$ hours) is given twice daily, the average amount of inhibitor

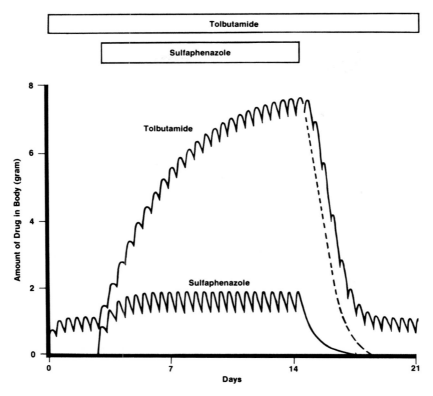

Fig. 17–6. Tolbutamide-sulfaphenazole interaction kinetics simulation when tolbutamide (0.5 gram, twice daily) is given in the absence and in the presence of sulfaphenazole (1 gram, twice daily). The bars denote the duration of each drug regimen. In the presence of sulfaphenazole, an inhibitor of tolbutamide oxidation, the amount of tolbutamide rises from one plateau to another, when output once again equals input. Upon cessation of sulfaphenazole, the decline of tolbutamide, whether continued (solid line) or stopped at the same time as sulfaphenazole (dotted line), is primarily controlled by the rate of removal of sulfaphenazole. Consequently, several days elapse before the level of tolbutamide once again falls into the accepted therapeutic range. (From Rowland, M., and Matin, S.B.: Kinetics of drug-drug interactions. J. Pharmacokin. Biopharm., *1*: 553–567, 1973.)

in the body at plateau, according to Equation 7, is 1.4 grams. This plateau is reached within two days. Substituting this amount of inhibitor into Equation 8 indicates that the new half-life of tolbutamide is eight times (1 + 1.4 grams/0.2 gram) longer than normal, that is, 32 to 64 hours. Accordingly, it takes approximately one week to reach a new plateau; the average amount of tolbutamide in the body is now eight times the average plateau value in the absence of the inhibitor (Eq. 7).

These data suggest that if tolbutamide and sulfaphenazole had to be given together, the dosing rate of tolbutamide would have to be reduced by a factor of 8 to maintain the normal amount of tolbutamide in the body at plateau. These data also explain why stopping tolbutamide at the same time as sulfaphenazole would not resolve a toxicity problem much quicker than stopping sulfaphenazole alone; the rate of decline of tolbutamide is determined by its half-life and that in turn is controlled by the rate of removal of sulfaphenazole. Interestingly, tolbutamide has no demonstrable effect on sulfaphenazole elimination; this sulfonamide is eliminated primarily by glucuronidation.

The influence of inhibition on tolbutamide kinetics is dramatic because this drug is eliminated by only one pathway, $fm_1 = 1$, instead of several, the more usual situation. Commonly, one pathway may only account for 50 percent ($fm_1 = 0.5$) or less of drug elimination. Then, even if this pathway is completely inhibited, the half-life of the drug increases by no more than twofold. Because the average amount of drug in the body would also not be raised more than twofold, no change in the dosage regimen of the drug may be warranted, unless the therapeutic index of the drug is small.

Inhibition of metabolism and secretion are examples of a chemically mediated pharmacokinetic interaction. The lower hepatic clearance of lidocaine when given together with propranolol, a β-adrenergic blocking drug, is an example of a physiologically mediated pharmacokinetic interaction. Propranolol diminishes cardiac output and hence hepatic blood flow, which, in turn, reduces the clearance of lidocaine, a drug highly extracted by the liver. Presumably, since the degree of β-adrenergic blockade is a graded response, the interaction with lidocaine is dependent on the plasma concentration of propranolol.

Beneficial Interactions

Penicillin-probenecid combination therapy is an example of the successful use of a drug interaction. Both of these acidic drugs are renally secreted by an anionic transport system. Probenecid competitively inhibits the renal secretion of penicillin thereby substantially reducing its renal clearance, the major component of total clearance. Consequently, in the presence of probenecid, higher than usual plasma concentrations of penicillin are achieved following a normal dosage regimen of the antibiotic. Of note is the lack of a major effect of penicillin on probenecid elimination. Although actively secreted into the kidney tubule, being lipophilic, unlike penicillin, probenecid is mostly reabsorbed. Consequently, the renal clearance of probenecid is low; metabolism is the major route of its elimination.

ELEVATED UNBOUND CLEARANCE

The unbound clearance of a drug can be increased in numerous ways. Raising urine pH by giving acetazolamide or sodium bicarbonate increases the renal clearance of salicylic acid and other acids whose renal clearance is pH sensitive. Giving ammonium chloride or ascorbic acid to make the urine more acidic increases the renal clearance of pH-sensitive basic drugs. Some drugs increase the metabolic clearance of other drugs. They do so most commonly by inducing the drug-metabolizing enzymes, but they may also activate enzymes or retard enzyme degradation. Occasionally, like glucagon, they increase hepatic blood flow and thereby increase the hepatic clearance of drugs that are highly extracted by the liver.

The resulting changes in the pharmacokinetic parameters and the kinetic consequences of an increased metabolic clearance were discussed in Chapters 11 and 12. The implications of these changes on dosage requirements and the events that follow the addition or the withdrawal of the drug causing the altered clearance are now presented.

In general, a dosage regimen adjustment is required only when the clearance of the affected pathway is or becomes a significant fraction of total drug clearance. Thus, a need to change the dose is anticipated if the clearance associated with a particular pathway, previously 20 percent of total clearance, were to increase sixfold, because total drug clearance is doubled. In contrast, a need to change the dose is not anticipated, even if metabolic clearance increased twentyfold, if this clearance usually contributes only 1 percent to the total clearance. An exception arises when the metabolite formed is either the active species or is toxic, because its plasma concentration can be greatly increased.

The events depicted in Figure 17–7 illustrate salient consequences of an increased clearance. It is assumed that a patient, stabilized on one drug, also receives another that doubles the value of the clearance of the first drug. If the dosing rate of the first drug is not changed, then the concentration of this drug will fall by one-half, at a rate determined by the half-life of the drug *in the presence of the second drug*. The fall in concentration can be avoided by doubling the rate of administration of the first drug for as long as the second drug is given. However, a problem of excessive accumulation of the first drug exists if the higher dosing rate is maintained when the second drug is withdrawn. Because the half-life of the first drug is generally longer when given alone, especially for a drug of low extraction ratio, it follows that the time taken to reach a plateau is longer in the absence than in the presence of the second drug.

Two major assumptions were made in constructing the curves in Figure 17–7, namely, that the effect of the second drug is achieved instantly and remains constant as long as it is administered, and that the effect immediately disappears upon withdrawing the second drug. In practice, both assumptions are invalid.

Enzyme induction was mentioned as the prime cause of increased metabolic clearance. However, a change in clearance is an indirect measure of the effect of an inducer; the direct effect is an increase in the synthesis rate of the drug-metabolizing enzyme. Accordingly, there is a delay between the direct effect and its reflection in the measured response. Thus, even if the plasma concentration of the inducer was attained instantly and then maintained constantly, the clearance of the drug would increase with time as the enzyme level rose

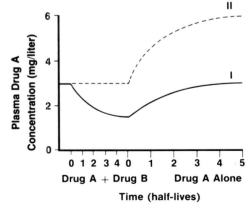

Fig. 17–7. When a patient stabilized on Drug A also receives Drug B, a drug which increases twofold the clearance of Drug A, the plasma concentration of Drug A falls (case I) unless the dosing rate is doubled (case II). The problem of excessive accumulation arises if the administration of Drug A is not reduced to the previous rate when the administration of Drug B is stopped. Note that the time to reach a plateau is less in the presence, than in the absence, of Drug B.

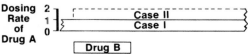

from one plateau value to another. Similarly, there would be a delay in the decrease of drug clearance on removing the inducer. The magnitude of the time delay depends, like other systems in the body, on where the rate-limiting step lies.

When elimination of enzyme is the rate-limiting step, then changes in the clearance of the drug may continue to occur even though the concentration of the inducer is relatively constant. When, however, elimination of the inducer is the rate-limiting step, changes in the concentration of inducer are then reflected relatively instantaneously by changes in the amount of enzyme and hence clearance of the affected drug. This last possibility may explain the effect of phenobarbital on the temporal changes in the plasma concentration of dicumarol and its prothrombin time, a measure of its anticoagulant effect, in a patient receiving dicumarol chronically (Fig. 17–8). Both the fall in the concentration and the drug's effect following phenobarbital treatment have been attributed to the barbiturate inducing the enzymes responsible for dicumarol metabolism. It took approximately 3 to 4 weeks for the plasma dicumarol both to fall to a minimum during phenobarbital administration and to return to the prebarbiturate value after phenobarbital was discontinued. Phenobarbital ($t_{1/2}$ of 5 days) also takes approximately the same period of time to reach a plateau in the body and to be eliminated. Thus, the observations are compatible with the hypothesis that the induced enzyme system responds relatively rapidly to changes in plasma phenobarbital concentration; that is, phenobarbital elimination rate-limits the process. For a further discussion of the kinetic aspects of induction, see Chapter 23, Turnover Concepts.

The data in Figure 17–8 suggest that the prothrombin time may be maintained at the prebarbiturate value by raising the dose of dicumarol during phenobarbital administration. An increased risk arises, however, if the dose of anticoagulant is not reduced when phenobarbital is discontinued. The plasma dicumarol concentration then rises insidiously, as phenobarbital is slowly eliminated, and may

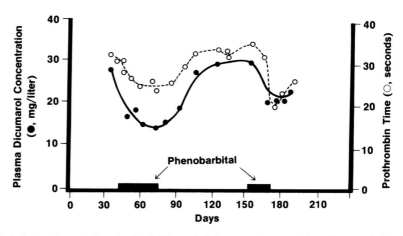

Fig. 17–8. Administration of phenobarbital (60 mg daily) to a patient receiving dicumarol chronically (75 mg daily) reduces the plasma concentration of the anticoagulant (●) and the prothrombin time (○), a measure of its effect on the concentration of the vitamin K_1-dependent clotting factors. (One mg/liter = 3.0 micromolar.) (Redrawn from Cucinell, S.A., Conney, A.H., Sansur, M.S., and Burns, J.J.: Lowering effect of phenobarbital on plasma levels of dicumarol and diphenylhydantoin. Clin. Pharmacol. Ther., 6:420–429, 1965.)

go unnoticed for several weeks after discontinuing the barbiturate until, perhaps, a hemorrhagic crisis occurs.

Study Problems

(Answers to Study Problems are in Appendix G.)

1. The usual dosage regimen of a drug (half-life of 13 hours) is 100 milligrams every 8 hours. Eighty percent is oxidized to a single inactive metabolite; the remainder is excreted unchanged. It is necessary to give the drug to a patient who is also taking another drug that is an inhibitor of this drug's oxidation pathway. Knowing that the oxidation proceeds at 20 percent of the normal value in the presence of the other drug (level is constant with time), suggest how the dosage regimen of the affected drug should be adjusted to maintain the usual average amount of drug in the body.

2. Drug B is a known plasma protein displacer and enzyme inducer of Drug A. A single intravenous dose of Drug A is administered alone and again several weeks later after Drug B is repeatedly administered, and steady state is achieved. The clearance, half-life, fraction unbound, and fraction excreted unchanged of Drug A, when given alone, are 0.5 liter/hour, 26 hours, 0.05, and 0.1, respectively. In the presence of Drug B the enzyme activity and the fraction unbound are approximately doubled. Prepare separate semilogarithmic graphs to illustrate the salient features of the effect of Drug B on the total and unbound concentrations and the urinary excretion rate of Drug A. On each graph show the time course of Drug A in the presence as well as in the absence of Drug B.

3. Drug A is given by infusion at a rate of 25 milligrams/hour to maintain a constant plasma concentration. The data in Table 17–4 are obtained in a subject who is infused at this rate in the absence and presence of Drug B (assume that it is at steady state when present).

Table 17–4.

Plateau Plasma Concentration of Drug B (mg/liter)	Plateau Plasma Concentration (mg/liter)	Urinary Excretion Rate at Steady State (mg/hour)	Fraction Unbound in Plasma	Half-life (hours)
0	10.0	15	0.1	12
20.0	6.7	4	0.3	8

Data for Drug A

Given this information and the observation that the creatinine clearance in this subject is 120 milliliters/minute,

(a) Determine if there is evidence for Drug A being secreted and/or reabsorbed in the kidneys.

(b) Determine the mechanism(s) by which Drug B interacts with Drug A.

(c) Discuss the therapeutic implications of coadministering Drug A with Drug B.

4. Table 17–5 contains pharmacokinetic values for an individual subject that typify what is known about the interaction between quinidine and digoxin.

Table 17–5.

	Availability	Clearance (ml/minute)	Renal Clearance (ml/minute)	Volume of Distribution (liters)	Fraction Unbound
Digoxin alone	0.75	140	101	500	0.77
Digoxin plus quinidine[a]	0.75	72	51	240	0.79

[a]When the $C_{ss,av}$ of quinidine is 1–3 mg/liter.

(a) Briefly comment on how quinidine affects the distribution of digoxin.

(b) Using the appropriate digoxin parameter values in Table 17–5, calculate the probable "loading" dose of digoxin needed when therapy with this drug is initiated in a patient who is undergoing antiarrhythmic therapy with quinidine. The therapeutic concentration range, 1 to 2 micrograms/liter, remains the same for digoxin.

(c) Knowing that the half-lives of digoxin and quinidine are about 2 days and 8 hours, respectively, briefly discuss in terms of the digoxin concentration the therapeutic consequence of administering quinidine to a patient who is receiving digoxin therapy. This is the more common situation in which the interaction is observed. Use the digoxin parameter values in Table 17–5 and consider the events upon both initiating and discontinuing quinidine coadministration.

(d) Do you think quinidine would affect the dosage requirements for digoxin in a patient with severe renal function impairment? Briefly discuss.

5. Normal values for the pharmacokinetic parameters: clearance, fraction unbound, and fraction excreted unchanged are listed in Table 17–6 for drugs A through G. Situations are presented that alter the kinetics of each of these drugs. On the right indicate whether the value of each parameter would be observed to increase (↑), decrease (↓), or show little or no change (↔). All drugs are administered orally and have volumes of distribution greater than 50 liters.

Table 17-6.

Drug	Normal Values				Observations				
	Clearance[a] (ml/minute)	Fraction[a] Unbound	Fraction Excreted Unchanged	Situations	Clearance[a]	Volume of Distribution[a]	Half-life	Fraction Excreted Unchanged	Availability
A	420	0.5	0.7	Simultaneous administration of a competitive inhibitor of renal secretion					
B (acid, renal clearance pH sensitive)	200	0.1	1.0	Urine pH increased by another drug					
C	1200	0.5	0.99	Simultaneous administration of a competitive inhibitor of metabolism of Drug C					
D	1200	0.05	0.01	Simultaneous administration of a drug that displaces Drug D from plasma proteins					
E	50	0.4	0.5	Simultaneous administration of a drug that displaces Drug E from tissue binding sites					
F	10	0.1	0.01	Simultaneous administration of a drug that displaces Drug F from plasma proteins					
G	1300	0.7	0.95	Simultaneous administration for several days of an inducer of enzymes that metabolize Drug G					

[a]Based on measurement of drug concentration in blood.

18

Plasma Drug Concentration Monitoring

Objectives

The reader will be able to:

1. **List the criteria for determining when monitoring of plasma drug concentrations and applying of target concentration strategy are appropriate.**

2. **Estimate the likely pharmacokinetic parameter values in an individual patient, based on both population and patient characteristics, for digoxin, gentamicin, phenobarbital, and theophylline.**

3. **Calculate the plasma drug concentration(s) expected at the time(s) of sampling, using the estimated pharmacokinetic parameter values and the dosing history of the patient.**

4. **Revise pharmacokinetic parameters from measured plasma concentration data acquired under either steady-state or nonsteady-state conditions.**

5. **Upon evaluation of a pharmacokinetic problem observed during chronic drug therapy, ascribe the problem to a change in availability, compliance, clearance, volume of distribution, or a combination of these values.**

Drugs are administered to achieve a therapeutic objective. Once this objective is defined, a drug and its dosage regimen are chosen for the patient (Chap. 13). Drug therapy is subsequently managed as shown schematically in Figure 18–1, together with the steps required to initiate therapy. This management is usually accomplished by monitoring the incidence and intensity of both the desired therapeutic effects and the undesired toxic and side effects. Examples of this method of individualizing therapy are given in Table 18–1.

Although preferable, it is not always possible to use a direct measure of the desired effect as a therapeutic end point. Sometimes, signs of toxicity are used as a dosing guide. The dose of salicylates, for example, when used in the treatment of rheumatic diseases, is often increased until tinnitus or nausea and vomiting intervene. In moderate to severe asthmatic cases, theophylline too is frequently titrated to a toxic end point. Excessive dryness of the mouth is a

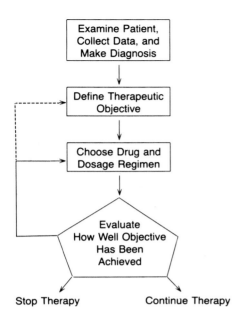

Fig. 18–1. General scheme for initiation and management of drug therapy. The major tasks are: defining the therapeutic objective, choosing the drug and its dosage regimen, and evaluating how well the objective has been achieved. Monitoring the plasma drug concentration often may assist in accomplishing the last two tasks through feedback (———), although it may assist in redefining the therapeutic objective as well (– – –).

Table 18–1. Examples of Monitoring Drug Therapy by the Effects Produced or by Alternative Tests

Drug	Condition	Observation Suggesting Increased Dosage	Observation Suggesting Holding or Decreasing Dosage	Severe Toxic Signs
		Group I. Drugs Monitored by Effects		
1. Salicylates	Rheumatoid arthritis or rheumatic fever	Inadequate reduction of inflammation and pain	Tinnitus, nausea, vomiting	Metabolic acidosis
2. Theophylline	Constrictive airway disease	Insufficient bronchodilation	Nausea, vomiting	CNS stimulation
3. Atropine	GIT spasms	Inadequate control	Dryness of mouth	Palpitations
4. Phenytoin	Convulsive disorders	Inadequate reduction of frequency of epileptic fits	Nystagmus	Ataxia and lethargy
5. Thiopental	Induction of anesthesia	Insufficient anesthesia	Anesthesia too deep	Respiratory failure
		Group II. Drugs Monitored by Effects and Alternative Tests		
6. Warfarin	Thromboembolic disease	Prothrombin time too short	Prothrombin time too long	Hemorrhage
7. Immunosuppressive agents	Renal transplantation	Rosette inhibition test; antibodies too high	Antibodies too low	Infection
8. Tolbutamide	Adult onset diabetes	Glucose in urine	No glucose in urine	Hypoglycemic shock
9. Uricosurics	Gout	Elevated serum uric acid	Decreased serum uric acid	Gastrointestinal irritation

common measure of the upper dosage of atropine when used as a spasmolytic agent.

The therapeutic effects of salicylates, theophylline, and atropine, although often subjective and vague, can be assessed and hence can be used in judging the success of therapy. This is not so readily accomplished for antiepileptic drugs; the therapeutic effect here is the nonoccurrence of seizures. Seizures may be infrequent, and as a result, delays and difficulties exist in assessing therapeutic success. Toxic effects that can be readily measured, nystagmus and ataxia for example, have therefore been used to assist in determining the upper limit of an epileptic patient's dosage requirement. A similar situation arises in the use of oral anticoagulants; the therapeutic objective is the prevention of thromboembolic complications. Again the therapeutic objective cannot readily be assessed, and therefore an alternative, simple, and rapid laboratory test, prothrombin time, which measures the tendency of blood to clot, is substituted as the therapeutic objective. Likewise, for immunosuppressive, hypoglycemic, and uricosuric agents, clinical laboratory tests are employed as alternative therapeutic end points. Clearly, to be useful, any alternative test must be graded and must always be closely related to the true therapeutic effect.

The seriousness of the first toxic effect observed is a major determinant of whether it can or cannot be used as an end point. The titration of young adults on salicylate therapy to the occurrence of tinnitus is relatively safe, as tinnitus is an easily measured mild toxicity, although it does not always occur before the advent of more serious toxicity; its presence may be particularly difficult to assess in young children and in patients with impaired hearing. In contrast, titrating the dosage of digoxin and related glycosides to cardiac toxicity is always unsafe.

Another approach is to monitor plasma concentrations. This approach may be especially useful if the concentration is closely related to the probability and severity of toxicity, and if the therapeutic effect is hard to evaluate, as is the case for antiepileptic drugs for which the desired response is the nonoccurrence of seizures. In this way, the plasma concentration serves as an intermediate therapeutic end point and as a prophylactic of toxicity. At a minimum, the plasma concentration can serve as an additional piece of information to guide and assess drug therapy.

The application of the plasma concentration of a drug to therapy involves *target concentration strategy*. The basic idea is to apply a strategy to achieve and maintain a target concentration or a target range of concentrations for an individual patient. This approach has been a theme throughout this book.

TARGET CONCENTRATION STRATEGY

This strategy is useful as an adjunct in initiating and monitoring drug therapy when a number of criteria listed below are satisfied. Some of the criteria are absolute in nature, others are relative. Most of them, however, must be met for the strategy to be routinely effective.

The plasma concentration of a drug must correlate quantitatively with both the intensity and the probability of therapeutic and toxic effects. A direct relationship between concentration and effect may be insufficient grounds for plasma concentration monitoring if the therapeutic effect itself is easily monitored. The strategy becomes particularly attractive when therapeutic end points are either difficult to quantify, as with the nonoccurrence of epileptic seizures, or are lacking, as in the prophylactic use of drugs. The strategy is most pertinent when the objective is to maintain the therapeutic effect, which most often requires the maintenance of a concentration within a limited range to optimize its utility (Chap. 5).

Target concentration strategy is also indicated when there is a high probability of encountering a therapeutic failure, that is, either a lack of effect or the occurrence of undue toxicity. A therapeutic failure is most likely to arise if the drug has a low therapeutic index and a great variability in its pharmacokinetics or if the patient is at particular risk because of genetic factors (Chap. 14), concurrent disease (Chap. 16), or multiple drug therapy (Chap. 17). A higher frequency of therapeutic failures is also anticipated when either noncompliance or erratic absorption is likely.

Examples of drugs for which target concentration strategy has been found to be appropriate and general information pertinent to their monitoring are listed in Table 18–2.

For some drugs the strategy is applied only when a problem arises. The problem may be a lack of response at usual or even higher dosages as a result of one or more of the following conditions: noncompliance, poor availability, unusually rapid elimination, or a pharmacodynamic resistance to the drug. Measurement of the plasma concentration permits a distinction to be made between pharmacokinetic and pharmacodynamic causes of the problem. Simi-

Table 18–2. Information Pertinent to the Plasma Concentration Monitoring of Selected Drugs

Drug	Concurrent Disease States	Plasma Protein Binding	Concurrent Drug Therapy	Active Metabolites	Other Pertinent Information
Digoxin	Renal disease, congestive cardiac failure, thyroid disease	—[a]	Diuretics	—	Distribution characteristics
Gentamicin	Renal disease	—	Some penicillins	—	Composed of three isomers
Phenytoin	Renal disease, chronic hepatic disease	Extensively bound to albumin	Dicumarol, isoniazid, phenylbutazone, some sulfa drugs	—	Saturable metabolism
Procainamide	Renal and hepatic diseases	—	—	N-acetyl procainamide	Acetylation polymorphism
Theophylline	Pneumonia, chronic obstructive pulmonary disease, congestive cardiac failure, hepatic cirrhosis, acute pulmonary edema	Moderately bound to albumin	Triacetyloleandomycin, erythromycin, phenobarbital	—	Available in many dosage and salt forms

[a]Therapeutically unimportant.

larly, the cause of a toxic or unusual response at customary or lower dosages may be ascertained.

Efficient use of the strategy requires prior knowledge of the pharmacokinetic parameters of the drug, the conditions in which these parameters and the target concentrations are likely to be altered, and if altered, the extents of the changes. The last two requirements are relative in that, by monitoring the concentration, adjustments in dosage can be made for altered pharmacokinetics.

A sensitive, accurate, and specific assay for the drug must be available. In addition, to be useful, the results must be available before the next therapeutic decision is made. The half-life is a useful index of this "turn-around" time because it is the time frame in which accumulation on multiple dosing and disappearance on discontinuing a drug occur.

THE TARGET CONCENTRATION

The target concentration initially chosen is the value or range of values with the greatest probability of therapeutic success (Table 5–2, p. 57), keeping in mind that the population value (or range) may be inappropriate for an individual. Higher concentrations may be appropriate when the condition is severe, and the converse may be true when the condition is mild. If altered plasma protein binding is anticipated, such as in uremia, after surgery, or when displacing drugs are also administered, then the target concentration should be adjusted to attain the same unbound concentration.

The principles for establishing a dosage regimen to achieve a desired concentration or to keep within concentration limits were presented in Chapter 7. Adjustment in the usual dosage regimen can often be anticipated based on the patient's age, weight, and clinical status, especially renal, hepatic, and cardiovascular functions (Chaps. 13 to 16). Yet, even after taking these factors into account, sufficient uncertainty often remains in the kinetics of the drug in the individual patient to warrant monitoring the plasma concentration. From such observations the patient's current pharmacokinetic parameters can be estimated, and a new dosage regimen can be designed to more closely achieve the target value(s).

The frequency of monitoring is a function of the presumed change in the factors that influence drug response. For example, the plasma concentration of phenobarbital in epileptic patients, whose state of health and drug therapy may remain stable, may need to be monitored only a few times a year; more frequent monitoring may be indicated if the patient's health deteriorates or if therapy with other drugs is altered. Daily or even more frequent monitoring of plasma theophylline concentrations may be needed for optimal use of theophylline in the treatment of an asthmatic patient in an intensive care unit, especially if congestive cardiac failure, pneumonia, hepatic cirrhosis, and smoking are all present. These conditions alter theophylline metabolism, which is likely to be quite variable in this situation.

PERTINENT INFORMATION NEEDED

Several kinds of information, given in Table 18–3, are needed to evaluate a measured plasma concentration efficiently. A history of drug administration,

Table 18–3. Data Collection

History of Drug Administration
  Drug, dose, dosage forms, routes of administration, times of administration, compliance, inpatient or outpatient

Time of Sampling (relative to dose)

Present and Previous (if any) Plasma Drug Concentrations

Clinical Status of Patient
  Weight, age, gender, condition being treated, concurrent disease states (especially cardiovascular, hepatic, and renal diseases)

Laboratory Data
  Renal function (serum creatinine, creatinine clearance)
  Hepatic function (prothrombin time, serum albumin, serum bilirubin)
  Protein binding (plasma proteins and albumin)

Concurrent Drug Therapy
  Interacting Drugs
  Assay interferences

Active Metabolites

Assay Method (reproducibility, sensitivity, and specificity)

Usual Pharmacokinetic Parameters Associated with Type of Patient in Question
  Availability, absorption rate constant, volume of distribution, unbound fraction in plasma, clearance, renal clearance

which includes the doses and the times of dosing, and of the times of sampling are mandatory.

Specific patient population pharmacokinetic information for monitoring digoxin, gentamicin, phenobarbital, and theophylline concentrations is given in Table 18–4. These four drugs are used throughout the remainder of this chapter as examples of the application of the principles of plasma drug concentration monitoring.

EVALUATION PROCEDURE

Using the dosing history and the time(s) of sampling, judgment is needed on whether the measured value(s) is a good estimate of the maximum, average, or minimum concentration at steady state on a fixed regimen or of a nonsteady-state concentration(s) obtained either shortly after starting dosing or following an erratic schedule. Having established the conditions and an appropriate kinetic model, a generally recommended procedure to evaluate one or more concentrations is as follows:

1. Estimate the likely values of the pharmacokinetic parameters (F, CL, V, and $t_{1/2}$) in the patient based on population parameters, taking into account the patient's age, weight, renal function, concurrent diseases, drug therapy, dosage form, route of administration, and any other information about the patient known to affect the kinetics of the drug. The major intent here is to identify the subpopulation to which the patient belongs (see Chap. 13).

2. Using the appropriate kinetic model and the parameter values above, estimate the plasma drug concentration(s) expected at the time(s) of sampling, taking into account the dosing history of the patient.

3. Compare the observed and expected concentrations. If they are in agree-

Table 18-4. Patient Population Pharmacokinetic Parameters of Digoxin, Gentamicin, Phenobarbital, and Theophylline[a]

Parameters	Digoxin	Gentamicin	Phenobarbital	Theophylline[b]
Salt form factor	1.0	1.0	1.0	0.85 hydrous amino-phylline
			0.9 (Na salt)	0.8 anhydrous amino-phylline (intravenous use)
Oral availability	0.75 tablets 0.8 elixir 0.95 liquid-filled capsules	<0.01	1.0	1.0
Volume of distribution (liters/kg)	c	0.22	0.55	0.5
Clearance (liters/hour per kg)	d	CL_{cr}[e]	0.0037	0.04[f]
Half-life (hours)	44[g]	h	103	8.7[i]
Fraction excreted unchanged	0.7	>0.95	0.3	0.13
Therapeutic window				
Milligrams/liter	0.0008–0.002	peak >6, trough <2[j]	10–30	10–20
Micromolar	0.001–0.0025	peak >11, trough <2[j]	43–130	55–110

[a]Adapted from data in Applied Pharmacokinetics, 2nd ed., Edited by W.E. Evans, J.J. Schentag, and W.J. Jusko. Spokane, Applied Therapeutics, 1986.
[b]Many controlled release dosage forms are available.
[c]V (liters/kg) = 3.8 + 52 CL_{cr}; CL_{cr} in liters/hour per kilogram for adults.
[d]In severe congestive cardiac failure patients, CL (liters/hour per kg) = 0.9 CL_{cr} + 0.02; in mild to moderate conditions, CL = CL_{cr} + 0.048, where CL_{cr} is in liters/hour per kilogram.
[e]Approximately the same as patient's creatinine clearance.
[f]Multiply 0.04 by the factor below to adjust for smoking, age, disease, and concurrent drugs. Consider the factors to be multiplicative when more than one condition is present.

Smoking	1.6	Concurrent Drugs		Age (years)		
Diseases		Phenytoin	1.5	Child	1–4	2.4
Cirrhosis	0.5	Rifampin	1.8	Child	5–17	1.6
Cor pulmonale	0.7	Cimetidine	0.6			
Pulmonary edema	0.5	Erythromycin	0.7			
Congestive		Phenobarbital	1.3			
cardiac failure	0.4	Troleandomycin	0.5			

[g]$t_{1/2}$ = 0.693 V/CL; V and CL estimated from footnotes c and d.
[h]$t_{1/2}$ = 0.15/CL_{cr}; CL_{cr} in liters/hour per kilogram.
[i]$t_{1/2}$ = 8.7/m; value of m is the factor determined in footnote f.
[j]Desired peak (30 minutes after the end of a 30-minute infusion) and trough concentrations are indicated.

ment, then one's confidence in knowing the parameters in the patient is increased. A clinical decision to modify the dosage in the patient depends on the concentration observed and on several other factors including, most importantly, the current response(s) of the patient.

4. If the observed and expected concentrations are judged to be different, then one may wish to revise the pharmacokinetic parameter estimates. Here it is necessary to weigh how much confidence one has in the initial parameter es-

timates from previous population studies relative to that in the estimates obtained from the measured plasma concentration(s) (Chap. 13).

5. A recommendation for dosage adjustment or patient education (noncompliance) may be appropriate. In addition, comments to the clinician could aid in the interpretation of the drug concentration. Such comments include the need to adjust the therapeutic window when altered protein binding is expected and when a change in time of sampling is appropriate.

DOSING SCENARIOS

Chapters 6 and 7 contained the basic relationships needed for evaluating concentrations obtained during a constant-rate infusion and a multiple-dose regimen of fixed doses and fixed intervals, respectively. These relationships are now supplemented with equations, which are useful for four additional, frequently occurring scenarios, namely: when one or more doses is missed; when a patient is on a four-times-a-day regimen in which the intervals are not equal, for example, 9 a.m., 1 p.m., 5 p.m., 9 p.m. (subsequently called a 9-1-5-9 regimen); when the drug is repeatedly infused over a period of time approaching the half-life of the drug; and when the doses vary and the dosing intervals are erratic. Unless otherwise noted, dosing and sampling times are subsequently based on the 24-hour clock.

For each of the scenarios, absorption is assumed to be much more rapid than elimination, that is, the intravenous bolus approximation applies. Absorption decreases fluctuation; it should be taken into account, when necessary, using the principles previously given in Chapter 7.

Missed Dose

Although it would seem that missed doses would greatly complicate the evaluation of a measured concentration, it is not necessarily so. Figure 18–2 shows a fixed dose, fixed interval multiple-dose regimen in which one dose is missed. To account for the missed dose one needs only to calculate the concentration expected if this dose had been given and then to subtract the concentration

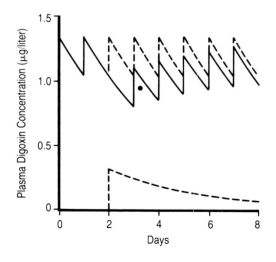

Fig. 18–2. A missed dose results in the lowering of the fluctuating concentrations from their steady-state values. The degree of this lowering is equivalent to the concentration remaining from the missed dose. The expected concentration at any time following the missed dose (——) can then be estimated by the difference between the value expected with no missed dose (----) and the concentration expected at that time had only the missed dose been given (bottom curve). The observed concentration on the day after the missed dose, 0.9 micrograms/liter, is superimposed (●). The parameters used in the figure are those expected in the patient in the digoxin example case history. (One mg/liter = 1.3 micromolar.)

expected at the time of sampling if only the "missed" dose had been given. This correction is based on the principle of the additivity of concentrations from each dose. For example, consider the measurement of a concentration at time t_1 within a dosing interval at steady state. In this case,

$$C_{ss,t_1} = \frac{F \cdot S \cdot D}{V} \cdot \frac{e^{-kt_1}}{(1 - e^{-k\tau})} \qquad 1$$

if absorption is instantaneous relative to elimination. The parameter S, salt form factor, is simply a coefficient correcting for the fractional content of drug in a salt form. Its use is unnecessary if the dose is expressed in millimoles. The concentration that would have occurred from the missed dose is

$$C_{(missed\ dose)} = \frac{F \cdot S \cdot D}{V} \cdot e^{-kt_2} \qquad 2$$

where t_2 is the time since the dose was missed. Therefore, the concentration expected is

★

$$C = \frac{F \cdot S \cdot D}{V} \left[\frac{e^{-kt_1}}{(1 - e^{-k\tau})} - e^{-kt_2} \right] \qquad 3$$

9-1-5-9 Regimen

In institutional settings many drugs are given in regimens similar to the one portrayed in Figure 18–3. Such regimens have a 24-hour repetitive or regular cycle, even though the dosing intervals within the day are unequal. The expected concentration at any time during the day can be viewed simply as the sum of the concentrations resulting from each of the four daily doses. When given once daily, the first dose of the day is expected to yield a concentration, C_1, at steady state, given by

$$C_1 = \frac{F \cdot S \cdot D}{V} \cdot \frac{e^{-kt_1}}{(1 - e^{-k\tau})} \qquad 4$$

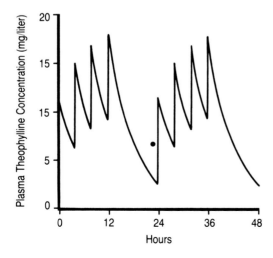

Plasma Theophylline Concentration (mg/liter)

Hours

Fig. 18–3. The plasma theophylline concentration varies extensively at steady-state (24-hour repeating pattern) with a "9-1-5-9" type of regimen. In this example the concentration, 2.1 milligrams/liter, at the time of the morning dose (9:00 = "zero" time) would be ineffective (therapeutic window = 7 to 20 mg/liter). An increase in the dose to overcome this low trough value, however, may cause toxicity, particularly during the evening hours after the dose at 21:00 (12 or 36 hours). The observed trough concentration of 6.3 milligrams/liter (●) is superimposed. The parameter values used are those in the theophylline case history. (One mg/liter = 5.5 micromolar.)

where t_1 is the time during the day between giving the dose and sampling the blood. The concentration resulting from giving only the second dose on a daily regimen is

$$C_2 = \frac{F \cdot S \cdot D}{V} \cdot \frac{e^{-kt_2}}{(1 - e^{-k\tau})} \qquad 5$$

and so on. Thus, the concentration expected on such a regimen is

★

$$C = \frac{F \cdot S \cdot D}{V} \cdot \left[\frac{(e^{-kt_1} + e^{-kt_2} + e^{-kt_3} + e^{-kt_4})}{(1 - e^{-k\tau})} \right] \qquad 6$$

where τ is 24 hours, the dosing interval in each of the once daily regimens.

Intermittent Infusion Model

The aminoglycosides, e.g., gentamicin, are often administered every 6 to 8 hours by a constant-rate infusion of each dose over 30 to 60 minutes. This form of administration is neither a multiple-dose intravenous bolus regimen nor a constant-rate infusion, but rather an *intermittent infusion* regimen. When the infusion time approaches the half-life of a drug, a multiple-dose intravenous bolus model is no longer adequate for predicting concentrations and revising parameter values. The appropriate steady-state model, shown in Figure 18–4, is

$$C = \underbrace{\frac{R_o \cdot (1 - e^{-kt_{inf}})}{CL}}_{A} \cdot \underbrace{\frac{1}{(1 - e^{-k\tau})}}_{B} \cdot \underbrace{e^{-k(t - t_{inf})}}_{C} \qquad \begin{array}{c} ★ \\ 7 \end{array}$$

where τ is the dosing interval; t_{inf} is the infusion time; $R_o = S \cdot Dose/t_{inf}$; and t is the time in the last dosing interval between the start of the infusion and the

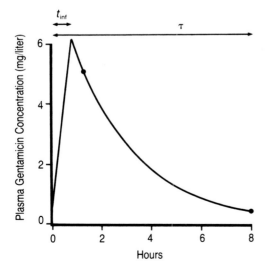

Fig. 18–4. The plasma concentration of gentamicin, predicted during an 8-hour dosing interval at steady state and following the repeated 45-minute constant-rate infusion of the drug, shows similarities with repeated intravenous boluses, except for there being less fluctuation. When the input time (infusion duration, t_{inf}) is a significant part of the half-life (1.9 hours here), the intermittent infusion can result in considerable error unless the *intermittent infusion model* is used to calculate expected concentrations within the interval. These calculations are based on the parameter values expected for the patient in the third case history. The two observed concentrations, 4.9 and 0.4 milligrams/liter, are superimposed (●). (One mg/liter = 1.8 micromolar.)

withdrawal of the blood sample. The model results from the accumulation of drug remaining from each of the successive doses. Part A of the equation is the concentration expected just at the end of the infusion, at rates $\cdot$ D/t_{inf}. Part B is the accumulation factor for repeated administration to steady state (see Appendix D), and Part C is the fraction remaining at postinfusion time, $t - t_{inf}$, after achieving the peak concentration, the product of A $\cdot$ B.

Unequal Dose and Interval

The situation in which neither the dose nor the interval have any degree of regularity is frequently observed in therapeutic monitoring. Another model is needed here to estimate expected concentrations and revise parameter values. In this situation, one can simply sum up drug that remains from previous doses with the realization that doses given more than four patient half-lives ago can be disregarded, since so little drug remains in the body from each of them. The plasma concentration expected after three doses, for example, is

$$C = \frac{F \cdot S}{V} (D_1 e^{-kt_1} + D_2 e^{-kt_2} + D_3 e^{-kt_3}) \qquad \bigstar \qquad 8$$

where D_1, D_2, and D_3 represent the doses taken at times t_1, t_2, and t_3 before sampling.

Confidence in Estimates

To revise pharmacokinetic parameter values properly, one must consider several pieces of information. Information about compliance, availability, times(s) of sampling (actual versus reported), assay reproducibility and specificity, and dosing history are of paramount importance. One must also weigh the relative confidence one has in the parameter values estimated from literature data, previous experience, and the concentration data. Recall (Chap. 13) that literature parameter values are those values estimated to apply to the subpopulation to which the patient belongs. Misassignment of the subpopulation and variability in the expected parameter values are, of course, concerns here.

There are additional kinetic factors that affect one's confidence in the use of a concentration value. Consider, for example, the case of sampling while drug accumulates during a constant-rate intravenous infusion. A plasma concentration obtained during such an infusion is a function of rate of administration, clearance, and volume of distribution (Chap. 6).

$$C = \frac{R_o}{CL} (1 - e^{-(CL/V)t}) \qquad 9$$

Evaluation of a plasma concentration requires knowing whether clearance or volume of distribution is the more variable and appreciating on which of these two parameters the concentration is more dependent. The latter may be considered from the events depicted in Figure 18–5 during the infusion of a drug in three separate situations. In Case A, the values of the clearance and volume parameters are those anticipated, the average values. In the other two situations, the half-life is three times greater than the average value, in Case B due to a

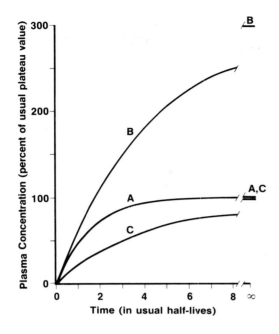

Fig. 18–5. Following a constant-rate infusion, monitoring the concentration at one usual half-life does little to distinguish between a patient with average values of clearance and volume of distribution, Case A, and one with a threefold reduction in clearance and an averge volume of distribution, Case B. Distinguishing between these patients, without producing undue toxicity, is probably best done by monitoring at four usual half-lives. Although a threefold increase in volume of distribution, Case C, is readily detected at one usual half-life, this observation provides little information on the final plateau concentration to be achieved.

threefold reduction in clearance and in Case C due to a threefold increase in volume of distribution.

With little drug having been eliminated, an early concentration is primarily a function of infusion rate and volume of distribution. Accordingly, there is little virtue in taking a sample before the usual half-life to estimate the dosage requirements needed to achieve therapeutic concentrations. A steady-state concentration depends only on the rate of administration and the value of clearance (Chap. 6). Accordingly, sampling at this time provides the most confidence in estimating dosing rate requirements.

Sampling between the time of initiating the infusion and steady state often leads to inconclusive information. At two usual half-lives, the observation of the concentration expected, Case A, does not mean that CL and V have the expected values. They may both differ and fortuitously give the expected concentration. The lower-than-expected concentration at two usual half-lives, Case C, could be due to either an increased clearance or an increased volume, as shown. In contrast, the observation of a concentration at this time equal to or above the expected steady-state value, Case B, is a clear indication that clearance is less than usual. Indeed, the greater this difference, the lower is the probable value of clearance and the greater the need to reduce the rate of administration to avoid toxicity.

In the region of two to six usual half-lives, a major consideration in interpreting a single observation is whether the clearance or the volume of distribution parameter is the more variable. For example, the clearance (in units of liters/hour per kg) of theophylline varies over an eightfold range or more, particularly if age and disease state are considered. The range of values for the volume of distribution (liters/kg) is only about twofold. Thus, estimates of the clearance of theophylline can be made from nonsteady-state values obtained within this time span.

Although the preceding concepts regarding estimates of parameters were developed for administration by infusion, they generally apply to all forms and schedules of drug administration intended to produce a plateau concentration.

CASE HISTORIES

To demonstrate the principles of plasma drug concentration monitoring, the subsequent case histories are evaluated by the procedure suggested above. The population parameter estimates for the drugs utilize the information given in Table 18–4. Included are values for select subpopulations of patients. For gentamicin and digoxin, several parameter values depend on an estimate of renal function, such as creatinine clearance (Chap. 16). Parameter estimates of theophylline are obtained by multiplicative factors. For example, the clearance of theophylline in a 62-year-old, 65-kilogram female smoker (1.6) with congestive cardiac failure (0.4) and concurrently taking phenytoin (1.5) is calculated as follows:

$$0.04 \times (1.6 \times 0.4 \times 1.5) \times 65 = 2.5 \text{ liters/hour}$$

No correction for the age of this adult is included. One expects a decrease in clearance with age, especially in the elderly patient. However, current methods for estimating parameter values for theophylline do not include such an adjustment. It is important to note that rules developed here are intended to be examples and not to summarize all that is currently known. Furthermore, as more information is obtained, new and more refined relationships will become available.

Case 1. *Digoxin*. Mrs D.H., a 53-year-old, 82-kilogram patient with congestive cardiac failure for the past three years, was admitted on April 16 to the hospital at 16:00 because of a worsening of her congestive cardiac failure symptoms. Her admission history indicated that she had taken her digoxin tablet (0.25 mg) that morning at the usual time (8:00–9:00), but had failed to take a tablet on Sunday (April 15). A plasma sample (blood withdrawn at 17:00) was obtained to see if the symptoms were consistent with noncompliance. A plasma digoxin concentration of 0.9 microgram/liter and a serum creatinine of 0.9 milligram/ deciliter were reported.

Step 1. *Estimation of Parameter Values.* From age, gender, weight, and serum creatinine, the creatinine clearance (Table 16–2, p. 247) is

$$CL_{cr} \text{ (milliliters/minute)} = \frac{(140 - 53) \times 82}{85 \times 0.9} = 93 \text{ milliliters/minute}$$
$$\text{(5.6 liters/hour or}$$
$$\text{0.068 liter/hour per kilogram)}$$

Clearance of digoxin (Table 18–4) is then

$$CL \text{ (liters/hour per day)} = 0.9 \times 0.068 + 0.02$$
$$\text{(0.0812 liter/hour per}$$
$$\text{kg or 6.66 liters/hour)}$$

and the volume of distribution is

$$V \text{ (liters/kg)} = 3.8 + 52 \times 0.068 \text{ (7.34 liters/kg or 602 liters)}$$

The elimination rate constant and half-life are then

$$k = CL/V = 0.011 \text{ hour}^{-1}$$
$$t_{1/2} = 63 \text{ hours}$$

The values of S and F for digoxin tablets are 1.0 and 0.75, respectively.

Step 2. *Estimation of Concentration at Time of Sampling.* The first question to be addressed is that of the appropriate kinetic model for evaluating this concentration. Presumably the patient has been taking digoxin for three years. The dosing history indicates a single, recently missed dose. Thus, a steady-state model incorporating the missed dose is appropriate. Since the expected half-life is 63 hours and the dosing interval is 24 hours, there should be minor fluctuation in concentration; a constant-rate infusion model would seem reasonable. Alternatively, a steady-state, multiple-dose model could be employed. Using the constant-rate infusion model, the concentration expected, C, (Fig. 18–2) is $C_{ss} - C_1$, where C_1 is the concentration expected 32 hours (t) after administration, had only the missed dose been given.

$$C = \frac{F \cdot S \cdot \text{Dose}}{CL \cdot \tau} - \frac{F \cdot S \cdot \text{Dose} \cdot e^{-kt_1}}{V}$$

Using a steady-state, multiple-dose model, the concentration expected is that 8 hours (t_1) into the 24-hour dosing interval (τ) minus C_1, as defined above ($t_2 = 32$ hours).

$$C = \frac{F \cdot S \cdot \text{Dose}}{V} \cdot \left[\frac{e^{-kt_1}}{1 - e^{-k\tau}} - e^{-kt_2} \right]$$

The values are 0.95 and 1.01 milligram/liter, a difference explained by the assumption of *average* steady-state concentration in the first model.

Step 3. *Comparison of Observed and Expected Concentrations.* The observed and expected values are virtually the same. Step 4, revision of parameter values, is unnecessary. Furthermore, the clinician now has some confidence that the patient is handling the drug as expected, but the concentration present may be inadequate to control her congestive cardiac failure. A decision must now be made on how much higher a concentration may be needed, or if therapy should be augmented with other drugs or be changed.

Case 2. Theophylline. J.T., a 6-year-old, 22-kilogram boy suffering from asthma and epilepsy, was taking 100-milligram aminophylline tablets ($S = 0.85$) four times a day at 8:00, 12:00, 16:00, and 20:00. Because of poor control of both his asthma and his seizures, a blood sample was obtained at 8:00, just before the next dose, for determination of theophylline and phenobarbital concentrations. The theophylline concentration was 6.3 milligrams/liter.

Step 1. *Estimation of Parameter Values.* To estimate the clearance of theophylline, the patient's age and concurrent drug therapy need to be considered. The clearance (Table 18–4) is then

$$CL = 0.04 \times 1.6 \times 1.3 \times 22 = 1.83 \text{ liters/hour}$$

Note that the clearance per kilogram in the 6-year-old boy is adjusted by a factor of 1.6; younger children (1 to 4 years of age) are adjusted by a factor of 2.4 (Table 18–4). These numbers are close to the values expected for adjustment based on surface area (Chap. 15). The factor 1.3 is an adjustment for the concurrent administration of phenobarbital, which induces theophylline metabolism. The volume of distribution (0.5 liter per kg times weight in kg) is 11 liters. The elimination rate constant and half-life are then 0.166 hour^{-1} and 4.2 hours, respectively. Values of other pertinent parameters are $F = 1$, $S = 0.85$.

Step 2. *Estimation of Concentration at Time of Sampling.* Using Equation 6, the concentration at 8:00 is

$$C = \frac{0.85 \times 100}{11} \times \left[\frac{e^{-k \cdot 24} + e^{-k \cdot 20} + e^{-k \cdot 16} + e^{-k \cdot 12}}{(1 - e^{-k \cdot 24})} \right]$$

$$= 2.1 \text{ milligrams/liter}$$

This situation is depicted in Figure 18–3.

Step 3. *Comparison of Observed and Expected Concentrations.* The observed concentration is 3 times greater than that expected, assuming that compliance, dosing and sampling histories, and assay are not questionable. Literature data on theophylline show that clearance is highly variable, much more so than volume of distribution.

Step 4. *Revision of Parameter Values.* Apparently, either volume or clearance, or both, needs revision. The questions are which one and how to revise. One approach would be to assume that the volume term is correct and change the value of k (or CL, since $k = CL/V$) in the equation above until the right side of the equation is equal to 6.3. The following values are determined:

k (hour^{-1})	Right Side of Equation (mg/liter)
0.166	2.1
0.12	4.3
0.10	6.2
0.08	9.1

This procedure, called *iteration*, is used frequently in clinical pharmacokinetics. Note that the most likely value of k, to explain an observation of 6.3 milligrams/liter, is about 0.10 hour^{-1}, a value not too different from that expected, 0.166 hour^{-1}.

A similar analysis could be carried out assuming that the value of clearance is that expected and the observation is a result of an unexpected volume of distribution. In this case,

$$C \text{ (mg/liter)} = \frac{0.85 \times 100}{V}$$

$$\times \left[\frac{e^{-1.83 \times 24/V} + e^{-1.83 \times 20/V} + e^{-1.83 \times 16/V} + e^{-1.83 \times 12/V}}{(1 - e^{-1.83 \times 24/V})} \right]$$

By iteration, the following values are determined:

V (liters)	Right Side of Equation (mg/liter)
11	2.1
20	4.0
40	5.7
60	6.4

Note that a large increase in the value of V is necessary to account for the observed concentration. As stated before, the volume of distribution of theophylline does not vary widely, whereas clearance does. The prudent decision is to adjust clearance and not volume of distribution in this patient. This general procedure, whereby the sensitivity of the observed measurement to changes in parameter values is assessed, is called *sensitivity analysis*. We conclude from it, and our general knowledge of the population pharmacokinetics of theophylline, that clearance ($k \cdot V$) in this patient is about 1.1 liters/hour, a small adjustment in the initial estimate for a threefold difference in observed and expected concentrations. We are reasonably confident in our new clearance estimate because the time elapsed, 24 hours, is more than 3 times the revised half-life.

Step 5. *Recommendation for Adjustment of Dosage.* The maximum concentration expected after the dose at 20:00 is the trough value times $e^{+k \cdot 12}$, a value derived from the maximum having decayed by a factor of $e^{-k \cdot 12}$. In this case, the best estimate of the maximum concentration is 20.9 milligrams/liter. The concentration range 6.3 to 20.9 is too great. A solution is to switch to a controlled-release dosage form. The patient's daily need is about 400 milligrams. A 200-milligram dose with an appropriate controlled-release product, to be taken twice daily, is recommended here.

Case 3. *Gentamicin.* Mr. B.G., a 23-year-old, 58-kilogram patient with a gram-negative pneumonia, was being treated with gentamicin and ampicillin. Gentamicin had been given as an intravenous infusion (80 mg) over 45 minutes every 8 hours. Blood samples were obtained just before and 30 minutes after the end of the fourth infusion to prevent toxicity and to evaluate his therapy. The gentamicin concentrations reported were 0.4 and 4.9 milligrams/liter. The serum creatinine in the patient was 1.2 milligrams/deciliter.

Step 1. *Estimation of Parameter Values.* The creatinine clearance in this patient, estimated from the patient's age, weight, gender, and serum creatinine (Table 16–2), is estimated to be 79 milliliters/minute (4.7 liters/hour). The clearance of gentamicin is approximated by creatinine clearance (Table 18–4). The volume of distribution is 12.8 liters (0.22 liter/kg $\cdot$ 58 kg). The elimination rate constant and half-life are then 0.37 hour^{-1} and 1.9 hours, respectively.

Step 2. *Estimation of Concentrations at Times of Sampling.* The samples are obtained under steady-state conditions (expected half-life = 1.9 hours), and the drug is constantly infused over a period of time, 45 minutes (0.75 hour), approaching the half-life. The intermittent infusion model (Eq. 7, $F = 1$) seems to be appropriate. The concentration just before the next infusion is equivalent to the value at the end of the dosing interval (see Fig. 18–4). Thus, the concentrations 30 minutes after the end of the infusion (1.25 hours after starting the infusion) and at the end of the 8-hour interval can be calculated from

$$C = \frac{80}{4.7 \times 0.75} \frac{(1 - e^{-0.37 \times 0.75})}{(1 - e^{-0.37 \cdot \tau})} \cdot e^{-0.37 (t - 0.75)}$$

The expected concentrations are 4.8 and 0.4 milligram/liter, respectively (Fig. 18–4).

Step 3. *Comparison of Observed and Expected Concentrations.* Since the observed and expected values are virtually the same, the estimated parameter values are assumed to apply to this patient.

Arguably, in all three of the preceding examples, dosage could have been adjusted solely by titrating to the effects observed. A point in favor of concentration measurement is that an assessment could be made as to why toxicity or a lack of effect occurred. These measurements also permitted facile and rapid estimation of the patient's dosage requirement, which otherwise might have required a considerable degree of readjustment from observing the effects alone. The fineness of the adjustment was also much greater with the plasma concentration data than it would have been without them.

Study Problems

(Answers to Study Problems are in Appendix G.)

1. List and briefly describe the criteria for performing drug concentration monitoring and applying target concentration strategy.

2. An 85-kilogram, 42-year-old female patient is receiving 120-milligram doses of gentamicin in short-term, constant-rate infusions over 45 minutes every 8 hours. The patient has a serum creatinine of 1.2 milligrams/deciliter. Plasma samples were obtained just before and 45 minutes after the end of the fourth dose.

    (a) Estimate the values of clearance, volume of distribution, and half-life expected in this patient.

    (b) Estimate the gentamicin concentration in plasma expected at the two sampling times.

3. **Mr. V.J. is a 70-kilogram, 65-year-old asthmatic patient with congestive cardiac failure. He is started on aminophylline tablets orally and has a plasma theophylline concentration measured as noted in Table 18–5. He smokes 2 packs of cigarettes a day.**

Table 18–5.   Dosing and Sampling History

Date	Time	Time Since Dose (hours)	Oral Dose (mg)
June 1	18:00	24	400
	22:00	20	200
June 2	8:00	10	300
	12:00	6	300
	18:00	Plasma sample obtained $C = 18$ milligrams/liter	

   (a) Estimate the values of clearance, volume of distribution, and half-life expected in this patient.

   (b) Estimate the concentration expected at the time of sampling.

   (c) Compare the observed and estimated concentrations.

   (d) State which parameters you think need to be revised and by how much to account for any difference between observed and estimated concentrations.

4. **Mr. D.W., a 68-year-old, 74-kilogram, alcoholic, epileptic patient, has been taking phenobarbital (200 mg at bedtime) for three years. He has been free of seizures for at least one year. He was admitted to the hospital on January 10 with ataxia and general central nervous system depression, without alcohol on his breath. A plasma phenobarbital concentration of 56 milligrams/liter was measured in a blood sample drawn at 11:00 of that day. The drug was discontinued (including no dose on January 10) and another blood sample was obtained on January 16 at 10:00 to**

determine if the patient was metabolizing the drug more slowly than expected, as the patient had signs of hepatic cirrhosis. The second concentration was 16 milligrams/liter.

(a) Evaluate the data in the sequential manner requested in Problem 3.

(b) Given that clearance of this drug is much more variable than volume of distribution (Table 13–2), state the likely cause of the observations made and provide a recommendation for his future antiepileptic therapy with phenobarbital.

5. Given the usual parameter values for theophylline (Table 18–4), provide a pharmacokinetic interpretation for each of the following theophylline concentrations, obtained in three different adult patients during an infusion of aminophylline at a constant rate of 0.8 milligram/hour per kilogram. No theophylline was present in the body at the start of the infusion. In your interpretations include both a comparison of observed and expected plasma concentrations and an estimation of the values of clearance and half-life in each patient. Assume that the volume of distribution (liters/kg) is the same in all three patients and that they are nonsmoking, healthy adults, except for their asthmatic condition.

Patient	Time of Sampling (hours into infusion)	Plasma Theophylline Concentration (mg/liter)
1	3	3.5
2	16	18
3	30	6

Selected Topics

19

Distribution Kinetics

Objectives

The reader will be able to:

1. State why the one-compartment model is sometimes inadequate to describe kinetic events within the body.

2. Name and compare the two common forms of representing pharmacokinetic data showing distribution kinetics.

3. Estimate the clearance and the half-life of the phase associated with the majority of elimination from plasma concentration-time data of a drug showing multiexponential disposition following an intravenous bolus dose.

4. Define and estimate the parameters: initial dilution volume (V_1), volume during the terminal phase (V), and volume of distribution at steady state (V_{ss}).

5. Explain the influence of distribution kinetics and duration of administration on the time-courses of concentration in plasma and amount in tissue during and after stopping a constant-rate infusion.

6. Explain the significance of distribution kinetics on the interpretation of plasma concentration-time data following drug administration.

7. Explain the influence of distribution kinetics on the fluctuations of plasma and tissue levels with time following a multiple-dose regimen.

8. Explain the effect of distribution kinetics on the interpretation of plasma concentration-time data and terminal half-life when clearance is altered.

The first four sections of the book have covered most of the fundamentals of pharmacokinetics. Section Five now expands on selected topics; it begins with chapters on distribution kinetics and pharmacologic response. Subsequent chapters deal with metabolite kinetics, dose and time dependencies, turnover concepts, dialysis, and kinetic consequences of a small volume of distribution. These topics do not build on each other as extensively as do the previous topics in the book. Notable exceptions to this statement are found in applications of distribution kinetic concepts in the chapters on pharmacologic response, turnover concepts, and dialysis.

Portraying the body as a single compartment is appropriate for establishing the fundamental principles of pharmacokinetics, but is an inaccurate representation of the events that follow drug administration. A basic assumption of the concept of a one-compartment representation of distribution is that equilibrium of drug between tissues and blood occurs spontaneously. In reality, distribution takes time. The time taken depends on tissue perfusion, permeability characteristics of the tissue membranes for the drug, and partitioning of drug between the tissues and blood (Chap. 10). Ignoring the kinetics of distribution is reasonable so long as the error incurred is acceptable. This error becomes unacceptable when: the one-compartment representation fails to adequately explain the observations following drug administration; there is a danger of significant misinterpretation of the observations; and major discrepancies occur in the calculation of drug dosage. Such situations are most likely to arise when substantial amounts are eliminated before distribution equilibrium is achieved and when the effect of the drug is directly related to its plasma concentration and the observation is made while distribution occurs. This chapter deals with the pharmacokinetic consequences of distribution kinetics. The impact of distribution kinetics on pharmacologic response is dealt with in the next chapter, Pharmacologic Response.

EVIDENCE OF DISTRIBUTION KINETICS

Evidence of distribution kinetics is usually inferred from the early rapid decline in the blood or the plasma drug concentration following an intravenous bolus dose, when little drug has been eliminated, and from the rapid onset and decline in the pharmacologic effect of some drugs during this early phase. Data in Figure 19–1, which show the concentration of thiopental in various tissues after an intravenous bolus dose of this preoperative general anesthetic to a dog, provide direct evidence of distribution kinetics. Thiopental is a highly lipid soluble drug for which distribution into essentially all tissues is perfusion rate-limited. The results seen with this drug are therefore typical of those observed with many other lipophilic drugs.

Notice that thiopental in the liver, a highly perfused organ, reaches distribution equilibrium with the drug in plasma by five minutes (the first observation), and thereafter, the decline of drug in the liver parallels that in the plasma. The same holds true for drug in other highly perfused tissues, including the brain and the kidneys.

Redistribution of thiopental from the well-perfused tissues to the less well-perfused tissues, muscle and fat, primarily accounts for the subsequent decline in plasma drug concentration over the next three hours; less than twenty percent of the dose is eliminated from the body during this period. Due to a combination of poor perfusion and high partitioning, even by three hours distribution equilibrium in adipose tissue has not been established. Analysis of the situation indicates that this does not occur for some hours, at which time the majority of thiopental remaining in the body is in fat. Recall: The greater the partition of a drug into fat, or into any tissue, the longer is the time required to achieve distribution equilibrium (Chap. 10). However, only if the apparent volume of distribution of tissue ($K_p \cdot V_T$) is a major fraction of the total volume of distribution, does uptake into that tissue substantially affect the events within plasma. With thiopental, which has an adipose-to-plasma partition coefficient of 10, fat

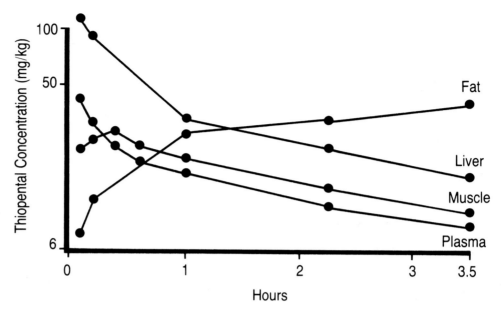

Fig. 19–1. Concentration of thiopental in various tissues following an intravenous bolus dose of 25 milligrams/kilogram to a dog. Note the early rise and fall of thiopental in the well-perfused tissues (e.g., liver) and in lean muscle tissue. After three hours much of the drug remaining in the body is in adipose tissue. (One mg/liter = 4.1 micromolar.) (Redrawn from Brodie, B.B., Bernstein, E., and Mark, L.: The role of body fat in limiting the duration of action of thiopental. J. Pharmacol. Exp. Ther., *105*: 421–426, 1952. © Williams & Wilkins (1952).)

(0.12 liter/kg) constitutes approximately 50 percent of the total volume of distribution (2.3 liter/kg). Accordingly, the plasma concentration of thiopental not only falls markedly, but the distribution phase in plasma is seen to take many hours. For other drugs, distribution may take even longer if the partitioning into tissues is more extensive than for thiopental. In contrast, the distribution phase in plasma is complete within thirty minutes after administration of the antiarrhythmic drug, procainamide (Fig. 3–1). Either procainamide does not partition into poorly perfused tissues or it does so readily, but the partition coefficients are very low. It is impossible to distinguish between these two possibilities by only measuring procainamide in plasma, since plasma poorly reflects the events that might occur within these tissues.

INTRAVENOUS BOLUS DOSE

Presentation of Data

Sum of Exponential Terms. The early rapid and subsequent slower decline in the plasma concentration of aspirin in an individual subject following a 650-milligram intravenous bolus dose (Fig. 19–2) is typical of many drugs. Had no samples been taken during the first ten minutes, the terminal linear decline of the plasma concentration when plotted on semilogarithmic graph paper would have been characterized by a monoexponential equation, and one-compartment disposition characteristics would have been applied to aspirin. Recall: The mono-

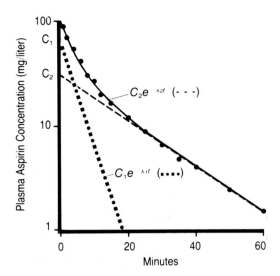

Fig. 19–2. When viewed on a semilogarithmic plot, the fall in the plasma concentration of aspirin is initially rapid, but then slows down after administering an intravenous bolus dose of 650 milligrams to a subject. The decline of the aspirin concentration (——) in plasma can be characterized by the sum of two exponential equations of the form: $C_1 e^{-\lambda_1 t}$ (●■●■) and $C_2 e^{-\lambda_2 t}$ (- - -). (One mg/liter = 5.5 micromolar.) (Redrawn from Rowland, M. and Riegelman, S.: Pharmacokinetics of acetylsalicylic acid and salicylic acid after intravenous administration in man. J. Pharm. Sci., *57*: 1313–1319, 1968.)

exponential equation is $C(0) \cdot e^{-kt}$, where k is the rate constant with an associated half-life, given by $0.693/k$, and $C(0)$ is the anticipated initial plasma drug concentration, given as the intercept on the plasma concentration axis when the line is extrapolated back to time zero. For aspirin the value of k is 0.050 minute^{-1}, the corresponding half-life is 14 minutes, and the value of $C(0)$ is 33 milligrams/liter. Going further, the volume of distribution [Dose/$C(0)$] is 20 liters and clearance ($k \cdot V$) is 0.98 liter/minute.

Notice, however, that the early plasma concentrations are higher than those anticipated by back extrapolation of the terminal slope, the difference being greater the earlier the time. When the difference at each sample time is plotted on the same graph, all the difference values fall on another straight line, which can be characterized by a monoexponential equation, $B(0)e^{-\alpha t}$, where α is the decay rate constant and $B(0)$ is the corresponding zero-time intercept. For aspirin, $\alpha = 0.23$ minute^{-1}, $t_{1/2} = 3.0$ minutes, and $B(0) = 67$ milligrams/liter.

Since all the plasma concentrations at the later times can be fitted by one equation, $C(0)e^{-kt}$ and since at the earlier times all of the difference values can be fitted by another equation, $B(0)e^{-\alpha t}$, it follows that the entire plasma drug concentration (C) versus time data can be fitted by the *sum* of these two exponential terms. That is

$$C = B(0)e^{-\alpha t} + C(0)e^{-kt} \qquad 1$$

For example, the biexponential equation $C = 67e^{-0.23t} + 33e^{-0.050t}$, where t is time in minutes, adequately describes the decline in the plasma concentration of aspirin following a 650-milligram bolus dose. Sometimes, when using this difference procedure, known commonly as the method of residuals, a sum of three and occasionally four exponential terms is required to adequately fit the observed concentration-time data. Since the principles in approaching such data are the same as those used to analyze and interpret events described by a biexponential equation, only the simpler case is considered further in this book.

Before proceeding, a more uniform set of symbols will be employed. Rather than using the different symbols α and k, the general symbol λ will be used to denote the exponential coefficient. Thus Equation 1 can be rewritten as

$$C = C_1 e^{-\lambda_1 t} + C_2 e^{-\lambda_2 t}$$

★

2

where the subscripts 1 and 2 refer to the first and second exponential terms respectively, and C_1 and C_2 refer to the corresponding zero-time intercepts, or coefficients. By convention, the exponential terms are arranged in order, starting with the largest value of λ. For example, in the case of aspirin $C_1 = 67$ milligrams/ liter, $\lambda_1 = 0.23$ minute^{-1}, $C_2 = 33$ milligrams/liter, and $\lambda_2 = 0.050$ minute^{-1}.

With aspirin, two exponential terms and hence two phases are seen when plasma concentration-time data are displayed on a semilogarithmic plot. Commonly, the last phase is called the *terminal phase*. With aspirin and many other drugs it is a correct description. Sometimes, however, there is an additional, still slower phase, which may have been missed because the assay procedure employed was insufficiently sensitive to measure the concentration of drug at these later times. This was certainly the case with the aminoglycosides and some amine drugs before the advent of more sensitive assays. This slower phase indicates that distribution equilibrium with all tissues had not previously been reached. In the subsequent discussion, however, the assumption is made that the observed terminal phase is correctly designated.

Initial Dilution Volume. At time zero the anticipated plasma concentration is, by reference to Equation 2, equal to the sum of the coefficients, $C_1 + C_2$. At that time the amount of drug in the body is the dose, no drug having been eliminated. Hence, by definition, the volume into which the drug appears to distribute initially, the *initial dilution volume* or initial volume of distribution, V_1, is given by

$$V_1 = \frac{\text{Dose}}{(C_1 + C_2)}$$

Initial volume
of distribution

★

3

For the aspirin example, the anticipated initial concentration is 100 milligrams/ liter, so that the initial dilution volume of aspirin is 6.5 liters.

A Compartmental Model. Although for the majority of situations in pharmacokinetics the desired information can be obtained either directly from or through modification of Equation 2, it is sometimes convenient to represent the events pictorially. Figure 19–3, a *two-compartment model*, is a common form of such a representation. Compartment 1, the initial dilution volume mentioned above, is also frequently called the central compartment because drug is administered into and distributed from it. As mentioned, the initial dilution volume of aspirin is 6.5 liters; for many other drugs it is much larger. These values are clearly greater than the plasma volume, 3 liters, and therefore this initial dilution volume must be composed of additional tissues into which drug distributes extremely rapidly. These tissues are the well-perfused ones, and since they include the liver and the kidneys, the major eliminating organs, elimination is usually depicted as occurring *directly* and *exclusively* from the central compartment. Drug distributes between this central compartment and a peripheral compartment, composed of tissues into which drug distributes more slowly.

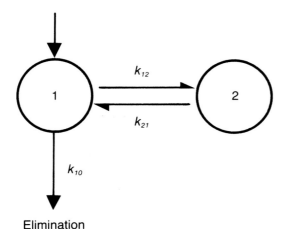

Fig. 19–3. A two-compartment model in which drug distributes between compartments one and two and is eliminated via compartment one.

Elimination

Several points are worth mentioning here. First, the minimum number of compartments or pools required to adequately describe distribution within the body equals the number of exponential terms needed to describe the plasma concentration-time data. Thus, a three-compartment model is needed when the data are best fitted by a triexponential equation. Next, the model depicted in Figure 19–3, or any other model where drug elimination is portrayed as occurring exclusively from the central compartment, is not unique. There are three two-compartment models that can adequately describe a biexponential plasma concentration decay curve: the one depicted in Figure 19–3, one with elimination occurring from both compartments, and one with loss occurring exclusively from the peripheral compartment. No distinction between these three possibilities can be made from plasma drug concentration-time data alone, and while the model depicted in Figure 19–3 is the most favored one, based on such physiologic considerations as the initial dilution volume exceeding the plasma volume, elimination can sometimes occur in tissues of the peripheral compartment. Moreover, occasionally the liver (and kidneys) is not part of the central compartment. For example, the initial dilution volume of indocyanine green, a dye used as a dynamic test of hepatic function, is only 3 liters, the plasma volume. The major peripheral tissue, in this instance the liver, is also the primary site of elimination via biliary excretion. A two-compartment model, with elimination occurring only from the peripheral compartment, therefore best describes the disposition kinetics of this dye. Lastly, drug distribution within a compartment is not homogenous. Although the concentrations of drug within and among such tissues usually vary enormously, tissues are lumped together in a compartment because the time taken for distribution equilibrium in each is similar. However, a small change in drug concentration in a region of a compartment should immediately reflect a proportional change elsewhere in that compartment.

In Figure 19–3 the movement of drug between the compartments can be characterized by the transfer rate constants, k_{12} and k_{21}, where k_{12} denotes the rate constant associated with the uptake of drug into compartment 2 from compartment 1, and k_{21} is the rate constant associated with the reverse process. The rate constant k_{10} is associated with the loss of drug from compartment 1 by metabolism and excretion. The unit of all rate constants is reciprocal time.

Rate equations can be written for the movement of amounts between the compartments and for drug elimination. Following an intravenous bolus dose these equations are

$$
\begin{array}{l}
\text{Rate of change} \\
\text{of amount of} \\
\text{drug in} \\
\text{compartment 1}
\end{array}
= \quad -k_{12}A_1 \quad - \quad k_{10}A_1 \quad + \quad k_{21}A_2 \qquad 4
$$

	Rate of movement from compartment 1 to compartment 2	Rate of elimination	Rate of movement from compartment 2 to compartment 1

$$
\begin{array}{l}
\text{Rate of change} \\
\text{of amount of} \\
\text{drug in} \\
\text{compartment 2}
\end{array}
= \quad k_{12}A_1 \quad - \quad k_{21}A_2 \qquad 5
$$

	Rate of movement from compartment 1 from compartment 2	Rate of movement to compartment 2 to compartment 1

where A_1 and A_2 are the amounts of drug in compartments 1 and 2, respectively. Solution of these rate equations provides a biexponential equation, of the same form as Equation 2, for the decline of drug from plasma, except the coefficients and exponents are recast in terms of the parameters defining the compartmental model. Although expressing the data in terms of a compartmental model and associated parameters may appear to give greater insight into the data, caution should be exercised in doing so. Remember that the compartmental model chosen is often not unique, and one can rarely assign a physical or physiologic meaning to the value of any of the rate constants. Accordingly, much of the subsequent discussion is related to the description of drug disposition by the sum of exponentials. However, the pharmacokinetic observations of a drug are discussed in terms of the compartmental model when this procedure facilitates general understanding. The equivalent relationships between the biexponential model and the two-compartment model are listed in Table 19–1.

Pharmacokinetic Parameters

Clearance. Elimination occurs at all times. Just as the plasma concentration is highest immediately following a bolus dose, so is the rate of elimination ($CL \cdot C$). Subsequently, both the plasma concentration and corresponding rate of elimination fall rapidly. To calculate the amount eliminated in a small unit of time, dt, recall that

$$
\text{Amount eliminated within interval } dt = \text{Clearance} \cdot C \cdot dt \qquad 6
$$

where $C \cdot dt$ is the corresponding small area under the plasma drug concentration-time curve within the interval dt. The total amount eliminated, the dose administered, is the sum of all the small amounts eliminated from time zero to time infinity. Therefore,

$$
\text{Dose} = \text{Clearance} \cdot AUC \qquad \bigstar \quad 7
$$

Table 19–1. Equivalent Relationships Between the Biexponential Model and the Two-compartment Model[a]

Parameters	Sum of Exponentials	Two-compartment Model
Plasma concentration (C)	$C_1 e^{-\lambda_1 t} + C_2 e^{-\lambda_2 t}$	$\left[\dfrac{Dose}{V_1} \cdot \dfrac{(k_{21} - \lambda_1)}{(\lambda_2 - \lambda_1)} \right] e^{-\lambda_1 t} + \left[\dfrac{Dose}{V_1} \cdot \dfrac{(k_{21} - \lambda_2)}{(\lambda_1 - \lambda_2)} \right] e^{-\lambda_2 t}$
	λ_1	$\frac{1}{2}\left[(k_{12} + k_{21} + k_{10}) + \sqrt{(k_{12} + k_{21} + k_{10})^2 - 4k_{21}k_{10}} \right]$
	λ_2	$\frac{1}{2}\left[(k_{12} + k_{21} + k_{10}) - \sqrt{(k_{12} + k_{21} + k_{10})^2 - 4k_{21}k_{10}} \right]$
	$(\lambda_1 + \lambda_2)$	$k_{12} + k_{21} + k_{10}$
	$\lambda_1 \cdot \lambda_2$	$k_{21} \cdot k_{10}$
Initial concentration	$C_1 + C_2$	$Dose/V_1$
Initial dilution volume (V_1)	$Dose/(C_1 + C_2)$	V_1
Clearance (CL)	$Dose/\left(\dfrac{C_1}{\lambda_1} + \dfrac{C_2}{\lambda_2} \right)$	$V_1 \cdot k_{10}$
Volume of distribution (V)	CL/λ_2	$V_1 \cdot k_{10}/\lambda_2$
Volume of distribution at steady state (V_{ss})	$\dfrac{Dose\left[\dfrac{C_1}{\lambda_1^2} + \dfrac{C_2}{\lambda_2^2} \right]}{\left[\dfrac{C_1}{\lambda_1} + \dfrac{C_2}{\lambda_2} \right]^2}$	$V_1 \cdot (1 + k_{12}/k_{21})$

[a]Assuming elimination takes place from the initial dilution volume only.

where AUC is the total area under the plasma drug concentration-time curve. Accordingly, as with the simpler one-compartment model, clearance (CL) is most readily estimated by dividing Dose by AUC. The area may be determined by using the trapezoidal rule (Appendix A) or, more conveniently, by realizing that the total area underlying a monoexponential term is the zero-time intercept divided by the corresponding exponential coefficient. Thus, the total area corresponding to Equation 2 is given by

$$AUC = \underbrace{\frac{C_1}{\lambda_1}}_{\substack{\text{Area asso-}\\\text{ciated with}\\\text{initial term}}} + \underbrace{\frac{C_2}{\lambda_2}}_{\substack{\text{Area asso-}\\\text{ciated with}\\\text{last term}}} \qquad ★ \qquad 8$$

When inserting the appropriate values for the aspirin example into Equation 8, the value of AUC associated with the 650-milligram dose is 957 milligrams · minutes/liter, so that the total clearance of aspirin in the individual is 679 milliliters/minute. Notice that this value of clearance is considerably smaller than the value calculated assuming a one-compartment model, 976 milliliters/minute. The latter is an overestimate of the true value, because elimination of drug during the attainment of distribution equilibrium was ignored. If instead of the first phase a later phase is missed, the error in estimating clearance will be large only if the missed area is a major fraction of the total area. Obviously, given the ease of estimating the total area and provided that blood sampling times are adequate, the true value for clearance should always be calculated.

Volume of Distribution. One purpose of a volume term is to relate the plasma drug concentration to the amount of drug in the body. The initial dilution volume fulfills this purpose. Subsequently, however, as drug distributes into the slowly equilibrating pool, the plasma concentration declines more rapidly than does the amount of drug in the body (A). Accordingly, as illustrated in Figure 19–4, the effective volume of distribution (A/C) increases with time until distribution equilibrium between drug in plasma and all tissues is achieved; this occurs during the terminal phase. Only then does decline of drug in all tissues parallel that

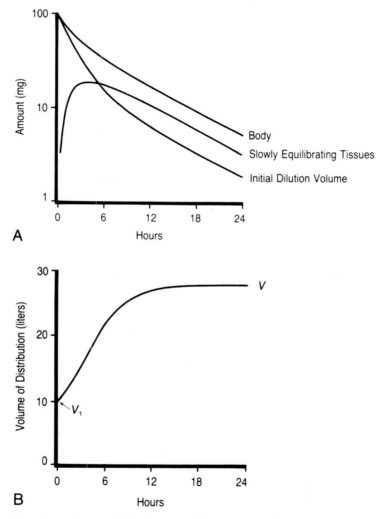

Fig. 19–4. Several events occur following a single intravenous bolus dose. As shown in Panel A, loss of drug from the initial dilution volume, of which plasma is a part, is due to both elimination from the body and distribution into the more slowly equilibrating compartment. The fall in amount of drug in the body, Panel A, is therefore initially less than the fall of drug in the initial dilution volume. Only when distribution equilibrium has been achieved do the falls in the amounts of drug in the initial dilution volume and in plasma parallel that in the body. Reflecting these events, the value of the apparent volume of distribution (A/C), which just after giving the dose equals the initial dilution volume (V_1), increases with time approaching a limiting value (V), which occurs when distribution equilibrium is achieved (Panel B).

in plasma and is proportionality between plasma concentration and amount of drug in the body achieved.

The value of the volume of distribution during the terminal phase (V) can be calculated as follows. During this phase the concentration is given by $C_2e^{-\lambda_2 t}$ (Fig. 19–2), and correspondingly,

$$\begin{array}{l}\text{Amount of drug}\\ \text{in body during} \quad = V \cdot C = V \cdot C_2e^{-\lambda_2 t} \qquad\qquad\qquad 9 \\ \text{terminal phase}\end{array}$$

Hence, extrapolating back to time zero, $V \cdot C_2$ must be the amount of drug needed in the body to give a plasma concentration of C_2, had it spontaneously distributed into the volume, V. It remains to calculate the amount, $V \cdot C_2$. When placed into the body, the amount, $V \cdot C_2$, is eventually matched by an equal amount eliminated. As the amount eliminated is the product of clearance and area, and as C_2/λ_2 is the associated area, it follows that

$$V \cdot C_2 \quad = \quad CL \cdot \frac{C_2}{\lambda_2}$$

$$\begin{array}{ccc}\text{Amount in} & & \text{Amount} \\ \text{body} & & \text{eliminated}\end{array} \qquad\qquad 10$$

or

$$V \quad = \quad \frac{CL}{\lambda_2} \qquad\qquad\qquad \bigstar$$

$$\begin{array}{cc} & \qquad\qquad 11\end{array}$$

$$\begin{array}{cc}\text{Volume of} & \dfrac{\text{Total clearance}}{\text{Terminal exponential coefficient}} \\ \text{distribution} & \end{array}$$

Returning to the example of aspirin, CL = 679 milliliters/minute and λ_2 = 0.050 minute^{-1}, therefore its volume of distribution is 13.6 liters. That is, if during the terminal phase the plasma concentration is 10 milligrams/liter, then the amount of drug in the body is 136 milligrams. Since 65 milligrams (10 mg/liter × 6.5 liters) is in the initial dilution volume, the remaining 71 milligrams must be in the tissues with which aspirin slowly equilibrates.

A comparison of Equation 11 with the one that has been used in all previous chapters to define the volume of distribution ($V = CL/k$) shows them to be the same, recognizing the equivalence of k and λ_2, the terminal exponential coefficient. The difference in the computed values for volume of distribution arises from a difference in the calculated clearance values; the residual area above that associated with the terminal slope is ignored when calculating clearance in the one-compartment model.

The ratio V_1/V gives an estimate of the degree of error in predicting the initial plasma concentrations using a one-compartment model. For example, for aspirin, with values for V_1 and V of 6.3 and 13.6 liters, respectively, the error in predicting initial concentrations from the plasma concentration-time data during the terminal phase can be large. The error can be even larger when predicting conditions beyond the measured final phase if a still slower one exists. This last error is only of concern if there is an appreciable accumulation of drug in this phase during chronic administration, a point considered subsequently in this chapter.

Distribution Kinetics and Elimination

During the distribution phase, more elimination occurs than would have been expected had distribution been spontaneous. The additional elimination is due to the particularly high concentrations of drug presented to the organs of elimination during this period. For many drugs this increased elimination is small and, with respect to elimination, viewing the body as a single compartment is adequate. For other drugs, the additional elimination represents a major fraction of the administered dose and approximation of the kinetics with a one-compartment model is inappropriate. A basis for making this decision rests on area considerations.

Recall from Equation 9 that elimination associated with the concentrations defined by the terminal exponential term, $C_2 e^{-\lambda_2 t}$, gives an amount equal to $CL \cdot C_2/\lambda_2$. Expressing this amount as a fraction of the administered dose, f_2, and utilizing the relationship in Equation 8 gives

$$\text{Fraction of elimination associated with last exponential term} = f_2 = \frac{C_2/\lambda_2}{AUC} \qquad 12$$

The remaining fraction, f_1, must therefore have been eliminated as a result of concentrations above those expected had spontaneous distribution occurred, that is, those concentrations defined by $C - C_2^{-\lambda_2 t}$ or $C_1 \cdot e^{-\lambda_1 t}$.

Applying Equation 12 to the case of aspirin, elimination of 70 percent of the dose is associated with the terminal slope; the remaining 30 percent eliminated therefore must be associated with plasma concentrations above those expected had spontaneous distribution occurred. Although distribution kinetics cannot be ignored, the majority of aspirin elimination is clearly associated with events defined by the terminal phase, which has a half-life of 14 minutes. Based on the same reasoning, the terminal half-life is the elimination half-life for the majority of drugs. There are some drugs, however, for which the calculated value of f_2 is very low. Gentamicin is an example. Over 98 percent of an intravenous bolus dose is eliminated before distribution equilibrium with all tissues of the body has been achieved. In this case, the reason lies in a permeability-limited distribution of gentamicin into certain tissues. Clearly, for gentamicin and similar drugs, the appropriate half-life defining elimination after a bolus dose is $0.693/\lambda_1$.

A Mathematical Aid

For all but the mathematically inclined, the analysis and prediction of plasma concentration-time data for a drug that displays multiexponential disposition characteristics are difficult. A useful mathematical aid to facilitate such analyses and predictions is to imagine that each exponential term arises from the independent administration of a different drug having one-compartment characteristics, and that the sum of their individual concentrations is the observed one. For example, imagine that a biexponential equation, $C_1 e^{-\lambda_1 t} + C_2 e^{-\lambda_2 t}$, arises from administration of two hypothetical drugs, Drug 1 and Drug 2; Drug 1 produces the curve $C_1e^{-\lambda_1 t}$ and Drug 2 produces the curve $C_2e^{-\lambda_2 t}$. Furthermore, assume that each hypothetical drug has the same clearance value, CL. Therefore, because the two drugs have different rate constants, λ_1 and λ_2, they have different volumes of distribution, which are given by CL/λ_1 and CL/λ_2, respectively. To complete the analysis, the doses of the hypothetical drugs are needed. These are obtained from area considerations as follows. Since dose is the product of clearance and area, the respective doses are $CL \cdot (C_1/\lambda_1)$ and $CL \cdot (C_2/\lambda_2)$. Furthermore, since $CL(C_1/\lambda_1 + C_2/\lambda_2)$ equals the total administered dose, it follows from Equation 12 that $f_1 \cdot$ Dose and $f_2 \cdot$ Dose are the corresponding doses. Hence, the total observed concentration is given by

$$C = \frac{f_1 \cdot \text{Dose } e^{-\lambda_1 t}}{(CL/\lambda_1)} + \frac{f_2 \cdot \text{Dose } e^{-\lambda_2 t}}{(CL/\lambda_2)} \qquad 13$$

Although the above equation is a devise that cannot, for example, predict the events in slowly equilibrating tissues, it readily permits calculation of the events in plasma under a variety of circumstances, as will be shown.

CONSTANT-RATE INFUSION

Figure 19–5 illustrates the anticipated effect of distribution kinetics on the plasma drug concentration upon stopping a constant-rate infusion at various times during the approach to plateau. At early times, a pronounced distribution phase is seen upon stopping the infusion, because distribution equilibrium has yet to be achieved between drug in blood and drug in many tissues. With a more prolonged infusion, more drug enters the tissues. The tendency of drug to move from blood to tissues is then much reduced, and the distribution phase appears much shallower upon stopping the infusion. Even at plateau, however, some distribution may still be seen upon stopping the infusion. At plateau, the

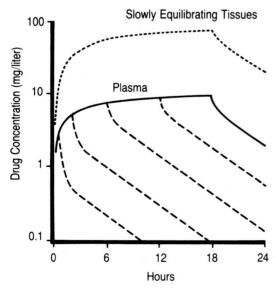

Fig. 19–5. Events in plasma (——) and in the slowly equilibrating tissues (----) during and after stopping a constant-rate infusion. As the concentration of drug in the slowly equilibrating tissues rises during the infusion, the net tendency of drug to enter these tissues decreases. Consequently, on stopping the infusion, the distribution phase in plasma (– – –) appears shallower the more prolonged the infusion. For simplicity, only the decline in tissue concentration when the infusion is stopped at plateau is shown. Equation 20 describes the plasma concentration during an infusion. At the end of an infusion of duration τ, the concentration, $C(\tau)$, is therefore $C_{ss}[f_1(1 - e^{-\lambda_1 \tau}) + f_2(1 - e^{-\lambda_2 \tau})]$. Furthermore, on stopping the infusion, the plasma concentration is given by $C_{ss}[f_1(1 - e^{-\lambda_1 \tau}) \cdot e^{-\lambda_1 t_{post}} + f_2(1 - e^{-\lambda_2 \tau}) \cdot e^{-\lambda_2 t_{post}}]$, where t_{post} is the time after stopping the infusion. The last equation can be derived using the mathematical aid (p. 307), recognizing, for example, that $f_1 \cdot C_{ss}(1 - e^{-\lambda_1 \tau})$ is the concentration at the end of the infusion associated with the first phase, and $e^{-\lambda_1 t_{post}}$ is the corresponding fraction remaining at time t_{post}.

rates of drug entry into and out of the tissues are equal. Upon stopping the infusion, the elimination of drug from plasma, with the subsequent fall in plasma concentration, creates a gradient for efflux of drug from the tissues. Initially, the rate of elimination of drug from plasma exceeds the rate of efflux from tissues, and the plasma concentration falls rapidly. Eventually, however, the rate of efflux of drug from the tissues limits the rate of elimination from the plasma. The body then acts, once again, as a single compartment; the plasma concentration and the amounts of drug in the tissues, and hence in the body as a whole, fall with a half-life equal to that seen during the terminal phase following an intravenous bolus dose.

The actual events seen after stopping an infusion at steady state depend largely on the kinetics of distribution. If distribution from the tissues is slow relative to elimination from the plasma, the plasma concentration falls substantially before the terminal phase is reached. Conversely, distribution may be so fast that, on stopping the infusion, only the terminal monoexponential decay is seen. The latter situation contrasts with events that would be seen following an intravenous bolus dose; a biexponential curve is invariably seen if blood is sampled early enough. As a guiding principle, a frank biphasic curve, on stopping an infusion at steady state, is only seen if f_2 is small, that is, when the majority of drug in plasma (and rapidly equilibrating tissues) is eliminated before distribution equilibrium is achieved.

Returning to events during infusion, the basic questions that remain are What controls the plateau concentration? and How long does it take to reach plateau?

Events at Plateau

Plateau Plasma Concentration. The plateau is reached when the rate of drug elimination matches the rate of infusion, R_o. The plasma drug concentration, C_{ss}, is therefore readily given by the familiar equation

★

$$C_{ss} = \frac{R_o}{\text{Clearance}}$$

14

Thus, as long as clearance is accurately determined, the rate of infusion needed to produce a given steady-state concentration can be calculated. Conversely, clearance can be determined from the concentration at steady state.

Volume of Distribution at Steady State. Although the volume of distribution, V, usefully relates amounts in body to plasma concentration during the terminal phase, its value is unfortunately influenced by the rate of elimination. As seen in Figure 19–6, the faster a drug is eliminated the greater is the ratio of drug in the slowly equilibrating tissues to that in plasma during the terminal phase and, correspondingly, the larger is the apparent volume of distribution. A need, therefore, exists to define a volume term to purely reflect distribution of drug within the body. The problem of elimination on estimating this volume term is overcome by infusing drug at a constant rate until steady state is reached. This volume term, volume distribution at steady state, V_{ss}, defined by

★

$$V_{ss} = \frac{\text{Amount of drug in body at steady state}}{\text{Plasma drug concentration at steady state}}$$

15

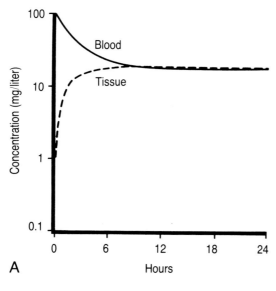

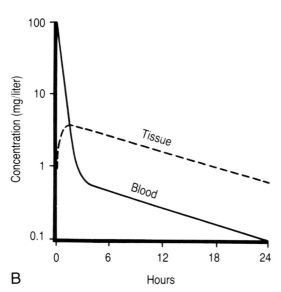

Fig. 19–6. Clearance of drug influences the volume of distribution during the terminal phase. To appreciate this statement, imagine the distribution of a drug between blood (volume, V_B, 5 liters) and a tissue (volume, V_T, 20 liters). Furthermore, let $K_p = 1$, so that the concentration in each compartment at equilibrium is equal if no elimination occurs (Panel A). The volume of distribution at equilibrium is then 25 liters. With elimination of drug, the concentration in the tissue (---) lags behind that in blood (——) during the terminal phase, thereby giving rise to a higher apparent value of K_p, $K_{p_{app}}$ (Panel B). Consequently, the apparent volume of distribution ($V_B + K_{p_{app}} \cdot V_T$) is increased above that expected under true equilibrium conditions, $V_B + K_P \cdot V_T$.

is a constant, whose value reflects drug distribution alone. Conceptualization of this volume may be helped by considering the two-compartment model depicted in Figure 19–3. At steady state, the rates of drug entering and leaving the slowly equilibrating tissues are exactly matched. It then follows from Equation 5 that the amount of drug in the slowly equilibrating compartment at steady state, $A_{2,ss}$ is given by

$$A_{2,ss} = \frac{k_{12}}{k_{21}} \cdot A_{1,ss}$$

16

The amount of drug in the body at steady state, A_{ss}, is the sum of $A_{1,ss}$ and $A_{2,ss}$. Therefore,

$$A_{ss} = A_{1,ss} \left[1 + \frac{k_{12}}{k_{21}} \right] \qquad 17$$

Finally, as $A_{1,ss} = V_1 \cdot C_{ss}$ and $A_{ss} = V_{ss} \cdot C_{ss}$, it follows that

$$V_{ss} = V_1 \left[1 + \frac{k_{12}}{k_{21}} \right] \qquad 18$$

Volume of
distribution at
steady state

In practice, as the amount of drug in the body cannot be determined physically, the value of V_{ss} is usually calculated from the disposition parameters (C_1, λ_1, C_2, and λ_2) following intravenous bolus administration (Table 19–1). The inter-relationships required are best understood from the concept of mean residence time (Chap. 24, Turnover Concepts, and Appendix F). The value of V_{ss} lies between the value of the initial dilution volume, V_1, and the volume of distribution, V. In general the difference between the values of V_{ss} and V is small and inconsequential. For aspirin, however, because appreciable elimination occurs before distribution equilibrium has been achieved, the value of V_{ss} (10.4 liters) is considerably smaller than the value of V (13.6 liters). In such circumstances estimating V_{ss} is worthwhile, especially if, for any reason, the disposition kinetics of aspirin were altered and one wished to assign the change to altered drug distribution or elimination, or both.

Time to Reach Plateau

Recall that for practical purposes the time to achieve plateau is that time required to reach 90 percent of the true value, recognizing that theoretically it takes an infinite time to reach steady state. Because of distribution kinetics, the time to reach plateau differs between plasma and tissue.

Events in Plasma. The terminal half-life of the immunosuppressive agent, cyclosporine A, is approximately 8 hours. Therefore, one would normally expect that 50 percent of the plateau plasma concentration is reached by 8 hours during a constant-rate infusion. Instead it takes only 2 to 3 hours, and instead of the expected 27 hours ($3.3 \cdot t_{1/2}$), the plateau is reached by approximately 12 hours (Fig. 19–7).

This difference arises because cyclosporine A's disposition kinetics are biphasic, with substantial drug eliminated occurring during the first phase, which has a half-life of approximately only 1 hour. The result is a rapidly rising initial curve followed by a much slower approach to plateau.

The importance of not just the half-lives, but also the relative rates of distribution and elimination, on the approach of the plasma concentration to plateau can be appreciated by the events depicted in Figure 19–8, where the values of λ_1 and λ_2 are fixed and the fractional term associated with the terminal phase, f_2, is varied between 0 and 1. When $f_2 = 1$, drug distributes spontaneously relative to elimination; the body acts as one compartment and, as expected, all

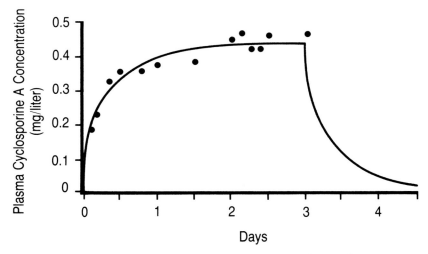

Fig. 19–7. By 2 hours into a 72-hour, constant-rate intravenous infusion of cyclosporine A (0.29 mg/kg per hour), the plasma concentration has risen to 50 percent of the plateau value, despite a terminal half-life of 8 hours in the patient. This rapid approach to plateau is a result of events in plasma being primarily controlled by an initial phase, with a half-life of 1 hour, during which time significant elimination occurs following a bolus dose. The solid line is the predicted plasma concentration on fitting a biexponential model to the data. (One mg = 0.83 micromolar.) (Redrawn from Gupta, S., Legg, B., Solomons, L., Johnson, R., and Rowland, M.: Pharmacokinetics of cyclosporin: Influence of dosing rate in renal transplant patients. Brit. J. Clin. Pharmacol., 24:519–526, 1987.)

the drug is eliminated during the terminal (and only) phase. In this case, it takes 1 terminal half-life $(0.693/\lambda_2)$ and 3.3 such half-lives to reach 50 percent and 90 percent of the plateau, respectively. However, as the value of f_2 falls, more drug is correspondingly eliminated before distribution equilibrium is established. As a result, the time to achieve 50 percent of the plateau, for example, occurs earlier until, when $f_2 = 0$; this time is the half-life of the first phase, $0.693/\lambda_1$, and the body once again acts as a single compartment, but with a smaller volume of distribution, V_1. For most drugs f_2 is close to 1, and so the terminal half-life

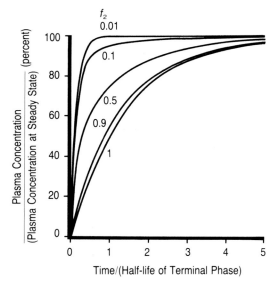

Fig. 19–8. The approach to plateau in plasma, during a constant-rate intravenous infusion, for a drug that displays biexponential disposition kinetics is determined primarily by the relative rates of distribution and elimination. In this example the values for the two exponential coefficients λ_1 and λ_2 are kept constant (with $\lambda_1 = 10\lambda_2$), and the value of the fractional elimination term associated with the terminal phase, f_2, is varied from 0.01 to 1. Only when drug distributes rapidly compared with elimination (f_2 approaches 1) does the terminal half-life control the time to approach plateau. When f_2 is very low, e.g., 0.01, implying elimination occurs much faster than distribution, the approach to plateau is determined primarily by λ_1. Included for reference is the expected curve when the drug exhibits one-compartment characteristics ($f_2 = 1$), in which case 50 percent and 90 percent of the plateau is reached by 1 and 3.3 terminal half-lives, respectively. Note that time is expressed in units of terminal half-life.

primarily determines the time to reach plateau. For cyclosporine A, significant elimination occurs before distribution equilibrium is achieved and hence the observation in Figure 19–5. For gentamicin, with f_2 close to 0, it is the half-life of the first phase, usually 2 to 4 hours, that primarily determines the time for this aminoglycoside to reach plateau in plasma.

Another view of the events in plasma is in relation to the expanding volume of distribution on approach to equilibrium (see Fig. 19–4). A plateau is reached when the rates of infusion and elimination are equal. When distribution into the tissue is slow, the effective volume of distribution remains close to the initial dilution volume, V_1, for some time, so that for a given rate of input the plasma concentration rises much faster than if rapid distribution into the tissue occurs. Therefore, as rate of elimination = $CL \cdot C$, it follows that, for a given clearance value, the approach to plateau occurs earlier the slower the distribution of drug into the tissue.

The plasma concentration at any time on approach to plateau can be calculated using concepts presented in Figure 19–8. Remember for a drug with one-compartment characteristics the concentration at any time during an infusion is given by

$$C = \frac{R_o}{CL} (1 - e^{-kt})$$

For a drug that exhibits biexponential disposition characteristics the corresponding equation is

$$C = \frac{f_1 R_o}{CL} (1 - e^{-\lambda_1 t}) + \frac{f_2 R_0}{CL} (1 - e^{-\lambda_2 t}) \qquad 19$$

or

$$C = C_{ss}[f_1(1 - e^{-\lambda_1 t}) + f_2(1 - e^{-\lambda_2 t})] \qquad \bigstar \qquad 20$$

These solutions follow by imagining that the total concentration is the sum derived from two hypothetical drugs, each with the same clearance value, infused at rates $f_1 \cdot R_o$ and $f_2 \cdot R_o$, respectively. Equations 19 and 20 emphasize the importance of f_2 (and hence C_1 and C_2) as well as λ_1 and λ_2 in determining the events in plasma following a constant-rate infusion. Equation 20 also permits ready calculation of the percent of plateau reached at any time. For example, if the half-lives associated with the first and terminal exponential terms are 1 and 12 hours, respectively, and $f_2 = 0.5$, then at 6 hours, the concentration will be 64 percent of the plateau concentration. The converse, that is, the time taken to reach a certain percent of plateau cannot be calculated directly, because there are two exponential terms containing the unknown time. However, the time can be determined by iteration (Chap. 18) by substituting different times into Equation 20 until the right answer is reached. In the example above, the time taken to reach 50 percent of plateau is 2.75 hours.

Events in Peripheral Tissue. As illustrated in Figure 19–9, the time to achieve plateau in the slowly equilibrating tissues is *always* determined by the terminal half-life, irrespective of the time required to achieve plateau in plasma. To appreciate this point, consider events in terms of the two-compartment model depicted in Figure 19–3. When distribution occurs rapidly, drug in tissue for most of the time is virtually at equilibrium with drug in plasma. That is,

$$k_{21}A_2 \simeq k_{12}A_1$$ 21

Rate of drug   Rate of drug
leaving tissue   entering tissue

and therefore

$$A_2 \simeq \frac{k_{12}}{k_{21}} \cdot A_1$$ 22

which shows that the amount of drug in the tissue parallels changes in plasma. When, however, distribution is slow relative to elimination, the concentration in plasma approaches its plateau before much drug has entered the slowly equilibrating tissue. The situation is then similar to a constant-rate input to the compartment from which loss occurs. Accumulation is determined by the elimination half-life, which in this case is associated with k_{21}, the exit rate constant from the tissue. In reality, the situation is somewhat more complex because of the reversible movement of drug between plasma and tissue. Nonetheless, under these circumstances, the slow rate constant for transfer out of the tissue is a major determinant of the terminal rate constant, $\lambda 2$.

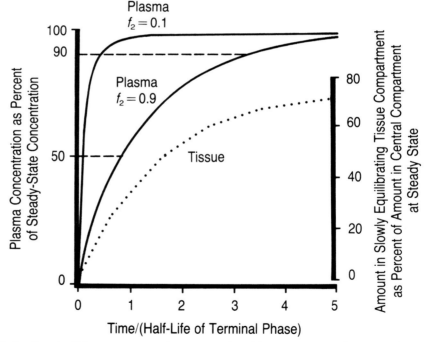

Fig. 19–9.   Despite differences seen in plasma, reproduced from Figure 19–8, the approach to plateau in the slowly equilibrating tissue (····) during a constant-rate intravenous infusion is controlled by the terminal half-life of the drug. Shown are events for two drugs that both display biexponential disposition kinetics. They have the same value for the exponential coefficients (λ_1 and λ_2), but differ in the importance of each phase to drug elimination, signified by the value of f_2. Note that time is expressed in units of terminal half-life. The horizontal dashed lines correspond to 50 percent and 90 percent of the plateau plasma concentration.

Bolus Plus Infusion

Lidocaine is used in the control of ventricular arrhythmias in emergency settings. A bolus is given to rapidly achieve an effective concentration and is followed by a constant-rate infusion to maintain the concentration. Although the infusion eventually achieves the last objective, initially it cannot match the fall in plasma concentration associated with distribution into the tissues, potentially leading to a period of ineffective concentrations. The events are depicted schematically in Figure 19–10. A larger bolus dose would overcome the problem, but would also increase the likelihood of toxicity because of the initially higher concentrations. A common solution is to give supplementary bolus doses or an initially higher rate of infusion during this period of potential deficiency. A more elegant solution lies in giving a supplemental, exponentially declining infusion. The object of the supplemental infusion is to match the net rate of movement of drug into the tissues. This rate is highest initially, when no drug is in the tissue. However, as the concentration in the tissue rises with time on approach to plateau, the net movement into the tissue progressively declines.

AN EXTRAVASCULAR DOSE

Often absorption is slower than distribution so approximating the body as a single compartment is reasonable. Occasionally it is not, as illustrated with digoxin in Figure 19–11. Following oral administration, digoxin is absorbed before much distribution has occurred, and consequently the distribution phase is still evident beyond the peak concentration. In this situation the peak concentration and the time of its occurrence are dependent on the kinetics of both absorption and distribution. The implication of these events to drug therapy and monitoring depends on whether the site of action resides in a rapidly or a slowly equilibrating tissue. Digoxin distributes slowly into the heart, the target organ. Accordingly, it is inappropriate to relate plasma concentration to effect until distribution equilibrium is achieved, approximately 6 hours for this drug. Before that time, even when plasma concentration is declining, response is increasing due to a rising cardiac concentration, making any interpretation of

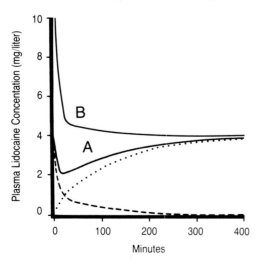

Fig. 19–10. Although a bolus (V_1C_d) can be given to initially achieve a desired plasma lidocaine concentration of 4 milligrams/liter, C_d, constant infusion at a rate required to maintain this value (rate = $CL \cdot C_d$) fails to do so in the early moments, owing to distribution kinetics. It should be noted that the observed plasma concentration (——, A) is the sum of that associated (– – –) with the bolus (Eq. 2) and that associated (– – –) with the constant-rate infusion (– – –) (Eq. 20). A larger bolus dose can be given, but the resulting high initial plasma concentrations (——, B) may increase the chance of toxicity. (One mg/liter = 4.3 micromolar.)

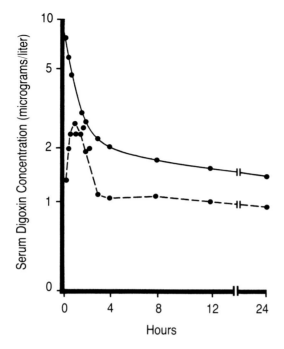

Fig. 19–11.   Depicted is a semilogarithmic plot of the mean concentration of digoxin (●) following 0.5 milligram administered orally (two 0.25-mg tablets, dashed line) and intravenously (solid line) to four volunteers. Because absorption is much faster than distribution, a biphasic curve is still seen after attainment of the peak concentration following the oral dose. (One mg/liter = 1.3 micromolar.) (Taken from Huffman, D.H. and Azarnoff, J.: Absorption of orally given digoxin preparations. JAMA, 222: 957–960, 1972. Copyright 1972, American Medical Association.)

the plasma concentration extremely difficult (Chap. 20). In contrast to digoxin, many drugs equilibrate rapidly with such highly perfused tissues as the heart and the brain; then plasma concentration correlates positively with response at all but the earliest of times.

As with the simple one-compartment model, availability is given by $F = CL \cdot AUC/$Dose, and relative availability is estimated by comparison of AUC values following different formulations or routes of administration, correcting for dose.

MULTIPLE DOSING

The impact that distribution kinetics can have on events during multiple dosing is illustrated by the data in Figure 19–12, obtained following an 8-hourly intramuscular regimen of gentamicin for 8 days to a patient for the treatment of a serious infection. Seen are the large fluctuation in plasma concentration resulting from this regimen and the long terminal half-life on stopping therapy. In common with other aminoglycosides, gentamicin is polar, and while it distributes rapidly into the extracellular water space, approximate volume of 15 liters, it enters cells very slowly. Accordingly, although gentamicin has a long terminal half-life, approximately 87 hours in the patient, the majority of a dose is eliminated by eight hours, associated with the 4-hour half-life of the first phase. Indeed, as a reasonable approximation, the terminal phase can be ignored with respect to events in plasma, as was the case when previously considering gentamicin dosing (Chap. 18, Drug Monitoring). The reasonableness of this approximation is borne out by the observed rapid establishment of a plateau in plasma and by the large degree of fluctuation in plasma concentration, which is expected for a drug with a half-life of 4 hours (in the patient) when it is given every 8 hours. Associated with this regimen, however, is a slow but continual

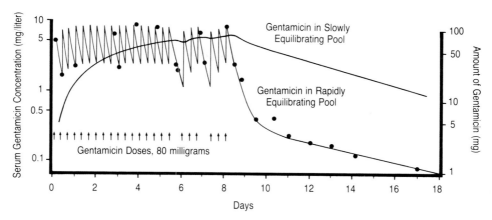

Fig. 19–12.   Depicted are semilogarithmic plots of the levels of gentamicin in the body occurring during and after intramuscular administration of gentamicin, 80 milligrams, almost every 8 hours (times indicated by arrows) to a patient for just over 8 days. The biphasic decline in serum drug concentration (●) when administration was stopped was fitted to a model that assumes that gentamicin distributes between a rapidly equilibrating compartment and a slowly equilibrating compartment, with elimination, entirely by renal excretion, occurring exclusively from the rapidly equilibrating compartment (see Fig. 19–3). The lines are the predicted serum gentamicin concentrations (left-hand ordinate), the amount of gentamicin in the rapidly equilibrating compartment (right-hand ordinate), a value obtained by multiplying the serum concentration by the estimated initial dilution volume, and the predicted amount of gentamicin in the slowly equilibrating compartment (right-hand ordinate). Little accumulation and large fluctuations of drug occur in the rapidly equilibrating pool. In contrast, the amount of gentamicin slowly, but extensively, accumulates in the slowly equilibrating pool during drug administration, with little fluctuation within a dosing interval; disappearance of drug from the slowly equilibrating tissues is also slow on stopping the drug. During administration, the concentration in plasma after the Nth dose can be calculated from the formula

$$C = \frac{D_M}{V_1} \left\{ f_1 \left[\frac{1 - e^{-N\lambda_1 \tau}}{1 - e^{-\lambda_1 \tau}} \right] e^{-\lambda_1 t} + f_2 \left[\frac{1 - e^{-N\lambda_2 \tau}}{1 - e^{-\lambda_2 \tau}} \right] e^{-\lambda_1 t} \right\}$$

where D_M is the maintenance dose given every τ, t is the time since giving the last dose, and V_1 is the initial dilution volume. This equation can be derived using the multiple-dosing equation (Appendix D), assuming instantaneous absorption, and the mathematical aid (p. 307). (One mg/liter = 1.8 micromolar.) (Adapted from Schentag, J.J. and Jusko, W.J.: Renal clearance and tissue accumulation of gentamicin. Clin. Pharmacol. Ther., 22: 364–370, 1977. Reproduced with permission of C.V. Mosby.)

accumulation of drug in the slowly equilibrating tissues, where it takes approximately 12 days (3.3 terminal half-lives) to reach plateau. However, at plateau accumulation is so extensive that there is more gentamicin in these tissues than exists, on average, in the rapidly equilibrating pool. Furthermore, because of slow distribution there is little fluctuation of drug in the slowly equilibrating pool.

Accumulation, both time-course and extent thereof, are clearly dependent on the site of measurement. For gentamicin there is little accumulation in plasma, and a plateau is reached soon after initiating therapy. In contrast, extensive accumulation occurs in the slowly equilibrating tissues, where it takes considerable time to attain plateau. In Chapter 7, based on consideration of the minimum amount of drug after the first dose and at plateau (p. 83), a proposed index of accumulation was $1/(1 - e^{-k\tau})$. As a reasonable approximation, this index can also be employed here using the appropriate rate constant. For example, in plasma ($\lambda_1 = 0.172$ hour^{-1}) with $\tau = 8$ hours, the accumulation index for gentamicin is only 1.33, whereas in the slowly equilibrating pool ($\lambda_2 = 0.008$ hour^{-1}) it is as much as 16.

The events on stopping gentamicin administration are predictable. The plasma concentration falls rapidly for the first two days, with a half-life controlled by the first phase. Eventually, however, elimination of drug from plasma is rate limited by egress of drug from the slowly equilibrating tissues. Except for the high degree of fluctuation in plasma, the events seen with gentamicin are those expected following a constant-rate infusion for any drug with a very low value of f_2 (Fig. 19–9).

Significant clinical implications arise from the distribution kinetics of gentamicin. Most organisms against which gentamicin is used reside in the rapidly equilibrating extracellular space, and so frequent administration is needed to maintain an adequate antimicrobial concentration. Unfortunately, ototoxicity and nephrotoxicity, associated with the accumulation of drug at slowly equilibrating sites within the ear and the kidneys, can eventually occur. Accumulation cannot be avoided if an effective plasma concentration is to be maintained. To minimize the problem, a prudent practice is to limit the total duration of gentamicin administration whenever possible. Monitoring the plasma concentration also may help. Of the measures in plasma, the trough value is the most sensitive indicator of the rising concentration in the slowly equilibrating tissues, although as illustrated in Figure 19–11, even this measurement is not that sensitive. Nonetheless, monitoring of trough concentrations is of value, particularly if the concentration continues to rise, indicating a greater-than-expected rise of drug in the slowly equilibrating pool with a corresponding increase in the potential for toxicity.

ALTERED CLEARANCE

When discussing the use of gentamicin in patients with renal insufficiency (Chap. 16), the terminal phase was ignored in adjusting dosing regimens to achieve therapeutic concentrations. Generally this is reasonable because renal impairment primarily affects the first phase. For example, as illustrated in Figure 19–13, only the initial half-life is altered among patients with varying degrees of renal insufficiency; the terminal half-life is virtually unaffected. The observation may be rationalized in the following manner. When renal function is normal most of gentamicin in the rapidly equilibrating pool is eliminated before distribution equilibrium is either achieved after administration of a bolus dose (Fig. 19–14) or re-established on stopping administration after chronic dosing (Fig. 19–13). Under these circumstances before distribution equilibrium is achieved, elimination may be viewed as occurring from volume V_1 with a clearance, CL. Hence the rate constant for decline of drug in the rapidly equilibrating pool (including plasma) approaches CL/V_1, with a corresponding half-life of $0.693 \cdot V_1/CL$. Reduction in clearance is then reflected by an almost proportional increase in half-life of the first phase. In contrast, during the terminal phase the loss of drug from plasma (and the rapidly equilibrating pool) is rate limited by efflux of drug out of the slowly equilibrating tissues and not by its clearance from plasma. Accordingly, the terminal half-life is unchanged. However, with a reduction in clearance, distribution equilibrium takes somewhat longer to be established and, because less drug is eliminated by then, the concentration of

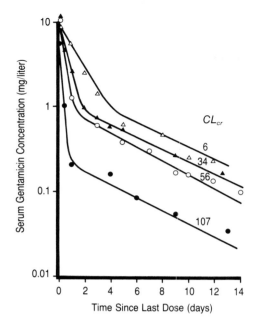

Fig. 19–13. Semilogarithmic plots of the decline in the serum concentration of gentamicin in four patients with different degrees of renal function, as assessed by creatinine clearance, CL_{cr}, after stopping gentamicin administration. Notice that renal function impairment primarily affects the half-life of the first phase and the depth of the decline in concentration before the terminal phase is reached. (One mg/liter = 1.8 micromolar.) (Redrawn from Schentag, J.J., Jusko, W.J., Plaut, M.E., Cumbo, T.J., Vance, J.W., and Abrutyn, E.: Tissue persistence of gentamicin in man. JAMA, *238*: 327–329, 1977. Copyright 1977, American Medical Association.)

gentamicin in plasma is higher compared with that in a patient with normal renal function (see Figs. 19–13 and 19–14). Ultimately, if renal function is sufficiently low, the terminal half-life is sensitive to renal function. Then the first phase primarily reflects distribution, as shown in Figure 19–14. To appreciate the last point, consider administration of a bolus dose of drug to a patient with no renal function. Drug in plasma would still decline initially with a half-life determined solely by distribution. Between this extreme and normal renal function is a range over which the terminal half-life changes noticeably with renal function. For gentamicin, calculation shows this to occur when renal function is less than 7 percent of normal. Then, albeit slowly for gentamicin, distribution

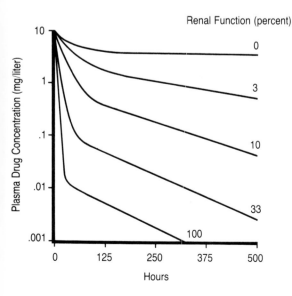

Fig. 19–14. Semilogarithmic plots of the simulated decline in the plasma concentration after intravenous bolus administration of a drug, with disposition characteristics similar to gentamicin, for different degrees of renal function from 0 to 100 percent of normal. Notice that renal function primarily affects the half-life of the first phase and the depth of decline in concentration before the terminal phase is reached, until renal function is very low. When renal function is very low, the initial decline is determined primarily by distribution, and the impairment is reflected by changes in the terminal half-life.

is achieved before much drug is eliminated, the condition that normally prevails for most drugs.

With gentamicin concern exists for excessive accumulation of drug in the slowly equilibrating tissues during chronic dosing, particularly in patients with renal insufficiency. However, provided that adjustment in dosing rate has been made to compensate for diminished renal function, there should be no greater risk of toxicity in patients with renal insufficiency than in patients with normal renal function. This conclusion is based on consideration of events at plateau. The amount in the slowly equilibrating tissues at steady state is the difference between the amount of drug in the body ($V_{ss} \cdot C_{ss}$) and that in the rapidly equilibrating pool ($V_1 \cdot C_{ss}$). That is,

$$\text{Amount of drug in slowly equilibrating tissues at steady state} = (V_{ss} - V_1) \cdot C_{ss} \qquad 23$$

From this last relationship it is seen that, provided dosing rate is adjusted to maintain a given steady-state plasma concentration, the amount in the slowly equilibrating tissues is unaltered, as both V_1 and V_{ss} are purely distribution terms that, at least for gentamicin, are unaltered by renal insufficiency.

Study Problems

(Answers to Study Problems are in Appendix G.)

1. Define the following terms: initial dilution volume, volume of distribution during terminal phase, and volume of distribution at steady state.

2. Comment on the following statements.

   (a) All drugs are expected to exhibit distribution kinetics.

   (b) For most drugs it is reasonable to represent the disposition kinetics by a compartmental model, with elimination occurring exclusively from the central compartment.

   (c) Following an intravenous bolus dose of drug, essentially all drug is eliminated from the body by 5 terminal plasma half-lives.

3. Hamilton *et al.* (reference in Table 19–2) assessed the effect of acetylator phenotype on the disposition kinetics of amrinone, a positive inotropic agent with vasodilatory properties. The acetylator status was determined for the subjects with isoniazid. Each subject then received a 75-milligram bolus dose intravenously (infused over 10 minutes). Table 19–2 lists the plasma concentration-time data in one fast and one slow acetylator. The drug is metabolized (probably in the liver) and is excreted unchanged. Assume that both subjects weigh the same and that the dose was given instantaneously.

Table 19–2.[a]

Time (hours)	Plasma Amrinone Concentration (mg/liter)[b]	
	Slow Acetylator	Fast Acetylator
0.16	1.30	1.20
0.25	1.03	0.93
0.33	0.89	0.76
0.5	0.72	0.54
0.67	0.64	0.42
1	0.59	0.31
2	0.52	0.19
3	0.47	0.13
4	0.42	N.D.[c]
8	0.27	N.D.[c]
12	0.17	N.D.[c]
15	0.12	N.D.[c]

[a]Problem adapted from data in Hamilton, R.A., Kowalsky, S.F., Wright, E.M., Cernak, P., Benziger, D.P., Stroshane, R.M., and Edelson, J. Clin. Pharmacol. Ther., 40:615–619, 1986.
[b]One mg/liter = 5.3 micromolar.
[c]N.D. Below detection limit of assay.

(a) Plot the data on two-cycle semilogarithmic graph paper and, using the method of residuals, determine the values of the parameters of the biexponential equations that fit each set of data: C_1, λ_1, C_2, and λ_2.

(b) From the values in (a), calculate CL, V_1, and V. Which of these parameters show(s) major differences between the fast and slow acetylator?

(c) Is the assumption that the liver and kidneys are part of the initial dilution volume reasonable?

(d) Had data been available from one hour onward, when only the terminal phase is evident, what values for V and CL would be expected? Would one conclude that the difference between the fast and slow acetylators was greater from these data?

(e) What fraction of the dose eliminated is associated with the terminal exponential term for each subject?

(f) Is it reasonable to conclude, for both subjects, that the terminal half-life will principally determine the time to reach plateau in plasma following a constant-rate infusion?

4. A moderately polar drug is eliminated entirely by renal excretion. Following a 50-milligram intravenous bolus dose to a 68-kilogram healthy subject, the plasma drug concentration was observed to decline biexponentially: C (mg/liter) $= 2.71e^{-0.19t} + 0.034e^{-0.0095t}$, where t is in hours. The fraction of the drug unbound in plasma is 0.37 and is independent of drug concentration over the range seen in plasma.

(a) Assuming that elimination occurs only from the initial dilution volume (central compartment), calculate the following pharmacokinetic parameters: V_1, CL, V (V_{ss}, optional).

(b) Comment on the mechanism of renal excretion of the drug and the appropriateness of the assumption that elimination occurs only from the central compartment.

(c) Optional: comment on the discrepancy between V and V_{ss}.

(d) Calculate the fractions of the dose eliminated that are associated with each exponential term, and comment on the question, "What is the half-life of the drug?"

(e) The drug is given by a constant-rate infusion.

1. Using an iterative procedure, calculate how long it takes for the plasma concentration to reach 50 percent and 90 percent of the steady-state value. Comment on the statement, "It takes 1 half-life to reach 50 percent of plateau and 3.3 half-lives to reach plateau."

2. Comment on why a pronounced biexponential curve is seen in the decline of plasma concentration postinfusion after steady state has been reached.

3. Would you expect to have detected a biexponential curve on stopping the infusion at steady state had the disposition kinetics of the drug following a 50-milligram bolus dose been defined by the equation $C(t) = 0.56e^{-0.19t} + 0.14e^{-0.0095t}$. That is, the same exponential coefficients, but different coefficients compared with the drug discussed above.

5. The fractions of drug normally excreted unchanged after intravenous administration of both the neuromuscular blocking agents d-tubocurarine and pancuronium are similar at approximately 0.65. Yet, as seen in Figure 19–15, the effect of compromised renal function on the disposition kinetics of these drugs is different. For pancuronium the terminal half-life is prolonged, whereas for d-tubocurarine the terminal half-life is unchanged. Briefly discuss the reason for the difference in the effect of renal dysfunction on these two drugs.

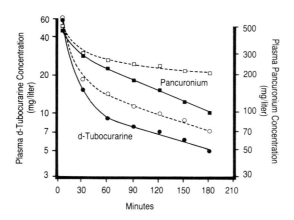

Fig. 19–15. The disposition kinetics of d-tubocurarine (○,●) and pancuronium (□,■) for patients with both normal (——) and impaired renal function (----). (Redrawn from Miller, R.D.: Pharmacokinetics of muscle relaxants and their antagonists. In Pharmacokinetics of Anesthesia. Edited by C. Pry-Roberts and C.C. Hug. Oxford, Blackwell Scientific Publications Limited, 1984, p. 255.)

6. In Figure 21–10 (Metabolite Kinetics) the plasma concentrations of the benzodiazepine halazepam are shown during and following an oral dosage regimen of 40 milligrams of the drug every 8 hours for 14 days.

(a) Why is the plasma concentration of halazepam fluctuating markedly even at steady state?

(b) Can the terminal half-life of halazepam be determined during administration of the dosage regimen?

20

Pharmacologic Response

The basic principles surrounding the establishment of an appropriate dosage regimen of a drug were presented in Chapter 5. These principles rest heavily on the assumption that a functional relationship, albeit sometimes complex, exists between the concentration of drug at the site(s) of action and the response produced. Some evidence supporting this view was presented in Chapter 5, together with short commentaries on such additional considerations as delays in drug response, role of active metabolites, and tolerance. In this chapter some of these aspects are considered in greater depth and the temporal relationship between dose (or concentration) and response is explored. The chapter begins with an examination of the concentration-response relationship and ends with a discussion of dosage regimen design based on response data.

CONCENTRATION AND RESPONSE

Because most sites of action reside outside the vasculature, delays exist between the placement of drug into blood and the response produced. This kinetic phenomenon can obscure underlying relationships between concentration and effect. One potential solution is to measure the concentration at the site of action. Although this is possible in an isolated organ system, it is not a practical solution for studies in man. Apart from ethical and technical issues that arise, many effects observed *in vivo* represent an integration of many different responses occurring at numerous sites. Another approach is to develop a model that takes into account the time-course of drug movement between the plasma and the site of action, thereby producing "effector site" concentrations that can then be related to response. Yet another approach is to examine response under steady-state conditions. Whatever the approach adopted, the resulting concentration-response relationships for most drugs have features in common. The response increases with an increase in concentration at low concentrations and tends to approach a maximum at high concentrations. Recall from Chapter 5 that this was observed for the relaxant effect of terbutaline in an isolated, contracted human bronchial muscle; it is also observed in man, as illustrated for two compounds in Figure 20–1. These compounds, R(−) − ketamine and S(+) − ketamine, are optical isomers which, as a 50–50 mixture or racemate, constitute the commercially available intravenous anesthetic agent, ketamine. Although both compounds have an anesthetic effect, they clearly differ from each other. Not only is the maximum effect (E_{max}) achieved less with R(−) − ketamine than with S(+) − ketamine, but the plasma concentration required to produce 50 percent of its E_{max}, referred to as the EC_{50} value, is also greater (1.8 mg/liter versus 0.7 mg/liter). Moreover, the response curve for R(−) − ketamine appears shallower than that for S(+) − ketamine. Although the reason for the differences are unclear, these observations stress the importance that stereochemistry can have in drug response.

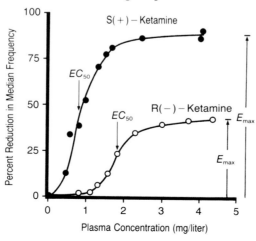

Fig. 20–1. Changes in the electroencephalographic median frequency were followed to quantify the anesthetic effect of R(−) − ketamine and S(+) − ketamine in a subject who received an infusion of these two optical isomers on separate occasions. Shown is the percent reduction in the median frequencies *versus* plasma concentration. Although characteristic S-shaped, or sigmoidal, curves are seen with both compounds, they differ in both the maximum effect achieved, E_{max}, and the concentration needed to produce 50 percent of E_{max}, the EC_{50}. These relationships may be considered direct ones as no significant time delay was found between response and concentration. (One mg/liter = 4.2 micromolar.) (Redrawn from Schuttler, J., Stoeckel, H., Schweilden, H., and Lauvan, P.M.: Hypnotic drugs. In Quantitation, modeling and control in anaesthesia. Edited by H. Stoeckel. George Thieme Verlag, Stuttgart, 1985, pp. 196–210.)

General Equation

A general equation has been found to describe the types of observations seen in Figures 5–1 and 20–1 adequately. It is

★

$$\text{Intensity of Effect} = \frac{E_{max} \cdot C^{\gamma}}{EC_{50}{}^{\gamma} + C^{\gamma}} \qquad 1$$

where E_{max} and EC_{50} are as defined above and γ is the *shape factor* that accommodates the shape of the curve. The intensity of response is usually a change in a measurement from its basal value. Although empirical, Equation 1 has found wide application. Certainly, it has the right properties.

Figure 20–2A shows the influence of γ on the shape of the concentration-response relationship. The larger the value of γ, the greater the change in response with concentration around the EC_{50} value. For example, if $\gamma = 1$ then, by appropriate substitution into Equation 1, the concentrations corresponding to 20 percent and 80 percent of maximal response are 0.25 and 4 times EC_{50}, respectively, a sixteenfold range. Whereas, if $\gamma = 2$ the corresponding concentrations are 0.5 and 2 times EC_{50}, only a fourfold range. Using the increase in the forced expiratory volume in one second (FEV_1) as a measure of the bronchodilatory effect produced by theophylline in patients with obstructive pulmonary disease, the average value of γ is close to 1 (Fig. 20–3). Generally the value of γ lies between 1 and 3. Occasionally it is much greater, in which case the effect appears almost as an all-or-none response, because the range of concentrations associated with minimal and maximal responses becomes so narrow.

Patients differ widely in their values of EC_{50} and γ, as illustrated for theophylline in Figure 20–3. Part of the variability in EC_{50} values may be due to differences in plasma protein binding, as response depends on unbound drug at the site of action. Even when based on unbound concentration, the EC_{50} value may still vary, indicating differences in sensitivities to the drug among patients. Variability may also exist in the E_{max} value, so that the maximal effect produced in one individual differs from that in another.

A common form of representing concentration-response data is a plot of the intensity of response against the *logarithm* of the concentration. Figure 20–2B shows this transformation of the curves in Figure 20–2A. This transformation is popular because it expands the initial part of the curve, where response is changing markedly with a small change in concentration, and contracts the latter part, where a large change in concentration produces only a slight change in response. It also shows that, between approximately 20 and 80 percent of maximum, response appears to be proportional to the logarithm of the concentration.

The reduction of exercise tachycardia by propranolol is proportional to the logarithm of its plasma concentration (Fig. 20–4). This straight-line relationship, instead of the expected S-shaped or sigmoidal curve seen in Figure 20–2, arises in part because the results were obtained in man, not in an isolated preparation. To illustrate this point, consider a drug that increases heart rate through sympathetic stimulation. In an isolated heart preparation, the baseline heart rate can be controlled precisely so that the response to a small concentration of drug can readily be measured. *In vivo*, in response to internal and external stimuli, the baseline heart rate is much more variable, making it more difficult to detect the minor changes in heart rate observed *in vitro*. Perhaps the response can only

A

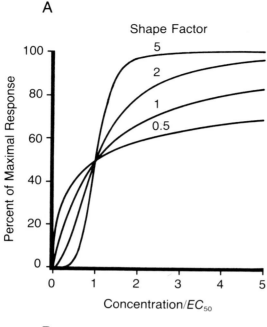

Shape Factor

Fig. 20–2. Cartesian (A) and semilogarithmic (B) concentration-response curves, predicted according to Equation 1, for three hypothetical drugs that have the same EC_{50} value, but different values of the shape factor, γ. At low concentrations the effect increases almost linearly with concentration (A), when $\gamma = 1$, approaching a maximal value at high concentrations. Between 20 and 80 percent of maximal effect, the response appears to be proportional to the logarithm of the concentration (B) for all values of γ.

B

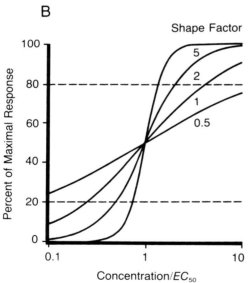

Shape Factor

be measured accurately when it is at least 10 to 20 percent different from the baseline rate, that is, in the linear part of the response-log concentration curve. At the other extreme, the greatest response that may be produced *in vivo* is often less than 80 percent of the maximum response. The entire cardiovascular system may deteriorate, and the animal (or the patient) may die long before the heart rate approaches the maximum rate capable of being produced. Other toxicities of the drug or metabolite(s) may further limit the maximally tolerated concentration *in vivo*.

Notwithstanding the visual appeal of the linear relationship produced by the

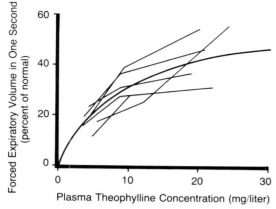

Fig. 20–3. Concentration-response curves for the-ophylline in patients with obstructive pulmonary disease. The effect is the one-second forced expiratory volume (FEV_1) expressed as a percent of the value predicted for a comparable person with normal pulmonary function. Both individual curves (points joined by straight lines) and curves predicted for the group using Equation 1 with $\gamma = 1$ (continuous line) are shown. Average values for the group are $E_{max} = 63$ percent of normal function and $EC_{50} = 10$ milligrams/liter, with considerable interpatient variability. (One mg/liter = 5.5 micromolar.) (Experimental data from Mitenko, P.A. and Ogilvie, R.I.: Rational intravenous doses of theophylline. Reprinted by permission of the New England Journal of Medicine, *289*: 600–603, 1973. Predicted line, obtained by regression analysis of the data using Equation 1, from Holford, N.H.G. and Sheiner, L.B.: Kinetics of pharmacologic response. Pharmacol. Ther., *16*: 143–166, 1982.)

logarithmic transformation of concentration-response data, its use in predicting the concentration needed to produce a given effect is to be discouraged. Extrapolation of the linear relationship predicts that a minimum concentration is needed to produce a response and that response will continue to increase progressively with an increase in concentration; both statements are incorrect.

All the examples above are graded responses. Equation 1 has also been found to describe concentration-response curves involving a quantal response. In such cases, the EC_{50} refers to the concentration that results in a 50 percent probability of response and the γ determines the shape of the cumulative probability versus the concentration curve within the population studied. Figure 20–5 shows not only the application of Equation 1 to describe probability data arising from a study with the opioid analgesic, alfentanil, but also that the concentration needed to produce an effect can vary with the specific application. Assessed in the study was the frequency of patients undergoing surgery who did not exhibit a series of clinical end points, indicative of less than optimal anesthetic control, when receiving alfentanil to supplement nitrous oxide anesthesia. Plotted in Figure 20–5 is the mean percent probability of attaining satisfactory control against the mean arterial alfentanil concentration for groups of patients undergoing breast,

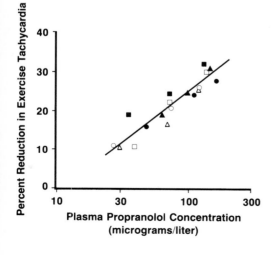

Fig. 20–4. The percent reduction in exercise tachycardia is proportional to the logarithm of the plasma concentration of propranolol. The line of best fit is shown. Each symbol denotes observations in a single subject. (From McDevitt, D.G. and Shand, D.G.: Plasma concentrations and the time-course of beta blockade due to propranolol. Clin. Pharmacol. Ther., *18*:708–713, 1975.)

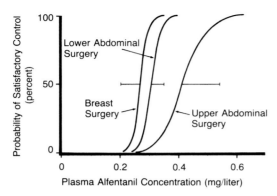

Fig. 20–5. Mean arterial concentration-response relationships obtained for alfentanil, an opioid analgesic, during the intraoperative period in each of three surgical groups of patients during nitrous oxide anesthesia. The lines are those predicted from Equation 1, using EC_{50} and γ values determined by averaging the estimates of individual patients. The respective mean values of EC_{50} and γ for the three surgical procedures are breast (0.27 milligram/liter; 21), lower abdomen (0.31 milligram/liter; 21), and upper abdomen (0.41 milligram/liter; 11). (−) is the standard deviation of EC_{50}. (One mg/liter = 2.0 micromolar.) (Redrawn from Ausems, M.E., Hug, C.C., Stanski, D.R., and Burm, A.G.L.: Plasma concentrations of alfentanil required to supplement nitrous oxide anesthesia for general surgery. Anesthesiology, 65:362–373, 1986. Reproduced by permission of J.B. Lippincott.)

lower abdominal, or upper abdominal surgery. In common with other opioids, the concentration-response curve is very steep in both the groups and the individual patients. In addition, the mean EC_{50} values for the three surgical procedures were in the order: upper abdominal > lower abdominal > breast, and all were greater than the EC_{50} value required for satisfactory spontaneous ventilation at the end of surgery. Collectively, these data not only indicate that different operative conditions require different drug concentrations, but also that alfentanil administration must be finely adjusted to the individual's need in order to maintain adequate anesthetic control, yet permit rapid recovery after surgery.

Time Effects

So far, a response has been assumed to be sustained as long as the concentration at the site of action is maintained. Although this is frequently the case, occasionally it is not. *Tolerance* can develop, whereby the response is diminished with time for a given concentration (Chap. 5). The time course of tolerance can vary from minutes to weeks. The mechanism for tolerance also varies. It may involve the depletion of either an endogenous transmitter or the number of receptors to which drug must bind to initiate a response. Tolerance may also be caused by a homeostatic mechanism whereby, through feedback control, the measurement returns toward the predrug value. When acute tolerance exists, the *rate* at which the concentration of drug is changing may be as important as the concentration itself. The effect of nifedipine on hemodynamics illustrates this last statement. Nifedipine, a calcium channel blocking agent, both increases heart rate (tachycardia) and lowers diastolic blood pressure when given to patients as a rapidly disintegrating capsule. Figure 20–6 shows the changes in heart rate and blood pressure, together with the plasma concentrations of nifedipine, following two schedules of intravenous administration to a group of normotensive subjects. When a regimen is employed that promptly attains and then maintains a constant plasma concentration, a sustained increase in heart rate but no fall in diastolic blood pressure is observed. In contrast, a fall in diastolic blood pressure but no tachycardia occurs when a constant-rate infusion is employed alone, despite a comparable steady-state concentration of nifedipine. Nifepidine's primary action is arteriolar vasodilation. This causes a reduction in

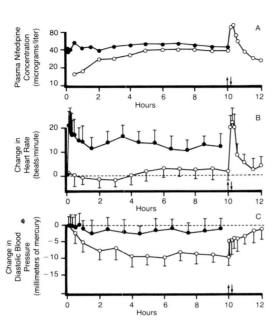

Fig. 20–6. The rate of change of plasma concentration can be a major determinant of response, as demonstrated here with the hemodynamic effects produced by nifedipine. Each of six subjects received nifedipine in distinct regimens on two different occasions. Regimen I—a constant-rate infusion of 1.3 milligrams/hour for 10 hours at which time the infusion rate was increased tenfold, to 13 milligrams/hour, for 10 minutes (the period denoted by ↑↓); or Regimen II—by means of a computer-controlled infusion pump, the rate was adjusted to immediately attain and then maintain a relatively constant plasma concentration for 9.5 hours. Panel A shows the plasma concentration in one subject associated with Regimens I (○) and II (●); Panels B and C show the corresponding mean group changes in heart rate and diastolic blood pressure, respectively. The slow approach to plateau associated with Regimen I caused a fall in diastolic blood pressure but no tachycardia, whereas with Regimen II the converse was obtained. Further supporting the importance of rate considerations is the sharp rise in concentration and heart rate when the infusion rate was increased sharply and momentarily at the end of Regimen I, prior to which time the plasma concentrations produced by the two regimens were comparable. The mechanism for this regimen-dependent difference produced by nifedipine is still not fully understood, but may be associated with the time needed for the baroreceptor reflex to respond to a change in arteriolar vasodilation produced by nifedipine. (One mg/liter = 2.9 micromolar.) (From Kleinbloesem, C.H., van Brummelen, P., Danhof, M., Faber, H., Urquhart, J., and Breimer, D.D.: Rate of increase in the plasma concentration of nifedipine as a major determinant of its hemodynamic effects in humans. Clin. Pharmacol. Ther., 41: 20–30, 1987. Reproduced with permission of C.V. Mosby.)

peripheral resistance and blood pressure, followed by an increase in cardiac output and heart rate through activation of the baroreceptor reflex. Apparently, if drug input is slow enough, the adaptive control system has sufficient time to respond and so maintains the basal heart rate. Further evidence supporting this hypothesis is the increase in heart rate produced when a small supplementary dose is administered at the end of the constant-rate-alone schedule, which momentarily raises the plasma nifedipine concentration above an already high steady-state concentration. The failure to observe a lowering of blood pressure with the constant-rate-alone regimen is at variance with the consistent lowering achieved in patients. These results only serve to underline the need to complement baseline studies in healthy subjects with studies in patients. Nonetheless, the observations described in Figure 20–6 may have a practical application. The primary use of nifedipine is to lower blood pressure; tachycardia is an undesirable side effect. The data suggest that the latter effect can be reduced by slowing the drug's rate of absorption.

TIME DELAYS

As mentioned previously, effect often lags behind plasma concentration. A striking example of such a delay is the rise in effect of digoxin on the heart,

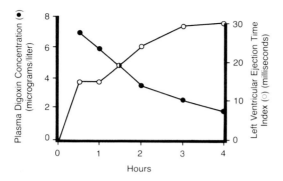

Fig. 20–7. The prolongation in the left ventricular ejection time index (○), a measure of effect, increases as the plasma digoxin concentration (●) declines for 4 hours after intravenous administration of a 1-milligram dose of digoxin. Average data from six normal subjects. (One mg/liter = 1.3 micromolar.) (Redrawn from data of Shapiro, W., Narahara, K., and Taubert, K.: Relationship of plasma digitoxin and digoxin to cardiac response following intravenous digitalization in man. Circulation, 42:1065–72, 1970. Reproduced by permission of the American Heart Association, Inc.)

while the plasma concentration falls during the first 4 hours after an intravenous bolus dose (Fig. 20–7). Certainly, these data do not mean that less drug is needed to produce a greater effect. Rather, the likely explanation is slow distribution of digoxin into cardiac tissue. Therefore to use plasma digoxin concentration as a guide to therapy it is necessary to wait until distribution equilibrium of drug with cardiac tissue is reached, which is 4 to 6 hours after a dose of digoxin.

A useful technique to help visualize the temporal features of drug effect is illustrated in Figure 20–8 for the intravenous opioid analgesic, alfentanil. Shown

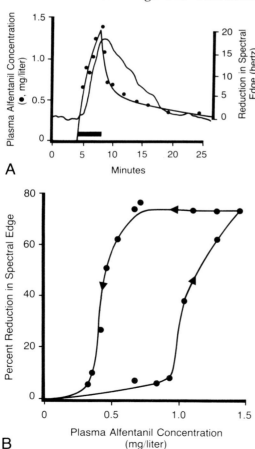

Fig. 20–8. Panel A, Time-course of the reduction in the spectral edge (an electroencephalographic measure of effect on the central nervous system) and the arterial plasma alfentanil concentration (●) in a subject during and following a 1.5-milligram/minute infusion of alfentanil for 5 minutes (solid bar). Panel B, Percent reduction of spectral edge versus plasma alfentanil concentration, demonstrating an anticlockwise hysteresis loop probably caused by delayed distribution of drug into the brain. The arrows indicate the time sequence of the observations. (One mg/liter = 2.0 micromolar.) (From Scott, J.C., Pongania, K.V., and Stanski, D.R.: EEG-quantitation of narcotic effect: The comparative pharmacodynamics of fentanyl and alfentanil. Anesthesiology, 62:234–241, 1986. Reproduced by permission of J.B. Lippincott.)

in Figure 20–8A are the plasma concentrations and the reduction of the spectral edge, an electroencephalographic measure of effect, in a subject during and after a 5-minute infusion of the drug. Although there is a suggestion of a time lag between plasma concentration and effect from this graph, the delay is much more apparent when the effect is plotted directly against the corresponding plasma concentration (Fig. 20–8B), yielding a characteristic *hysteresis* loop. Initially, during the infusion, effect lags behind the rise of alfentanil in plasma. Subsequently, while the plasma concentration falls rapidly there is little change in effect. Only after 10 minutes does effect follow the fall in plasma concentration. Notice that the chronologic sequence of the paired concentration-response observations moves in an anticlockwise direction.

With alfentanil, as with many other drugs, this anticlockwise hysteresis is most likely caused by delayed distribution into the site of action. More generally, other explanations for delayed response include the formation of an active metabolite, which takes time to reach an adequate concentration (see Chap. 21, Metabolite Kinetics); the observed effect is an indirect measure of the true effect (see Chap. 24, Turnover Concepts); and the drug reduces the concentration of an endogenous material, but only when the concentration falls below a critical value does this material become rate limiting in a reaction that produces the observed response.

Many drugs are lipophilic and equilibrate rapidly across well-perfused tissues, such as the heart and the brain, which are often target organs. For these tissues, because the period of observation in clinical practice is often hours if not days, any time delay in effect is likely to be minimal and drug in plasma can be correlated directly with effect. This was the case in the experiment from which the propranolol data in Figure 20–4 were obtained. Propranolol was given orally, and measurements were made over several hours, particularly after the peak plasma concentration had been reached. The statements above are true even if drug distribution throughout the body has not been achieved; all that is required is that distribution equilibrium of drug between plasma and the target organ be reached.

A special setting is an emergency or a surgical procedure during which responses are frequently measured in minutes rather than hours. Here, delays in effect after drug administration are almost always noticed. Even though plasma concentration monitoring is unlikely to be employed in these circumstances, it is still important to delineate the determinants of the time-course of effect in order to improve general understanding and aid optimal drug use.

ONSET-DURATION-INTENSITY RELATIONSHIPS

Two features of the temporal pattern of response are shared by all drugs following their administration: the onset of effect is delayed; and the effect has limited duration, unless drug administration is continued. However, because of the many complexities that determine the temporal pattern of drug response, it is difficult to develop concepts that have universal application. The subsequent discussion is restricted to drugs that act reversibly and directly at the site of action to produce a response described by Equation 1. Furthermore, metabolites are considered to be either inactive or not to reach a sufficiently high concentration to contribute to the response.

Before proceeding, it is important to realize that the amount of drug involved in producing an effect is usually only a minute fraction of the total amount in the body. Consequently, drug so involved has no effect on its own pharmacokinetics, except, for example, in the rare instance in which the effect is a reduction in both the cardiac output and the hepatic blood flow and the drug has a high hepatic extraction ratio.

Onset of Effect

An effect occurs when the concentration at the site of action reaches a critical value. The time of onset of an effect depends on many factors: the release rate of drug from its dosage form, its route of administration, the distribution kinetics of drug into the target site, and other time delays, which have been discussed previously in this chapter and elsewhere in the book. Additional factors affecting the time of onset are the dose and the concentration-response relationship.

Increasing the dose shortens the onset of effect by shortening the time required for the critical concentration at the site of action to be achieved. For the same dose, the time of onset of effect is also shortened in an individual with a low EC_{50} value, because less time is needed to reach the concentration producing the effect. The value of γ may also influence the time of onset.

Duration

An effect lasts as long as the minimum effective concentration at the site of action is exceeded. The duration of effect is, therefore, a function of both dose and rate of drug removal from the site of action. Removal can result from either elimination of drug from the body or its redistribution from the site to more slowly equilibrating tissues. Initially, the first situation (where elimination solely controls loss of drug from the site of action) is discussed. Subsequently, the case of redistribution is considered.

Spontaneous Distribution. In this situation, drug is assumed to distribute spontaneously into all tissues of the body including the site of action and response is assumed to spontaneously reflect the changing drug concentration at the site of action. Duration following single bolus doses and following doses repeated every time the response falls to a minimum value are considered.

Single Bolus Dose. Consider a drug that distributes into a volume V, is eliminated by first-order kinetics, and is characterized by rate constant k (Fig. 20–9). After a bolus dose, the plasma concentration falls exponentially, that is

$$C = \frac{\text{Dose}}{V} \cdot e^{-kt} \qquad\qquad 2$$

Eventually a time is reached, the duration of effect (t_d), when the plasma concentration falls to a value (C_{min}) below which the response is less than that minimally desired. The relationship between C_{min} and t_d is given by appropriately substituting into the preceding equation; thus,

$$C_{min} = \frac{\text{Dose} \cdot e^{-k \cdot t_d}}{V} \qquad\qquad 3$$

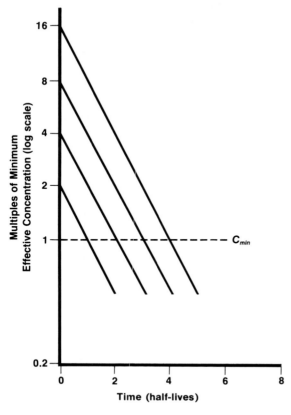

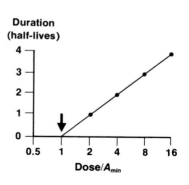

Fig. 20–9. The duration of effect increases by one half-life with each doubling of the dose. Duration is proportional to the logarithm of the dose (inset).

Upon rearrangement and taking logarithms, an expression for t_d is obtained,

★

$$t_d = \frac{1}{k} [\log \text{Dose} - \log (C_{min} \cdot V)]$$ 4

where $C_{min} \cdot V$ is the minimum amount of drug needed in the body, A_{min}. According to Equation 4 a plot of duration of effect against log dose should yield a straight line with a slope of $1/k$ and an intercept, at zero duration of effect, of log A_{min} (Fig. 20–9, inset). Evidence supporting these expectations is forthcoming. Thus, the duration of effect of many local anesthetics is proportional to the logarithm of the injected dose. The muscle relaxant effect of succinylcholine conforms to this last equation. Figure 20–10 shows the times to 10 (T_{10}), 50 (T_{50}), and 90 (T_{90}) percent recovery of muscle twitch (a measure of neuromuscular block) after the intravenous injection of 0.5-, 1-, 2-, and 4-milligram/kilogram bolus doses of succinylcholine in man. As expected, the slope, $1/k$, is independent of the end point chosen; the choice of end point only influences the value of A_{min}. The value of k, estimated from the slope, is 0.2 min^{-1}; the half-life is 3.5 minutes.

To further appreciate the last equation, consider the following statement: "The

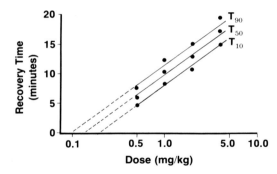

Fig. 20–10.   The time to recover from succinylcholine paralysis is proportional to the logarithm of the dose injected. T_{90}, T_{50}, and T_{10} indicate 90, 50, and 10 percent recovery of muscle twitch (a measure of the degree of return of muscular function). (Redrawn from the figure by Levy, G.: Kinetics of pharmacologic activity of succinylcholine in man. J. Pharm. Sci., 56:1687–1688, 1967. The original data are from Walts, L.F. and Dillon, J.B.: Clinical studies of succinylcholine chloride. Anesthesiology, 28:372–376, 1967.)

duration of effect increases by one half-life with each doubling of dose." This must be true. To prove that it is, let a dose produce a duration of effect, t_d. When twice the dose is given the amount of drug in the body falls by one-half in one half-life, that is, to Dose; the duration of effect beyond one half-life must be t_d. The total duration of effect produced by the larger dose is, therefore, $t_{1/2}$ + t_d. The increase in the duration of effect on doubling the dose is, therefore, one half-life. For example, since a dose of 0.5 milligram/kilogram of succinylcholine results in a T_{10} of approximately 4.5 minutes, the duration of effect following 1 milligram/kilogram is 8 minutes (Fig. 20–10). The increase in the time to recover, 3.5 minutes, is the half-life of succinylcholine at the site of action. Confirm that the same value is obtained with each doubling of dose on either the T_{10}, the T_{50}, or the T_{90} curve.

Multiple Bolus Doses. As noted previously, one way of extending the duration of effect is to increase the dose. This approach, however, rapidly results in a condition of diminishing returns, especially for a drug with a short half-life and a narrow therapeutic index. For example, when the duration of effect is extended by two half-lives, the quadrupled dose required may produce too great a response or substantially increase the chance of toxicity.

Instead of increasing the dose, a safer approach is to give the same dose each time the effect reaches a predetermined level, for example, just when the effect is wearing off (Fig. 20–11). With the alternative approach, an increase in duration of effect and, if the response is graded, an increase in intensity of effect is expected with the second dose. The reason is readily apparent. Immediately after giving the second dose, the amount of drug in the body is not the dose, but Dose + A_{min}. How much the intensity or the duration of effect increases, therefore, depends upon the magnitude of the dose and A_{min}. If A_{min} is small relative to the dose, very little remains from the first dose when the second dose is given, and little increase in effect, or duration of effect, is expected. In contrast, large increases in both effect and duration are expected when the effect from the first dose wears off before much drug is lost.

No further increase in intensity or in duration of effect is anticipated with the third and subsequent doses, because the amount of drug in the body always returns to the same value, A_{min}, before the next dose is given. Stated differently, from the second dose onward, during each dosing interval, the amount lost equals the dose given.

Distribution Kinetics. The impact of distribution kinetics on the duration and intensity of effect of a drug depends on two factors: the speed of equilibration of drug at the site of action and the size of the dose. Remember that the amount

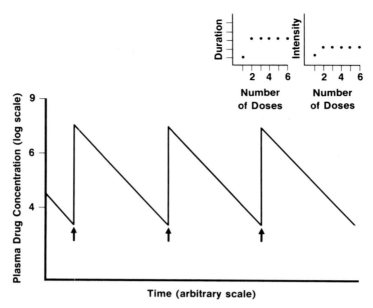

Fig. 20–11.   Both the duration and the intensity of a graded response increase with the second, but not with subsequent bolus doses when each dose is given, indicated by an arrow, at the time the effect (or concentration) reaches a predetermined level.

of drug involved in producing the response does not affect the pharmacokinetic parameters of the drug.

Single Bolus Dose. Consider first the situation in which the site of action is in a rapidly equilibrating, and hence well-perfused, tissue. The peak effect is seen almost immediately after an intravenous bolus dose, and thereafter the effect is directly related to the plasma concentration. Typical plasma concentration-time curves observed after various bolus doses are shown in Figure 20–12A; the curves only become linear on this semilogarithmic plot when distribution equilibrium is achieved in all tissues. If the dose is small (less than 10 units), the plasma concentration falls to the minimum effective value, and the effect wears off, during the distribution phase. In that case, on increasing the dose, the duration of effect increases disproportionally with the logarithm of the dose (Fig. 20–12B), because it takes disproportionally longer to reach the minimum effective concentration due to a slowing in the rate of decline of the plasma concentration with time. Only when the effect wears off well into the terminal phase in which the body acts as a single compartment, is the duration of effect proportional to the logarithm of the dose.

Supporting these expectations are the times of recovery to 10 (T_{10}), 50 (T_{50}), and 90 (T_{90}) percent of normal muscle twitch after intravenous injection of bolus doses (between 4 to 16 mg per square meter of body surface area) of the neuromuscular blocking agent, d-tubocurarine (Fig. 20–13A). The plasma concentration-time profile displays pronounced distribution kinetics; it takes an hour before the plasma concentration reaches the terminal exponential phase (Fig. 20–13B). Relative to this time frame, drug equilibrates quite rapidly between plasma and the neuromuscular junction, the site of action. The increase in recovery time should only begin to increase proportionally to the logarithm of

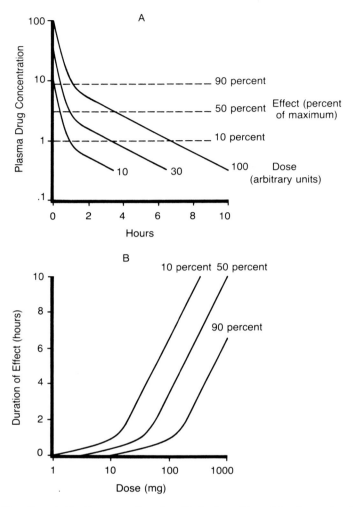

Fig. 20–12. Duration of effect increases linearly with the logarithm of the dose only when the effect wears off well into the terminal phase of a drug for which the site of action is in a rapidly equilibrating tissue. When the effect wears off during the distribution phase of a drug, because either the dose is small or substantial response still exists at the predetermined end point, the duration of effect increases disproportionally for small increases in dose. Shown are semilogarithmic plots of simulated plasma concentration-time profiles for different intravenous bolus doses of a drug that displays pronounced multiexponential disposition kinetics (Panel A), and the corresponding duration of effect-versus-log dose plots for predetermined end points corresponding to different degrees of maximal effect (Panel B).

the dose when the duration of effect is well in excess of one hour. This condition begins to be met only at the highest doses of d-tubocurarine and when a small response, T_{90}, is chosen as the end point. At lower doses and when a greater response, T_{10}, is chosen, the duration of effect is seen to increase disproportionally with the logarithm of the dose.

Multiple Dosing. Figure 20–14 illustrates the expected results when the same size dose is administered each time the pharmacologic effect falls to a predetermined level, or when the effect of the drug has just worn off. The second dose produces a higher concentration of drug in plasma and all tissues of the

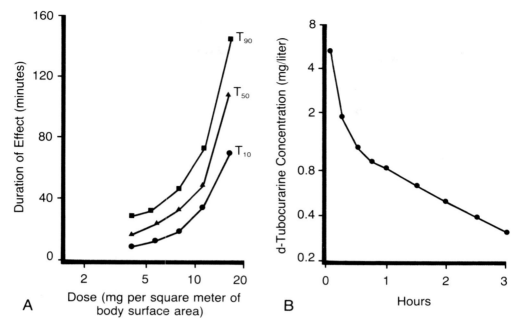

Fig. 20–13.   Panel A, Relationship between the median duration of effect and the size of the bolus dose of d-tubocurarine given intravenously to a group of subjects. T_{90}, T_{50}, and T_{10} indicate 90, 50, and 10 percent recovery of muscle twitch (a measure of the degree of return of muscle function). Panel B, Semilogarithmic plot of estimated mean population plasma d-tubocurarine concentration time profile following 0.5-milligram/kilogram dose of drug to a group of 10 subjects. (A: Redrawn from the figure by Gibaldi, M., Levy, G., and Hayton, W.: Kinetics of elimination and neuromuscular blocking effect of d-tubocurarine in man. Anesthesiology, 36: 213–218, 1972. The original data from Walts, L.F. and Dillon, J.B.: Duration of action of d-tubocurarine and gallamine. Anesthesiology, 29: 498–504, 1968. Reproduced with permission of J.B. Lippincott. B: Redrawn from the data of Sheiner, L.B., Stanski, D.R., Vozeh, S., Miller, R.D., and Harm, J.: Simultaneous modeling of pharmacokinetics and pharmacodynamics: Application to d-tubocurarine. Clin. Pharmacol. Ther., 25: 358–371, 1979. Reproduced with permission of C.V. Mosby.)

body and a correspondingly more intense response than that achieved after the first dose. Also, since the tendency for drug to move out of tissues is also reduced, the duration of effect is greater than after the first dose. Up to this point the result is the same as expected for a drug displaying one-compartment characteristics (Fig. 20–10), but differences do emerge on administering the third and successive doses. On repeating administration and as drug in the slowly equilibrating tissues rises, the tendency to distribute out from blood and other rapidly equilibrating tissues diminishes. Accordingly, the duration of effect becomes progressively longer until, within a dosing interval, the amount eliminated from the body equals the dose administered. Only then are the concentrations of drug in any tissue the same at the beginning and end of the dosing interval. In contrast to duration, the intensity of effect does not increase beyond the second dose because the concentration at the site of action just before the next dose is always the same.

The events shown in Figure 20–15 with thiopental are illustrative of dosing to a minimum effect. Following repetitive intravenous dosing, the plasma concentration declines more slowly and the effect lasts longer after the second and third doses, even though these doses were smaller than the first to prevent too

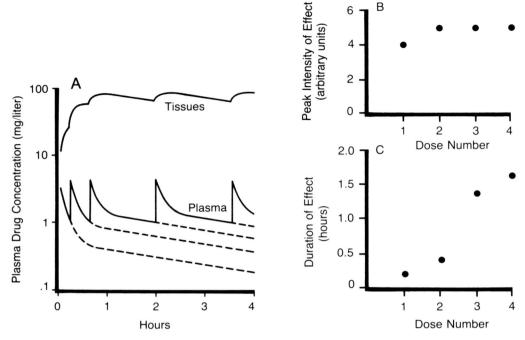

Fig. 20–14.   Panel A, When the same dose size is administered repeatedly each time the effect wears off and the effect is directly related to the plasma concentration, the duration of effect (time above a predetermined value following each successive dose) increases for a drug showing distribution kinetics. The increase is explained by the accrual of drug in the tissues, which reduces the tendency for net movement from plasma into tissue, with a resultant slowing in the decline of the plasma concentration on repetitive dosing (——). Also shown is the plasma concentration expected had the successive doses not been given (– – –). Panel B, Note that the peak intensity of effect is expected to increase only with the second dose. Panel C, This is in contrast to duration of effect. Notice how the duration increases dramatically when the time the effect wears off moves into the terminal phase.

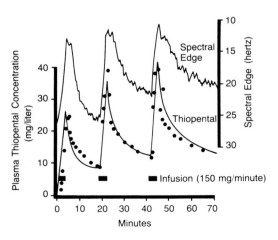

Fig. 20–15.   Both the plasma concentration of thiopental (●) and the spectral edge (jagged line), an electroencephalographic measure of effect, were monitored in a subject who received three successive short-term intravenous infusions of thiopental. The tendency for the concentration to fall in plasma and in rapidly equilibrating tissues such as the brain diminishes, and the effect is prolonged on the second and third doses, associated with the rise of drug concentration in slowly equilibrating tissues. To minimize the increase in maximal effect, above that produced with the first dose (8.4 mg/kg), the sizes of the two successive doses were reduced (to 5.7 mg/kg). The solid line close to the plasma concentration values is the predicted concentration after fitting a biexponential disposition model to the plasma concentration-time data. Because thiopental produces a diminution in the spectral edge, the spectral edge scale is inverted for clarity. (One mg/liter = 4.1 micromolar.) (Redrawn from Hudson, R.J., Stanski, D.R., Saidman, L.J., and Meathe, E.: A model for studying depth of anesthesia and acute tolerance to thiopental. Anesthesiology, 59: 301–308, 1985. Reproduced with permission of J.B. Lippincott.)

great a response. The data with thiopental also indicate that the brain is a rapidly equilibrating site, with a minimal delay in effect. In addition, these data do not support an earlier suggestion that tolerance to the hypnotic effect of thiopental occurs acutely. If tolerance had occurred, the sensitivity to thiopental would have decreased; it would have been expressed as a higher EC_{50} value. No increase in the EC_{50} value with time was observed, however.

Major differences between rapidly and slowly equilibrating sites of action are apparent on administering a drug on a fixed dose, fixed interval regimen, as illustrated in Figure 20–16. When drug at the effector site equilibrates rapidly, the effect follows the plasma concentration with minimal delay. When, however, equilibration is slow, it may take several doses before the maximal effect is seen, even though the plasma concentration is at virtual steady state. In addition, upon stopping drug administration, the effect will wear off slowly and may remain noticeably long after the plasma concentration as fallen below detection. In the absence of such insight, there may be a temptation to mistakenly classify the drug as one with hit-and-run characteristics.

Along similar lines, binding of drug at the site of action can conceivably be so tight that its removal, and subsequent decline in effect, is slower than the overall decline of drug in the body. Plasma concentration then correlates poorly with the temporal pattern of drug effect. Clearly, a failure to detect drug in plasma does not mean it is absent from the site of action.

LEVEL-INTENSITY-TIME RELATIONSHIPS

An effect subsides when the concentration of drug at the site of action falls. How the intensity of effect varies with time therefore depends, as does the

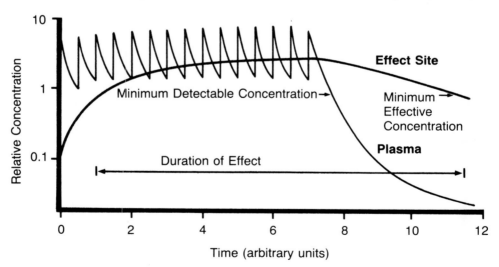

Fig. 20–16. When distribution to and from the tissues where the drug acts is slow relative to elimination, the drug in the tissues accumulates slowly on multiple dosing of drug. This delays the onset of effect, even when the drug is given intravenously. After discontinuing drug administration, the plasma concentration may quickly fall below the detectable limit, but the concentration at the site of action may persist for some time. Clearly, it is a mistake here to regard the action of this drug as hit-and-run. The duration of effect is simply a consequence of slow distribution. (Modified from Gibaldi, M., Levy, G., and Weintraub, H.: Drug distribution and pharmacologic effects. Clin. Pharmacol. Ther., *12*:734–742, 1971. Reproduced with permission of C.V. Mosby.)

duration of effect, on the dose and the rate of removal of drug from the active site. The intensity also depends on the region of the concentration-response curve covered during the decline. Here, the discussion is limited to the situation in which the concentration-response relationship is maintained at all times and in which the drug is distributed in a single compartment and is eliminated by first-order kinetics.

To appreciate the relationships among dose, intensity of effect, and time, consider the events, depicted in Figure 20–17, that follow the intravenous administration of a 10-milligram bolus dose of a drug that has a half-life of 1 hour. A plot of the intensity of the response against the logarithm of the plasma concentration is shown in the inset.

A complete description of the entire time-course of effect can be gained by substituting the equation defining the relationship between concentration and time into Equation 1. However, for didactic purposes it is convenient to divide the plot into three regions.

In *region 1*, up to 20 percent maximal response, the intensity of response is proportional to the plasma concentration; in *region 2*, covering 20 to 80 percent maximal response, it is proportional to the logarithm of the concentration; and in *region 3*, the response slowly approaches the maximal value despite large changes in the concentration. Since initial concentration lies in region 3, despite

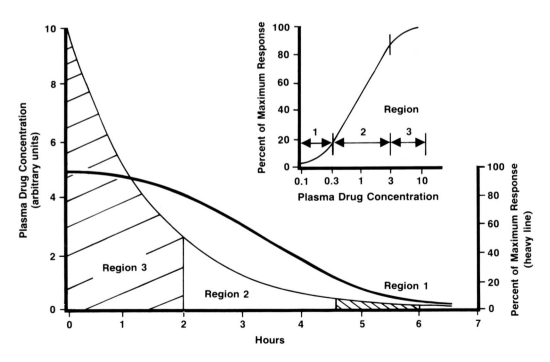

Fig. 20–17.   The decline in the intensity of pharmacologic effect with time, following a single large dose, has three parts corresponding to the regions of the concentration-response curve (inset). Initially, in region 3, the response remains almost maximal despite a 75 percent fall in the concentration. Thereafter, as long as the concentration is within region 2, the intensity of response approximately declines linearly with time. Only when the concentration falls into region 1 does the decline in response parallel that of drug in the body. The concentration-response relationship is defined by Equation 1, with $EC_{50} = 1$ and $\gamma = 1$.

the rapid fall in concentration in the first hour, the intensity of response remains almost constant and maximal. Only after 2 hours, when the concentration falls below 3 units and response falls below 80 percent of maximal response, does response begin to decline more rapidly. Then, for the next $2\frac{1}{2}$ hours, on passing through region 2 response declines at an almost constant rate of 22 percent/hour. The reason for this constant decline in response, while the plasma concentration declines exponentially, is apparent from the inset of Figure 20–17, because in region 2

$$\text{Intensity} = m \cdot \log C + b \qquad\qquad 5$$

where m is the slope of the intensity-log concentration curve. The value of the constant, b, is obtained by extrapolating the linear regression of the intensity versus the logarithm of the concentration, C, to zero intensity. The constant is the intercept on the log C axis and may be defined as the minimum effective concentration, assuming that the intensity of response is always proportional to the logarithm of the concentration.

Substituting $C_o \cdot e^{-kt}$ for C in Equation 5, where C_o is the concentration upon entering region 2 from region 3, and collecting terms therefore yields:

$$\text{Intensity} = (m \cdot \log C_o + b) - m \cdot k \cdot t \qquad\qquad 6$$

Letting E_o be the intensity of response when the concentration is C_o gives

$$\text{Intensity} = E_o - m \cdot k \cdot t \qquad\qquad 7$$

Thus, *the intensity of effect falls linearly with time* in region 2. It should be noted that the rate of decline, $m \cdot k$, depends on both the slope of the intensity-log concentration curve and the half-life of the drug. In this instance, for example, $m = 72$ (in region 2 the intensity of response changes by 72 percent of the maximal response for a 1-log change in C), and since $k = 0.7$ hour^{-1}, a constant rate of 22 percent/hour in the decline of activity is anticipated.

Beyond 5 hours, when the concentration has fallen below 0.3 unit and entered region 1, the fall in response parallels that of the drug. In theory, the drug's half-life can be determined from the intensity of response-time data in this region; it is the time for the intensity of a response to fall by one-half. In practice, however, measurements in this region are often too imprecise, being too close to a variable baseline, to permit accurate assessment of the half-life.

The foregoing equations are expressed in terms of concentration. The corresponding equations using dose administered and amount of drug in the body are obtained by multiplying each respective concentration term by the volume of distribution. The numerical value of b also changes. The concepts developed above are now illustrated with two examples: the degree of muscle paralysis produced by succinylcholine and the lowering of blood pressure produced by minoxidil.

Changes in the degree of muscle paralysis with time, following a 0.5-milligram/kilogram bolus dose of succinylcholine to a patient, are shown in Figure 20–18. The one-minute delay before onset of effect is probably accounted for in part by the time taken for the drug to circulate from the injection site to the muscle and in part by the time taken for succinylcholine to diffuse into the neuromuscular junction. Once at the site, however, full response ensues promptly; the time between onset and total paralysis is less than one minute. Total paralysis is then maintained for a full two minutes despite the continual rapid hydrolysis of this agent. Subsequently, the effect subsides. As predicted, between 20 and 80 percent of maximal response, the effect declines at a constant rate: in this instance, 22 percent/minute. At higher doses, the duration of effect is longer (Fig. 20–19), but once 80 percent of maximal response is reached, the amount

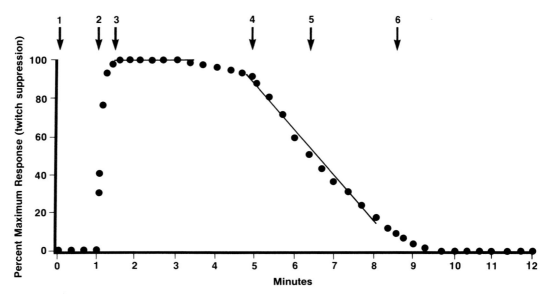

Fig. 20–18.   Changes in the degree of muscle paralysis (assessed as the suppression of a twitch produced in response to ulnar nerve stimulation) following an intravenous bolus dose of 0.5 milligram/kilogram succinylcholine to a subject. 1, Time of injection; 2, onset of twitch suppression; 3, complete twitch suppression; 4, 5, and 6, recovery of twitch to 10 percent (T_{10}), 50 percent (T_{50}), and 90 percent (T_{90}) of the maximum twitch height. The straight lines cover the regions of maximum response (horizontal line) and where the response declines (between 4 and 6) essentially linearly with time. (Modified from Walts, L.F. and Dillon, J.B.: Clinical studies on succinylcholine chloride. Anesthesiology, *28*:372–376, 1967.)

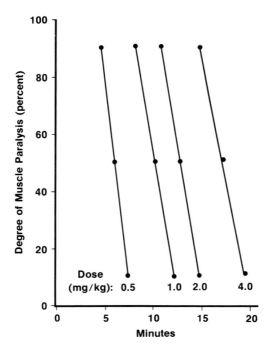

Fig. 20–19.   Irrespective of the dose of succinylcholine administered, once 90 percent of maximal paralysis is reached, the rate of decline in muscle paralysis is constant at 22 percent/minute. (Redrawn from the figure by Levy, G.: Kinetics of pharmacologic activity of succinylcholine in man. J. Pharm. Sci., 56: 1687–1688, 1967. The original data are from Walts, F. and Dillon, J.B.: Clinical studies on succinylcholine chloride. Anesthesiology, *28*:372–376, 1967.)

of drug in the body should be the same and should be independent of the dose administered; the subsequent rate of decline in the intensity of effect should be constant. This is indeed so. Knowing the rate of decline $(m \cdot k)$ and also the value of k (from the duration-log dose plot, Fig. 20–10), the value for m, the slope of the intensity of the response-log (amount of drug in the body) curve, can be calculated; for succinylcholine, $m = 250$. It is the short half-life (3.5 minutes) and the steep response-dose curve that makes succinylcholine such a useful agent clinically. Changes in muscle paralysis can be produced within a few minutes of changing the infusion rate, which allows fine and continuous control of the effect. Also once the infusion is stopped, the patient promptly recovers.

Figure 20–20 shows the lowering of the mean arterial blood pressure (MAP) in a patient with a baseline MAP of 157 millimeters of mercury following 10- and 25-milligram oral doses of minoxidil, a potent antihypertensive drug. A constant decay in the effect, given by the return of the MAP toward the baseline value of approximately 1 millimeter of mercury/hour, is evident following each dose; the intensity of the response lies between 20 and 80 percent of the maximal value.

DOSAGE REGIMENS AND RESPONSE

Regimens are designed to maintain a therapeutic response for the duration of therapy. Several schemes for determining the appropriate regimen have been discussed (Chaps. 5 to 7). These schemes use pharmacokinetic information derived initially from single-dose studies. A similar approach may be taken using only pharmacologic data. For illustrative purposes only, consider the previous information derived for minoxidil. For example, assume that the objectives of minoxidil therapy are to give an initial dose to immediately reduce the MAP to 95 millimeters of mercury and then to give supplementary doses at a frequency that maintains the MAP between 95 and 105 millimeters of mercury. A dosage

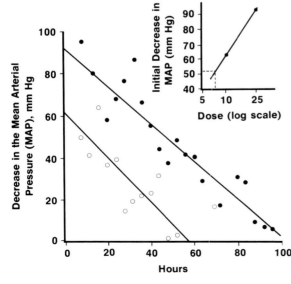

Fig. 20–20. The degree of lowering of the mean arterial blood pressure (MAP) in a patient with a baseline MAP of 157 millimeters of mercury falls at a constant rate following 10- (○) and 25- (●) milligram single oral doses of minoxidil. In the inset, the extrapolated value for the initial lowering of the MAP is plotted against the logarithm of the dose. (From Shen, D., O'Malley, K., Gibaldi, M., and McNay, J.L.: Pharmacodynamics of minoxidil as a guide for individualizing dosage regimens in hypertension. Clin. Pharmacol. Ther., 17:593–598, 1975.)

regimen to meet these objectives can be estimated using the limited information in Figure 20–20. The baseline MAP in the patient is 157 millimeters of mercury. The initial dose must lower the MAP by approximately 60 millimeters of mercury, which is achieved by giving 10 milligrams of minoxidil orally. Since the effect wears off at the rate of approximately 1 millimeter of mercury/hour, by 12 hours the MAP has risen to the upper limit of 105 millimeters of mercury. A supplementary dose must then be given to reduce the MAP by 10 millimeters of mercury back down to 95 millimeters of mercury. The required supplementary dose may be estimated from the response-log dose plot, admittedly constructed with limited data, shown in the inset in Figure 20–20. By interpolation, it can be seen that the amount of drug in the body at 105 millimeters of mercury, that is, when the MAP is depressed by 52 millimeters of mercury, is 7.5 milligrams. Thus, the supplementary dose is 2.5 milligrams, and it must be given every 12 hours if the MAP is to be maintained between 95 and 105 millimeters of mercury. Based on clinical experience, the generally recommended daily doses of minoxidil are higher than calculated here. There are many possible reasons for this difference, among them are interpatient variability in response and a change in response with time with long-term administration. One interesting specific feature of minoxidil is the discrepancy between the 4-hour half-life based on pharmacokinetic data and the half-life of one day calculated from the pharmacologic response data, which was derived from the slope of the duration-log dose relationship and the decline in response with time. The reason remains unclear. Although extensively metabolized, the metabolites are either inactive or too weakly active to contribute to response. Slow release from the effector site has been proposed, but not confirmed.

On chronic dosing, the average plateau plasma concentration of the drug is independent of the frequency of administration for a given dosing rate; only the degree of fluctuation around the average value is affected. This is not necessarily so with average response; much depends on the region of the concentration-response curve produced by the regimen. Examination of the concentration-response relationship (Fig. 20–2A) shows that below 30 percent of maximal response, response is almost proportional to concentration. Accordingly, provided that maximal response achieved with even the most infrequently administered regimen does not produce a response greater than 30 percent of the full effect possible, the average response, like average concentration, should be independent of either the dosing frequency or the dosage form used. However, as the average plasma concentration rises, so that response approaches or exceeds 50 percent of the full effect, the response does not increase proportionally with concentration. When this occurs, the average response at plateau tends to decrease the greater the degree of fluctuation in the plasma concentration. These predictions, of course, apply to both desired and unwanted effects, so that the relative value of any particular dosing schedule must be evaluated for the specific drug.

Study Problems

(Answers to Study Problems are in Appendix G.)

1. Indicate whether the following statements are true (T) or false (F).

   (a) For a drug showing first-order disposition kinetics and producing a graded response, the duration of effect increases linearly with dose.

   (b) A hysteresis loop in a response versus plasma drug concentration curve is not expected to be observed after intravenous administration of a bolus dose.

   (c) For a graded response, the EC_{50} is the plasma drug concentration at steady state that produces 50 percent of the maximum response.

   (d) For responses less than 20 percent of the maximum, the response is directly proportional to drug concentration only when γ of Equation 1 equals one.

   (e) One should wait for distribution equilibrium between drug in plasma and that at the site of action to be established before attempting to use plasma monitoring as a guide to therapy.

2. The concentration-response relationship for a drug that produces a graded response is characterized by an EC_{50} of 10 milligrams/liter and a γ of 2.5. To be effective, the response to the drug must be kept between 20 and 80 percent of the maximal value. Calculate the range of concentrations that are needed to achieve this objective. Assume that drug at the site of action equilibrates rapidly with drug in plasma.

3. An experimental anesthetic agent, CI-581, produces coma in human subjects. Table 20–1 shows the mean duration of coma as a function of the intravenous dose of CI-581 administered (Domino, E.F., Chodoff, P., and Corssen, G.: Clin. Pharmacol. Ther., 6:279–291, 1965.)

Table 20–1.

Dose (mg/kg)	0.5	1.0	1.5	2.0
Duration of coma (minutes)	1.7	5.8	9.0	10.0

Several subjects, immediately after the initial coma had ended following the 1.0-milligram/kilogram dose, received a second 1.0-milligram/kilogram dose. The duration of coma associated with this second dose was 8.0 minutes. Assuming a one-compartment model,

   (a) Determine the minimum dose of CI-581 required to produce coma.

   (b) Is the increase in duration of coma seen with the second dose consistent with the information obtained following the single dose?

4. A compound is given as an intravenous bolus to a patient requiring a minimum plasma concentration of 40 milligrams/liter for a therapeutic effect. Given that: Dose = 1000 milligrams; $k = 0.10$ hour^{-1}; $V = 8$ liters, and assuming a one-compartment model,

   (a) Calculate how long the clinical effect will last with this dose.

   (b) Calculate how long the clinical effect will last following a 2000-milligram dose.

(c) Determine the duration of effect following a 1000-milligram dose, if $k = 0.05$ hour^{-1} and the change in the k is a result of (1) a two-fold decrease in clearance; and (2) a doubling of the volume of distribution by increased nonspecific tissue binding.

(d) Does doubling the dose of a drug yield the same change in duration of clinical effect as doubling the half-life?

5. Assuming that the data presented in Figure 20–20 are applicable, design a suitable dosage regimen of minoxidil to immediately reduce a patient's MAP of 180 milliliters of mercury to 95 millimeters of mercury and then to maintain the MAP between 95 and 105 millimeters of mercury.

6. Table 20–2 lists the duration of effect achieved with the neuromuscular blocking agent pancuronium following the administration of a 0.02-milligram/kilogram intravenous dose each time the response returned to 10 percent of maximal effect. Assume that drug at the site of action rapidly equilibrates with drug in plasma.

Table 20–2. Neuromuscular Blocking Effect of Successive Doses[a] of Pancuronium

Dose Number	1	2	3	4
Duration of Effect (minutes)[b]	14	20	36	>54

Abstracted from summary in Gibaldi, M., Levy, G., and Weintraub, H. Clin. Pharmacol. Ther., *12*:734–742, 1971. Original data from Norman, J., Katz, R.C., and Seed, R.F. Br. J. Anaesth., *42*:702–710, 1970.

[a]0.02 milligram/kilogram intravenously.
[b]Time to recover 90 percent of normal function.

(a) Briefly discuss why the duration of effect progressively increases each time a dose is administered.

(b) Will the duration of effect continue to increase if drug administration continues to be administered in the same manner?

7. McDevitt, D.G. and Shand, D.G. (Clin. Pharmacol. Ther., *18*:708–715, 1975) observed a linear relationship between effect (percent reduction in exercise tachycardia) and the logarithm of plasma concentration of propranolol (Fig. 20–4). The slope of the line is 11.5 percent. Table 20–3 lists the effect with time after intravenous administration of 20 milligrams propranolol.

Table 20–3.

Time (hours)	0.25	1	2	4	6
Percent reduction in exercise tachycardia	28	25.5	22	15	8

(a) Estimate the apparent half-life of propranolol in plasma.

(b) Calculate how long the reduction in exercise tachycardia is expected to remain above 15 percent (1) after a 40-milligram intravenous dose and (2) after a 60-milligram intravenous dose.

21

Metabolite Kinetics

Objectives

The reader will be able to:

1. State the pharmacokinetic parameters that influence the plasma metabolite concentration and the amount of metabolite in the body following drug administration.

2. Determine if the elimination of a metabolite is rate-limited by its formation.

3. Determine if the total clearance of a metabolite is less than that of its parent drug, given plasma concentration-time data of drug and metabolite following drug administration.

4. Describe the consequence of hepatic extraction on plasma metabolite concentrations following oral administration of a drug.

5. State the pharmacokinetic parameters that control the amount and concentration of metabolite at plateau following administration of drug as either a constant-rate intravenous infusion or a multiple-dose regimen.

6. Describe why the elimination half-life of metabolite is the determinant of accrual of metabolite, when a constant amount of drug is maintained in the body.

7. Describe why the elimination half-life of the slowest step, drug elimination or metabolite elimination, controls the accrual of metabolite following either a constant-rate drug infusion or a multiple-dose regimen.

8. Calculate the average plateau concentration of metabolite following an oral multiple-dose drug regimen, given the area of the metabolite after a single dose of the drug and the dosing interval.

9. Suggest a mechanism whereby the half-life of a drug, which is renally excreted unchanged to only a small extent, can increase substantially in patients with renal function impairment.

The reason for our interest and concern with metabolites can be summed up in four words: action, toxicity, inhibition, and displacement. All too often metabolites are thought of as weakly active or inactive waste products. For many this is so, but as seen in Table 21–1, for many others it is not. Some drugs, prodrugs, are inert and depend on metabolism for activation. Some metabolites have pharmacologic properties in common with the parent drug and augment

347

its effect. Some have a different pharmacologic profile and may even be the cause of toxicity. Some are inactive but may, by acting as inhibitors, prolong or enhance the response to a drug. Still others may affect the disposition of a drug by competing for plasma and tissue binding sites. It is not sufficient, however, to know that a metabolite possesses the potential for any or all of these properties. Unless a sufficient concentration exists at the appropriate site, the presence of a metabolite is of little therapeutic concern.

This chapter examines the factors that influence the kinetics of metabolites in the body. It begins with a few comments on pathways and sites of metabolism. For purposes of clarity, it is assumed that the body acts as a single compartment for both drug and metabolites, that all kinetic processes are first-order, and that no change in plasma protein binding occurs, unless stated otherwise.

The most common routes of drug metabolism are oxidation, reduction, hydrolysis, and conjugation. Frequently, a drug simultaneously undergoes metabolism by several competing pathways. The amount of each metabolite formed depends on the relative rates of each of the parallel pathways. The metabolites may undergo further metabolism. For example, oxidation, reduction, and hydrolysis are often followed by a conjugation reaction. These reactions occur in series or are said to be *sequential.*

Table 21–2 contains representative drugs whose pathways of biotransformation are classified by chemical alteration and by site of metabolism. Several metabolic transformations occur in the endoplasmic reticulum of the liver and of certain other tissues. On homogenizing these tissues the endoplasmic reticulum is disrupted with the formation of small vesicles called microsomes. For this reason, metabolizing enzymes of the endoplasmic reticulum are called microsomal enzymes. Drug metabolism, therefore, may be classified as microsomal and nonmicrosomal.

The liver is often thought of as *the* site of drug metabolism; often it is. However, some metabolizing enzymes are located in other tissues. For example, glucuronide formation occurs in the kidneys, in the membranes of the gastrointestinal tract, and in the skin as well as in the liver. The blood contains esterases; these enzymes are also found in many other tissues. The blood clearance, under these circumstances, is theoretically no longer limited by hepatic blood flow. The lungs are also rich in some enzymes, and since essentially all the cardiac output passes through these organs, clearance can potentially also be extremely high. The activity of some drug-metabolizing enzymes in the human placenta is high. In

Table 21–1. Representative Therapeutically Important Metabolites

Compound Administered	Metabolite	Compound Administered	Metabolite
Acetylsalicylic acid	Salicylic acid	Lidocaine	Desethyllidocaine
Amitriptyline	Nortriptyline	Meperidine	Normeperidine
Carbamazepine	Carbamazepine-10,11-epoxide	Phenacetin	Acetaminophen
		Phenylbutazone	Oxyphenbutazone
Chlordiazepoxide	Desmethylchlordiazepoxide	Prednisone	Prednisolone
Codeine	Morphine	Primidone	Phenobarbital
Diazepam	Desmethyldiazepam	Procainamide	N-Acetylprocainamide
Glutethimide	4-Hydroxyglutethimide	Propranolol	4-Hydroxypropranolol
Imipramine	Desipramine	Sulindac	Sulindac sulfide
Isosorbide dinitrate	Isosorbide 5-mononitrate	Verapamil	Norverapamil

Table 21–2. Patterns of Biotransformation[a] of Representative Drugs[b]

Prodrug	Drug	Active Metabolite	Inactive Metabolite[c]
	Acetohexamide $\xrightarrow{(R)}$ Hydroxyhexamide		
Acetylsalicylic Acid[d] $\xrightarrow{\quad(H)\quad}$ Salicylic Acid			$\xrightarrow{(C)}$ Salicyl (acid) glucuronide $\xrightarrow{(C)}$ Salicyl (phenolic) glucuronide $\xrightarrow{(C)}$ Salicyluric acid $\xrightarrow{(O)}$ Gentisic acid
Glutethimide $\xrightarrow{(O)}$ Hydroxyglutethimide		$\xrightarrow{(C)}$ Hydroxyglutethimide glucuronide	
6-Mercaptopurine		$\xrightarrow{(C)}$ 6-Mercaptopurine ribonucleotide $\xrightarrow{(O)}$ 6-Thiouric acid	
Phenacetin $\xrightarrow{(O)}$ Acetaminophen			$\xrightarrow{(C)}$ Acetaminophen glucuronide $\xrightarrow{(C)}$ Acetaminophen sulfate
Phenytoin			$\xrightarrow{(O)}$ p-Hydroxyphenytoin
Prednisone $\xrightarrow{(R)}$ Prednisolone			
Succinylcholine			$\xrightarrow{(H)}$ Succinylmonocholine
Theophylline			$\xrightarrow{(O)}$ 1-Methylxanthine $\xrightarrow{(O)}$ 1,3-dimethyluric acid
Tolbutamide $\xrightarrow{(O)}$ Hydroxy-tolbutamide			$\xrightarrow{(O)}$ Carboxytolbutamide

[a]Classification: microsomal, $\longrightarrow$; nonmicrosomal, $- - \rightarrow$; (O), oxidation; (R), reduction; (H), hydrolysis; (C), conjugation.

[b]For each drug only representative metabolic pathways are indicated.

[c]Inactive at concentrations obtained following the therapeutic administration of the parent drug.

[d]Its status as a prodrug or drug for anti-inflammatory activity is not well established.

some instances the activity is equal to or greater than that in the liver on a weight basis. The therapeutic importance of placental drug metabolism is, however, basically unknown.

SINGLE DOSE OF DRUG

Rate-Limiting Step

To appreciate the factors that influence the amount of metabolite in the body, $A(m)$, with time following a single intravenous dose of drug, consider the scheme:

$$A \xrightarrow[k]{\text{Metabolism}} A(m) \xrightarrow[\text{Elimination } k(m)]{\text{Metabolite}} Ae(m)$$

Drug   Metabolite   Eliminated
in body   in body   metabolite

in which drug is metabolized to a single species that, in turn, is eliminated unchanged. The two steps are characterized by the respective first-order rate constants k and k(m). Also, at any time

$$\text{Rate of change of amount of metabolite in body} = \underset{\substack{\text{Rate of} \\ \text{formation}}}{k \cdot A} - \underset{\substack{\text{Rate of} \\ \text{elimination}}}{k(m) \cdot A(m)} \qquad \bigstar \; 1$$

Strictly speaking $k \cdot A$ refers to the rate of entry of the metabolite into the general circulation. Sometimes, metabolite formed in the liver can be further metabolized there, so that only a fraction of the formed metabolite is measured in blood. In the subsequent discussion, however, it is assumed that the rate of metabolite formation is its rate of entry into the general circulation.

In the scheme above, either step can be rate-limiting; the rate-limiting step has the smaller rate constant. Figure 21–1, two semilogarithmic plots of the amount at the various sites against time following a single dose of drug, shows the consequence of a rate limitation in each step.

A rate limitation in drug disposition, the most common situation, has a number of consequences. First, the half-life of the drug disposition step is longer than that of the metabolite. Second, there is always more drug than metabolite in the body. Last, *metabolite elimination is formation rate-limited;* that is, the metabolite is cleared so rapidly that during the decline phase of metabolite whatever is formed is almost immediately eliminated. Approximately, therefore

$$\underset{\substack{\text{Elimination rate} \\ \text{of metabolite}}}{k(m) \cdot A(m)} \approx \underset{\substack{\text{Formation rate} \\ \text{of metabolite}}}{k \cdot A} \qquad\qquad 2$$

and on rearranging,

$$\text{Amount of metabolite} \approx \left(\frac{k}{k(m)}\right) \cdot \text{Amount of drug} \qquad\qquad 3$$

In this case, the metabolite declines with the same half-life as the drug.

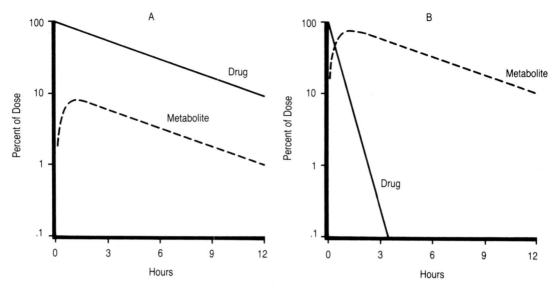

Fig. 21–1.   Consequences of a rate limitation. When the elimination rate constant of the drug is smaller than that of the metabolite, the metabolite declines in parallel with the drug (A). Conversely, when the elimination rate constant of the metabolite is smaller than that of the drug, the metabolite declines more slowly than the drug (B). In the former case (A), the half-life of the metabolite decline is rate-limited by the elimination of the drug and, in the latter case (B), by the elimination of the metabolite. The graphs were simulated using k and $k(m)$ values of 0.2 and 2 hour^{-1} in the former case, and 2 and 0.2 hour^{-1} in the latter.

A metabolite builds up substantially in the body only when its elimination is the slower step. That is, the half-life of the metabolite is longer than that of the drug. When this occurs, most of the drug has been eliminated by the time the peak metabolite level is reached; decline of the metabolite is then controlled by its elimination half-life.

In the foregoing simplified scheme the rate of metabolite formation is the rate of drug elimination. This need not be the case. Equations 1 to 3 are valid no matter what fraction of drug is converted to the metabolite. Thus, if k_f denotes the rate constant for formation of a metabolite, the rate of metabolite formation is $k_f \cdot A$, which does not alter the direct proportionality between amount of metabolite in the body, $A(m)$, and the amount of drug, A, when metabolite elimination is formation rate-limited. The decline of drug does, however, depend on the overall elimination rate constant, k, which is the sum of k_f plus the rate constants associated with other routes of elimination; these include renal excretion of unchanged drug and other routes of metabolism. In Equations 1–3, $k(m)$ refers to the rate constant for metabolite elimination. Just how many pathways are involved in metabolite elimination is not important. What is important is knowing where the rate-limiting step lies. In any sequence, substances formed beyond the rate-limiting step decline proportionally with the half-life of this slowest step. To emphasize this point consider the following scheme:

$$C \qquad\qquad F$$

$$A \xrightarrow[\ 0.2\ ]{} B \xrightarrow[\ 1.5\ ]{} E \xrightarrow[\ 8.2\ ]{} G \xrightarrow[\ 0.05\ ]{} H \xrightarrow[\ 0.5\ ]{} I \xrightarrow[\ 2.0\ ]{} J$$

with branches $0.1 \nearrow C$, $0.3 \searrow D$ from A, and $2.2 \nearrow F$ from E.

$$D$$

in which A refers to the drug, B through I refer to metabolites, J is the excreted metabolite I, and the number above each arrow is the value of the respective rate constant in hour^{-1}.

Q. What is the rate-limiting step in the entire sequence?

A. Elimination of metabolite G, $t_{1/2} = 0.693/0.05 = 13.9$ hours.

Q. What are the half-lives for decay of A, B, E, H, and I from the body following administration of drug?

A. Disposition of A rate limits B and E, $t_{1/2} = 0.693/(0.1 + 0.2 + 0.3) = 1.16$ hours for A, B, and E. Elimination of G rate limits H and I, $t_{1/2} = 13.9$ hours.

Occasionally, the half-lives of drug and metabolite are comparable and then neither step is rate-limiting. However, metabolite will decline more slowly than anticipated from its half-life alone because, for much of metabolite elimination, some drug remains to sustain the level of metabolite.

Plasma Concentration

The preceding discussion, helpful in realizing the importance of rate-limiting steps, dealt with amounts of drug and metabolite in the body. However, plasma concentrations are measured and are of greater interest. Furthermore, in most cases, metabolite has not been given independently to permit determination of its volume of distribution, and therefore, the amount in the body cannot be calculated. Our attention therefore turns to clearance, the most important parameter determining plasma concentrations. Several examples are discussed to illustrate the application of the clearance concept to metabolite kinetics.

The first example concerns the potential contribution of a metabolite to drug toxicity. Management of the coma induced by large overdoses of the sedative hypnotic, glutethimide, is complicated by a poor correlation between the plasma concentration of glutethimide and the clinical course of the patient. The duration of the coma is longer than expected and the depth is greatest long after the plasma concentration of glutethimide has reached a maximum value. As illustrated in Figure 21–2, substantial accumulation of a metabolite, 4-hydroxyglutethimide (Table 21–1), seems to be the explanation. Notice that the coma is deepest at the time of the peak metabolite concentration. Although these data do not extend long enough to determine whether the elimination of 4-hydroxyglutethimide is rate-limited by its formation or disposition, they do permit the conclusion to be drawn that the high concentration of this metabolite is due to its clearance being much lower than that of glutethimide in this patient. The argument is as follows:

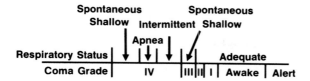

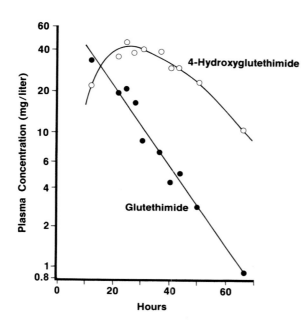

Fig. 21–2. A male patient was admitted to hospital in coma following a 12-gram dose of glutethimide ingested about 11 hours previously. His respiratory status and grade of coma worsened, which correlated with a substantial accumulation of an active metabolite, 4-hydroxyglutethimide. Only when this metabolite declined did the patient's status improve. The accumulation of 4-hydroxyglutethimide is caused by its total clearance being much lower than that of glutethimide. (Glutethimide: one mg/liter = 4.6 micromolar; 4-hydroxyglutethimide: one mg/liter = 4.3 micromolar.) (Modified from Hansen, A.R., Kennedy, K.A., Ambre, J.J., and Fischer, L.J.: Glutethimide poisoning: A metabolite contributes to morbidity and mortality. N. Engl. J. Med., 292:250–252, 1975. Reprinted by permission.)

At any time,

Rate of change
of amount of $= CL_f \cdot C \qquad - CL(m) \cdot C(m)$
metabolite in body

                                               Rate of   Rate of   4
                                               metabolite   metabolite
                                               formation   elimination

where CL_f is the clearance associated with the oxidation of glutethimide to hydroxyglutethimide, sometimes referred to as the formation clearance, $CL(m)$ is the total clearance of this metabolite, and C and $C(m)$ are the respective plasma concentrations of drug and metabolite.

Integrating the foregoing equation gives the amount of metabolite in the body at any time. However, since no 4-hydroxyglutethimide is present in the body at zero or at infinite time, it follows, upon integrating Equation 4 between these time limits, that

★

$$\frac{AUC(m)}{AUC} = \frac{CL_f}{CL(m)}$$ 5

where $AUC(m)$ and AUC are the total areas under the drug and metabolite concentration-time profiles, respectively. Substituting $fm \cdot CL$ for CL_f, where fm

is the fraction of an intravenous dose of drug converted to the metabolite, the following relationship is obtained:

★

$$\frac{AUC(m)}{AUC} = fm \cdot \frac{\text{Clearance of drug}}{\text{Clearance of metabolite}}$$ 6

Returning to Figure 21–2, it is apparent that, even though the plot is semilogarithmic, the area under the metabolite concentration-time curve is much greater than that under the glutethimide curve. This greater area would be even more apparent were the data plotted on ordinary graph paper. Accordingly, since the value of *fm* cannot exceed unity, the clearance of the metabolite must be less than that of glutethimide. If the ratio of areas had been less than 1, then, unless the value of *fm* is known, the relative total clearance values cannot be assessed. Because no knowledge of the amount of drug in the body is necessary to arrive at the above conclusion, this area method of interpreting metabolite data can be extremely useful, especially in cases of drug poisoning in which the amounts ingested and absorbed are frequently unknown.

The second example deals with propranolol. Based on the data in Figure 21–3A, obtained after giving propranolol intravenously, the drug has the following characteristics: total clearance, 1.1 liters/minute; volume of distribution, 380 liters; and elimination half-life, 4 hours. Other data suggest that almost the entire dose is metabolized in the liver. Metabolites of propranolol include one or more glucuronides and naphthoxylactic acid, which was measured specifically in this study. What can be learned from the data in Figure 21–3A?

From considerations of areas of drug and metabolite one must conclude that the clearance of naphthoxylactic acid is much lower than that of propranolol. However, the parallel decay of metabolite and drug indicates that elimination of this metabolite is rate-limited by its formation. Hence, the elimination half-

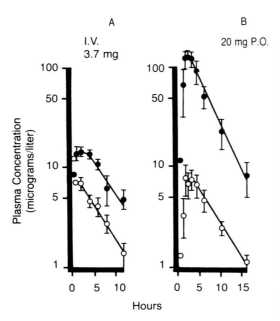

Fig. 21–3. A, Semilogarithmic plot of the plasma concentrations of propranolol (○) and of one of its metabolites, naphthoxylactic acid (●), (mean ± SEM) after a single intravenous dose of 3.7 milligrams propranolol to 3 subjects. Note that the elevated metabolite concentration, which declines in parallel with parent drug, is due to a lower total clearance and a smaller volume of distribution of naphthoxylactic acid compared with propranolol. B, Semilogarithmic plot of the plasma concentrations of propranolol (○) and naphthoxylactic acid (●) (mean ± SEM) after a single 20-milligram oral dose of propranolol to 5 subjects. As a consequence of extensive hepatic clearance, only a small fraction of the dose is absorbed intact. The remainder appears as metabolites, such as naphthoxylactic acid, which reach a peak value at the same time as propranolol, 1.5 to 2 hours after drug administration. For a strict comparison, the naphthoxylactic acid should be expressed in propranolol equivalents, but the difference in their molecular weights (260 and 284, respectively) is small. (One mg /liter of propranolol = 3.9 micromolar.) (Redrawn from Walle, T., Conradi, E.C., Walle, K., Fagan, T.C., and Gaffney, T.E.: Naphthoxylactic acid after single and long-term doses of propranolol. Clin. Pharmacol. Ther., 26:548–554, 1979. Reproduced with permission of C.V. Mosby.)

life of this more polar metabolite must be shorter, and the amount in the body aways lower, than that of the parent drug (see Fig. 21–1A).

The only explanation consistent with these observations is that volume of distribution of the metabolite, $V(m)$, must be smaller than that of the parent drug by a factor even greater than the ratio of the clearance values. This conclusion follows from a comparison of the elimination rate constants for metabolite and drug:

$$\frac{k(m)}{k} = \frac{CL(m)/CL}{V(m)/V} \qquad\qquad 7$$

For $k(m)/k$ to be much greater than one, the ratio $V(m)/V$ must be much lower than the ratio $CL(m)/CL$. Confirming this conclusion is a concentration of metabolite much higher than that of the parent drug (Fig. 21–3A), despite a much lower amount of metabolite in the body. The findings with propranolol are quite commonly encountered, particularly with amine drugs that are converted to acidic metabolites. The volume of distribution of many basic drugs is often in excess of 100 liters, whereas that of their acidic metabolites is closer to 10 to 20 liters. These metabolites are not only more polar and tend to bind less to tissue constituents than the parent drug, but also many of them bind strongly to albumin, thereby further restricting their distribution.

Kinetically, giving an intravenous bolus of drug and measuring the plasma metabolite concentration is the same as giving an oral dose of drug and measuring its plasma concentration. In both situations, one monitors the appearance and disappearance of a species (metabolite in one case, drug in the other) after placing a bolus dose in the preceding compartment, thus

Metabolism

$$A \quad \xrightarrow[\text{Metabolism}]{k} \quad A(m) \quad \xrightarrow[\text{Elimination of metabolite}]{k(m)}$$

Drug in   Metabolite
body   in body

Absorption

$$Aa \quad \xrightarrow[\text{Absorption}]{ka} \quad A \quad \xrightarrow[\text{Elimination of drug}]{k}$$

Drug at   Drug
absorption   in
site   body

Recall from Chapter 4 that the peak plasma concentration of a drug given extravascularly reflects the balance between the rates of drug absorption and elimination. Correspondingly, the 1.5 to 2 hours taken for naphthoxylactic acid to reach a peak in Figure 21–3A reflects the balance between the rates of formation and elimination of metabolite.

The last example is a comparison of tolbutamide and acetohexamide, two effective hypoglycemic agents. Both are extensively metabolized to the following products,

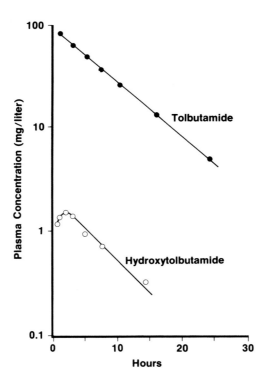

$$CH_3-\!\!\!\bigcirc\!\!\!-SO_2NHCONHCH_2CH_2CH_2CH_3 \xrightarrow{\text{Oxidation}}$$

Tolbutamide

$$\boxed{HOCH_2-}\!\!\!\bigcirc\!\!\!-SO_2NHCONHCH_2CH_2CH_2CH_3$$

Hydroxytolbutamide

Both metabolites are active, but only hydroxyhexamide is therapeutically important. The explanation lies in the differences in their clearances relative to those of their parent drugs. As seen in Figure 21–4, the concentrations of hydroxytolbutamide are always so low that they never augment the effect of tolbutamide. In the case of tolbutamide, almost all of the drug is converted to the metabolite, that is, fm is close to one. Accordingly, the twentyfold difference between the drug and metabolite areas reflects a corresponding difference in total clearance values, with that of hydroxytolbutamide being the much larger of the two. In contrast, hydroxyhexamide is cleared more slowly than acetohexamide, and so accumulates substantially and depresses blood glucose long after the majority of acetohexamide has been eliminated (Fig. 21–5).

Tolbutamide elimination clearly rate limits the elimination of hydroxytolbutamide. Under these circumstances, the metabolite-to-drug plasma concentration

Fig. 21–4. A subject received a 1-gram intravenous bolus of tolbutamide. The concentration of tolbutamide in plasma fell with a half-life of 4 hours. Although oxidation to hydroxytolbutamide is almost obligatory for tolbutamide elimination, the plasma concentration of this metabolite is always very low owing to its extremely high clearance value. As a consequence, since the volumes of distribution are similar (0.15–0.30 liter/kg), oxidation of tolbutamide rate limits hydroxytolbutamide elimination. (Tolbutamide: one mg/liter = 3.7 micromolar; Hydroxytolbutamide: one mg/liter = 3.5 micromolar.) (Redrawn from Matin, S.B., and Rowland, M.: Determination of tolbutamide and metabolites in biological fluids. Anal. Letters, 6:865–876, 1973, by courtesy of Marcel Dekker, Inc.)

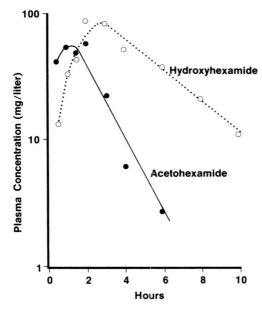

Fig. 21–5. A subject received 1 gram of acetohexamide orally. The lower total clearance of hydroxyhexamide explains why the plasma concentration of this metabolite of acetohexamide is soon higher than that of the parent drug. Furthermore, the disposition, rather than the formation, of hydroxyhexamide must also be rate-limiting since the concentration of this metabolite declines more slowly than does that of the drug. (Acetohexamide: one mg/liter = 3.1 micromolar; Hydroxyhexamide: one mg/liter = 2.9 micromolar.) (Redrawn from Galloway, J.A., McMahon, R.E., Culp, H.W., Marshall, F.J., and Young, E.C.: Metabolism, blood levels and rate of excretion of acetohexamide in human subjects. Diabetes, 16:118–123, 1967. Reproduced with permission from the American Diabetes Association.)

ratio is fixed during metabolite decay by the ratio of $fm \cdot CL$ to $CL(m)$. Thus, substituting for both clearance and concentration in Equation 1 gives

$$
\underset{\substack{\text{Rate of metabolite} \\ \text{elimination}}}{CL(m) \cdot C(m)} \approx \underset{\substack{\text{Rate of metabolite} \\ \text{formation}}}{fm \cdot CL \cdot C} \qquad 8
$$

and rearranging, yields

$$
\frac{\text{Metabolite concentration}}{\text{Drug concentration}} \approx fm \cdot \frac{CL}{CL(m)} \qquad 9
$$

For example, the twentyfold difference in the total clearance between hydroxy-tolbutamide and tolbutamide is reflected by the plasma concentration of metabolite being only a small percent of that of tolbutamide.

Impact of Hepatic Extraction

Ingesting drugs that are cleared by the liver is like taking a mixture of drug and metabolite. The reason, as mentioned in Chapter 2, is that all ingested drug must pass through the liver before entering the general circulation. The composition of the mixture varies with the hepatic extraction ratio of the drug. When the extraction of the drug is high, metabolism during absorption is extensive and the situation comes close to administering just metabolite. Table 21–3 lists some drugs undergoing extensive first-pass hepatic elimination and forming active metabolites. For them, caution must be taken against attempting to relate plasma drug concentration alone to effect following oral administration.

To appreciate the impact of first passage of drug through the liver on the plasma concentration of metabolite, consider the data in Figure 21–3B, obtained following oral administration of propranolol. Compared to the situation following an intravenous dose (see Fig. 21–3A), the naphthoxylactic acid-to-propran-

Table 21–3.   Representative Drugs Undergoing Extensive First-Pass Hepatic Elimination and Forming-Active Metabolites

Drug	Active Metabolite[a]	Drug	Active Metabolite[a]
Alprenolol	4-Hydroxyalprenolol	Lorcainide	Norlorcainide
Amitriptyline	Nortriptyline	Meperidine	Normeperidine
Codeine	Morphine	Metoprolol	α-Hydroxymetoprolol
Dextropropoxyphene	Norpropoxyphene	Naloxone	6-β-Hydroxynaloxone
Dihydroergotamine	8'-Hydroxydihydroergotamine	Phenacetin	Acetaminophen
Encainide	0-Demethylencainide	Propranolol	4-Hydroxypropranolol
Imipramine	Desipramine	Quinidine	3(S)-Hydroxyquinidine
Isosorbide dinitrate	Isosorbide 5-mononitrate	Verapamil	Norverapamil

[a]For some drugs more than one active metabolite is formed.

olol concentration ratio is much higher and the metabolite concentration peaks as early as the parent drug. These observations are understood by examining the following scheme:

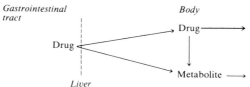

As anticipated from its high hepatic clearance, and confirmed by comparing the areas under the oral and intravenous propranolol concentration-time curves with correction for differences in dose, only 21 percent of the orally administered dose of propranolol filters past the liver. The remainder enters the body directly as metabolites. The small fraction of propranolol absorbed is then handled like an intravenous dose of the drug. Thus, the observed metabolite concentrations is the sum of the concentrations derived from the two sources (Fig. 21–6). Recall that, when propranolol is given intravenously, the accrual of metabolite (Fig. 21–3A) is dependent on the elimination half-lives of both drug and metabolite. In contrast, the concentration of metabolite peaks as early as drug and is higher after oral propranolol administration, because absorption of this drug (and hence entry of the majority of metabolites) is rapid.

The therapeutic implications of the preceding discussion depend on the activities of the drug and the metabolite. A shorter onset and a more intense response may be seen by giving a dose of drug orally rather than parenterally if the drug is inactive, passes readily and completely across the gastrointestinal wall, is highly extracted by the liver, and hepatic metabolism is required to generate the active species. In this case, a low availability of drug does not mean a poor therapeutic effect following oral drug administration. On the other hand, if the metabolites are inactive, a larger oral than parenteral dose is required to achieve an equivalent therapeutic response. The situation with propranolol appears to lie somewhere between these two extremes. Following a single oral dose, the pharmacologic effect is maximal at the peak propranolol concentration, but for a given plasma concentration of propranolol the effect seen after an oral dose is greater than that observed following an intravenous dose. The explanation appears to be the presence of a significant concentration of one or more pharmacologically active metabolites, formed on the first pass through the liver.

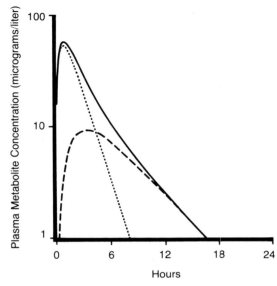

Fig. 21–6. Following an oral dose of drug the observed plasma concentration of metabolite (——) is the sum of metabolite from two sources: that formed during the absorption of drug (· · · ·) and that formed from absorbed drug (– – –). Note, on this semilogarithmic plot, the decline of metabolite formed during absorption is determined by the elimination half-life of the metabolite; whereas, decay of metabolite formed from the absorbed drug is determined by the half-life of the drug, the rate-limiting step here. If the hepatic extraction ratio of the drug is high, then most of the dose is converted to metabolite during the absorption of drug, and the decline phase appears biphasic. In this simulation, drug and metabolite have half-lives of 3.5 and 1.1 hours, respectively, and 90 percent of the drug is converted to metabolite during absorption of drug.

Certainly, one identified metabolite, 4-hydroxypropranolol, is as active as propranolol.

In Chapter 9 (Table 9–2), examples of drugs stated to be partially metabolized within the gastrointestinal tract are given. For some, evidence favoring this site of metabolism is the failure to detect a metabolite when drug is given parenterally, yet significant concentrations of this metabolite are measured after oral drug administration. Were metabolism to occur primarily within the liver, then the fraction of the dose converted to the metabolite should be independent of the route of drug administration. Thus, assuming that ingested drug entirely traverses the gastrointestinal wall and that only hepatic metabolism occurs, drug, whether given orally or parenterally, is equally and fully available to the liver for metabolism. The oral availability of the drug may be low if its hepatic extraction ratio is high, but the fraction of dose converted to a metabolite must be independent of the route of drug administration. The data in Figure 21–7 support this last point. Nortriptyline is highly and almost exclusively cleared by the liver. Using area as a measure of the amount of material entering the body, the availability of nortriptyline is low, but the availability of the metabolite 10-hydroxynortriptyline is the same, when comparing results of oral and intramuscular drug administrations. Likewise, the equality of areas of naphthoxylactic acid following oral and intravenous administration of propranolol (Fig. 21–3), appropriately correcting for differences in dose administered, supports the formation of this metabolite in the liver.

CONSTANT-RATE DRUG INFUSION

In Chapter 6, the kinetics of a constant-rate intravenous infusion was examined. Recall that infusion rate and clearance determine the plateau concentration

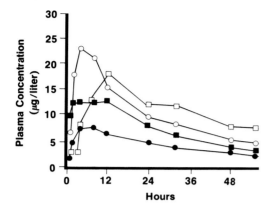

Fig. 21–7. Patients received 40 milligrams nortriptyline hydrochloride orally and 42.5 milligrams nortriptyline hydrochloride intramuscularly on separate occasions. Plasma concentration of drug (●-oral, ■-I.M.) and a metabolite, 10-hydroxynortriptyline, (○-oral, □-I.M.) were measured; average data in 6 patients are shown. As a consequence of extensive hepatic metabolism, the oral availability of the drug is reduced (F = 0.66). The same amount of metabolite, however, enters the systemic circulation, as judged by the equality of areas associated with the metabolite following the two routes of drug administration. (One mg/liter = 3.8 micromolar.) (Redrawn from Alvan, G., Borga, O., Lind, M., Palmer, L., and Siwers, B.: First pass hydroxylation of nortriptyline: Concentrations of parent drug and major metabolites in plasma. Eur. J. Clin. Pharmacol., 11:219–224, 1977.)

and that half-life alone determines the time to approach plateau. These observations can be extended to the accumulation of metabolite following constant-rate drug infusion. The essential features can be understood by considering the scheme:

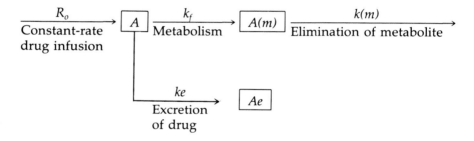

and the events depicted in Figure 21–8.

The Plateau

At any time during drug infusion,

$$\text{Rate of change of metabolite in body} = k_f \cdot A \quad - \quad k(m) \cdot A(m) \qquad 10$$

| | Rate of metabolite formation | Rate of metabolite elimination | |

or expressing the equation in terms of plasma concentrations of drug and metabolite,

$$\text{Rate of change of metabolite in body} = CL_f \cdot C - CL(m) \cdot C(m) \qquad 11$$

When the plateau or steady state is reached for both drug and metabolite, the

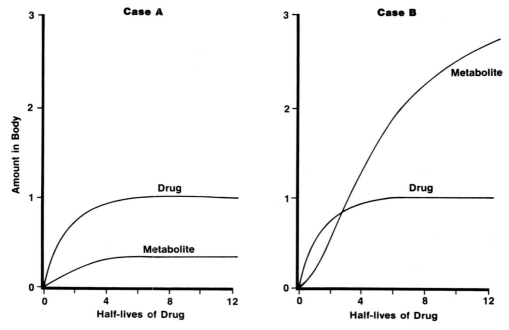

Fig. 21–8. Two situations following constant-rate drug infusion are depicted. In case A, the more usual situation, the metabolite half-life is shorter than that of the drug. Throughout most of drug accumulation, metabolite elimination is formation rate-limited; therefore, the approach to the metabolite plateau is determined by the half-life of the drug. In the less common situation, case B, the half-life of the drug is less than that of the metabolite. The drug is at steady state well before the metabolite has accumulated appreciably, and the approach of the metabolite to plateau is now determined by the metabolite half-life.

rate of drug elimination matches the rate of infusion and the rate of metabolite elimination matches its rate of formation. Then Equations 10 and 11 simplify to

$$\text{Amount of metabolite in body at steady state} = \frac{k_f}{k(m)} \cdot A_{ss} \qquad 12$$

and

$$\text{Concentration of metabolite in plasma at steady state} = \frac{CL_f}{CL(m)} \cdot C_{ss} \qquad 13$$

However, since fm is the fraction of an intravenous dose of a drug converted to the metabolite, the term $fm \cdot R_o$ must be equal to the rate of metabolite formation at the plateau, namely $k_f \cdot A_{ss}$ or $CL_f \cdot C_{ss}$, so

$$\text{Amount of metabolite at steady state} = \frac{fm \cdot R_o}{k(m)} \qquad 14$$

and

$$\text{Concentration of metabolite at steady state} = \frac{fm \cdot R_o}{CL(m)} \qquad 15$$

The only factors controlling the amount of metabolite at plateau are therefore the rate of drug infusion, the fraction of the drug converted to the metabolite, and the elimination rate constant of the metabolite. Only the first two factors and the total clearance of the metabolite control the plateau plasma concentration of the metabolite. Suppose, for example, that a drug is infused at 5 milligrams/hour, that the fraction of drug converted to metabolite, fm, is 0.5, that the elimination rate constant of the metabolite, $k(m)$, is 0.1 hour^{-1}, and that the total clearance of metabolite, $CL(m)$, is 1.0 liter/hour. Then,

$$\text{Amount of metabolite at plateau} = \frac{0.5 \times 5 \text{ milligrams/hour}}{0.1 \text{ hour}^{-1}} = 25 \text{ milligrams}$$

$$\text{Plasma concentration of metabolite at plateau} = \frac{0.5 \times 5 \text{ milligrams/hour}}{1.0 \text{ liter/hour}} = 2.5 \text{ milligrams/liter}$$

Time to Plateau

The time required for a metabolite to reach a plateau depends on whether or not a bolus of drug is given at the start of the constant-rate drug infusion. If a bolus is given and the infusion maintains that amount of drug in the body, then the approach of the metabolite toward plateau depends only on the metabolite's half-life. This point becomes apparent when one realizes that at constant drug concentration, metabolite is formed at a constant rate, $fm \cdot R_o$. As this is analogous to giving a constant-rate infusion of metabolite, it follows (from Chap. 6) that the approach to plateau is governed *solely* by the metabolite's half-life. Thus, one-half of the value at plateau is reached in one metabolite half-life. By approximately 3.3 metabolite half-lives, plateau is reached. Hence metabolites with short half-lives reach plateau quickly.

If no bolus is given, the situation is more complicated. The time to reach plateau can now be governed primarily by either the drug's or metabolite's half-life, whichever is the longer. To appreciate this point, consider two situations, both shown in Figure 21–8. In the more prevalent situation, case A, the drug has the longer half-life. As expected, the amount of drug in the body reaches plateau in approximately 3.3 drug half-lives. The amount of metabolite and hence the rate of metabolite elimination also rises. However, because elimination of the metabolite is a much faster process than that of the drug, the rate of metabolite elimination soon becomes limited by and approximately equal to its rate of formation. The metabolite is then at virtual steady state with respect to, and cannot rise any faster than, the drug. This follows, since under this condition (Eq. 3)

$$\text{Amount of metabolite} \approx \left(\frac{k}{k(m)} \right) \cdot \text{Amount of drug}$$

and the amount of metabolite proportionally reflects the amount of drug. Therefore the metabolite reaches plateau in approximately 4 drug half-lives.

In case B, the kinetics of the drug are faster than those of the metabolite. Now the drug reaches steady state before the metabolite level has barely risen. From then on the rate of metabolite formation is constant and, as observed previously, the accumulation of metabolite to plateau is controlled by the metabolite half-life. An example of case A is the oxidation of tolbutamide to hydroxytolbutamide, and of case B is the reduction of acetohexamide to hydroxyhexamide.

Postinfusion

As should now be anticipated, on stopping an infusion, the decline of metabolite is governed by the longer half-life, i.e., drug or metabolite. For example, on stopping a tolbutamide infusion, hydroxytolbutamide declines by one-half each tolbutamide half-life, whereas hydroxyhexamide's decline is determined by its half-life after stopping an infusion of acetohexamide.

MULTIPLE-DOSE DRUG REGIMEN

The concepts that apply to events following administration of a drug as a single dose and a constant-rate infusion can readily be applied to the most common situation of a multiple-dose oral drug regimen. As with the infusion of drug, the accumulation of metabolite to plateau depends as much on its half-life as on that of the parent drug. For example (Fig. 21–9), the accumulation of N-desalkylhalazepam, a metabolite of the benzodiazepine, halazepam, lags behind the parent compound during drug administration and falls more slowly after administration is stopped. Both observations occur because this metabolite has the longer half-life. In addition, the plateau concentration of N-desalkyl-halazepam is higher than that of halazepam, signifying that the metabolite has the lower clearance. The only noticeable difference expected between an infusion and a multiple-dose regimen is the fluctuation in the plasma concentrations of both drug and metabolite; the degree of fluctuation depends on the dosing frequency and half-lives of drug absorption, drug elimination, and metabolite elimination.

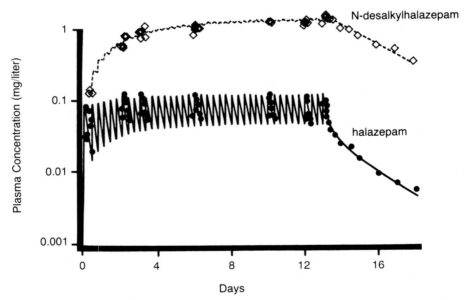

Fig. 21–9.   Because it has the longer half-life, the metabolite, N-desalkylhalazepam ($\diamond$), both accumulates and falls more slowly than the parent drug, halazepam ($\bullet$), during and after stopping the ingestion of 10 milligrams halazepam every 8 hours for 14 consecutive days. The metabolite also has a lower clearance, indicated by its higher plateau concentration, and undergoes less fluctuation compared with the parent drug (Halazepam: One mg/liter = 2.8 micromolar; Desalkylhalazepam: One mg/liter = 3.7 micromolar.) (Redrawn from Chung, M., Hilbert, J.M., Gural, R.P., Radwanski, E., Symchowicz, S., and Zampaglione, N.: Multiple-dose halazepam kinetics. Clin. Pharmacol. Ther., 35:838–842, 1984. Reproduced with permission of C.V. Mosby.)

As with that of drug, the concentration of metabolite during an oral multiple-dose drug regimen can readily be calculated from the plasma metabolite concentration-time profile after a single oral dose of drug. The concentration at any time into the regimen is obtained by adding the concentrations expected from each of the previous doses; there is no need to know the availability of drug, the fraction of drug converted to metabolite, the clearance of metabolite, or the respective half-lives of drug and metabolite. For example, if four doses of drug are given at 0, 12, 24, and 36 hours, then the concentration of metabolite at 48 hours is equal to the sum of the metabolite concentrations at 48, 36, 24, and 12 hours after a single dose of drug. The average concentration of metabolite at plateau can also be readily calculated from metabolite data after a single dose of drug. The area under the metabolite concentration-time curve after a single dose, $AUC(m)_{single}$, is then given by

$$AUC(m)_{single} = \frac{F_m \cdot \text{Dose}}{CL(m)} \qquad 16$$

where F_m is the fraction of the administered dose of drug that enters the general circulation as metabolite. At plateau, what metabolite is formed is lost within a dosing interval, τ, so that the average metabolite concentration, $C(m)_{ss,av}$, is

$$C(m)_{ss,av} = \frac{F_m \cdot \text{Dose}}{\tau \cdot CL(m)} \qquad 17$$

Substituting Equation 16 into Equation 17 gives

★

$$C(m)_{ss,av} = \frac{AUC(m)_{single}}{\text{Dosing interval}} \qquad 18$$

For example, if the $AUC(m)_{single}$ is 120 milligrams × hours/liter after a 100-milligram dose of drug, then the expected plateau metabolite concentration is 12 milligrams/liter when this dose is given every 12 hours. Obviously, if the observed plateau metabolite concentration differs from the expected value, then either F_m or clearance of metabolite, or both have been altered during the course of chronic drug administration.

VARIABILITY

As with parent drugs, the pharmacokinetics of metabolites vary widely among the patient population. Coupled with the additional variability in clearance of metabolite formation this often means that the variability in metabolite concentration can be even greater than that seen with parent drug concentration. The sources of variability in metabolite kinetics are the same as those affecting parent drug and include genetics, age, disease, and interacting drugs. Differences exist among patients in both metabolite clearance and volume of distribution, and as with a drug itself, it would seem preferable to relate everything to the unbound species.

Concern about metabolites is greatest when they significantly affect therapeutic response or toxicity. Frequently, the concentration of metabolite is too low to produce an effect, because only a small fraction of the dose is converted to a particular metabolite and because it has a high clearance. Situations can

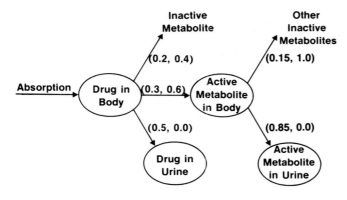

Fig. 21–10. Model for the absorption and disposition of a hypothetical drug and the disposition of its active metabolite. The first number in parentheses refers to the fraction of the elimination of the drug or metabolite that normally occurs by the pathway shown with an arrow. The second number refers to the same fraction when there is no renal function.

arise, however, in which metabolites reach concentrations high enough to be of concern. This occurs particularly in patients with renal insufficiency, because many metabolites are relatively polar and are primarily excreted unchanged. For example, the elimination of N-acetylprocainamide, a metabolite of procainamide, is reduced in patients with renal dysfunction. This metabolite is also effective, but perhaps less toxic than the drug itself.

Prediction of the total activity of the drug and of the dosage adjustment needed in patients with renal insufficiency is therefore more complex than usual. There are ways of treating such situations. The most useful is by the steady-state approach. To illustrate the use of this approach, consider the scheme in Figure 21–10, which shows the input and the disposition of a hypothetical drug and its active metabolite under normal renal function conditions. Table 21–4 lists the normal average values for several pharmacokinetic parameters of this drug and its active metabolite.

Assume that the drug and its active metabolite are equipotent and equitoxic in terms of plasma concentration. Further, assume that the rate of administration of the drug is 100 milligrams/hour.

At steady state, the plasma concentration of the drug may be calculated from the average rate of absorption and the total clearance,

$$C_{ss,av} = 0.8 \times \frac{100 \text{ milligrams/hour}}{30 \text{ liters/hour}} = 2.7 \text{ milligrams/liter}$$

The rate of formation of the active metabolite is 0.3 times the rate of absorption of the drug; therefore,

$$C(m)_{ss,av} = \frac{0.3 \times 0.8 \times 100 \text{ milligrams/hour}}{10 \text{ liters/hour}} = 2.4 \text{ milligrams/liter}$$

Table 21–4. Normal Average Pharmacokinetic Parameters of the Hypothetical Drug and Its Active Metabolite

Parameter	Drug	Active Metabolite
Total clearance	30 liters/hour	10 liters/hour
Renal clearance	15 liters/hour	8.5 liters/hour
Fraction excreted unchanged	0.5	0.85
Availability	0.8	0.3[a]

[a]Fraction of drug converted to active metabolite.

In an anuric patient the total clearance is the extrarenal clearance. For this drug, the extrarenal clearance is 15 liters/hour; for the metabolite, it is 1.5 liters/hour. Therefore, the predicted steady-state concentration of the drug in the anuric patient, $C(d)_{ss,av}$, is

$$C(d)_{ss,av} = \frac{0.8 \times 100 \text{ milligrams/hour}}{15 \text{ liters/hour}} = 5.3 \text{ milligrams/liter}$$

Because 0.6 of the total elimination, $[CL_f/(CL - CL_R)]$, goes to the active metabolite in the anuric patient, the steady-state concentration of the metabolite, $C(m,d)_{ss,av}$, is

$$C(m,d)_{ss,av} = \frac{0.6 \times 0.8 \times 100 \text{ milligrams/hour}}{1.5 \text{ liters/hour}} = 32 \text{ milligrams/liter}$$

Note that the average drug concentration is two times as great in the anuric patient, while the active metabolite concentration is increased thirteen times. If the drug and the active metabolite are equipotent and additive in their activities, then in the anuric patient the rate of administration should be $(2.7 + 2.4)/(5.3 + 32)$ or 0.14 that of normal. Thus, the anuric patient would require only 14 milligrams/hour. Although the metabolite makes a minor contribution to the total activity in patients with normal renal function, in the anuric patient it is primarily responsible for the activity.

ADDITIONAL CONSIDERATIONS

There are four other aspects of metabolite kinetics that warrant consideration. One is response, another is interconversion between metabolite and drug, and the other two are the use of metabolite data to quantify metabolic clearance and to identify possible causes of a change in pharmacokinetics.

Response

When all activity or toxicity resides with a particular metabolite, relating response to metabolite concentration is relatively straightforward. The problem is more difficult when both drug and metabolite contribute to activity or toxicity. Occasionally, it may be possible to relate the response to a linear combination of the plasma concentrations of drug and metabolite. More often, however, the relationship between response and concentrations is more complicated, and no simple relationship exists. For example, if the response produced by the drug alone approaches the maximum, E_{max}, the response will change little with increases in the concentration of a metabolite that acts as a competitive agonist. Although there are mathematical approaches to this problem, based for example on modification of Equation 1 in Chapter 20, they are unlikely to be used clinically. Nonetheless, measurement of the concentration of an active metabolite can help in explaining an observation and accounting for variability in drug response. Therefore, such measurements can serve as a useful semiquantitative guide to therapy.

Interconversion

Among the list of therapeutically important metabolites in Table 21–1 are some that are enzymatically converted back to the administered drug substance; they include prednisolone, the metabolite of prednisone, and sulindac sulfide, the metabolite of sulindac. Both drugs are prescribed as anti-inflammatory agents, but in each case the activity resides with the metabolite. These and other examples of drug-metabolite pairs that undergo interconversion are listed in Table 21–5.

Figure 21–11 illustrates some common features of interconversion. Shown are the plasma concentrations of prednisolone and prednisone after administration of each steroid on separate occasions. Notice, irrespective of which is administered, both steroids are present in plasma. Also, the ratio of prednisolone to prednisone rapidly reaches a fixed value of 10:1, after which the steroids decline in parallel on semilogarithmic graph paper. How quickly the equilibrium is established and where the ratio lies depends not only on the kinetics of interconversion but also on the irreversible loss of each species from the body, as can be visualized in the scheme below.

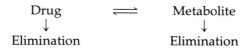

Each pathway is characterized by an associated clearance, and each species may differ in its volume of distribution. The terminal half-life of the interconverted pair is a hybrid of all these parameters. This scheme resembles the two-compartment distribution model discussed in Chapter 19 (Fig. 19–3), except now the two compartments represent drug and metabolite. The difference between the two models is that with interconversion loss can also occur from the

Table 21–5. Representative Drugs that Undergo Metabolic Interconversion

Drug	Metabolite[a]	Compound that Predominates at Equilibrium in Plasma	Comment
Dapsone	Monoacetyldapsone	Dapsone	Acetylation shows genetic polymorphism; metabolite is less active
Clofibrate[b]	Glucuronide	Clofibric acid	In renal impairment glucuronide elimination is reduced; this causes reduced apparent clearance of clofibric acid
Cortisol	Cortisone	Cortisol	Cortisone is inactive
Prednisone[c]	Prednisolone	Prednisolone	Prednisone is inactive
Sulindac	Sulindac sulfide	—[d]	Sulindac (a sulfoxide) is inactive, and therefore acts as prodrug for sulindac sulfide
Vitamin K	Vitamin K-epoxide	Vitamin K	Epoxide is inactive; oral anticoagulants work by blocking reduction of epoxide back to vitamin K, which is needed for blood clotting

[a]Definition of drug and metabolite somewhat arbitrary; the term drug tends to be reserved for administered compound.
[b]Clofibrate is ethyl ester of active clofibric acid; ester rapidly hydrolyzed *in vivo*.
[c]Commercially available as a drug substance.
[d]Situation complicated by enterohepatic cycling of sulindac and sulindac sulfide.

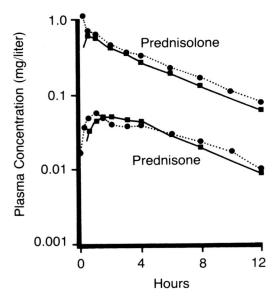

Fig. 21–11.   Once equilibrium is established, the concentrations of prednisone and prednisolone in plasma are independent of which drug is administered. Data are obtained after a single oral dose of 50 milligrams prednisone (■—■) and an intravenous dose of prednisolone (●· · ·●), as prednisolone succinate (40 mg), to a subject on separate occasions. Prednisolone succinate, not shown, is hydrolyzed very rapidly to prednisolone. (One mg/liter = 2.8 micromolar.) (Redrawn from Rose, J.Q., Yurchak, A.M., Jusko, W.J., and Powell, D.: Bioavailability and disposition of prednisolone tablets. Biopharm. Drug Disp., 1:247–258, 1980. Reprinted by permission of John Wiley & Sons, Ltd.)

"peripheral" (metabolite) compartment. Indeed, if no such loss occurs then, viewed from drug in plasma, the metabolite is effectively a component of drug distribution since, under these circumstances, no drug is irreversibly lost via this pathway.

The therapeutic importance of interconversion varies with the drug and the circumstance. For example, interconversion between sulindac and its sulfide helps to moderate and sustain the concentration of the active sulfide. In contrast, interconversion between the antileprotic drug dapsone and its less active metabolite monoacetyldapsone has no therapeutic relevance; the equilibrium is always strongly toward dapsone, which is primarily eliminated via pathways other than N-acetylation. Normally, the interconversion between clofibric acid (derived from the rapid hydrolysis of the administered ethyl ester, clofibrate) and its inactive glucuronide is not of concern; the glucuronide is excreted so rapidly that glucuronidation can be regarded as a pathway of irreversible loss of clofibric acid. Consequently, as only 6 percent of clofibric acid is usually excreted unchanged and all the activity resides with clofibric acid, no change in its pharmacokinetics is anticipated in patients with renal insufficiency. However, as shown in Figure 21–12, the unbound clearance of clofibric acid is markedly reduced, and its half-life is prolonged, as renal function decreases. The explanation lies in the reduction of the clearance of the glucuronide, which then accumulates and is hydrolyzed back to the parent acid; effectively, a major route of elimination of clofibric acid is increasingly blocked. To what extent the phenomenon seen with clofibric acid occurs with other drugs that depend heavily on glucuronidation for elimination is not known. Clofibric acid glucuronide is an ester; many other drugs form more stable ether glucuronides. Whether this

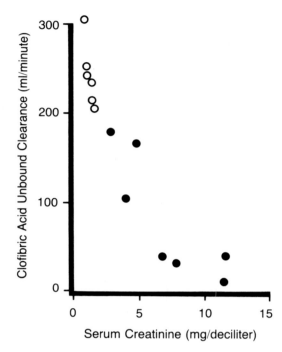

Fig. 21–12.   Although little clofibric acid is excreted unchanged ($fe(n) = 0.06$ to 0.1) when renal function is normal, the unbound clearance of clofibric acid decreases markedly with an increase in serum creatinine, an inverse measure of renal function. The apparent dependence of clofibric acid's unbound clearance on a patient's renal function is explained by its interconversion to a polar metabolite, whose loss from the body is dependent on renal function. Unbound clearance values in patients with normal (○) and compromised (●) renal function are shown. (One mg/liter = 4.7 micromolar.) (Redrawn from Gugler, P., Kurten, J.W., Jensen, C.J., Klehr, U., and Hartlapp, J.: Clofibrate disposition in renal failure and acute and chronic liver disease. Europ. J. Clin. Pharmacol., *15*:341–347, 1979.)

difference in the type of glucuronide formed is an important factor remains to be seen.

Estimation of Metabolic Clearance

Many metabolites are polar and are eliminated almost exclusively by renal excretion. The elimination (excretion) of these metabolites is frequently formation rate-limited for much of drug elimination, either because they have a much higher clearance, smaller volume of distribution, or both, compared with parent drug. Recall, when formation is rate-limiting, as a reasonable approximation during the terminal phase,

$$\text{Rate of metabolite excretion} \simeq CL_f \cdot C$$
$$\text{Rate of metabolite formation}$$

19

Thus, by measuring the rate of excretion of the metabolite and the corresponding plasma drug concentration, clearance associated with the formation of the metabolite may be estimated. This approach may be particularly useful for investigating drug interactions; it forms the basis for phenotyping genetically determined metabolic polymorphism in acetylation. In addition, it should be noted that when Equation 19 applies, the fall in metabolite excretion rate is determined by, and can be used to estimate, the half-life of the drug. Obviously, Equation 19 is more accurate at steady state than during the terminal phase following discrete doses.

Detection of Changes in Pharmacokinetics

Comparisons between drug and metabolite areas are helpful in identifying the organ of drug metabolism (i.e., gastrointestinal tract, liver) when drug is administered by different routes (p. 359). Area analysis can also be used to examine possible causes of any change in the pharmacokinetics of a drug. Suppose, for example, that the plasma concentrations of a drug of low clearance are reduced on Occasion B compared to the values on Occasion A when given orally. Possible explanations are reduced availability, increased clearance, or both. Examination of drug data alone might give a clue, but the situation is helped considerably by simultaneous use of metabolite data. The area ratios for drug are

$$\text{Occasion A:} \quad F_A \cdot \text{Dose} = CL_A \cdot AUC_A \tag{20}$$

$$\text{Occasion B:} \quad F_B \cdot \text{Dose} = CL_B \cdot AUC_B \tag{21}$$

and for metabolite the corresponding equations are

$$\text{Occasion A:} \quad fm_A \cdot F_A \cdot \text{Dose} = CL(m)_A \cdot AUC(m)_A \tag{22}$$

$$\text{Occasion B:} \quad fm_B \cdot F_B \cdot \text{Dose} = CL(m)_B \cdot AUC(m)_B \tag{23}$$

So that, by appropriate division,

$$\frac{AUC_B}{AUC_A} = \frac{F_B}{F_A} \cdot \frac{CL_A}{CL_B} \tag{24}$$

$$\frac{AUC(m)_B}{AUC(m)_A} = \frac{F_B \, fm_B \cdot CL(m)_A}{F_A \, fm_A \cdot CL(m)_B} \tag{25}$$

and since $fm \cdot CL = CL_f$, then

$$\left[\frac{AUC(m)}{AUC} \right]_A = \frac{CL_{f,A}}{CL(m)_A} \tag{26}$$

$$\left[\frac{AUC(m)}{AUC} \right]_B = \frac{CL_{f,B}}{CL(m)_B} \tag{27}$$

Now consider the various possibilities.

Possibility 1. Reduced availability due to incomplete dissolution of drug ($F_B < F_A$). If this is so, as clearance of neither drug nor metabolite is altered, it follows from Equations 24 and 25 that

Expectation:

$$\frac{AUC_B}{AUC_A} = \frac{AUC(m)_B}{AUC(m)_A}$$

That is, the ratio of areas of drug and areas of metabolite should be equal to each other, but be less than 1. Of course, the reason could also be due to the patient failing to take the dose as instructed, a compliance problem.

Possibility 2. Increased clearance of drug ($CL_B > CL_A$). If this is the reason for the decreased drug concentration, then the expected outcome for the metabolite depends on the mechanism responsible for the increase in drug clearance, namely, decreased binding of drug, enzyme induction, or increased renal clearance.

a. *Decreased binding of drug (fu ↑).*
If this occurs, CL_f is increased but *fm* is unaltered, because the clearance by all pathways of drug elimination are equally affected. As neither availability nor metabolite clearance is altered,

Expectation:

$$\frac{AUC(m)_A}{AUC(m)_B} = 1$$

$$\left[\frac{AUC(m)}{AUC}\right]_A > \left[\frac{AUC(m)}{AUC}\right]_B$$

b. *Enzyme Induction.*
If this occurs, CL_f may or may not change depending on whether or not the metabolic pathway is induced. Remember, there is often more than one enzyme responsible for drug metabolism, and all are not equally susceptible to induction by a given inducing agent.

b1. *Metabolite pathway induced.*
Since CL_f is increased, it follows that

Expectation:

$$\left[\frac{AUC(m)}{AUC}\right]_B > \left[\frac{AUC(m)}{AUC}\right]_A$$

Whether the metabolite area ratio changes depends on whether or not the metabolite is the only pathway of drug elimination. If it is, then, since *fm* = 1 and cannot increase further, no change in the metabolite area ratio is expected. Otherwise,

Expectation:

$$\frac{AUC(m)_B}{AUC(m)_A} > 1$$

b2. *Metabolite pathway not induced.*
Since CL_f is not changed but *fm* is decreased (as *CL* is increased), it follows that

Expectation:

$$\left[\frac{AUC(m)_B}{AUC(m)_A}\right] < 1$$

$$\left[\frac{AUC(m)}{AUC}\right]_B = \left[\frac{AUC(m)}{AUC}\right]_A$$

c. *Increased renal clearance* $(CL_R \uparrow)$.

The outcome in terms of the metabolite is the same as that predicted for case b2, because CL_f is unaltered and *fm* is decreased.

Expectation:

$$\left[\frac{AUC(m)_B}{AUC(m)_A}\right] < 1$$

$$\left[\frac{AUC(m)}{AUC}\right]_B = \left[\frac{AUC(m)}{AUC}\right]_A$$

From the above analyses it is apparent that metabolite data help to narrow the number of likely reasons for the reduced plasma concentrations of a drug. Giving the drug intravenously would have resolved the issue, but it is not always possible or practical to do so. Measurement of protein binding and of drug in urine would certainly have helped distinguish between the various possibilities. Of course it is possible that both availability and clearance of drug had changed, and metabolite clearance too; all of which complicate the interpretation. Notwithstanding such complications, it is often possible to make reasonable conclusions as to the likely cause of a change in drug pharmacokinetics from combined drug and metabolite data.

Study Problems

(Answers to Study Problems are in Appendix G.)

1. Elson *et al.* (Elson, J., Strong, J.M., Lee, W-K., and Atkinson, A.J. Clin. Pharmacol. Ther., *17*:134–140, 1975) determined the ratio of the plasma concentration of the active metabolite N-acetylprocainamide (see Table 21–1) to that of procainamide in patients on long-term procainamide therapy. The histogram (Fig. 21–13) on the next page shows the results of 33 patients; there is considerable variation. Assuming, as is likely, that these values are reasonable estimates of the ratio at plateau, comment on which pharmacokinetic parameters of drug and metabolite contribute to the observed variability in the ratio.

2. Which (if any) of the explanations offered below are consistent with the following statement? An increase in the ratio of area under the metabolite concentration-time profile to area under the drug concentration-time profile, *AUC(m)/AUC*, suggests that any of the following could have happened.

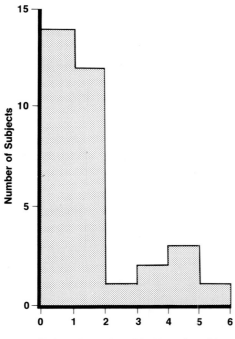

Fig. 21–13.

    (a) Induction of the metabolite formation pathway.

    (b) Reduction of the volume of distribution of the metabolite.

    (c) Increase in the dose of drug absorbed.

    (d) Reduction in the clearance of an alternative pathway of elimination of the drug.

3. Glycine conjugation, with the formation of salicyluric acid, is one of the major pathways for the elimination of salicylic acid in man. Salicylic acid is cleared slowly from the body, whereas salicyluric acid is cleared so rapidly and completely into the urine that the plasma concentration of this metabolite is very low. Discuss why measuring salicyluric acid in the urine could be successfully used to assess its rate of formation.

4. In common with chlorpromazine and some other phenothiazines, promethazine is oxidized to form a sulfoxide. There has been speculation that sulfoxide formation of phenothiazines occurs predominantly in the gastrointestinal tract. Taylor *et al.* (Taylor, G., Houston, J.B., Shaffer, J., and Mawer, G. Brit. J. Clin. Pharmacol. *15*: 287–293, 1983) administered promethazine, as its hydrochloride salt, intravenously (12.5 mg) and orally (25 mg) on separate occasions to a group of seven subjects. The corresponding mean *AUC* values for the sulfoxide were 7.2 and 11.5 milligrams-hour/liter. Knowing that approximately 10 percent of promethazine is converted to its sulfoxide and that essentially all oral promethazine is available to the gastrointestinal tract, do these data support a prominent role of the gastrointestinal tract in the formation of the sulfoxide?

5. Shown in Figure 21–14 are semilogarithmic plots of the plasma concentrations of propranolol (○) and its active metabolite, 4-hydroxypropranolol (●) after oral administration of propranolol (80 mg) to six healthy subjects. Discuss why the plasma concentration of 4-hydroxypropranolol peaks earlier and initially declines more rapidly than that of propranolol.

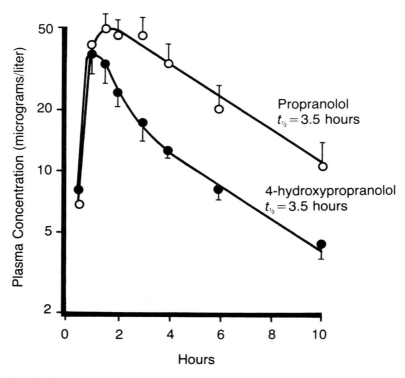

Fig. 21–14.

6. Listed in Table 21–6 are the plasma concentrations of a drug and one of its metabolites following oral administration of one gram of drug to a subject. For the following calculations assume that the drug is fully available orally, that absorption of the drug is rapid relative to its elimination, and that the volumes of distribution of drug and metabolite are equal. The molecular weight of the drug is 308, that of the metabolite is 326.

Table 21–6.

Time (hours)	0	0.5	1	1.5	2	3	4	6	8	12
Drug (mg/liter)	0	25	32	30	32	16	9	4	1.2	–
Metabolite (mg/liter)	0	10	22	31	44	42	32	25	16	8.5

(a) Calculate the fraction of drug converted to metabolite, the formation clearance of metabolite, and the disposition kinetics of the metabolite.

(b) The recommended dosage regimen of the drug is one gram orally every eight hours. The pharmacokinetics of both drug and metabolite do not change with time on chronic dosing.

1. Calculate the average concentrations of drug and metabolite at plateau.

2. Calculate the concentration-time profiles of drug and metabolite within a dosing interval at plateau.

3. Calculate the times required to reach their plateaus.

22

Dose and Time Dependencies

Objectives

The reader will be able to:

1. **List at least 10 sources of dose (or time) dependence in drug absorption, distribution, or elimination.**

2. **Recognize dose- (or time-) dependent kinetics from either plasma or urine data that show such behavior.**

3. **Graphically depict the kinetic behavior of a drug when the situation and the cause of a dose (or time) dependence is given.**

4. **On analyzing data in which a dose (or time) dependence occurs, identify the pharmacokinetic parameters that are affected and assign probable causes to the observed dependence.**

5. **Demonstrate the kinetic consequences at steady state of a change in the rate of input, *Vm* or *Km*, of a drug showing Michaelis-Menten metabolism.**

6. **Define saturable first-pass metabolism, describe how it can occur, and discuss its kinetic consequences.**

An epileptic patient who has not responded to phenytoin after two weeks on 300 milligrams/day is observed to have a plasma concentration of 4 milligrams/liter. Fifteen days after increasing the daily dose to 500 milligrams, the patient develops signs of toxicity, nystagmus, and ataxia; the plasma concentration of phenytoin is now 36 milligrams/liter. Why should only a 67 percent increase in daily dose give rise to a ninefold increase in the plasma concentration? The answer lies in the dose-dependent kinetic behavior of this drug.

Normally the plasma (or blood) concentration, the unbound concentration, and the amount of drug and its metabolites excreted in urine at any given time all increase in proportion to dose, whether drug is administered as a single dose or as multiple doses. Therefore, on correcting such observations for the dose administered, the values should superimpose at all times. This is referred to as the *principle of superposition.* When superposition occurs, the pharmacokinetics of a drug is said to be *dose-* and *time-independent.*

There are many reasons why the principle of superposition may not hold. Among them are the administration of a drug by different routes, in different dosage forms, or by different methods (bolus or infusion). In these cases, although the time profile may differ between treatments, the pharmacokinetic parameters may not change with dose or time. Other reasons for lack of superposition include changes in the pharmacokinetic parameters themselves with size of dose administered or with time, when all the other factors mentioned are held constant. The pharmacokinetics of such drugs are said to be *dose* or *time-dependent*. Such dose-dependent and time-dependent kinetics are sources of variability in drug response. Although relatively uncommon, they occur frequently enough in drug therapy to warrant special consideration. In drug overdose, they are more the rule than the exception.

This chapter deals with the identification and the consequences of dose-dependent and time-dependent kinetics. The major intent is to establish a general awareness of this topic, which can become both mathematically and conceptually complex.

EVIDENCE

Five pharmacokinetic parameters (F, ka, V, CL_R, and CL_H) basically define and summarize the time-course of a drug in the body. Usually none of these parameters systematically changes with time or dose in the same individual. But in *dose-dependent* and *time-dependent kinetics*, any one or a combination of these parameters changes with the administration of different doses or with time.

Table 22–1. Representative Causes of Dose- (or Time-) Dependent Kinetics and Selected Drug Examples

	Example	Parameter Affected[a]	
I. *Absorption*			
A. Saturable transport in gut wall	Riboflavin	F	↓
B. Drug comparatively insoluble	Griseofulvin	F	↓
C. Saturable gut wall or hepatic metabolism on first pass	Alprenolol	F	↑
II. *Distribution*			
A. Saturable plasma protein binding	Disopyramide	V, fu	↑
B. Saturable tissue binding	Cyclosporine A (blood cells)	V_b, fu_b	↑ [b]
III. *Excretion*			
A. Active secretion (saturable)	Penicillin G	CL_R	↓
B. Active reabsorption (saturable)	Ascorbic acid	CL_R	↑
C. Decrease in urine pH	Salicylic acid	CL_R	↓
D. Saturable plasma protein binding	Disopyramide	CL_R	↑
E. Nephrotoxicity (time)[c]	Aminoglycoside	CL_R	↓
F. Increase in urine flow (time)[c]	Theophylline	CL_R	↑
IV. *Metabolism*			
A. Capacity-limited kinetics, cofactor limitation, etc.	Phenytoin	CL_H	↓
B. Enzyme induction (time)[c]	Carbamazepine	CL_H	↑
C. Hepatotoxicity (time)[c]	Acetaminophen	CL_H	↓
D. Saturable plasma protein binding	Prednisolone	CL_H	↑
E. Decreased hepatic blood flow	Propranolol	CL_H	↓
F. Inhibition by metabolite (time)[c]	Lidocaine	CL_H	↓

[a]Direction of change: ↑ increase, ↓ decrease.
[b]V tends to decrease, but the effect is minor because the fraction of drug in body in blood cells is small.
[c]Time-dependent as well as dose-dependent.

Table 22–1 lists examples of representative causes of dose and time dependencies together with the pharmacokinetic parameters affected.

ABSORPTION

Dose or time dependencies in the absorption of a drug may be reflected by a change in either the availability or the rate constant of absorption with dose or time. These dependencies most often arise from three sources, following oral administration. The first is solubility and dissolution limitations in the release of drug from a dosage form in the gastrointestinal tract. The second is saturability in a transport mechanism for passage across the gastrointestinal membranes. The third is saturability in the metabolism of drug during its first pass through the gut wall and the liver.

Dissolution can be the cause of dose dependency in availability for drugs with low aqueous solubility, when given orally in relatively large doses. Recall that the rate of absorption, when there is an essentially saturated solution of drug at the absorption site, is relatively constant (Chap. 4, p. 34). Accordingly, with a fixed contact time of drug in the gastrointestinal tract, the amount of drug absorbed is unlikely to increase in proportion to the dose administered. An example is griseofulvin (Fig. 22–1). For this sparingly soluble drug (solubility is 10 mg/liter), availability decreases as the dose is increased from 250 to 500 milligrams.

Vitamin B_{12} is absorbed by a facilitated transport mechanism. Table 22–2 demonstrates how dramatically the absorption of vitamin B_{12} decreases as the dose is increased. The transport process exhibits saturability as a result of a maximum capacity to facilitate absorption. The availability of an intrinsic factor produced in the stomach is the specific limitation here.

Lorcainide, an antiarrhythmic agent, is an example of a drug with dose dependence in oral availability because of saturability in its metabolism on the first pass through the liver. The area under the blood lorcainide concentration-time curve, relative to dose, increases when the single oral dose of lorcainide is increased from 100 to 500 milligrams (Fig. 22–2).

SATURABILITY OF PLASMA PROTEIN AND TISSUE BINDING

There are a limited number of binding sites on plasma proteins. Recall from Table 10–3 that the plasma concentration of albumin is usually 43 grams/liter or 0.6 millimolar (molecular weight = 67,000). At one binding site per albumin molecule there is then a maximum concentration of 0.6 millimolar for the bound drug. If a drug primarily binds to α_1-acid glycoprotein, the limitation occurs at about 0.015 millimolar, a much lower concentration. The sites to which drugs bind in the tissues may similarly be limited. Consequently, the volume of distribution may depend on the plasma concentration, a *concentration-dependent* behavior.

For drugs that show saturable binding to plasma proteins, the volume of distribution is expected to increase with the plasma concentration (Chap. 10). Conversely, for drugs that show saturability in binding to tissues, the volume of distribution decreases as the plasma concentration is increased. Because of the potential dependence on the fraction unbound in plasma and the dependence

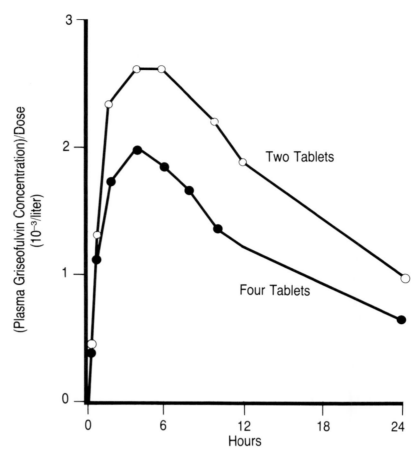

Fig. 22–1. Plasma concentration, normalized to dose, as a function of time following the oral administration of two tablets (upper curve, ○) and four tablets (lower curve, ●) of ultramicronized griseofulvin (125 mg/tablet). (One mg/liter = 2.8 micromolar.) (Adapted from data in Barrett, W.E. and Bianchine, J.R.: The bioavailability of ultramicronized griseofulvin (GRIS-PEG®) tablets in man. Curr. Ther. Res., *18*:501–509, 1975.)

Table 22–2. Gastrointestinal Absorption of Vitamin B_{12}

Dose (micrograms)	Amount Absorbed (micrograms)	Percent of Dose Absorbed
0.5	0.4	80
2.0	0.9	45
5.0	1.3	26
10	1.5	15
50	2.0	4
200	3.3	1.6
500	6	1.1

Adapted from the figure on p. 484, Documenta Geigy, Scientific Tables, 7th Ed., 1970.

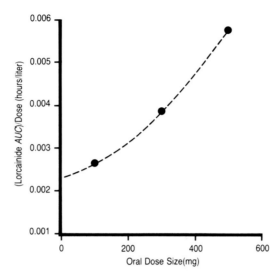

Fig. 22–2.   Area under the blood concentration-time curve, normalized to dose, after the oral administration of various doses of the antiarrhythmic agent, lorcainide, to an individual subject. The area-to-dose ratio following intravenous administration was constant at 0.0137 hour/liter, a value much higher than that observed when the drug was given orally. This difference indicates that the availability is low for all these oral doses. (Adapted from data in Jähnchen, E., Bechtold, H., Kasper, W., Kersting, F., Just, H., Heykants, J., and Meinertz, T.: Lorcainide. I. Saturable presystemic elimination. Clin. Pharmacol. Ther., 26:187–195, 1979.)

of half-life on both clearance and volume of distribution, dose dependence in distribution may be difficult to identify and to quantify, unless plasma protein binding is measured. Consider the following example of phenylbutazone.

As seen in Panel A of Figure 22–3, the steady-state plasma concentration of phenylbutazone relative to the dose administered decreases with the daily dose when given at therapeutic rates of 200 to 400 milligrams/day. Consider how one might interpret these data given the additional knowledge that only negligible amounts of the drug appear in urine and feces.

Since the phenylbutazone was administered orally, the steady-state concentration could reflect either a decreased availability, an increased clearance, or a change in both parameters on increasing the dose. This conclusion is based on the relationship:

$$\frac{C_{ss,av}}{(\text{Dose}/\tau)} = \frac{F}{CL} \qquad\qquad 1$$

where the symbols are as usually defined. Because only negligible amounts of the drug are detected in urine or feces, it is tempting to conclude that absorption is always complete. However, availability can decrease with an increased oral dose, even though no drug appears in the feces, if unabsorbed drug is degraded by the microflora in the lower intestines. Dose dependence in absorption could be proven unambiguously by parenteral administration, but an intravenous formulation of phenylbutazone is not available. One example of an increased clearance, elevated organ blood flow, can be immediately excluded. Clearance, estimated by appropriately substituting the data in Figure 22–3 into Equation 1, is low and so is not expected to change with blood flow. As drug was not detected in urine, a change in clearance must occur by an extrarenal route, presumably by hepatic metabolism. Another possible explanation for an increased clearance is an increased ability to metabolize the drug. This possibility might arise from enzyme activation, a dose-dependent mechanism, or from induction of the

A

B

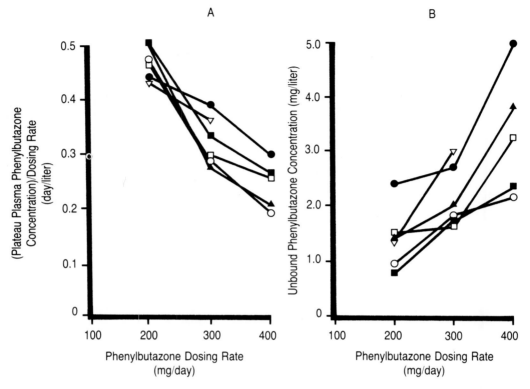

Fig. 22–3. Conditions at plateau for phenylbutazone, a drug of low extraction ratio. The events at plateau were monitored in patients receiving increasing daily doses (200–400 mg) of phenylbutazone; each dose was maintained for a minimum of three weeks. Evidence of concentration dependence is seen by the decrease in the plateau plasma concentration, normalized to the daily dose administered (A). This concentration dependence arises from saturation of plasma protein binding sites. When corrected for differences in binding, the unbound concentration increases linearly with dosing rate (B), indicating that the unbound clearance is unchanged. Each symbol corresponds to data from one patient. (One mg/liter = 3.2 micromolar.) (Redrawn from Higham, C., Aarons, L.J., Holt, P.J.L., Lynch, M., and Rowland, M.: A chronic dose-ranging study of the pharmacokinetics of phenylbutazone in rheumatoid arthritic patients. Brit. J. Clin. Pharmacol., *12*: 123–129, 1981. Reproduced with permission of Blackwell Scientific Publications.)

drug's own metabolic enzymes, a dose- and time-dependent mechanism. The data do not permit distinction between these possibilities.

The actual cause of the dose-dependent observation is apparent when plasma protein binding is measured. Clearance is increased because of the saturability of phenylbutazone binding to plasma proteins. The unbound clearance of phenylbutazone is constant (slope of unbound drug in Panel B of Figure 22–3); the total clearance $((Dose/\tau)/C_{ss,av})$ changes with concentration. Furthermore, saturation of binding to albumin is expected at bound (total minus unbound) concentrations of 80 to 120 milligrams/liter or 0.3 to 0.4 millimolar (molecular weight = 308), values approaching the molar concentration typical of plasma albumin (0.6 millimolar).

The therapeutic consequence of decreased binding to plasma proteins at higher daily doses of a drug of low extraction ratio dramatically differs from that of increased enzyme activity. When the binding is decreased, the total concentration in plasma is not increased much on doubling the rate of administration, but the unbound concentration is, a consequence of no change in the unbound clearance. The toxic and therapeutic responses are expected to increase accordingly. An increase in enzyme activity would affect both unbound and total concentrations proportionally. Thus, if induction were responsible, only a minor increase in the responses to the drug would be expected at the higher rates of administration.

Although the approach toward saturation of binding sites in the tissues has no effect on the clearance of a drug, it does have an effect on volume of distribution and therefore on elimination half-life. Following a single dose sufficiently large to approach saturation of tissue binding sites, the total and unbound plasma drug concentrations would decline, with half lives that increase, at lower concentrations as shown in Panel A of Figure 22–4.

The expected change in the time-course of a drug in plasma when plasma protein binding is saturated is more complex. Changes occur in both the volume of distribution (Chaps. 10 and 25) and clearance (Chap. 11). The magnitude of the changes depends on both the volume of distribution and the extraction ratio of the drug. To demonstrate the effect of altered binding, a drug with a low extraction ratio and large volume of distribution is assumed. For this drug, the unbound concentration declines linearly on a semilogarithmic plot (Panel B, Fig. 22–4), as expected when its unbound volume and unbound clearance are constant. The total concentration, however, appears to decline in a downward convex manner, a result of the decrease in fu as the unbound concentration declines with time.

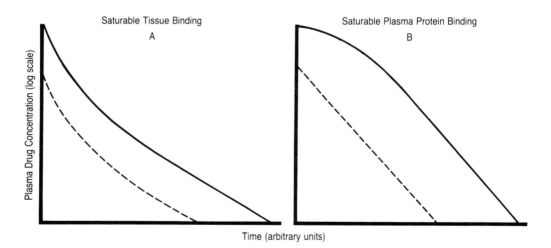

Fig. 22–4.   Simulation of the effect of saturable binding on the time-course of the total (——) and unbound (– – – –) plasma drug concentrations following a single intravenous dose. Distribution equilibrium is assumed to occur instantaneously. Panel A, As drug is eliminated, saturable tissue binding results in an increasing apparent volume of distribution and therefore an increasing half-life for both the total and the unbound concentrations, which fall in parallel. Panel B, As drug is eliminated, saturable binding to plasma proteins for a drug with a large volume of distribution and a low clearance results in the total concentration declining more slowly than the concentration of the unbound drug, a consequence of an increasing fraction unbound in plasma with time (see text).

CONCENTRATION-DEPENDENT RENAL EXCRETION

Renal clearance can vary with plasma concentration. Both filtration and reabsorption are usually passive processes, the rates of which are directly related to the plasma concentration. Active secretion and active reabsorption are saturable processes, that is, they have a maximum capacity. This is shown in Figure 22–5 for active secretion. The maximum rate of tubular secretion is often called the T_M value. The rate of transport increases in direct proportion to the plasma concentration until the transport approaches its capacity. Further increases in the drug concentration then produce little change in the rate of transport. Consequently, the clearance by secretion decreases as the plasma concentration increases.

Secretion never occurs alone; filtration is always a component and passive reabsorption may or may not be. Figure 22–5 also demonstrates how the rate of excretion of a drug that undergoes filtration and secretion, but no reabsorption, such as penicillin, always increases with plasma concentration. As the rate of secretion approaches a maximum, the rate of filtration increases in direct proportion to the plasma concentration. These events are shown in curve B in Figure 22–6.

There may be little to no excretion at low plasma concentrations for a drug that is actively reabsorbed, for example, glucose and water-soluble vitamins. Drug appears in urine when its rate of filtration (plus secretion, if any) exceeds the capacity of the active reabsorption process. This condition occurs when the plasma concentration exceeds what is sometimes called the threshold concentration.

Renal clearance is the rate of drug excretion divided by its plasma concentration. A drug that is only filtered, and is not bound in plasma, has the same renal clearance at all concentrations, as shown schematically in curve A of Figure 22–6. Curve B depicts the events that occur for a drug that is actively secreted. In the region of plasma concentrations well below those required to approach saturation, renal clearance is highest and is relatively insensitive to changes in drug concentration. The therapeutic concentrations of most actively secreted drugs lie within this region. At higher plasma concentrations, renal clearance decreases; the lower limiting value is that contributed by both filtration and passive reabsorption. The same limitation applies to a drug that is actively reabsorbed, curve C. However, at low concentrations the renal clearance of an actively reabsorbed drug is less, not more.

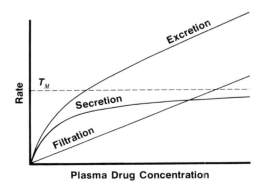

Plasma Drug Concentration

Fig. 22–5. The rate of renal secretion has a limiting value, the maximum transport rate (T_M), whereas the rate of filtration increases in direct proportion to the plasma concentration of a drug. Consequently, the rate of excretion of a drug that is both filtered and secreted increases with its plasma concentration, but not in direct proportion. Reabsorption is assumed not to occur.

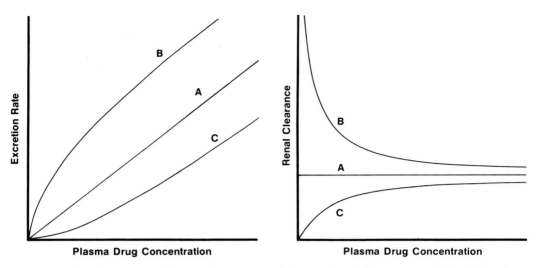

Fig. 22–6.   The relationships of the rate of excretion (on left) and of renal clearance (on right) with the plasma concentration depend on whether the drug undergoes filtration only (curve A), filtration and secretion (curve B), or filtration and active reabsorption (curve C).

Renal clearance may also show concentration dependence when the drug produces changes in pH and its tubular reabsorption is pH-dependent, e.g., salicylate; is a diuretic and the clearance is flow-dependent, e.g., theophylline; or causes nephrotoxicity, e.g., an aminoglycoside. The mechanisms of the last two drugs are also time-dependent. Theophylline produces diuresis soon after its administration, but this effect, and consequently its renal clearance, decrease with time. The nephrotoxic effect of aminoglycosides, on the other hand, develops with time of exposure to the drug.

CAPACITY-LIMITED METABOLISM

Perhaps the most dramatic dose-dependent kinetic mechanism is that of *capacity-limited metabolism*, a characteristic typical of enzymatic reactions. Recall from Chapter 11 (Eq. 7) that

$$\text{Rate of metabolism} = \frac{Vm \cdot Cu}{Km + Cu} \qquad 2$$

for a drug showing Michaelis-Menten kinetics. Also, recall that in this case

$$\text{Unbound metabolic clearance} = \frac{Vm}{Km + Cu} \qquad 3$$

The therapeutic consequences of Michaelis-Menten kinetics are subsequently explored.

Alcohol

The metabolism of alcohol to acetaldehyde by alcohol dehydrogenase is a prime example of capacity-limited metabolism. The values of the maximum rate of metabolism, Vm, and the Michaelis constant, Km, are approximately 10 grams/hour and 100 milligrams/liter, respectively. The pharmacologic effect of alcohol, which does not bind to plasma proteins, become apparent when the plasma concentration is about 250 milligrams/liter; concentrations above 5000 milligrams/liter are potentially lethal. Thus, the concentration range in which alcohol exerts its pharmacologic effects is well above the value of its Km. At high concentrations, the rate of elimination approaches Vm and is therefore independent of concentration. When the rate is constant at all concentrations, the kinetics are said to be zero-order (Chap. 4, p. 34).

Table 22–3 shows the calculated rate of metabolism and clearance of alcohol as a function of the concentration at the metabolic site, using the values given for Vm and Km and Equations 2 and 3. Note that the rate of metabolism of alcohol is essentially constant, zero-order, throughout the range of concentrations associated with activity of the drug and, accordingly, clearance decreases at high concentrations. At low concentrations, the intrinsic clearance (Vm/Km) approaches 100 liters/hour or 1.6 liters/minute, a value in excess of hepatic blood flow. Thus, at very low concentrations the extraction ratio is high and the rate of metabolism of alcohol is partially limited by hepatic perfusion.

The consequences of zero-order elimination can be dramatic. The usual size drink, one jigger (45 ml), of 80 proof (40 percent, volume/volume) whiskey contains about 14 grams of alcohol. Drinking this quantity of alcohol each hour exceeds the eliminating capacity of the body. Consequently, alcohol accumulates until ultimately either coma or death occurs.

Alcohol distributes evenly throughout total body water spaces; its volume of distribution is therefore 42 liters. Accordingly, approximately 200 grams of alcohol in the body are needed to achieve a concentration, about 5000 milligrams/liter, that can produce coma or, occasionally, death. But, since the rate of ingestion, 14 grams/hour, exceeds the rate of metabolism, 10 grams/hour, by only 4 grams/hour, this rate of drinking must be maintained for at least two days before 200 grams of alcohol have accumulated in the body. However, this degree

Table 22–3. Calculated Rate of Metabolism and Clearance of Alcohol as a Function of the Concentration at the Metabolic Site

Concentration at Site (mg/liter)	Rate of Metabolism[a] (grams/hour)	Clearance[b] (liters/hour)
7000	9.9	1.4
5000	9.8	2.0
3000	9.7	3.2
1000	9.1	9.1
500	8.3	17
200	6.7	33
100	5.0	50
50	3.3	67
10	0.91	91

[a]Rate of metabolism $= Vm \cdot Cu/(Km + Cu)$, $Vm = 10$ grams/hour, $Km = 100$ milligrams/liter.
[b]Clearance $= Vm/(Km + Cu)$.

of accrual can occur within five hours if four jiggers are consumed every hour, because this rate of ingestion, 56 grams/hour, exceeds the maximum metabolic capacity by 46 grams each hour.

If the rate were reduced to one-half jigger or (7 grams) per hour, then, with respect to the effect of alcohol, one can drink with virtual impunity as now shown. By definition, at steady state the rate of administration (or input), R_o, must equal the rate of elimination.

$$R_o = \frac{Vm \cdot Cu_{ss}}{Km + Cu_{ss}} \qquad\qquad 4$$

or on rearrangement

$$Cu_{ss} = \frac{Km \cdot R_o}{Vm - R_o} \qquad\qquad 5$$

Using the previously mentioned values for Km and Vm and an R_o value of 7 grams/hour, the plateau concentration of alcohol is 230 milligrams/liter, a value below that showing much of an effect.

Reflect on the calculations above. Chronically drinking one-half jigger per hour produces little or no effect, but drinking one jigger per hour becomes lethal. There can be no standard dosage to maintain the effects of alcohol.

The consequence of capacity-limited metabolism on the time-course of a drug in the body when the input rate is changed is also demonstrated with alcohol. When alcohol is administered 10 minutes after ingesting water, light cream, or a glucose solution (80 grams/240 ml), the plasma concentration-time profiles differ (Fig. 22–7). Compared to water, administration of light cream and glucose, materials that delay gastric emptying, lower both the AUC and the peak concentration and increase the time to reach the peak. These observations can be explained by the nearly zero-order metabolism of alcohol. To emphasize the point, assume that both elimination and input are strictly zero-order, as shown in Figure 22–8. The effect of decreasing the input rate, for a given total dose administered, is to lower the AUC and the peak concentration as well as to increase the peak time. Clearly, assessment of availability of a drug with zero-order elimination and variable input rates cannot be done by conventional area ratio methods.

Phenytoin

Therapeutic problems encountered with capacity-limited metabolism are classically exemplified by phenytoin. Typical Vm and Km values of this drug are 500 milligrams/day and 0.4 milligram/liter, although the values vary widely. The value of Km is usually expressed in terms of the total, rather than the unbound, plasma drug concentration. Since fu is normally 0.1, the apparent Km for the total concentration, Km', is equal to 4 milligrams/liter.

Plateau. Perhaps the most striking consequence of the kinetics of this drug is the relationship observed between steady-state plasma concentration and rate of administration, as shown in Figure 22–9. A greatly disproportionate increase in concentration is observed in, and above, the therapeutic plasma concentration range, 10 to 20 milligrams/liter. As a result, the difference between the daily

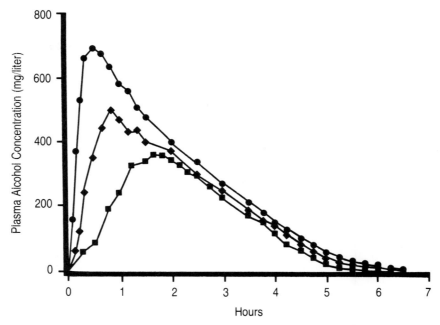

Fig. 22–7. A decrease in the absorption rate of alcohol, produced by slowing gastric emptying, causes the peak concentrations and the AUC to decrease and the time to reach the peak to increase. The effect differs from that expected of first-order kinetics by the observed decrease in AUC. This observation is explained by a constant rate of elimination at almost all concentrations, as illustrated schematically in Figure 22–8. Alcohol, 45 milliliters of 95 percent ethanol in 105 milliliters of orange juice, was administered 10 minutes after 240 milliliters of tap water (●); 240 milliliters of light cream (◆); or 240 milliliters of a 33 percent glucose solution (■). (One mg/liter = 22.0 micromolar.) (Redrawn from data of Sedman, A.J., Wilkinson, P.K., Sakmar, E., Weidler, D.J., and Wagner, J.G.: Food effects on absorption and metabolism of alcohol. Reprinted by permission, from Journal of Studies on Alcohol, Vol. 37, pp. 1197–1214, 1976. Copyright by Journal of Studies on Alcohol, Inc., Rutgers Center of Alcohol Studies, New Brunswick, NJ 08903.)

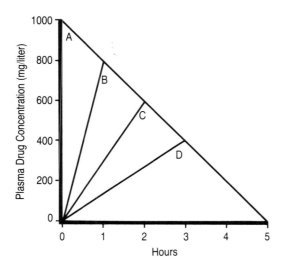

Fig. 22–8. As a consequence of zero-order elimination, the plasma concentrations at the end of a 50-gram dose by bolus injection (A) and constant-rate infusions of 1- (B), 2- (C), and 3- (D) hour durations are quite different from those expected with first-order kinetics. The amount in the body at the end of each infusion is the difference between the dose and the amount lost during the infusion period. Consequently, the concentration at the end of each of the infusions is the same as that expected at that time following the intravenous bolus dose. Note that the slower the input rate, the smaller is the AUC and the lower is the peak concentration. The time of the peak is, of course, increased. Indeed, if the dose had been infused over a 5-hour period, i.e., at 10 grams/hour, output would have matched input and there would not have been any AUC at all in this hypothetical example.

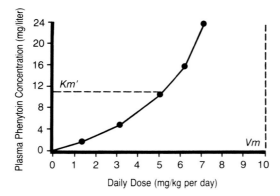

Fig. 22–9. The steady-state plasma phenytoin concentration increases disproportionately with the rate of administration (given twice daily) of phenytoin, a drug that is eliminated by a single metabolic pathway, exhibiting typical Michaelis-Menten enzyme kinetics. The estimated Vm, the maximum rate of metabolism, and Km', the plasma concentration at which the rate is half of the maximum, are shown. All the data were obtained in the same individual. (One mg/liter = 4.0 micromolar.) (Adapted from Martin, E., Tozer, T.N., Sheiner, L.B., and Riegelman, S.: The clinical pharmacokinetics of phenytoin. J. Pharmacokin. Biopharm., 5:579–596, 1977. Reproduced with permission of Plenum Publishing Corp.)

dose giving ineffective therapeutic concentrations, less than 10 milligras/liter, and that producing potentially toxic concentrations, above 20 milligrams/liter, is narrow.

The observed increase in concentration can be explained by rearrangement of Equation 5.

$$\frac{Cu_{ss}}{Km} = \frac{C_{ss}}{Km'} = \frac{R_o}{Vm - R_o} \qquad\qquad 6$$

Then, one can say that the consequences of Michaelis-Menten metabolism are caused by either the desired steady-state concentrations being above Km (Km' for total concentration) or the rate of administration required to achieve these concentrations approaching Vm.

Because of its kinetics, only small changes in phenytoin input caused, for example, by a change in salt form (acid and sodium salt are used) or in availability can produce large changes in the steady-state concentration. To illustrate this point, consider a male patient with Km' and Vm values of 3 milligrams/liter and 425 milligrams/day, respectively, who has an average steady-state concentration of 12 milligrams/liter when taking 200 milligrams orally every 12 hours. On switching from his current dosage form (availability = 0.85) to one with an availability of 0.95, it is seen, by setting $R_o = F \cdot D/\tau$ in Equation 4 and letting $fu = 0.1$, that the average steady-state concentration is expected to increase to 25 milligrams/liter. A minor change in availability causes a major change in the steady-state concentration when the dosing rate (in this case 400 milligrams/day) approaches the Vm value.

Time to Plateau. Because of capacity-limited metabolism, the time to reach steady state varies with the concentration desired and the rate of administration. Figure 22–10 shows the approach to plateau during each of four dosing rates, which increase by small increments from 300 to 425 milligrams/day, in a patient with typical Vm and Km' values. Note that the time to reach 90 percent of plateau increases with the rate of administration. These disproportionate changes in the steady-state concentration and the time required to reach them are major problems in interpreting phenytoin concentrations.

Alterations in Metabolism. Another therapeutically important facet of the kinetics of phenytoin is that of alterations in metabolism brought about by other drugs and disease states. Either Km' or Vm can be altered, but the effect on

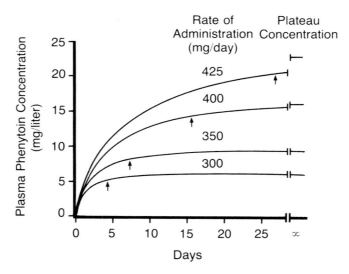

Fig. 22–10. Following administration (intravenous infusion is simulated) of phenytoin at constant rates of 300, 350, 400, and 425 milligrams/day, the plasma concentration approaches steady-state values of 6, 9.3, 16, and 22.7 milligrams/liter, respectively. Not only are the steady-state concentrations disproportionately increased, but so is the time required to approach the plateau. The arrows indicate the time required to reach 90 percent of the plateau value. The following parameter values were used: Km', 4 milligrams/liter; Vm, 500 milligrams/day; V, 50 liters. (One mg/liter = 4.0 micromolar.) (Reproduced by permission from Applied Pharmacokinetics: Principles of Therapeutic Drug Monitoring, 2nd edition, edited by William E. Evans, Jerome J. Schentag, and William J. Jusko, published by Applied Therapeutics, Inc., Spokane, Washington, 1986.)

plasma concentration is very different. From Equation 6 it can be seen that the phenytoin concentration at steady state is directly proportional to Km'. Thus, conditions, such as competitive inhibition of metabolism, which theoretically affects the Km' value, produce corresponding changes in the steady-state phenytoin concentration. For example, when cimetidine inhibits phenytoin metabolism to the extent that Km' is increased from 0.4 to 0.6 milligram/liter, then the steady-state unbound and total phenytoin concentrations are expected to increase by 50 percent as well.

In contrast, an increase in Vm, brought about by enzyme induction, or a decrease in Vm, caused by the presence of hepatic cirrhosis, brings about a disproportionate change in the steady-state phenytoin concentration. This can be seen by taking the ratio of the two different concentrations, $Cu_{ss,1}$ and $Cu_{ss,2}$ (Eq. 6), that result from the normal, Vm_1, and altered, Vm_2, values respectively.

$$\frac{Cu_{ss,2}}{Cu_{ss,1}} = \frac{Vm_1 - R_o}{Vm_2 - R_o} \qquad 7$$

For example, when R_o = 300 milligrams/day, Vm_1 = 500 milligrams/day, and Vm_2 = 400 milligrams/day, the unbound concentration at steady state is doubled, $Cu_{ss,2}/Cu_{ss,1}$ = 2. If Vm is increased to 600 milligrams/day, the ratio is 0.67. Thus, a 20 percent decrease in Vm doubles the steady-state concentration; a 20 percent increase in Vm reduces the steady-state concentration by 33 percent. Note that a reduction of Vm to 300 milligrams/day results in a concentration approaching infinity, and on decreasing Vm below 300 milligrams/day, steady state can never be achieved. The input rate would then always exceed the Vm, and Equations 2 to 7 would not be applicable.

Estimation of Vm and Km. Given plateau concentration data one can calculate Vm and Km, either graphically or numerically, for an individual. When more than three plateau values are available, a suitable graphic method is to plot R_o versus R_o/C_{ss}, as shown in Figure 22–11 for the data in Figure 22–9. By rearrangement of Equation 6

★

$$R_o = Vm - Km' \cdot \frac{R_o}{C_{ss}} \qquad\qquad 8$$

This plot is seen to give a straight line of slope $-Km'$ and an intercept of Vm when $R_o/C_{ss} = 0$. For this subject, $Vm = 10.0$ milligrams/kilogram per day and $Km' = 10.6$ milligrams/liter. Often only two plateau values are available. When this is so, the values of Vm and Km can be calculated numerically by solving the two simultaneous equations obtained by substituting the values of paired R_o and C_{ss} values into either Equation 6 or Equation 8. For example, taking the two plateau concentrations of 4.8 and 10.5 milligrams/liter obtained at daily dosing rates of 3.04 and 4.9 milligrams/kilogram per day (Fig. 22–11), Equation 8 yields the following:

$$3.04 = Vm - Km' \cdot \frac{3.04}{4.8}$$

$$4.9 = Vm - Km' \cdot \frac{4.9}{10.5}$$

Solving simultaneously, values of Vm (10.1 mg/kg per day) and Km (11.2 mg/liter) are obtained. The differences between these estimates and those determined graphically arise primarily from using only two of the five pairs of observations.

Although the computation to estimate both Vm and Km and their use to predict a dosing rate to achieve a specific plateau concentration (using either Eq. 6 or Eq. 8) is trivial, a word of caution is in order. The basic assumption made is that

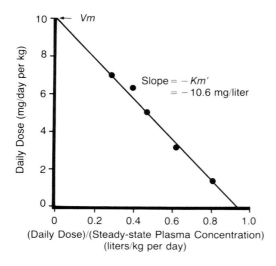

Fig. 22–11. Estimates of Vm and Km' can be gained graphically by a plot of dosing rate against (dosing rate)/C_{ss}. Illustrated here is such a plot of the transformed data given in Figure 22–9. The estimated values for Vm and Km' in the subject are 10 milligrams/kilogram per day and 10.6 milligrams/liter, respectively.

a plateau is reached, but as discussed previously it may take a long time to get there, especially if the dosing rate is close to the individual's Vm value. Even though the approach to plateau is usually quicker on reducing doses than on increasing them (Fig. 22–10), it can still take a long time, as shown in Figure 22–12.

Alcohol and phenytoin represent extreme cases in that almost all of each drug is eliminated by a single saturable pathway. For alcohol it is formation of acetaldehyde. For phenytoin it is formation of an epoxide, which is subsequently converted to hydroxylated products which, in turn, are primarily conjugated with glucuronic acid and excreted as such in the urine. More commonly, a drug is metabolized by several pathways, and only one or two of them becomes saturated. In this situation, saturation has only a minor effect on drug clearance. The extent of the effect depends on the value of fm, the fraction of drug eliminated by the saturable pathway at low drug concentrations. Only if fm is 0.5, or greater, under nonsaturating conditions is drug clearance materially affected by saturation of the pathway. Fortunately, this situation does not arise too often.

TIME-DEPENDENT DISPOSITION

The area of pharmacology that deals with changes in response to a single dose with time of day, month, or year or with effect with time on repeated drug administration is *chronopharmacology*. The pharmacokinetic component is *time-dependent kinetics*. Carbamazepine shows time dependence in its disposition (Fig. 22–13). The decrease in its peak concentration on repetitive administration indicates that either the availability decreases or the clearance increases with time. The latter has been shown to explain the observation, probably as a result of the drug inducing its own metabolism. This *autoinduction* is also dose- and concentration-dependent, a property common to most time-dependent phenomena.

The rate at which the clearance of carbamazepine increases with time is a function of the turnover of the enzymes that metabolize the drug. To illustrate this point, consider the metabolism to occur by a single enzyme and that the increase in its synthesis is the same for a wide range of carbamazepine concentrations. Assume also that the enzyme is eliminated by a first-order process. A threefold increase in synthesis rate triples the steady-state enzyme concentration (and hence clearance of drug), but the time required to get there depends on

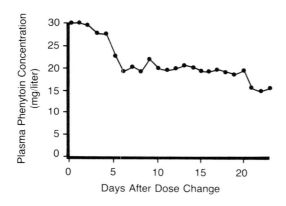

Fig. 22–12. On decreasing the daily dose from 250 to 200 milligrams/day, the plasma phenytoin concentration (obtained daily just before the morning dose) declines slowly toward a new steady state. Note that a 20 percent reduction in the daily dose leads to a 50 percent decrease in the concentration at steady state (the concentration stabilized after Day 23). (One mg/liter = 4.0 micromolar.) (Redrawn from Theodore, W.H., Qu, Z.-P., Tsay, J.-Y., Pitlick, W., and Porter, R.J.: Phenytoin: The pseudosteady-state phenomenon. Clin. Pharmacol. Ther., 35:822–825, 1984. Reproduced with permission of C.V. Mosby.)

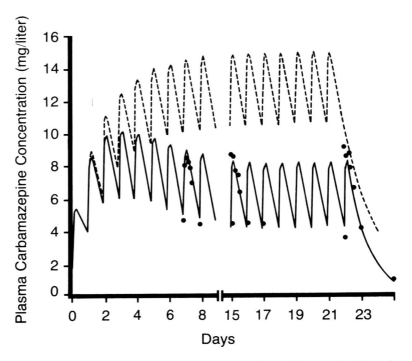

Fig. 22–13.   Carbamazepine undergoes autoinduction as evidenced by the declining plasma concentration (●), assessed on days 7, 8, 15, 16, 22, and 23 of an oral multiple-dose regimen of 6
milligrams/kilogram taken by a subject once daily in the morning for 22 consecutive days. Predictions
based on single-dose pharmacokinetic data, obtained previously in the subject and based on the
assumption that no induction occurs, are shown by the *stippled line*. Predictions assuming an autoinduction model for carbamazepine, in which the turnover time of the affected enzyme is approximately 5 days, are indicated by the *solid line*. (One mg/liter = 4.2 micromolar.) (Copyright 1976
by the American Pharmaceutical Association, *Clinical Pharmacokinetics: Concepts and Applications*,
Second Edition. Reprinted with permission of the American Pharmaceutical Association.)

the turnover of the enzyme (Chap. 23). For carbamazepine the turnover time
appears to be about 5 days. That is, it takes approximately 3 weeks for the full
effect of autoinduction of carbamazepine to be seen.

Although enzyme induction is perhaps the most common cause of time-dependent kinetics, there are many other reasons for this behavior. For example,
diurnal variations in renal function, urine pH, plasma globulin, α_1-acid glycoprotein concentrations, and cardiac output all occur. Chronic effects of a drug
on its own renal and hepatic elimination have also been seen, as previously
mentioned.

SATURABLE FIRST-PASS METABOLISM

The fraction of drug entering the body that is extracted by the liver, or intestinal
wall, during the first-pass increases with dose for several high hepatic extraction
ratio drugs, for example, 5-fluorouracil, hydralazine, lorcainide, phenacetin, and
propranolol. Figure 22–2 illustrates this phenomenon.

For several of these drugs availability shows dose dependence, but clearance
does not. The pertinent question is "How can this occur when the liver is the

principal if not the only organ of elimination?" To answer this question consider the following reasonable assumptions: instantaneous distribution; all the oral dose of drug reaches the liver intact; first-order input from gastrointestinal tract to portal vein; an absorption rate constant, ka, of 0.05 minute^{-1} (14-minute half-life); an availability at low doses of 0.1; a volume of distribution of 250 liters; and a total hepatic flow, Q_H, of 1.35 liters/minute.

The initial rate of input into the portal vein, $ka \cdot$ Dose, is also the initial rate of entry of drug into the liver, $Q_H \cdot C_{initial}$. Consequently, after a 100-milligram dose,

$$C_{initial} = \frac{ka \cdot \text{Dose}}{Q_H} = 3.7 \text{ milligrams/liter} \qquad 9$$

The concentration in the blood returning from the rest of body would have a maximum value of

$$C_{max} = \frac{F \cdot \text{Dose}}{V} = 0.04 \text{ milligram/liter} \qquad 10$$

The actual value should be less than 0.04 milligram/liter because elimination occurs during the absorption period.

The answer to the question is now apparent. The concentration entering the liver during the first pass can greatly exceed that recycling from the rest of the body. Given an average value of 0.1 for F, the ratio of $C_{initial}$ to C_{max} is

★

$$\frac{C_{initial}}{C_{max}} = \frac{ka \cdot V}{F \cdot Q} = 92 \qquad 11$$

This relationship indicates that the larger the value of ka or V or the smaller the value of F, the greater the value of the ratio and the more likely there is to be a separation in the saturation of metabolism during input and elimination phases. All the aforementioned drug examples that show saturable first-pass metabolism have pharmacokinetic parameters that favor a much higher portal concentration than a recirculating concentration during drug input.

SALICYLATE—AN EXAMPLE OF MULTIPLE SOURCES

Salicylic acid is eliminated from the body by several different routes. Dose dependence in its elimination is apparent from changes in the fraction of single

Table 22–4. Urinary Recovery of Salicylic Acid and Its Metabolites as a Percent of a Single Oral Dose[a]

Dose (mg)	Salicylic Acid	Salicyluric Acid	Salicyl Phenolic and Acyl Glucuronides
192	3	83	17
767	5	70	24
1533	17	59	24
3000	14	50	30

[a]Dose and recovery expressed in equivalents of salicylic acid. (Adapted from Levy, G.: Pharmacokinetics of salicylate elimination in man. J. Pharm. Sci., 54:959–967, 1965.)

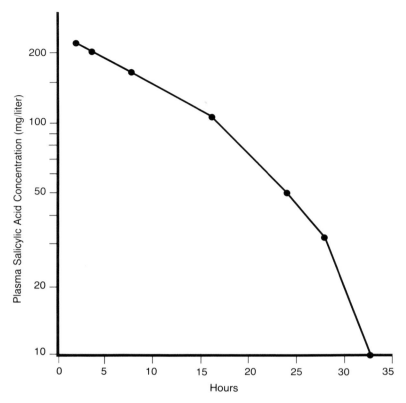

Fig. 22–14.   Semilogarithmic plot of the plasma concentration of salicylic acid in a human subject following a single oral dose of 3 grams of sodium salicylate. (One mg/liter = 7.2 micromolar.) (Adapted from data in Salassa, R.M., Bollman, J.L., and Dry, T.J.: The effect of para-aminobenzoic acid on the metabolism and excretion of salicylate. J. Lab. Clin. Med., 33: 1393–1401, 1948.)

Table 22–5.   Apparent Volume of Distribution and Fraction Unbound of Salicylic Acid

Intravenous Dose[a] (grams)	Plasma Concentration Extrapolated to Zero Time (mg/liter)	Volume of Distribution[b] (liters)	Fraction Unbound[c]
0.25	28	9.0	0.07
0.50	48	9.5	0.08
1.3	156	12	0.11
3.0 (oral)	220	15	0.13
8.5	400	21	–
17	570	30	–

[a]In salicylic acid equivalents.
[b]Composite data from Rubin, G.M., Tozer, T.N., and Øie, S.: Concentration dependence of salicylate distribution. J. Pharm. Pharmacol., 35:115–117, 1982.
[c]Estimated from data in Figure 22–15.

doses recovered in the urine as metabolites and unchanged salicylic acid (Table 22–4). A semilogarithmic plot of plasma salicylic acid concentration after a single intravenous dose, Figure 22–14, shows a fractional rate of elimination slower at high than at low concentrations, a characteristic of capacity-limited elimination.

The apparent volume of distribution of salicylic acid is also concentration-dependent. This is apparent from the data in Table 22–5 in which the volume of distribution is obtained from the extrapolated initial plasma concentration following an intravenous bolus dose. The reason for this dependence is related to the plasma concentrations observed at these doses. Salicylic acid binds to plasma albumin, and the fraction unbound increases, even at therapeutic concentrations of 100 to 300 milligrams/liter, owing to a limited capacity for binding. The impact of this change in binding on clearance and half-life is complicated by capacity-limited elimination.

At low concentrations, the apparent half-life of salicylic acid is close to 3 hours and the volume of distribution is approximately 9 liters; the clearance is therefore about 2 liters/hour. Since elimination is primarily metabolic (Table 22–4) and the metabolism is presumably in the liver, the drug must have a low hepatic extraction ratio and hence the unbound clearance is expected to remain unchanged

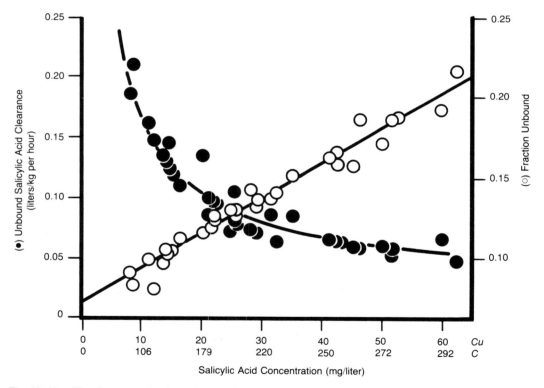

Fig. 22–15. The clearance of unbound drug (●), determined under steady-state conditions, and the fraction unbound in plasma (○) vary inversely with each other as the salicylic acid concentration is increased. The corresponding total plasma salicylic acid concentrations are superimposed on the linear scale of the concentration of unbound drug. (One mg/liter = 7.2 micromolar.) (Redrawn from Furst, D.E., Tozer, T.N., and Melmon, K.L.: Salicylate clearance: The result of protein binding and metabolism. Clin. Pharmacol. Ther., 26:380–389, 1979. Reproduced with permission of C.V. Mosby.)

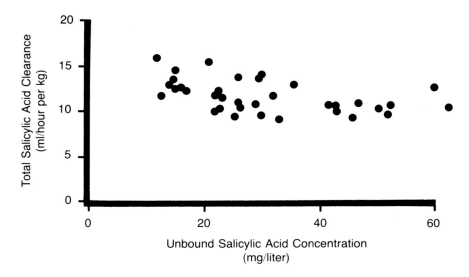

Fig. 22–16.   The total clearance of salicylic acid, determined under steady-state conditions, remains essentially constant within the range of therapeutic concentrations; a fortuitous consequence of the essentially equivalent and opposing effects of saturable plasma protein binding and saturable metabolism (One mg/liter = 7.2 micromolar.) (See Fig. 22–15.)

when the fraction unbound increases. To the contrary, the unbound clearance is observed to decrease dramatically with an increase in the concentration (Fig. 22–15), while the fraction unbound increases. The former is a result of the capacity-limited metabolism; the latter is a result of saturable protein binding. The consequence of these opposing tendencies is that (total) clearance remains relatively constant within the anti-inflammatory therapeutic range of unbound

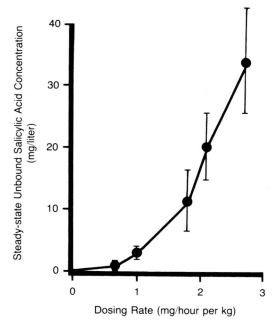

Fig. 22–17.   The steady-state unbound concentration of salicylic acid in plasma (mean ± S.D.) increases disproportionately with the dosing rate of aspirin. Aspirin is completely converted to the measured metabolite, salicylic acid. The disproportionate increase reflects the saturability of two of salicylic acid's major pathways of elimination, formation of salicyl phenolic glucuronide and salicyluric acid. (One mg/liter = 7.2 micromolar.) (Redrawn from Tozer, T.N., Tang-Liu, D.D.-S., and Riegelman, S.: Linear vs. nonlinear kinetics. In Topics in Pharmaceutical Sciences. Edited by D. Breimer and P. Speiser. Elsevier, 1981, pp. 3–17.)

concentrations, 10 to 60 milligrams/liter (Fig. 22–16). The decrease in the unbound clearance, the consequence of saturability in two major pathways of elimination of salicylic acid leads to a disproportionate increase in the unbound concentration with increasing dosing rate (Fig. 22–17).

THERAPEUTIC CONSEQUENCES

The therapeutic consequences of dose-dependent kinetics are perhaps best considered under steady-state conditions. Here, dose dependence in the rate constant of absorption is of little or no consequence unless availability is also altered. Alterations in the availability are important in that the unbound concentration and the amount in the body at steady state may change disproportionately on increasing the dose. Conditions that cause dose dependence in availability may also produce increased variability in the parameter at the same dose. For example, consider two drugs, a dissolution rate-limited one, such as griseofulvin, and one that is highly extracted on passing across the gastrointestinal membranes or through the liver, such as alprenolol. Changes in gastric emptying and in other physiologic factors can produce large variations in the availability of these drugs because of the varied differences in concentrations entering the liver. The effect of rapid gastric emptying may be a decrease in the availability of griseofulvin because of less mixing, but an increase in the availability of alprenolol because of saturability in intestinal and hepatic metabolism.

Clinically, the most dramatic source of dose dependence is capacity-limited metabolism. Only small changes in the rate of administration, or availability, can produce large changes in the steady-state concentration and hence careful titration of an individual patient's dosage requirement is mandatory with drugs that exhibit such kinetic behavior, especially if they have a narrow therapeutic index. Moreover, this source of dose-dependence also produces large interpatient and intrapatient variability in the steady-state concentration, as observed for phenytoin in Figure 1–5.

Time-dependent kinetics has been observed in humans. It is perhaps best typified by autoinduction. Another cause is decreased renal function on continued administration of a nephrotoxic drug. If the drug is primarily renally eliminated, the therapeutic consequence of the latter cause is clear and opposite to that of autoinduction.

In general, if there are two drugs equivalent in all respects except for one showing either a dose- or time-dependent kinetic behavior, then the one showing first-order kinetics is the drug of choice.

Study Problems

(Answers to Study Problems are in Appendix G.)

1. The intestinal absorption of both riboflavin and thiamine is saturable. Consequently, the oral availability of these vitamins given in solution is expected to (circle the appropriate answer):

    (a)   ↑   ↓   ↔* with dose.

    ---
    * ↑ increase, ↓ decrease, ↔ show little or no change.

(b) ↑   ↓   ↔ with hastening of gastric emptying.

(c) ↑   ↓   ↔ with increasing gastrointestinal transit time.

(d) ↑   ↓   ↔ when taken 2 hours before, rather than just after, a heavy meal.

2. For *each* of the tables below indicate *all* of the possibilities in the following list that might explain the dose-dependent kinetics observed for each drug.

List of Explanations

I. Saturable hepatic metabolism
II. Saturable renal tubular reabsorption
III. Saturable renal active secretion
IV. Saturable plasma protein binding with extraction ratio approaching one in organs of elimination
V. Saturable plasma protein binding with extraction ratio approaching zero in organs of elimination
VI. Saturable metabolism during first pass of drug through the intestines or the liver
VII. Saturable gastrointestinal transport

(a)

Table 22–6.

Single Oral Dose (mg)	300	600	900
Area Under Blood Concentration-time Curve (mg-hour/liter)	3	10	19

(b)

Table 22–7.

Rate of Intravenous Infusion (mg/hour)	5	10	15
Steady-state Plasma Concentration (mg/liter)	2	6.5	14

(c)

Table 22–8.   One-compartment drug

Single Intravenous Dose (mg)	50	100	200	400
Initial Blood Concentration (mg/liter)	1.1	2.0	4.3	8.7
Area Under Blood Concentration-time Curve (mg-hour/liter)	20	55	160	410

(d)

Table 22–9.

Urinary Excretion Rate at Steady State (mg/hour)	20	60	160	250	440	620
Blood Concentration at Steady State (mg/liter)	4	12	40	100	250	450

(e)

Table 22–10.

Single Oral Dose (mg)	500	1000	1500
Total Amount Excreted Unchanged (mg)	30	118	213

(f)

Table 22–11.

Daily Total Oral Dose (mg)	30	60	90	120
Average Steady-state Blood Concentration (mg/liter)	5	13	28	53

3. The relationship between glucose excretion rate and its plasma concentration in a healthy individual is displayed in Table 22–12. Prepare either a table or a graph of glucose renal clearance in milliliters/minute as a function of its plasma concentration, and briefly explain the observation.

Table 22–12.   Glucose Excretion Rate at Various Plasma Glucose Concentrations

Excretion Rate (mg/minute)	5	66	151	256	400	520	631
Plasma Glucose Concentration (mg/100 ml)	200	301	398	503	605	708	799

4. Stiripentol is an antiepileptic agent. Its pharmacokinetics are typified by the data for one subject in Table 22–13.

Table 22–13[a].

Steady-state Plasma Concentration, $C_{av,ss}$ (mg/liter)	0.42	1.3	9.2
Dosing Rate (mg/8 hours)	200	400	800

[a]Data from Levy, R.H., Loiseau, P., Guyot, M., Biehant, H.M., Tor, J., and Moreland, T.A. Clin. Pharmacol. Ther. 36:661–669, 1984.

Is this drug eliminated by Michaelis-Menten kinetics? If so, explain your conclusion and calculate the Vm and Km values.

5. Define saturable first-pass metabolism, and describe how it can be seen without observing dose-dependent kinetic behavior after an equivalent intravenous bolus dose.

6. Table 22–14 is intended to summarize the direction of change expected in the disposition parameters and in total and unbound steady-state blood concentrations of a drug, relative to the rate of intravenous administration, when there is dose dependency in absorption, distribution, or elimination. Complete the table by indicating ↑ for increase, ↓ for decrease, or ↔ for little or no change.

Table 22–14. Disposition Kinetics and Total and Unbound Steady-state Blood Drug Concentrations as a Function of Dose Dependency in Each of Several Sources Following Oral and Intravenous Administrations

Source of Dose Dependency	Direction of Change[a] with Increased Total Daily Dose	Volume of[b] Distribution	Clearance	Half-life	Concentration[c] Rate of Administration Total	Unbound
Oral Administration						
Availability	↓	↔				
Absorption Rate Constant	↓	↔				
Intravenous Administration						
Fraction Unbound in Blood						
Low extraction ratio drug	↑	↑				
High extraction ratio drug	↑	↑				
Fraction Unbound in Tissue	↑		↔			
Metabolic Clearance	↑		↑			
Renal Clearance	↓		↓			

[a]Only one example of each direction of change is shown.
[b]A volume of distribution at least ten times the blood volume is assumed.
[c]The average steady-state total and unbound blood drug concentrations relative to the rate of administration.

23

Turnover Concepts

Objectives

The reader will be able to:

1. Define turnover and turnover rate and the following parameters: turnover time, fractional turnover rate, and mean residence time.

2. Determine values for the turnover parameters and the turnover rate of a one-compartment, first-order system when its steady state is perturbed.

3. Distinguish between alterations in turnover rate and fractional turnover rate when provided with appropriate data. Also know what data are appropriate to do so.

4. Know what can and cannot be concluded from data obtained at a single time point when the turnover of a system is altered.

5. Determine the turnover rate and the mean residence time of a tracer or drug in a multicompartmental system in which elimination occurs only from the central sampling compartment, when data after a single bolus dose are provided.

6. Quantify the relationship between the turnover rate of an endogenous substance and the plasma concentration of an inhibitor of its production, given appropriate data.

CONCEPT OF TURNOVER

Many drugs act by affecting the concentration of a normal (endogenous) constituent of the body. Examples are the oral anticoagulants, which lower the plasma concentrations of certain clotting factors by inhibiting their synthesis, and uricosuric agents, which lower the plasma concentration of uric acid by increasing its renal clearance. Some endogenous compounds are also used to assess various body functions. Thus, creatinine is commonly used to assess renal function, and bilirubin is used to assess hepatic function. Accordingly, to be able to sensibly relate the pharmacokinetics of a drug to its pharmacologic effect when an endogenous compound is involved or to interpret the concentration of an endogenous compound in order to assess body function, the kinetics of the endogenous compound must be understood.

401

The amounts of many endogenous compounds remain fairly constant with time. This does not mean, however, that they are in a static state. Indeed, they are often being replaced or synthesized at a rapid rate; they are said to be "turning over." The concept of *turnover* can be applied to plasma proteins, enzymes, neurohormones, electrolytes, total body water, and in fact to virtually every substance in the body. The term *turnover*, however, does not indicate how rapidly the renewal process occurs. It only indicates the nature of the process.

Turnover implies that a substance is at steady state. Thus, the rate of renewal equals the rate of elimination. This rate, the *turnover rate*, does not fully convey the speed of the process. To do that, the turnover rate must be related to the amount of substance present, frequently called the *pool size*. The ratio of the turnover rate, R_t, to the pool size, A_{ss}, is called the *fractional turnover rate*, k_t, that is,

$$k_t = \frac{R_t}{A_{ss}} \qquad ★ \qquad 1$$

A second useful parameter for measuring turnover is *turnover time*, t_t. It is the time required to renew the amount in the pool. Complete renewal actually requires an infinite period of time because of the continuous mixing of newly entering substance with that already in the pool. Turnover time can be readily defined, however, by the time required to bring into the pool the amount that is in it, therefore,

$$t_t = \frac{A_{ss}}{R_t} \qquad ★ \qquad 2$$

Consequently, the relationship between turnover time and fractional turnover rate is

$$t_t = \frac{1}{k_t} \qquad ★ \qquad 3$$

The input may be either synthetic or may involve a transfer of substance into the pool from elsewhere, or both. A good example is total body water, which is both imbibed and synthesized by catabolism of foodstuffs.

Figure 23–1 schematically shows the turnover of water in the body. Using the data in the figure and Equations 1 to 3, the following average turnover values for water are obtained:

Turnover rate = 2.5 liters (or kg)/day

Fractional turnover rate = 0.06 day^{-1}

Turnover time = 17 days

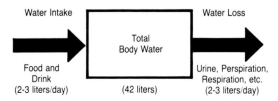

Water Intake

Water Loss

Total Body Water

Food and Drink (2-3 liters/day)

(42 liters)

Urine, Perspiration, Respiration, etc. (2-3 liters/day)

Fig. 23–1. Illustration of the turnover of total water in the body.

The fractional turnover rate used throughout the rest of the chapter is synonymous with the elimination rate constant. Although the turnover rate (2.5 kg/day) is a large value, the actual turnover of body water is unusually slow when reflected by the fractional turnover rate (6 percent per day) or turnover time (17 days). Clearly, these two parameters characterize turnover better than turnover rate alone.

The output may involve several pathways. For body water, urinary excretion, perspiration, and respiration are the major routes of elimination. In a hot, dry desert climate, the last two pathways, especially perspiration, may increase dramatically. Intake must then be increased to compensate for increased loss. The pool size remains essentially constant, although the turnover rate may be increased to 21 liters/day under these extreme conditions. In this situation, the fractional turnover rate and the turnover time of water become 0.5 day^{-1} and 2 days, respectively.

In contrast to water, the pool size, rather than fractional turnover rate or turnover time, of most endogenous substances usually changes when the turnover rate is altered. This results in a change in the concentration of the substance. Selected examples of this situation follow.

APPLICATIONS

Turnover concepts have a wide range of applications, as exemplified below.

Renal Function Tests

One of the best examples of the application of turnover concepts in clinical pharmacokinetics is the estimation of renal function from measurements of creatinine in plasma. Creatinine, an end-product of muscle catabolism, is eliminated from the body by renal excretion. Under normal circumstances, the plasma concentration and the amount of creatinine in the body are at steady state. When renal function is impaired, the plasma concentration rises until a new steady state is reached, provided both renal function and production rate remain reasonably stable with time.

Since plasma concentration, rather than amount in the body, is measured and since the rate of elimination at steady state is the product of renal clearance and concentration, then

$$\text{Plasma concentration of creatinine at steady state} = \frac{\text{Production rate}}{\text{Renal clearance}} \qquad 4$$

As long as muscle mass, the primary source of creatinine, remains unchanged, the production rate is constant. The steady-state plasma creatinine concentration then reflects changes in renal clearance.

The fractional turnover rate (k_t), or elimination rate constant, of creatinine depends on both its total clearance and volume of distribution, V, (Chap. 11). Accordingly, for creatinine

$$k_t = \frac{\text{Renal clearance}}{V} \qquad 5$$

Therefore, changes in either renal clearance or volume of distribution, or both, result in an altered half-life. For creatinine, its volume of distribution (close to total body water) is relatively unaffected when renal function is reduced, so its half-life varies inversely with renal function.

Uric Acid

The long-term treatment of gout involves the sustained lowering of plasma uric acid concentration. This lowering is accomplished in two ways. One is to decrease the synthesis of uric acid by giving a xanthine oxidase inhibitor, such as allopurinol. The other is to increase the renal clearance of uric acid by inhibiting its renal tubular reabsorption with a uricosuric drug, such as probenecid. Thus, the respective treatments involve controlling the production rate and the elimination rate constant of uric acid. The change in uric acid concentration in plasma is a means of quantifying the response since, unlike that for body water, the pool size of uric acid is not homeostatically controlled.

Enzyme Induction

Enzyme induction refers to an increased synthesis (turnover rate) of an enzyme. Enzyme induction is often implied in drug metabolism when the enzyme concentration is increased. The increased enzyme concentration could also be a result of stabilization of the enzyme (decreased fractional turnover rate). Distinction between increased synthesis and stabilization is difficult. Furthermore, other explanations are also possible, such as enzyme activation (conversion to a more active form) or increased concentration of a cofactor. Thus, enzyme induction should not be the sole conclusion when only an increase in enzyme activity is measured.

Onset and Duration of Pharmacologic Response—Warfarin

Sometimes the response to a drug is the result of an alteration in the turnover of an endogenous compound. The anticoagulant effect of warfarin, caused by decreased synthesis of several of the clotting factors, is an example. The onset of the observed response, a prolonging of the clotting time, therefore, is a function of the half-life of these clotting factors.

The duration of drug response may also be related to the turnover of an endogenous compound. A drug may be eliminated, but the response persists. Many phenomena such as "hit-and-run" action, dependence, and tolerance could be explained on the basis of the turnover of endogenous compounds.

Body Burden of Pesticides and Other Environmental Substances

The principles of turnover are also helpful in quantifying the body burdens, or the steady-state concentrations, of substances to which we are constantly exposed. Included among such compounds are pesticides, found ubiquitously in water, phthalate esters, used as softeners in many plastics, and the toxic metals, lead and mercury. The daily input rate and the elimination half-life determine the extent of accumulation of these substances in the body. Recall

(Chap. 6, Constant-Rate Regimens) that half-life determines how rapidly the concentration rises when the body is exposed to the substance and how rapidly it falls when the exposure is removed.

PERTURBATION OF STEADY STATE

The turnover parameters of a system may be obtained if two of the following three are measured: turnover rate, amount in the pool, and the fractional turnover rate. None can be obtained from the measurement of the steady-state plasma concentration of a substance alone. The turnover rate can be measured in some circumstances, e.g., the daily renal excretion of creatinine, but again, the other parameters remain unknown. Except through the use of tracer amounts of isotopically labeled substances, which can be measured independently of the substance in the pool, the fractional turnover rate can only be measured by perturbing the steady state.

To appreciate the consequences of altering the fractional turnover rate of an endogenous substance, consider the events in Figure 23–2 (upper graph) in which elimination is immediately and completely blocked. The input rate is assumed to be unaltered. The rate at which the substance accumulates depends on its normal turnover. The time required for the amount to increase by that

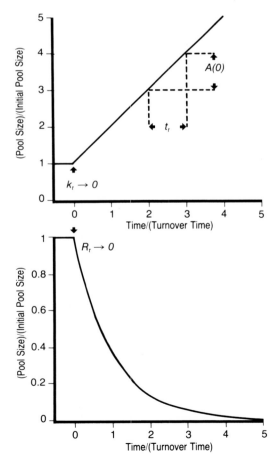

Fig. 23–2. *Upper graph,* The pool size increases linearly with time when (at arrow) elimination is completely blocked and input rate remains unchanged. The slope is the original turnover rate, $A(0)/t_t$. *Lower graph,* The pool size decreases with time when (at arrow) the input is completely blocked. The decline is exponential when first-order elimination and one-compartment distribution pertain. The rate constant for the decline (slope of semilogarithmic plot) is the fractional turnover rate. In both graphs, pool size is expressed relative to the original value, and time is related to the original turnover time.

amount present under normal turnover conditions, $A(0)$, is the turnover time, by definition. Similarly, if concentration is measured, the turnover time is the time taken for the concentration to increase to twice its usual steady-state value. This last calculation assumes that the system acts as a single compartment within the time frame of the measurements. To determine the turnover rate, the steady-state amount in the body must be known or the converse.

The consequences of immediately and completely blocking input under conditions in which elimination is first-order and the body acts as if it were a single compartment are depicted in Figure 23–2 (lower graph). The situation is equivalent to the stopping of a constant-rate intravenous infusion of drug at steady state. Recall that the amount of drug in the body (or plasma concentration) then falls exponentially by one half each half-life. Recall also that the fractional rate of elimination is the elimination rate constant k, and since $t_t = 1/k_t$, it follows that:

$$t_t = \frac{1}{k_t} = \frac{1}{0.693/t_{1/2}} = 1.44 \cdot t_{1/2} \qquad\qquad 6$$

or

$$t_{1/2} = 0.693 \cdot t_t \qquad\qquad 7$$

As an example of the equations above, consider measurement of the turnover of serotonin, a neurotransmitter. This endogenous compound, oxidatively deaminated to 5-hydroxyindoleacetic acid, has long been associated with central nervous system activities, especially brainstem functions. Figure 23–3 shows the kinetic behavior of this polar metabolite of serotonin in rat brain when (right

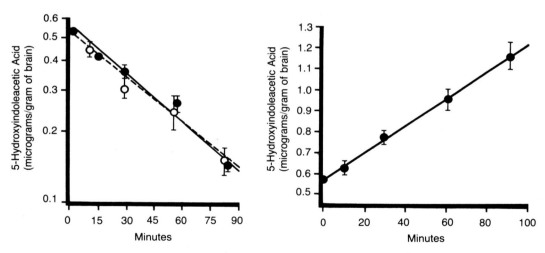

Fig. 23–3. Concentration of 5-hydroxyindoleacetic acid, a polar metabolite of serotonin, in rat brain at various times after the administration, on separate occasions, of agents that block the formation and elimination of this acid. Left Panel, Pargyline (75 mg/kg, i.p.(○)) or tranylcypromine (10 mg/kg, i.p. (●)). administered at time zero, causes the concentration of the acid to drop monoexponentially when it is no longer being formed. Right Panel, Probenecid (200 mg/kg, i.p.) causes the concentration of the acid to rise with time when transport out of the brain is blocked. Bars represent the mean ± standard error of five or six animals. (One mg/liter = 5.2 micromolar.) (Adapted from Neff, N.H. and Tozer, T.N.: *In vivo* measurement of brain serotonin turnover. Adv. Pharmacol., 6:97–109, 1968. Reproduced with permission of Academic Press.)

panel) its elimination, transport out of brain, is inhibited by probenecid and when (left panel) its formation is blocked by a monoamine oxidase inhibitor. The normal turnover rate of this acid, and presumably its precursor, serotonin, can be calculated from the rate of accumulation in the former case and from the initial rate of its decline ($k \cdot A(0)$) in the latter case. The turnover rates of serotonin, 0.40 and 0.44 microgram/gram of tissue per hour, so calculated, are in close agreement.

ESTABLISHMENT OF A NEW STEADY STATE

Instead of the two extreme cases of complete inhibition considered above, input or elimination is usually only partially affected. Quantitation of such a situation is difficult. When either the input rate or fractional turnover rate is immediately shifted to a new constant value, it takes time for the pool size to reach a new steady state and therefore to reflect the shift in turnover, as illustrated below.

Turnover Rate Altered to a New Constant Value

Changes in the pool size with time on increasing or decreasing the input (turnover rate) by a factor of four are shown, respectively, by the solid lines in Figure 23–4. The new steady states reflect the changes in turnover rate. As the elimination half-life is unaltered, the time to reach the new steady state is the same. This is seen by the time required to reach one-half the way to the new steady state. Had the turnover time been one hour, then it would have taken 42 ($0.693 \cdot t_t$) minutes to reach this point; if it had been one week, then it would have taken about five days.

Fractional Turnover Rate Altered to a New Constant Value

The consequences of changing the elimination rate constant (fractional turnover rate) are quite different from changing the input (turnover) rate. The difference is shown by the stippled lines in Figure 23–4. It can be seen that a fourfold decrease in the elimination rate constant quadruples the pool size, but it takes four times as long to reach the same new steady state as it did after quadrupling the turnover rate. A fourfold increase in the elimination rate constant, on the other hand, reduces the pool size by a factor of four and the new steady state is reached much more quickly than by the former mechanism. Examples of situations in which either or both the turnover rate and the fractional turnover rate are altered are listed in Table 23–1.

DISTINCTION BETWEEN ALTERATIONS IN TURNOVER RATE AND FRACTIONAL TURNOVER RATE

Distinction between an increased turnover rate and a decreased fractional turnover rate requires kinetic analysis. As shown in the upper graph of Figure

Table 23–1. Selected Examples of Altered Turnover

Observation	Cause	Turnover Rate (R_t)	Fractional Turnover Rate (k_t)	Turnover Time (MRT)	Example
I. Change in Pool Size					
Increased pool size (or concentration)	Increased synthesis or input	↑[a]	N/C[c]	N/C	Induction of the cytochrome P_{450} enzyme system by phenobarbital
	Decreased ability to eliminate	N/C	↓[b]	↑	Plasma creatinine in acute renal function impairment
Decreased pool size (or concentration)	Decreased synthesis or input	↓	N/C	N/C	Decrease in concentration of certain clotting factors after oral anticoagulants
	Increased ability to eliminate	N/C	↑	↓	Decreased renal tubular reabsorption of serum uric acid by a uricosuric agent
II. Little or No Change in Pool Size					
Increased output (or elimination)	Increased input	↑	↑	↓	Increased water consumption in hot weather
Decreased output (or elimination)	Decreased input	↓	↓	↑	Sodium in urine on a low salt diet

[a] ↑ = increase.
[b] ↓ = decrease.
[c] N/C = little or no change.

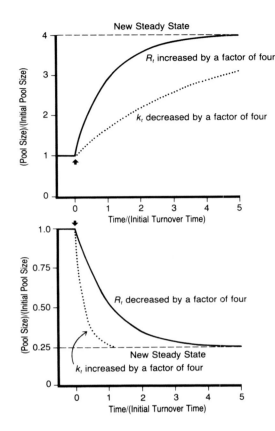

Fig. 23–4. *Upper graph,* The pool size increases to a value four times the original when (at arrow) the turnover rate (solid line) increases by four. A fourfold decrease in the fractional turnover rate (stippled line) gives the same end result; however, it takes four times as long to reach the new steady-state. *Lower graph,* The pool size decreases to a value one-fourth of the original when (at arrow) the turnover rate decreases (solid line) by a factor of four. A fourfold increase in the fractional turnover rate (stippled line) again produces the same new steady state; however, the new value is approached four times more rapidly.

23–5, the time to approach steady state when measured by the time to get halfway to the new value is the same no matter how much the turnover rate has been increased. When the fractional turnover rate is decreased, however, the time to reach the new steady state is increased, as shown in the lower graph of the figure. The principle here is illustrated by plasma creatinine. If renal function drops immediately to a value that is 50, 33, 25, or 20 percent of normal, the plasma creatinine concentration rises to a new steady state that is 2, 3, 4, or 5 times the normal value, respectively, as shown in the lower graph of Figure 23–5. The new steady-state concentration increases to a value that is directly proportional to the turnover time. The turnover time and the half-life of creatinine elimination at various degrees of renal function are shown in Table 23–2.

When there is no renal function, the plasma creatinine concentration, C, is expected to rise at a constant rate (dC/dt) of about 3.5 milligrams/100 milliliters (0.31 millimolar) per day in a young adult in whom the creatinine production is about 1500 milligrams/day and the volume of distribution is 42 liters/70 kilograms, because creatinine distributes into total body water space and is unbound

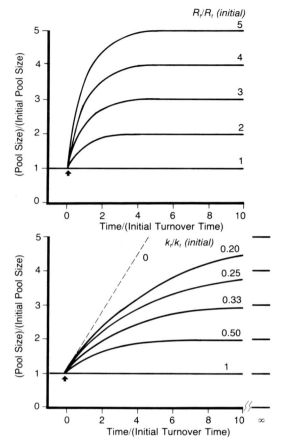

Fig. 23–5. *Upper graph,* The pool size is increased from one to five times its original value when (at arrow) the turnover increases by the factor $R_t/R_t(initial)$. The time (half-life, turnover time) to approach each new steady state is the same. *Lower graph,* The approach to the new steady state is prolonged when (at arrow) the fractional turnover rate decreases by the factor $k_t/k_t(initial)$. When the value of k_t approaches zero (stippled line), steady state is never achieved. The prolonged approach to the new steady state for the other conditions can be expressed by the time (half-life) required to reach the pool size that is the average of the initial and final values.

Table 23–2.   Calculated Turnover Time and Half-Life of Creatinine when Renal Function Is Decreased

Renal Function (percent of "normal")[a]	Turnover Time (hours)	Half-life (hours)
100	6	4
50	12	8
33	18	12
25	24	17
20	30	21
10	60	42

[a]Based on an expected creatinine clearance of 7 liters/hour for a 20-year-old, 70-kg male and a creatinine volume of distribution of 0.6 liter/kilogram.

in the body. The normal turnover time can be calculated from the rate of increase and the normal pool size, $V \cdot C(0)$, that is

$$t_t = \frac{A(0)}{R_t} = \frac{V \cdot C(0)}{V \cdot dC/dt} = \frac{C(0)}{dC/dt} \qquad 8$$

where $C(0)$ is the normal plasma concentration, about 0.9 milligram/100 milliliters (0.08 millimolar), in a patient with normal renal function. The usual turnover time is then 6 hours.

The time required for a plasma creatinine concentration to reflect a change in renal function can be greatly prolonged with severe renal function impairment. Interpretation of a plasma creatinine value in a clinical situation is therefore dependent on the acuteness of the change in renal function and on the degree to which renal function is impaired. Furthermore, in bedridden or only partially ambulatory patients with severe renal dysfunction, the muscle mass is typically decreased, leading to a reduced production rate of creatinine and a rise of only about 1 to 3 milligrams/100 deciliters (0.09 to 0.27 millimolar) per day in plasma creatinine between hemodialysis treatments (used to remove accumulated polar substances, see Chap. 24).

Distinction between decreased turnover rate and increased fractional turnover rate has similarities with the analysis above, but here the pool size decreases, as shown in Figure 23–6. The time required to approach the new steady state is the same when the production rate is decreased (upper graph), but is shortened when the fractional turnover rate is increased (lower graph). The rate of attainment of the new steady state is related to its new value; the lower the value the more quickly it is achieved, as shown in the lower graph of the figure.

The rate of decline in pool size, on decreasing the turnover rate, is limited by the fractional turnover rate itself. The decline in the clotting factors, on administering warfarin, serves as a good example. This system is examined in greater detail, as it is representative of many other such systems in the body.

THE ANTICOAGULANT EFFECT OF WARFARIN

In common with other endogenous substances, the amount of each clotting factor in the body, X, is a result of a difference between its rates of synthesis, R_{syn}, and degradation, $k_t \cdot X$. And, at any moment, whether at steady state or not,

$$\frac{dX}{dt} = R_{syn} - k_t \cdot X$$

Rate of change   Rate of   Rate of   9
of clotting factor   synthesis   degradation

where k_t is the degradation rate constant of the clotting factor. Normally, the system is at steady state, $dX/dt = 0$, with synthesis matching degradation. However, in the presence of warfarin the synthesis is inhibited, and the clotting factor concentration (or amount) falls at a rate that depends on both the degree of inhibition of synthesis and the value of k_t.

Either a steady-state or a kinetic approach can be used to assess the more direct relationship between synthesis rate and the plasma warfarin concentra-

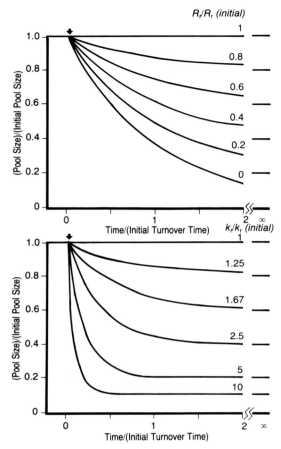

Fig. 23–6. *Upper graph,* The pool size decreases to a new steady state that corresponds to the factor $R_t/R_t(initial)$, by which the turnover rate decreases. The new steady state is approached with the same half-life when (at arrow) the input decreases. *Lower graph,* The pool size also decreases when (at arrow) the fractional turnover rate increases by the factor $k_t/k_t(initial)$, but the time (half-life) to achieve the new steady state is shortened.

tion. Each approach has its own merits. With the steady-state approach, the entire clotting system is allowed to reach a new steady state in the presence of a constant concentration of warfarin. Then, once again $dX/dt = 0$, so that $X_{ss} = R_{syn}/k_t$, and as the value of k_t is unaffected by warfarin, the steady-state amount of X is directly proportional to R_{syn}. The procedure is then repeated for different plateau concentrations of warfarin to elucidate the relationship between R_{syn} and plasma warfarin concentration. Although this sounds easy, it may take a long time to establish steady state. Recall that the time required to go from one plateau to another depends solely on the elimination half-life of the substance; the degradation half-life of the clotting factors affected by warfarin vary from hours to days, with an average effective half-life (for prothrombin complex activity) of about one day. It takes, therefore, nearly a week to reach each new steady state.

The kinetic approach, which uses data obtained following a single bolus dose, is more rapid, but requires an estimate of the value of k_t. This value can be obtained by giving a dose of warfarin that completely blocks synthesis initially ($R_{syn} = 0$). The prothrombin complex activity then falls exponentially (Eq. 9), so that a semilogarithmic plot of the prothrombin complex activity, X, against time gives a straight line with a slope of k_t. Subsequently, as the plasma concentration of warfarin falls, the degree of inhibition of clotting factor synthesis decreases and the concentration of the prothrombin complex rises (see Fig. 5–6), eventually returning to its pre-warfarin value. The synthesis rate, R_{syn}, with time is calculated from simultaneous measurement of warfarin and prothrombin complex activity on return to pre-warfarin value, as follows.

If X_1 and X_2 are the prothrombin complex activities at the beginning and end of a time interval, Δt, then the rate of change of activity is estimated from $(X_2 - X_1)/\Delta t$ and the average activity within the interval is given by $(X_1 + X_2)/2$. R_{syn} is then calculated from rearrangement of Equation 9.

$$R_{syn} = (X_2 - X_1)/\Delta t + k_t \cdot (X_1 + X_2)/2 \qquad 10$$

The percent inhibition of synthesis can be approximated from

$$\text{Percent inhibition of synthesis} = 100 \cdot [R_{syn}(n) - R_{syn})/R_{syn}(n)] \qquad 11$$

where $R_{syn}(n)$ is the normal synthesis rate. The normal rate is given by $k_t \cdot X(n)$, where $X(n)$ is the normal activity of the clotting factor. A plot of the percent inhibition of synthesis against the logarithm of the warfarin concentration gives the classic effect versus concentration relationship, as shown in Figure 23–7.

The responses to standard doses of warfarin change in disease states and following the coadministration of other drugs. By ascertaining the relationship between the plasma concentration and the direct effect, distinctions can be made between changes in the pharmacokinetics of warfarin and changes in the responsiveness of the clotting system to this drug. For example, the diminished response to doses of warfarin, when coadministered with heptabarbital, was found to be caused by increased elimination of and not by a change in the direct response to the drug (Fig. 23–7).

INTERPRETATION OF NONSTEADY-STATE OBSERVATIONS

The problem of using a plasma creatinine concentration to assess renal function when function changes acutely has been presented. Similarly, the prothrombin

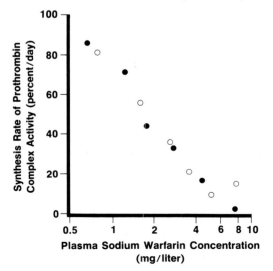

Fig. 23–7. Pretreatment with heptabarbital (400 mg daily for 15 days, starting 10 days before warfarin) decreased the response to a standard dose of warfarin, but failed to alter the linear relationship between the synthesis rate of prothrombin complex activity and the logarithm of the concentration of warfarin in a 21-year-old normal subject; control experiment (○), with heptabarbital (●). (One mg/liter = 3.0 micromolar.) (From Levy, G., O'Reilly, R.A., Aggeler, P.M., and Keech, G.M.: Pharmacokinetic analysis of the effect of barbiturate on the anticoagulant action of warfarin in man. Clin. Pharmacol. Ther., 11:372–377, 1970.)

activity five hours after a dose of warfarin is hardly a measure of the effect of the drug in blocking the synthesis of the clotting factors. To further illustrate the problem of interpreting nonsteady-state observations, consider the following situation:

A study is conducted to see if the drug metabolizing enzymes X and Y are inducible by phenobarbital. Homogenates of rat livers are obtained from untreated rats and from rats pretreated with phenobarbital to attain and maintain a constant concentration. The activity of each of the enzymes is determined in both groups of rats 12 hours after initiating phenobarbital administration. The average activity of enzyme X is increased to 250 percent of control. The average activity of enzyme Y is about 120 percent of control, but the value is not statistically different from the control value.

There is a tendency to conclude that enzyme X is induced whereas enzyme Y is not. Actually, enzyme Y may have been more induced than enzyme X. This condition is shown in Figure 23–8. Although induction is virtually instantaneous on administering phenobarbital, the enzymes have different turnover characteristics. Consequently, on sampling at 12 hours, t_1 in the figure, one sees a larger change in enzyme X activity because this enzyme has a shorter half-life. Enzyme Y takes much longer to express its increased synthesis rate because it normally turns over slowly. Had the phenobarbital treatment continued to t_2, the degree of induction would have appeared to be equal, whereas at t_3 a more accurate estimate of the actual degree of induction would have been obtained. Clearly, the time of sampling is critical to any interpretation. Furthermore, had different steady-state concentrations of phenobarbital been studied, the threefold

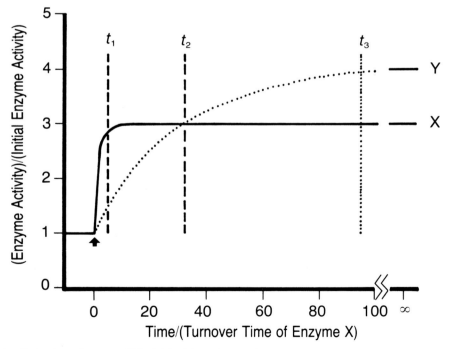

Fig. 23–8. Induction of enzyme X (solid line) by a factor of three and enzyme Y (dotted line) by a factor of four occurs. The turnover time of enzyme Y is 20 times as large as for enzyme X. The relative enzyme levels at the times indicated (dashed lines) are different, because of the differences in the turnover times of the two enzymes. Time is expressed in terms of the turnover time of enzyme X.

increase in the synthesis of enzyme X might have been the maximum value possible, whereas enzyme Y might have been maximally induced to a value ten times the normal one.

TURNOVER IN MULTICOMPARTMENTAL SYSTEMS

Endogenous compounds, like drugs, show distribution kinetics within the body (Chap. 19). This distribution is not apparent from the plasma concentration measurement of the endogenous compound under the usual steady-state conditions, but becomes so when a *tracer* dose of the compound, in an isotopically labeled form, is administered. A tracer dose, an amount small compared to the amount of endogenous compound so that it does not disturb the endogenous pool, permits determination of the turnover parameters of the endogenous compound. The two major assumptions are that the disposition of the tracer is identical to that of the endogenous substance and that input (formation) and elimination occur in the central (sampling) compartment. Unlike for most drugs, these restrictions are more problematic for endogenous compounds as they are often formed and destroyed in many tissues, some of which may not rapidly equilibrate with material in plasma.

Mean Residence Time

When the assumptions above hold, then a tracer molecule, on average, resides in the body the same length of time as a newly formed endogenous molecule. This time is called the *mean residence time (MRT)*; it is identical to the turnover time (t_t) of the endogenous substance.

A tracer bolus dose is the preferred method for measuring turnover. As derived in Appendix F, there are two procedures to estimate the mean residence time (turnover time). One method uses the area-under-the-(first)-moment versus the time curve, $\int_0^\infty t \cdot C^* \cdot dt$ or $AUMC$, and the area-under-the-concentration versus the time curve, AUC, namely

★

$$MRT = \frac{AUMC^*}{AUC^*}$$
12

where * refers to the labeled tracer. In the other method, the MRT is obtained from the urinary excretion of the unchanged tracer substance. Provided that fe remains constant with time, the MRT (turnover time) is then

★

$$MRT = \frac{\int_0^\infty (Ae^*_\infty - Ae^*)dt}{Ae^*_\infty}$$
13

where Ae_∞^* and Ae^* are the cumulative amounts of the labeled tracer in the urine to time infinity and to any previous time, respectively.

Steady-state Volume of Distribution

Remembering that: MRT (turnover time) is the ratio of the pool size to the turnover rate; input rate is the product of clearance and steady-state concentration, C_{ss}; and pool size is the product of volume of distribution at steady state and steady-state concentration, it follows that

$$MRT = \frac{A_{ss}}{R_t} = \frac{V_{ss} \cdot C^*_{ss}}{CL \cdot C^*_{ss}}$$
14

Thus, one arrives at the conceptually important relationship among the apparent volume of distribution under steady-state conditions, clearance, and *MRT* namely

$$MRT = V_{ss}/CL$$

★
15

The value of V_{ss} can be estimated using the plasma tracer concentration, realizing that $CL = \text{Dose}^*/AUC^*$ and combining Equation 12 with Equation 15, that is

★

$$V_{ss} = \frac{\text{Dose}^*}{AUC^*} \cdot \frac{AUMC^*}{AUC^*}$$

16

To illustrate the use of a tracer to determine turnover parameters and volume of distribution of an endogenous substance, consider the following biexponential equation, which summarizes the experimental observations after a 10-mega-Becquerel intravenous bolus dose of a tracer.

$$C^* = 1.2\, e^{-1.2t} + 0.2\, e^{-0.01t}$$

17

where C^* is the plasma concentration in units of megaBecquerels/liter and t is in minutes. The area under the concentration-time curve is

$$AUC^* = \int_0^\infty C^* \cdot dt = \frac{1.2}{1.2} + \frac{0.2}{0.01} = 21 \text{ megaBecquerel-minutes/liter}$$

The area under the first moment curve (Appendix F) is

$$\int_0^\infty t \cdot C^* \cdot dt = \frac{1.2}{(1.2)^2} + \frac{0.2}{(0.01)^2} = 2{,}001 \text{ megaBecquerel-minutes}^2\text{/liter}$$

The mean residence time (Eq. 12) is 95.3 minutes and the steady-state volume of distribution (Eq. 16) is then 45.4 liters (see Chap. 19 for the meaning of this volume term).

Calculation of the turnover rate requires knowledge of the concentration of the endogenous substance; assume 9 milligrams/liter. The amount of substance in the body (pool size) is then 9 milligrams/liter × 45.4 liters = 409 milligrams, and from the turnover time, the turnover rate (A_{ss}/MRT) is 4.3 milligrams/minute and the fractional turnover rate is 0.0105 minute^{-1}. The turnover of this substance is now completely quantified.

Study Problems

(Answers to Study Problems are in Appendix G.)

1. Define the following terms:

Turnover	Fractional turnover rate
Turnover rate	Mean residence time
Turnover time	

2. The "usual" plasma concentrations of urea and creatinine are 15 milligrams/100 milliliters (2.5 millimolar) and 1 milligram/100 milliliters (0.09 millimolar), respectively, in young adult patients with normal renal function. The renal clearances of the two compounds are 70 milliliters/minute and 120 milliliters/minute, respectively;

the volumes of distribution at steady state are about the same (40 liters). Assume that both compounds are eliminated only by renal excretion.

(a) Calculate the "usual" fractional turnover rates of both compounds.

(b) Were the rates of production of these compounds to remain "usual," how long would it take for the plasma urea concentration to increase by 30 milligrams/100 milliliters (5.0 millimolar) and the plasma creatinine concentration to increase by 2 milligrams/100 milliliters (0.18 millimolar) in an anephric patient?

(c) Urea is an end product of protein metabolism. Its formation can be reduced by decreasing protein in the diet. What is the total amount of urea ingested and produced in the body in 24 hours under steady-state conditions?

3. Consider two enzymes, A and B, both suspected of being subject to induction by a steroid hormone. Administration of the steroid to give nearly constant plasma concentrations for 24 hours results in a doubling of the activity of enzyme A, but enzyme B activity increases insignificantly (less than 20 percent). Based on this observation the statement is made—"The steroid has a much greater effect on the synthesis of enzyme A than on the synthesis of enzyme B." Is this conclusion warranted? Briefly discuss.

4. If the turnover time of an enzyme is 4 days and its synthesis rate is instantly increased to a constant value that is three times the normal rate, how long will it take for the enzyme activity (concentration) to double?

5. (a) Prior to an episode of acute renal failure, a patient (Height — 165 cm; Weight — 60 kg) had a daily renal excretion of 1.6 grams (14.2 millimoles) of creatinine and a plasma concentration of 1 milligram/100 milliliters (0.9 millimolar). During acute renal failure, the plasma creatinine concentration rose by 3 milligrams/100 deciliters (0.27 millimolar) per day and the daily renal excretion of creatinine was virtually nil—anuria. Calculate the "normal" mean residence time (MRT) of creatinine in this patient.

(b) Assume that acute renal insufficiency had resulted in an immediate drop in creatinine clearance to 10 percent of normal and that this functional state continued for an indefinite period of time. How long would it take for the plasma creatinine concentration to reach a value within 10 percent of the difference between that reflecting the degree of renal dysfunction and the initial value?

6. The turnover of albumin has been studied using tracer techniques (Sterling, K., J. Clin. Invest. 30:1228–1237, 1951). In one of the subjects, who received 6.75 megaBecquerels of ^{131}I-labeled albumin intravenously, the concentration of radioactivity was observed to decline according to the following relationship (1 Becquerel = 1 disintegration per second):

$$C \qquad = 1.5\, e^{-1.4t} + 1.2\, e^{-0.06t}$$
$$\text{(in megaBecquerels/liter)} \qquad (t \text{ in days})$$

Knowing that the plasma albumin concentration was 4.2 grams/deciliter in this subject and making the assumption that both the labeled and unlabeled albumin show the same kinetic behavior (observed to be a good approximation using other techniques), calculate the following:

(a) The turnover time and fractional turnover rate of albumin.

(b) The amounts of albumin in intravascular (initial dilution volume) and extravascular fluids.

(c) The synthesis rate of albumin.

7. A drug acts directly by inhibiting the synthesis of an endogenous substance (uric acid production, for example); the effect of the drug is measured indirectly, namely, by measurement of the plasma concentration of the endogenous substance, S. The scheme of events can be depicted as follows:

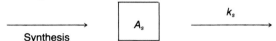

where A_s is the amount of S in the body and k_s is the elimination rate constant. In this scheme, the rate of synthesis of S responds instantaneously to changes in the concentration of drug.

The times and corresponding plasma concentrations of drug and S when a subject is challenged with a 100-milligram i.v. bolus dose of drug are presented in Table 23–3. The pharmacokinetics of the drug are characterized by a one-compartment model in which $k = 0.05$ hour^{-1} and $V = 10$ liters. As expected, there is a delay in the maximum lowering of the plasma concentration of S.

Table 23–3.

Time (hour)	0	2	4	6	8	10	12	16	24	30	36	48	60	72	84
Plasma concentration of drug (mg/liter)	10	9.0	8.2	7.4	6.7	6.1	5.5	4.5	3.0	2.2	1.7	0.91	0.5	0.27	0.15
Plasma concentration of endogenous substance, S (percent of normal)	100	72	53	40	31	25	21.5	19.1	24.5	32	48	72	88	96	99

Challenging the subject with a 200-milligram bolus dose on another occasion did not shorten the time taken for the concentration of S to initially fall by 50 percent; it did, of course, cause a deeper and more prolonged depression in the plasma concentration of S.

(a) Plot the time course of S on linear graph paper.

(b) Based on the scheme above and the information given, construct a direct response (inhibition of synthesis) versus plasma drug concentration curve. (Hint. Write the rate of equation for S and rearrange it to express the synthesis rate of S as a function of its plasma concentration and its elimination rate constant; you will need to estimate k_s to solve the problem.)

(c) From the curve drawn in part (b), estimate the EC_{50} value and comment on the most likely value of γ in the relationship

$$E = \frac{E_{max}\ C^{\gamma}}{EC_{50}^{\gamma} + C^{\gamma}}$$

(d) If a concentration of S, 30 percent of the normal value, is needed to achieve a desired therapeutic response, design a schedule (composed of a bolus dose and a constant-rate infusion) that will, as rapidly as possible, achieve this objective. For the purposes of these calculations let the bolus dose promptly achieve the desired plateau plasma concentration of the drug.

24

Dialysis

Objectives

The reader will be able to:

1. Define dialysis, hemodialysis, continuous ambulatory peritoneal dialysis, dialysis clearance, dialyzer, dialyzer efficiency, and clinical dialyzability.

2. Calculate the changes in clearance and half-life of a drug brought about by hemodialysis, continuous ambulatory peritoneal dialysis, or hemoperfusion given the clearance by the procedure, the total (body) clearance, and the half-life in the absence of the treatment.

3. Anticipate when a supplementary dose of a drug is required during dialysis or postdialysis, and determine what the supplementary dose should be.

4. Make a rational decision on the dialyzability of a drug in overdose situations from a pharmacokinetic point of view.

Dialysis procedures have become established treatments for patients with end-stage renal disease. These procedures are designed to remove toxic waste products that accumulate in patients with this disease. However, they also remove drugs. Thus, such procedures may require adjustment of drug administration in these patients. This chapter provides information needed to decide when and how to make an adjustment. Continuous ambulatory peritoneal dialysis is also discussed, because it is regarded as the treatment of choice for many patients. The last part of this chapter is devoted to the use of dialysis and a special procedure, hemoperfusion, to treat an overdosed patient.

HEMODIALYSIS

Basically, dialysis involves the separation of diffusible from less diffusible substances by the use of a semipermeable membrane. When the semipermeable membrane is that of the peritoneal cavity, the dialysis is termed peritoneal dialysis. Another dialysis procedure is to allow blood to pass through a system containing an artificial semipermeable membrane. Because of the large area of membrane required, such a system is, by necessity, outside the body. Accordingly, this method is termed *extracorporeal dialysis* or, more commonly, *hemodialysis*. The dialysis system itself is called a *hemodialyzer* or an *artificial kidney*. The most prevalent kind of system used today is the hollow fiber dialyzer. It contains hundreds of hollow fibers bundled within a compact cylinder. Blood flows through the semipermeable hollow fibers while dialysate fluid flows outside the fibers in a countercurrent direction. These systems are small, efficient, relatively easy to use, and are sometimes reused. In the following discussion on quantitative procedures, *dialysis* and *dialyzer* are terms used to describe the general method and the apparatus of hemodialysis, respectively.

The length of each dialysis treatment has been diminishing in recent years. A typical period has been reduced from 8 to about 3 to 4 hours at the present time. Efforts are being made to reduce the time further, perhaps even to 2 hours. The actual time required is a compromise between the time needed to adequately remove fluids and metabolic waste products from the body and the comfort and convenience to patients in general. Increased efficiency of the dialyzer is the major determinant of the shortened period.

The quantitative principles that are used for removal of endogenous substances apply to drugs as well. These principles follow.

Dialysis Clearance

As with many other applications of pharmacokinetics, the most useful concept when dealing with dialysis of drugs is clearance. Dialysis clearance is a measure of how effectively a dialyzer can remove a substance from blood. It is the rate of removal relative to the concentration in the blood entering the dialyzer. The use of the concentration in blood, rather than in plasma, has an advantage in relating blood clearance to blood flow and in relating rate of removal to rate of presentation to the dialyzer, principles previously developed for hepatic and renal extraction (Chap. 11). The use of unbound concentration is preferred when plasma protein binding is altered; however, most of the literature contains plasma concentration data.

To appreciate how dialysis clearance is measured, consider the schematic representation of a dialyzer shown in Figure 24–1. At steady state, that is, when there is no net change in the amount of substance in the dialyzer, the rate of removal of drug from the blood can be determined in three ways.

Extraction from Blood. One method is by taking the difference between the rates at which the substance enters ($Q_{b,in} \cdot C_{b,in}$) and leaves ($Q_{b,out} \cdot C_{b,out}$) the dialyzer, where $Q_{b,in}$ and $Q_{b,out}$ are the blood flows and $C_{b,in}$ and $C_{b,out}$ are the concentrations in the blood entering and leaving the dialyzer.

As clearance is the rate of removal relative to the entering drug concentration, dialysis blood clearance, CL_{bD}, can be calculated at steady state from measurement of drug in blood,

★

$$CL_{bD} = \frac{(Q_{b,in} \cdot C_{b,in} - Q_{b,out} \cdot C_{b,out})}{C_{b,in}} \qquad 1$$

Dialysis clearance, CL_D, based on drug concentration in plasma entering the dialyzer, C_{in}, can then be determined from $CL_D = CL_{bD} \cdot C_{b,in}/C_{in}$.

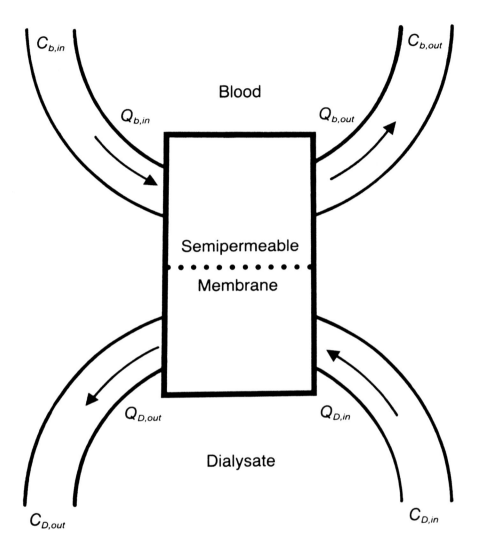

Fig. 24–1. Schematic representation of a hemodialysis system. Drug is delivered to the system at the rate $Q_{b,in} \cdot C_{b,in}$ and is returned to the body at the rate $Q_{b,out} \cdot C_{b,out}$. The difference between these rates is the net rate of loss into the dialyzing fluid. This rate of removal is the same as the difference between the rate leaving, $Q_{D,out} \cdot C_{D,out}$, and that entering, $Q_{D,in} \cdot C_{D,in}$, the dialyzer in the dialysate. Within the dialyzing system the blood and dialysate flows may be essentially concurrent, countercurrent, or crosscurrent, depending on the system design. The flows in the most common dialyzer, hollow fiber, are countercurrent as shown. $C_{b,in}$; $C_{b,out}$ = drug concentrations in blood entering and leaving dialyzer, respectively. $C_{D,in}$; $C_{D,out}$ = drug concentrations in dialysate entering and leaving dialyzer, respectively. $Q_{b,in}$; $Q_{b,out}$ = blood flows (usually 200 to 400 ml/minute) entering and leaving the dialyzer. $Q_{D,in}$; $Q_{D,out}$ = dialysate flows (usually 300 to 600 ml/minute) entering and leaving the dialyzer.

The values of $Q_{b,in}$ and $Q_{b,out}$ are not equal, as there is often a 2- to 3-liter loss of fluid during a typical 3- to 6-hour dialysis period. The value of $Q_{b,in}$ is often determined in research situations by measuring the movement of an air bubble in an input line of known dimensions. The value of $Q_{b,out}$ is calculated by multiplying $Q_{b,in}$ by the ratio of the hematocrit values across the dialyzer or by volumetric techniques.

Rate of Recovery in Dialysate. A second method uses the net rate at which the substance leaves the dialysate fluid, $Q_{D,out} \cdot C_{D,out} - Q_{D,in} \cdot C_{D,in}$, where $Q_{D,out}$ and $Q_{D,in}$ are the dialysate flows and $C_{D,out}$ and $C_{D,in}$ are the concentrations leaving and entering the dialyzer, respectively.

$$CL_{bD} = \frac{(Q_{D,out} \cdot C_{D,out} - Q_{D,in} \cdot C_{D,in})}{C_{b,in}} \qquad 2$$

The loss of water to the dialysate is accounted for here. With the common nonrecirculating (single pass) hollow fiber dialysis system, $C_{D,in} = 0$; calculation of clearance then requires knowing only the concentration of the substance in the dialysate, the dialysate flow, and the drug concentration entering the dialyzer, that is,

★

$$CL_{bD} = \frac{Q_{D,out} \cdot C_{D,out}}{C_{b,in}} \qquad 3$$

Amount Recovered in Dialysate. The third, and generally the most accurate and preferred, method of determining dialysis clearance is obtained from the recovery of amount of drug in the dialysate ($V_D \cdot C_D$) and the area under the blood concentration-time curve within the collection period, that is,

★

$$CL_{bD} = \frac{V_D \cdot C_D}{\int_0^\tau C_{b,in} \cdot dt} \qquad 4$$

Here, V_D is the volume of dialysate collected during the interval, τ, and C_D is the concentration of substance in the pooled dialysate.

As a rule, the value of dialysis clearance depends on the dialysis system, the fraction unbound in blood, and the molecular size of the substance as illustrated in Figure 24–2. As an approximation,

$$\frac{\text{Dialysis}}{\text{clearance}} = \frac{\text{Dialysis clearance}}{\text{of creatinine}} \cdot \sqrt{\frac{113}{\text{M.W.}}} \cdot fu_b \qquad 5$$

or

$$\frac{\text{Unbound}}{\text{dialysis clearance}} = \frac{\text{Dialysis clearance}}{\text{of creatinine}} \cdot \sqrt{\frac{113}{\text{M.W.}}} \qquad 6$$

where fu_b is the fraction unbound in blood (fu is pertinent if the clearances are based on drug concentration in plasma), M.W. is the molecular weight of the substance (a measure of molecular size), and unbound dialysis clearance is the proportionality constant between the rate of removal and the unbound concentration. With current dialyzers, dialysis clearance values for creatinine are usually between 80 and 150 milliliters/minute. The unbound dialysis clearance for drugs and most other substances are usually less than this because their molecular weights are greater than that of creatinine (M.W. = 113 daltons) and, in the case of (total) dialysis clearance, because they are often bound to plasma proteins or blood cells.

There is usually little, if any, correlation of dialysis clearance with either ionization or lipophilicity because the membranes used are ultrafilters rather than lipoidal barriers.

One observes a large range of dialysis clearance values. Part of this variability is caused by differences in binding of drug to plasma proteins, as shown in the figure. Molecular weight differences, even though relatively small in the range observed for most drugs, also contribute to this variability. When both of these sources are accounted for, there is still considerable variability in dialysis clearance owing, in large part, to the wide range of dialyzers and dialysis conditions used to acquire the information shown. Relating the dialysis clearance of a drug to that of creatinine should adjust for much of this remaining variability. In the absence of such information, Equations 5 and 6 can be used, but should be treated as rough approximations.

Dialysis Efficiency

Under steady-state conditions, the rate of removal relative to the rate of presentation is a measure of the efficiency of a dialysis system. By this definition, efficiency is the dialyzer extraction ratio, and its value can be calculated from the dialysis blood clearance and blood flow, that is,

$$\text{Efficiency} = \frac{CL_{bD}}{Q_{b,in}} \qquad 7$$

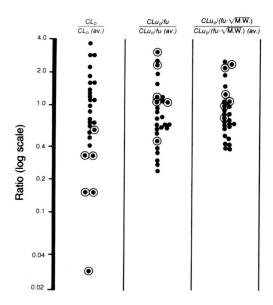

Fig. 24–2. Dialysis clearance and unbound dialysis clearance with an adjustment for molecular size for 27 different drugs show considerable variability. The variability is greatest for (total) dialysis clearance. On correcting for protein binding to give unbound dialysis clearance, the variability is decreased and those drugs that are highly bound (⊙) are brought into the range of unbound clearance values of the other drugs. Correction of unbound clearance with the square root of the molecular weight (M.W.) appears to diminish the variability further, but the prediction using both molecular weight and fraction unbound is still not too accurate. Presumably, further adjustment for dialyzer and dialysis conditions by relating the dialysis clearance of the drug to that of creatinine should be helpful. For comparative purposes, in each column the value for a drug has been expressed relative to the average value for all 27 drugs on a logarithmic scale. (Data from Lee, C.C. and Marbury, T.C.: Drug therapy in patients undergoing haemodialysis: Clinical pharmacokinetic considerations. Clin. Pharmacokin., 9:42–66, 1984.)

where CL_{bD} can be calculated from Equations 1, 2, or 4. Dialysis clearance and efficiency are measures of the ability of the dialyzer to remove a drug from blood, but they do not indicate how readily a drug is removed from the body. The terms dialyzable and nondialyzable are used to describe whether or not a drug or other substance is removed from the body in a clinically significant amount during a standard 3- to 4-hour period of dialysis treatment. Although dialyzability can be applied to the ability of a drug to pass through a semipermeable membrane, the clinically useful term refers to the ability of the dialysis system to remove a drug from the body.

Pharmacokinetic evaluation of hemodialysis and related procedures requires information on the parameters CL_b, CL_{bD}, and V_b (or the corresponding sets of values based on unbound drug CLu, CLu_D, and Vu; or on drug in plasma CL, CL_D, and V) and the duration of the procedure, τ. In the following derivation and throughout the remainder of this chapter, for convenience, only the set of parameter values based on measurement of drug in blood is used.

Drug Elimination

During dialysis, the dialysis clearance adds to the existing clearance; therefore,

$$\text{Rate of elimination from body during dialysis} = (CL_b + CL_{bD}) \cdot C_b \qquad 8$$

If the clearance values are constant during dialysis, then on integration the blood concentration at any time t since starting dialysis is

$$C_b = C_b(0) \cdot e^{-k_D t} \qquad 9$$

where $C_b(0)$ is the drug concentration in blood at the start of dialysis and k_D is the elimination rate constant during dialysis. Thus, $e^{-k_D \cdot \tau}$ is the fraction of drug remaining at the end of a dialysis period τ, and so

$$\text{Fraction lost from body during a dialysis period} = 1 - e^{-k_D \cdot \tau} \qquad 10$$

The contribution of dialysis to total drug elimination remains to be determined. Of the total drug eliminated during a dialysis period, the fraction removed by dialysis, f_D, is

$$f_D = \frac{CL_{bD}}{(CL_b + CL_{bD})} \qquad 11$$

Fraction of total elimination occurring by dialysis

The fraction of drug in the body at the start of dialysis that is eliminated by the dialysis procedure depends on the fraction of total elimination that dialysis represents, Equation 11, and the fraction of drug lost by all routes of elimination, Equation 10. Therefore,

$$\text{Fraction of drug initially in} \atop \text{body eliminated by dialysis} = f_D \cdot [1 - e^{-(CL_b + CL_bD)\tau/V_b}]$$

$$= f_D \cdot [1 - e^{-k_D \cdot \tau}]$$

★

12

Evaluation of Procedure

Figure 24–3 demonstrates the effectiveness of hemodialysis as a function of the unbound clearance and the unbound volume of distribution of a drug (Eq. 12, with respect to unbound drug) for a typical 4-hour dialysis period. An unbound dialysis clearance of 100 milliliters/minute, a common value for drugs, is used. It is apparent from this figure that hemodialysis is ineffective if the

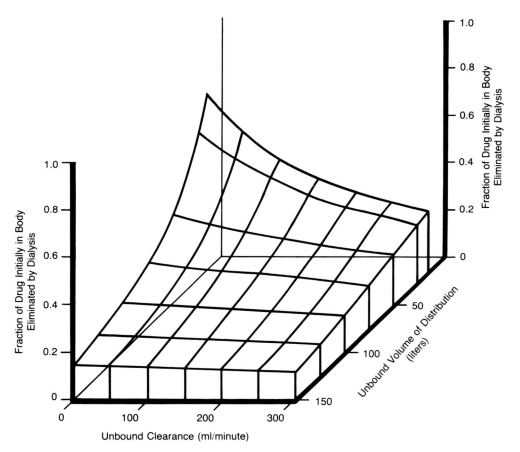

Fig. 24–3. Surface diagram of the fraction of drug initially in the body that is eliminated by 4 hours of dialysis as a function of the unbound clearance and the unbound volume of distribution. Dialysis clearance is assigned a value of 100 milliliters/minute, a high value for this parameter for current dialysis systems. For lower dialysis clearance values the total surface would be depressed. Note that for all values of unbound clearance, the fraction lost during dialysis is small (<0.2) if the unbound volume of distribution exceeds 150 liters. Also note that no surface is shown for an unbound volume of distribution less than 15 liters, the extracellular fluid volume and the lower limit of its value (see Chap. 25). The surface was calculated using Equation 12 and parameters based on unbound drug rather than whole blood.

unbound volume of distribution is large (greater than 150 liters), regardless of the clearance of a drug. Also, if the unbound clearance of a drug is much greater than the unbound dialysis clearance, dialysis becomes less effective in eliminating the drug.

The effectiveness of dialysis may also be evaluated by comparing a drug's half-lives on and off dialysis, as follows. The value of k_D, the overall elimination rate constant during dialysis, is given by

$$k_D = \frac{(CL_b + CL_{bD})}{V_b} \qquad 13$$

where V_b, the volume of distribution based on measurements in blood, is assumed to be constant with time. The corresponding half-life during dialysis is then

$$t_{1/2 \ on} = \frac{0.693 \cdot V_b}{(CL_b + CL_{bD})} \qquad 14$$

The change in the half-life during dialysis is a function of how much dialysis clearance contributes to the body's own clearance of a drug, that is,

$$\frac{t_{1/2 \ on}}{t_{1/2}} = \frac{CL_b}{(CL_b + CL_{bD})} = 1 - f_D \qquad 15$$

For digoxin, which has an unbound clearance of about 40 milliliters/minute in end-stage renal disease and an unbound dialysis clearance of 20 milliliters/minute, the half-life is shortened by 33 percent during dialysis. Furthermore, using Equation 12 (based on unbound drug) and an unbound volume of distribution of 400 liters, it is apparent that only about 2 percent of the drug initially present is lost by dialysis in 4 hours. Clearly, from a clinical point of view, this drug is not dialyzable.

A dramatic reduction in half-life during dialysis does not guarantee that the procedure is effective. For example, using an unbound dialysis clearance of 60 milliliters/minute and a volume of distribution of 50 liters, the half-life of phenobarbital is reduced from the usual 5 days to approximately 10 hours on dialysis, and 25 percent of the drug initially present (Eq. 13) is removed from the body during a 4-hour dialysis period. Thus, even though the half-life of phenobarbital is decreased 13-fold, the fraction removed in the dialysis period is much less than that initially expected based on the half-life change, because the half-life during dialysis is still longer than the period of dialysis.

PERITONEAL DIALYSIS

Peritoneal dialysis is accomplished by the insertion of a catheter into the abdomen and the introduction of dialysate through the catheter into the peritoneal cavity. After a period of time, referred to here as the *dwell time,* the fluid is drained and discarded. Table 24–1 lists the three kinds of chronic peritoneal dialysis procedures used clinically. The one that has become the most popular is continuous ambulatory peritoneal dialysis, CAPD. The subsequent discussion is largely restricted to this dialysis modality.

Table 24–1.   Chronic Peritoneal Dialysis Procedures

Procedure	Dialysis Time	Frequency of Procedure
Intermittent peritoneal dialysis	1-hour exchanges of dialysate for 10 to 12 hours	2 to 4 times a week
Continuous cycling peritoneal dialysis	Recycling of dialysate with varied dwell times	Nightly, while patient sleeps
Continuous ambulatory peritoneal dialysis (CAPD)	4 to 6 hours	Continuous

Dialysis Clearance

In CAPD, dialysis clearance, CL_{PD}, is most frequently expressed as the amount of a drug or substance recovered in the drained dialysate relative to the AUC during the dwell time, τ, after intravenous administration. Analogous to Equation 4 and with the subscript PC meaning peritoneal cavity,

$$CL_{PD} = \frac{C_{PC} \cdot V_{PC}}{\int_0^\tau C \cdot dt} \qquad 16$$

where V_{PC} is the dialysate volume in the peritoneal cavity. The plasma and dialysate concentrations of the cephalosporin, cefsulodin, during a 5-hour dwell time after intravenous and intraperitoneal administrations are shown in Figure 24–4. At the end of the dwell time, the peritoneal concentration approaches that of plasma after intravenous administration and the plasma concentration approaches that of dialysate after intraperitoneal administration. The clearance value obtained by Equation 16 then reflects the net movement of the drug during

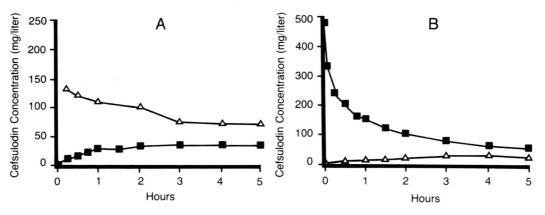

Fig. 24–4.   The plasma (△) and dialysate (■) concentrations of cefsulodin, a cephalosporin antibiotic that is virtually unbound in plasma, after intravenous administration (Panel A) and intraperitoneal administration (Panel B) to a patient with end-stage renal disease tend to approach an equilibrium within a 5-hour dialysate dwell time. The concentration in plasma after intravenous administration does not decline much because of the patient's renal disease and because the amount distributing into the 2-liter dialysate volume from the 16-liter extracellular fluid volume of distribution is small. In contrast, the concentration in the dialysate drops dramatically as it distributes from the 2-liter volume into the 16-liter volume. (One mg/liter = 1.9 micromolar.) (Data from Brouard, R., Tozer, T.N., Merdjan, H., Guillemin, A., and Baumelou, A.: Transperitoneal movement and pharmacokinetics of cefotiam and cefsulodin in patients on continuous ambulatory peritoneal dialysis. Clin. Nephrology, in press, 1988.)

the dwell time. Thus, this value of clearance decreases with dwell time in contrast to the clearance term for hemodialysis.

The unbound dialysis clearance value for most drugs lies between 2 and 7 milliliters/minute. The reason for this low value can be explained as follows. There is negligible protein in the dialysate fluid (1 to 2 grams per 2 liters) at the end of the dwell. Consequently, when equilibrium is achieved ($C_{PC} = Cu$), the amount in the dialysate is $Cu \cdot V_{PC}$, where Cu is the unbound concentration in plasma and C_{PC} is the unbound concentration in dialysate. If the plasma concentration is constant with time, then the unbound AUC is $Cu \cdot \tau$. Thus, the unbound dialysis clearance value is $Cu \cdot V_{PC}/Cu \cdot \tau$ or V_{PC}/τ. With a usual dialysate volume of 2000 milliliters and a τ of 300 minutes, the net clearance value is 6.7 milliliters/minute. This low clearance means that drug elimination by dialysis is not a major consideration for patients on CAPD. When CAPD is the only route of elimination and the drug is distributed in extracellular fluids (0.25 liter/kg, the smallest volume possible for unbound drug), the half-life is then 1810 minutes ($t_{1/2}$ = 0.693 [250 ml/kg × 70 kg]/6.7 ml/minute) or 1.26 days. Clearly, other routes of elimination or therapeutic maneuvers are generally of greater importance than CAPD.

Dialysis clearance values for intermittent peritoneal dialysis and continuous cycling peritoneal dialysis can be 10 to 40 milliliters/minute, values much greater than those for CAPD, because sink conditions tend to be maintained when using short dwell times. For this reason, removal of a significant fraction of drug in the body can occur during a treatment period just as with hemodialysis. The methods of analysis and prediction of drug removal are the same as for hemodialysis.

Route of Administration

Although little drug is lost from the body during CAPD after parenteral administration, most (50 to 90 percent) of a dose administered into the peritoneal cavity is absorbed into the body during a typical 4- to 6-hour dwell time. Because of the continuous nature of CAPD, this route of administration has a potential application for systemic purposes, especially for drugs that cannot be absorbed when taken orally, as is the case for many antibiotics, insulin, and heparin.

Peritonitis is the major drawback to CAPD. A major question here is whether direct administration of an antibiotic into the peritoneal cavity to treat the peritonitis might be more effective than systemic administration. Although the former mode of administration would appear to be superior, drug may be delivered to the site of infection more readily via the capillaries than through the peritoneum.

DRUG ADMINISTRATION IN HEMODIALYSIS PATIENTS

For selected drugs, direct information is known on the adjustment of dosage regimens needed in patients undergoing hemodialysis. For situations in which such information is not available, pharmacokinetic principles can be applied to predict and evaluate the appropriate dosage adjustment.

One approach to dosage adjustment is to replace the amount lost in the dialysate during the treatment period, which can be calculated from Equation

12, knowing the amount of drug in the body at the start of dialysis, $V \cdot C(0)$. A more appealing approach is to restore the amount of drug in the body at the end of the dialysis interval to the level that would have occurred had the patient not been dialyzed; this procedure permits the patient's existing regimen to be maintained (Fig. 24–5). Had no dialysis been employed, the fraction expected to remain at time τ is $e^{-k \cdot \tau}$; the fraction remaining when both dialysis and the body's own elimination processes are present is $e^{-kD \cdot \tau}$. The difference between these two terms is the fraction of the drug initially present needed to return the amount in the body to the level at which it would have been present had dialysis not occurred, that is,

★

$$\begin{array}{l}\text{Fraction of drug initially in body} \\ \text{required to cancel the loss by dialysis}\end{array} = e^{-k \cdot \tau} - e^{-kD \cdot \tau} \qquad 17$$

From the volume of distribution and the plasma concentration just before dialysis, $C(0)$, the required supplementary dose is

$$\text{Supplementary dose} = V \cdot C(0) \cdot [e^{-k \cdot \tau} - e^{-kD \cdot \tau}] \qquad 18$$

Drug therapy is complicated in patients who are functionally or anatomically without kidneys and who undergo hemodialysis treatment. Consideration must be given not only to the adjustment of drug administration because of the anephric condition, but also to the potential loss of drug during the dialysis treatment. If an appropriate adjustment has been made for the lack of renal function (Chap. 16), the subsequent considerations are: Is a significant amount of drug removed during a dialysis session? If so, how much drug must one administer to replace what is lost by dialysis and should the supplementary dose be given during dialysis or postdialysis?

To answer whether or not a significant loss occurs within the period of treatment, one needs to know how the anephric patient handles the drug and the dialysis clearance value. Using estimates of the clearance and volume of distribution in the anephric patient, the change in the half-life (Eq. 11) and the fraction

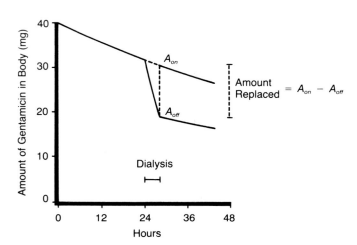

Fig. 24–5. The dose of gentamicin needed to return the amount in the body at the end of dialysis to the value that would have been present at that time, had the patient not been dialyzed, is the difference between the amounts in the body at the end of the interval in the presence (A_{on}) and absence (A_{off}) of dialysis. The dose (12 mg) in this example of an anephric patient is close to the amount in the dialysate because little has been lost by the body's own mechanisms during the dialysis interval.

of drug lost by dialysis in the dialysis interval (Eqs. 12 through 15) can be calculated. Using gentamicin as an example, let us first determine what the regimen of the drug should be in a functionally anephric patient.

The pharmacokinetic parameters of gentamicin in the typical 55-year-old adult are (Table 18–4) CL = 5.1 liters/hour per 70 kilograms, V = 15 liters/70 kilograms, $t_{1/2}$ = 2 hours, fe = >0.95. It is immediately apparent that as fe is greater than 0.95 and probably close to 1.0, the kinetics of this drug are drastically altered in a patient without renal function. From the relationship $t_{1/2}(d) = t_{1/2}(n)/(1 - fe(1 - RF))$ (Eq. 9, Chap. 16), the half-life of this drug in anephric patients is seen to be greater than 40 hours. Needless to say, administration of this drug to an anephric patient requires extreme caution. In practice, such long half-lives are less common because anephric patients on gentamicin are often concurrently administered a penicillin that may cause decomposition of gentamicin in the body by a direct chemical reaction. For purposes of the example below, assume a half-life of 72 hours in an individual anephric patient on gentamicin alone. This half-life corresponds to a clearance of 2.4 milliliters/minute; the rate of administration should therefore be 36 times less than usual. A common regimen of gentamicin for a patient with normal renal function is 80 milligrams (1.2 mg/kg), intramuscularly or intravenously, every 8 hours; the initial dose and the maintenance doses are the same. But a strong argument exists for reducing the initial dose of drug for an anephric patient, when the dosing interval is much shorter than the half-life (Chap. 16). Accordingly, an appropriate recommendation for an anephric patient might be a 40-milligram loading dose followed by 12 milligrams every other day.

The expected amount of drug in the body with time following this recommended regimen, in the absence of dialysis, is shown as Curve A in Figure 24–6. The anephric patient is dialyzed for 4 hours on days 1, 3, and 5 between doses on days 0, 2, and 4. Consideration of a supplementary dose requires an estimate of the fraction lost in the dialysate during each treatment period. The dialysis clearance of gentamicin, a drug not bound in plasma, in a common dialyzer is 30 milliliters/minute. The combined clearance in this patient is therefore 32.4 milliliters/minute. The corresponding elimination rate constant, k_D, is 0.13 hour^{-1}. Using Equation 10, the fraction lost during a 4-hour dialysis period is 0.4.

Thus, hemodialysis every 2 or 3 days would result in very little drug being in the anephric patient (Curve B, Fig. 24–6) if the suggested regimen above were not adjusted. Clearly, a supplementary dose at the end of each dialysis period is needed.

The amount of the supplementary dose should be sufficient to return the amount in the body to the value that would have occurred had the patient not been dialyzed, the condition simulated in Curve C of Figure 24–6. The amount continues to decline with dialysis every other day after a loading dose of 40 milligrams. The amount in the body at the time of the first dialysis on day 2 (40 × $e^{-0.693 \times 24/72}$) is 32 milligrams. The supplementary dose is then 12 milligrams (Eq. 18). Table 24–2 shows representative drugs for which supplementary doses might be considered.

For a drug that is readily dialyzed and is required by the patient at all times, consideration might be given to administering it during the dialysis treatment. Another approach is to use a therapeutic (unbound) concentration of the drug

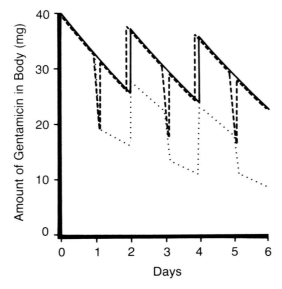

Fig. 24–6.   Sketch of the amount of gentamicin in the body with time in an anephric patient on an intramuscular dosage regimen of 40 milligrams initially and 12 milligrams every other day. Curve A (———)—patient not dialyzed. Curve B (· · · · ·)—patient undergoing dialysis (for 4 hours) on days 1, 3, and 5. Curve C (– – – –)—patient undergoing dialysis is given a supplementary dose of 12 milligrams just after each dialysis period. A one-compartment model for gentamicin is assumed.

in the dialysate. Although theoretically more logical, the latter approach may be very expensive. The total volume used is 144 liters if a usual dialysate flow rate of 600 milliliters/minute is continued for 4 hours. For gentamicin, a therapeutic concentration of 2 milligrams/liter in the dialysate would therefore require an addition of almost 300 milligrams. If the drug is an antibiotic, one might argue that doing this would help to prevent peritonitis.

Although only about 25 percent of phenobarbital initially present was previously calculated to be removed in a single dialysis session, the steady-state phenobarbital concentration may be considerably reduced during repeated sessions. The amount of phenobarbital in a patient who has a half-life of 5 days and a volume of distribution of 50 liters is decreased by 13 percent ($e^{-CL \cdot \tau/V}$) during the dosing interval (1 day). The additional loss of 25 percent every other day (on dialysis) would result in a doubling of the average percent lost (13 percent off dialysis, about 38 percent on dialysis). In this patient, the dosage would have to be doubled to keep the same average amount in the body. Clearly, the effect of dialysis should also be examined at steady state, the therapeutically relevant situation for phenobarbital.

Table 24–2.   Representative Drugs for Which Supplemental Doses Postdialysis may be Required in Patients Undergoing Hemodialysis[a]

Aminoglycosides	*Cephalosporins*	*Penicillins*
Amikacin	Cefamandole	Amoxycillin
Gentamicin	Cefazolin	Ampicillin
Kanamycin	Cefsulodin	Carbenicillin
Tobramycin	Cephalexin	Penicillin-G
Other Antimicrobial Agents	*Immunosuppressive Agents*	*Miscellaneous*
Chloramphenicol	Cyclophosphamide	Disopyramide
Isoniazid	5-Fluorouracil	Phenobarbital
Flucytosine	Methotrexate	Theophylline

[a]Lee, C-S.C. and Marbury, T.C.: Drug therapy in patients undergoing haemodialysis: Clinical pharmacokinetic considerations. Clin. Pharmacokin., 9:42–66, 1984.

DIALYSIS IN DRUG OVERDOSE

Assessment of the contribution of hemodialysis to the reduction of the morbidity and mortality of drug intoxication requires concurrent quantitative information on drug removal. Measurement of the amount of drug in the dialysate alone is inadequate. For example, a recovery of ten grams in the dialysate may be unimportant if more than 100 grams were in the body at the start of the dialysis procedure. Required to be known is the fraction of the amount initially in the body that is eliminated by dialysis. Currently, only a limited amount of such information is available.

There are several factors associated with the overdosed patient that may affect the pharmacokinetics of a drug, for example, anoxia, metabolic acidosis, carbon dioxide retention, hypotension, depressed renal function, and hypothermia. Furthermore, complications may arise because of slow tissue distribution of a drug (Chap. 19) and because of the concentrations of drug and active metabolites attained (Chap. 21). Comments on a few of these complications are in order.

Drug Redistribution

An important consideration in evaluating the potential use of dialysis in an overdose situation is drug redistribution. For certain drugs, dialysis may remove drug more readily from the plasma than it can be replaced from tissue stores, thereby resulting in a rebound of the plasma drug concentration when dialysis is stopped. Two primary mechanisms account for this slow return of drug from the tissues: slow diffusion through the tissue membranes and limited vascular perfusion of the tissues (Chap. 10).

Lithium (Fig. 24–7) is an example of a drug that exhibits postdialysis rebound due to slow diffusion from cells. Dialysis clearance adds substantially to the total body clearance (virtually all renal clearance) of this drug. Lithium disappears rapidly from plasma during dialysis, and a large fraction of drug in the body is expected to be removed into the dialysate. The slow return from tissue stores, however, limits the total amount removed and produces the rebound of the plasma drug concentration after dialysis treatment. In this case, assessment of the fraction of the initial amount of drug removed by dialysis is relatively simple, since virtually all the drug eliminated by the body is excreted into the urine. The fraction is the amount recovered in the dialysate divided by the sum of the amounts in the dialysate and the urine during the dialysis period.

Another method of assessing the contribution of dialysis to total elimination is to extrapolate the terminal part of the curve, when equilibrium has been reestablished, back to the beginning of dialysis (see Fig. 24–7). The difference between the initial concentration (3.0 mg/liter) and the extrapolated value (1.6 mg/liter) relative to the initial value is the fraction eliminated by dialysis.

Concentration-dependent Kinetics

An additional consideration in the dialysis of drugs in the overdose situation is concentration-dependent kinetics (Chap. 22), whereby either the volume of distribution or the total clearance, or both, depends on the concentration of drug in the plasma. Ethchlorvynol shows such concentration-dependent kinetic be-

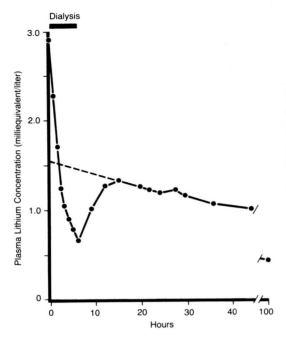

Fig. 24–7. During 6.5 hours of hemodialysis (solid bar) of a patient poisoned with lithium, the plasma concentration of lithium (●) drops dramatically; however, on discontinuing dialysis the plasma concentration rises with a redistribution of drug from tissue cells to plasma, so that only about one-half of the lithium initially in the body is removed by dialysis. The rough estimate of the actual fraction lost can be obtained by extrapolating (– – – –) the terminal curve back to the time dialysis was started. A semilogarithmic plot should be used for the extrapolation in those situations in which the postdialysis concentration declined linearly on such a plot. (Redrawn from data of Amdisen, A. and Skjoldborg, H.: Haemodialysis for lithium poisoning. Lancet, 2:213, 1969.)

havior (Fig. 24–8). At normal therapeutic doses the half-life is 25 hours; in overdose cases it is increased to more than 100 hours, probably because of a decreased metabolic clearance at the higher concentrations. Similar to lithium, ethchlorvynol also shows plasma rebound after dialysis. The redistribution here is a consequence of the affinity of the drug for fat, a poorly perfused tissue.

As stated in Chapter 22, concentration-dependent kinetics is perhaps more the rule than the exception in drug overdose. Assessment of the dialyzability of drugs under this circumstance is more difficult than at therapeutic concentrations.

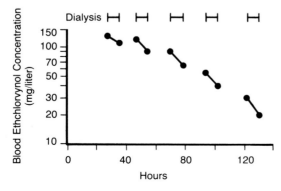

Fig. 24–8. The overall decline of ethchlorvynol concentration in blood on this semilogarithmic plot shows concentration dependence in an intoxicated patient. During each 8-hour dialysis period (⊢——⊣), the concentration (●—●) was reduced but tended to rise again when dialysis was discontinued, indicative of redistribution. (One mg/liter = 6.9 micromolar.) (Redrawn from Tozer, T.N., Witt, L.D., Gee, L., Tong, T.G., and Gambertoglio, J.: Evaluation of hemodialysis for ethchlorvynol (Placidyl) overdose. Amer. J. Hosp. Phar., 31:986–989, 1974. Original data from Gibson, P.F. and Wright, N.: Ethchlorvynol in biological fluids: Specificity of assay methods. J. Pharm. Sci., 61:169–174, 1972.)

Toxic Metabolites

Little correlation may exist between the drug concentration and the patient's clinical status for drugs for which a metabolite(s) is primarily responsible for the toxicity. The clinical response is then expected to be more closely related to the blood concentration of the metabolite(s). The dialyzability of the active metabolite(s), as well as the unchanged drug, should be kept in mind. The formation of the toxic metabolite hydroxyglutethimide from glutethimide (Chap. 21) in the overdose situation is an example; however, in this case both compounds contribute to the toxicity. Generally, there is a paucity of information of this nature.

Other Considerations

Determination of the overall benefit-to-risk ratio of hemodialysis requires the consideration of many factors. The severity of the poisoning, the value of other procedures such as forced diuresis (Chap. 11), the control of urine pH and good supportive care, and the risks of the procedure to the patient, in addition to pharmacokinetic considerations, must all be weighed. Table 24–3 lists representative substances for which hemodialysis may be of potential value in treating severely intoxicated patients.

HEMOPERFUSION

A final system, which operates on principles different from those of peritoneal dialysis and hemodialysis, is hemoperfusion. In this system, whole blood is passed through a charcoal or a resin bed. Molecules that are adsorbed are retarded; blood cells and plasma proteins readily pass through. This system can have a high efficiency for removing certain drugs. As virtually all the drug can be extracted from the blood and, as blood flows through the hemoperfusion cartridge can be 200 to 400 milliliters/minute, clearances of greater than 200 milliliters/minute can be obtained for substances that strongly adsorb to the system. This system appears to have potential in the treatment of drug overdose. It is, however, not without its own set of limitations, including the removal of platelets, white blood cells, various endogenous steroids, and other substances. The pharmacokinetic principles discussed for assessing the effectiveness of hemodialysis also apply here, except that drug removed by hemoperfusion is determined from the amount within the cartridge instead of the amount recovered in the dialysate.

Table 24–3. Representative Substances for Which Hemodialysis may be of Potential Value in Treating Severe Intoxication[a]

Aminoglycosides	Lithium
Bromide	Methanol
Chloral Hydrate	Meprobamate
(trichloroethanol)	Phenobarbital
Ethylene Glycol	Salicylic Acid

[a]Cutter, R.E., Forland, S.C., Hammond, P.G.S.J., and Evans, J.R.: Extracorporeal removal of drugs and poisons by hemodialysis and hemoperfusion. Ann. Rev. Pharmacol. Toxicol., 27:169–191, 1987.

Study Problems

(Answers to Study Problems are in Appendix G.)

1. Define dialysis, hemodialysis, continuous ambulatory peritoneal dialysis, dialysis clearance, dialyzer, dialyzer efficiency, and clinical dialyzability of a drug.

2. In a study of the removal of phenytoin by hemodialysis (Adapted from Martin, E., Gambertoglio, J.G., Adler, D.S., Tozer, T.N., Roman, L.A., and Grausz, H., JAMA, *238*:1750–1753, 1977), the following data were obtained in one of the subjects. Sodium phenytoin (350 mg of acid form of drug) was administered intravenously over 30 minutes 2 hours before hemodialysis treatment. The average blood and dialysate flows through the dialyzer were 305 and 267 milliliters/minute, respectively. The plasma phenytoin concentration dropped from 3.9 to 3.5 milligrams/liter during the 6-hour dialysis treatment. The fraction unbound was 0.21, and the amount of phenytoin collected in the 6-hour dialysate was 14 milligrams. The dialysis clearance of creatinine was 83 milliliters/minute. The concentrations in blood and plasma were virtually identical.

   (a) Calculate the dialysis clearance of phenytoin.

   (b) What is the efficiency of the dialyzer used?

   (c) The blood concentrations into and out of the dialyzer could have been used to determine dialysis clearance. If they had been used, what would the ratio (out/ in) have been to give the clearance observed in (a)? Assume no net loss of fluid from the body into the dialysate. Do you think clearance could have been determined accurately from the blood concentrations into and out of the dialyzer?

   (d) Calculate the fraction of drug initially in the body that is eliminated by dialysis.

   (e) Is the observed dialysis clearance of phenytoin (M.W. = 252 daltons) close to the value predicted by Equation 5 in the text?

3. The data in Table 24–4 on vancomycin were acquired in patients receiving CAPD treatment. Vancomycin was given intravenously and intraperitoneally in doses of 10 milligrams/kilogram on separate occasions. The first dwell time after vancomycin administration was 4 hours. Two additional 4-hour exchanges and an overnight 12-hour dwell time were used.

Table 24–4[a].

Route of Administration	Clearance[b] (ml/minute)	Peritoneal Dialysis Clearance (ml/minute)
Intravenous	9	1.5[c]
Intraperitoneal instillation	15	2.5[d]

[a]Bunke, C.M., Aronoff, G.R., Brier, M.E., Sloan, R.S., and Luft, F.C., Clin. Pharmacol. Ther., *34*:631–637, 1983.
[b]Includes peritoneal dialysis clearance. Calculated from Dose/AUC.
[c]Amount in dialysate between 0 and 72 hours divided by AUC within the same interval.
[d]Amount in dialysate between 4 and 72 hours divided by AUC within the same interval.

   (a) The authors claim that the value of vancomycin peritoneal dialysis clearance, calculated after intraperitoneal instillation, differs from that after intravenous administration. Do you agree? Defend your answer.

(b) Can you explain the differences observed in the estimates of clearance from the two routes of administration?

4. Table 24–5 contains the value of several pharmacokinetic parameters and the recommended dosage regimen for adults with normal renal function for digitoxin and theophylline. In addition, their approximate values for dialysis clearance are given.

Table 24–5. Selected Pharmacokinetic Parameters, Dosage Regimens, and Dialysis Clearances of Digitoxin and Theophylline[a]

Parameters	Digitoxin	Theophylline
Half-life (hours)	160	8
Volume of distribution, plasma (liters)	38	35
Fraction excreted unchanged	0.3	0.13
Route of administration	oral	oral
Usual maintenance dosage regimen	0.1 milligram daily	240 milligrams every 6 hours
Dialysis clearance, plasma (liters/hour)[b]	<0.1	2.5
Fraction unbound	0.03	0.44

[a]In patients with normal renal function.
[b]Estimates from Equation 5. Dialysis clearance of creatinine on the dialyzer used is assumed to be 120 milliliters/minute.

In answering the following questions, assume: metabolites are inactive and nontoxic; nonrenal clearance, volume of distribution, and availability in normal and anuric patients are the same; the pharmacokinetic parameter values are independent of concentration; and distribution to the tissues is instantaneous. Also, assume that theophylline is essential to the therapeutic management of an anephric (no renal function) patient who is undergoing repeated hemodialysis treatment every other day.

(a) Based on pharmacokinetic principles, indicate whether or not a supplementary dose might be appropriate at the end of a 4-hour dialysis period. Show how you come to your conclusion.

(b) What supplemental dose would you suggest for postdialysis administration?

(c) Fully delineate the dosage regimen that you would recommend for initiating and maintaining theophylline therapy in the anephric patient undergoing hemodialysis?

5. From a pharmacokinetic point of view, is digitoxin (see Table 24–5) a candidate for hemodialysis (24-hour duration) detoxification of a severely overdosed patient with normal renal function?

25

Small Volume of Distribution

Objectives

The reader will be able to:

1. Calculate the fraction of drug in the body that is:
   a. unbound
   b. in the extracellular fluids
   c. outside the extracellular fluids
   d. bound to plasma proteins
   e. bound to plasma proteins in the extracellular fluids
   f. bound intracellularly (in or on tissue cells)

   from knowledge of the volume of distribution and the fraction unbound in plasma.

2. Quantify the value of the extravascular/intravascular distribution ratio of a plasma protein from the volume of distribution of a drug that is virtually only bound to this protein in the body.

3. Calculate the values given in objective 1 for conditions, such as pregnancy and hepatic cirrhosis, in which the extravascular/intravascular distribution ratio of albumin, or any other plasma protein, is altered.

4. Anticipate the effect of altered plasma protein binding on the half-life of a drug with a volume of distribution less than 0.2 liter/kilogram.

Changes in the binding of drugs to either plasma proteins or to components outside plasma produce changes in both the apparent volume of distribution and the kinetics of drugs in the body. The consequences of changes in binding in these two locations are quite different, but unfortunately, since drug binding in the tissues cannot be readily measured, changes in tissue binding must be inferred from measurements made in plasma.

In the model presented in Chapter 10 (Eq. 22), drug in the body is accounted for by that in plasma and that outside plasma, that is,

$$V \cdot C \;=\; V_p \cdot C \;+\; V_{TW} \cdot C_{TW}$$

$V \cdot C$	$V_p \cdot C$	$V_{TW} \cdot C_{TW}$
Amount in body	Amount in plasma	Amount outside plasma

1

From the definitions of fu and fu_T and under the distribution equilibrium condition, $Cu = Cu_T$, it was shown that

$$V = V_P + V_{TW} \cdot \frac{fu}{fu_T} \qquad 2$$

It is apparent that on measuring V and fu in a control and in an altered state (hypoalbuminemia, renal failure, drug interaction, and saturable binding), changes in V_{TW}/fu_T can be inferred, since V_P is simply the plasma volume, about 3 liters, and V_{TW} is a physiologic aqueous volume into which drug distributes. This is a useful model; however, it does not take into account the fact that plasma proteins are distributed throughout the extracellular fluids. Any alteration in binding to a plasma protein is expected to be reflected both in and outside plasma. A model is therefore needed to distinguish, in tissues, between binding to the plasma proteins and binding to other constituents. This need is particularly great for drugs with small (less than 0.2 liters/kg) volumes of distribution. The purpose of this chapter is to present such a model and to discuss its applications.

MODEL

The distribution of albumin is used in this chapter as a prototypic model for any plasma protein that distributes throughout the extracellular fluids. In developing this model, the body is represented as having three aqueous compartments, as shown in Figure 25–1. The amount of drug in plasma is the product of the volume of plasma and the plasma drug concentration. The amount of drug in the extracellular fluids outside plasma is the product of the aqueous volume of this space and the average concentration within this space that accounts for the total amount of drug there. The amount outside the extracellular

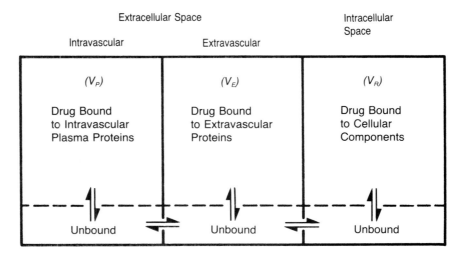

Fig. 25–1. Drug distributes among plasma (volume = V_P), the extracellular fluids outside plasma (volume = V_E), and the remainder of the body water (volume = V_R). Equilibrium is achieved when the unbound concentrations in the three spaces are the same. The bound concentrations in the three spaces are functions of the affinities of the drug for the substances in these spaces to which the drug binds. Throughout the extracellular fluids (V_P and V_E) drug is bound to the same protein(s).

space (in or on cells or bound to connective elements) is accounted for, as in the model in Chapter 10, by the product of the aqueous volume into which the drug distributes outside the extracellular fluids and an average concentration in this compartment.

Using the symbols defined in Table 25–1,

$$V \cdot C \quad = V_P \cdot C \quad + V_E \cdot C_E \quad + \quad V_R \cdot C_R$$

| Amount in body | Amount in plasma | Amount in extracellular fluids outside plasma | Amount in the remainder of the body | 3 |

Defining fu_R as Cu/C_R, fu as Cu/C, and Cb_E as the average concentration of bound drug in the extracellular space outside plasma and dividing by C, yields

$$V = V_P + V_E \cdot fu \cdot \frac{(Cu + Cb_E)}{Cu} + V_R \cdot \frac{fu}{fu_R} \qquad 4$$

To be useful, it is necessary to solve for C_{bE} in Equation 4. This is accomplished as follows. For a given protein with one class of binding sites, the law of mass action gives

$$Ka = \frac{Cb_P}{Cu \cdot (P)_P} = \frac{Cb_E}{Cu_E \cdot (P)_E} \qquad 5$$

where Cb_P and Cb_E are the bound drug concentrations and $(P)_P$ and $(P)_E$ are the

Table 25–1. Symbols and Their Definitions

Symbol	Definition
C	Total concentration of drug in plasma
Cb_P	Concentration of bound drug in plasma
Cb_E	Average concentration of bound drug in extracellular fluids outside plasma
Cb_R	Average concentration of drug bound outside the extracellular fluids
C_E	Average total concentration of drug in extracellular fluids outside plasma
C_R	Average total concentration of drug outside the extracellular fluids
Cu	Concentration of unbound drug in plasma and, presumably, throughout aqueous spaces into which drug distributes
C_{TW}	Average concentration of drug in aqueous volume outside plasma into which drug distributes
fu	Fraction unbound to protein in plasma, Cu/C
fu_R	Fraction unbound outside the extracellular fluids, Cu/C_R
fu_T	Fraction unbound outside plasma, Cu/C_{TW}
K_a	Association or affinity constant between drug and protein
$(P)_P$	Concentration of available binding sites on protein in plasma
$(P)_E$	Average concentration of available binding sites on plasma protein in extracellular fluids outside plasma
$(Pt)_P$	Total concentration of binding sites on protein in plasma
$(Pt)_E$	Average concentration of binding sites on protein in extracellular fluids outside plasma
$R_{E/l}$	Ratio of the total binding sites (or amount of protein) in the extracellular fluids outside plasma to the total binding sites in plasma
V	Apparent volume of distribution of drug
V_{bw}	Volume of total body water, average value = 42 liters/70 kilograms
V_P	Plasma volume, average value = 3 liters/70 kilograms
V_E	Extracellular fluid volume minus plasma volume, average value = 12 liters/70 kilograms
V_R	Aqueous volume outside extracellular fluids into which drug distributes
V_{TW}	Aqueous volume outside plasma into which drug distributes

concentrations of unoccupied protein binding sites in the plasma and in the other extracellular fluids, all expressed in equivalent units, respectively, and Ka is the association or affinity constant between drug and protein. If the unbound drug concentrations are identical in both fluids ($Cu_E = Cu$), then

$$\frac{Cb_P}{(P)_P} = \frac{Cb_E}{(P)_E} \qquad 6$$

Also,

$$(Pt)_P = (P)_P + Cb_P \qquad 7$$

and

$$(Pt)_E = (P)_E + Cb_E \qquad 8$$

where $(Pt)_P$ and $(Pt)_E$ are the average total concentrations of binding sites in the plasma and in the other extracellular fluids, respectively. It follows that $(Pt)_P/(P)_P = (Pt)_E/(P)_E$ (obtained by dividing Eq. 7 by $(P)_P$ and Eq. 8 by $(P)_E$). Consequently,

$$Cb_E = Cb_P \cdot \frac{(Pt)_E}{(Pt)_P} \qquad 9$$

or

$$Cb_E = Cb_P \cdot R_{E/I} \cdot \frac{V_P}{V_E} \qquad 10$$

where $R_{E/I}$ is the ratio of the total number of binding sites, or amount of protein, in extracellular fluids outside plasma (extravascular) to that in plasma (intravascular). This relationship, Equation 10, can also be shown to be valid when there is more than one class of binding sites on a protein or when saturation is approached. Substituting Equation 10 into Equation 4 gives

$$V = V_P + fu \cdot \left[\frac{V_E \cdot Cu + Cb_P \cdot V_P \cdot R_{E/I}}{Cu}\right] + \frac{V_R \cdot fu}{fu_R} \qquad 11$$

However, since by dividing by C,

$$Cb_P/Cu = (1 - fu)/fu \qquad 12$$

then

★

$$V = V_P(1 + R_{E/I}) + (V_E - V_P \cdot R_{E/I}) \cdot fu + \frac{V_R \cdot fu}{fu_R} \qquad 13$$

The extracellular fluids outside plasma are, on average, 12 liters and the plasma volume is 3 liters in a normal 70-kilogram man. Furthermore, as about 60 percent of the total body albumin is usually found outside plasma (Table 25–2), its extravascular/intravascular distribution ratio, $R_{E/I}$, is approximately 1.5. Using these normal values, Equation 13 becomes

$$V = 7.5 + 7.5 \cdot fu + V_R \cdot \frac{fu}{fu_R} \qquad 14$$

or

Table 25–2.   Distribution of Albumin in the Body[a]

Organ	Amount (grams/70-kg man)	Concentration (grams/kg organ)
Intravascular		
Plasma	140	43
Extravascular		
Muscle	50	2.3
Skin	40	7.7
Liver	2	1.4
Gut	8	5
Other tissues	110	3
Total:	210	
Total body	350	

[a]Adapted from compilation of data of Peters, T.: Serum albumin. In The Plasma Proteins. 2nd Ed., Vol. 1, Edited by F.W. Putnam, New York, Academic Press, 1975, p. 162.

★

$$V = 7.5 + \left[7.5 + \frac{V_R}{fu_R}\right] \cdot fu \qquad\qquad 15$$

These equations state that if a drug is distributed only in the extracellular fluids, e.g., if it cannot enter the cells ($V_R = 0$), the smallest apparent volume of distribution it can have is

$$V = 7.5 + 7.5 \cdot fu \qquad\qquad 16$$

Thus, at distribution equilibrium, the observed apparent volume of distribution of any drug cannot be less than 7.5 liters, the volume of distribution of albumin, no matter how tightly the drug is bound to albumin. For a drug that is restricted to the extracellular fluids only ($V_R = 0$) and is not plasma protein bound ($fu = 1$), the apparent volume of distribution is limited to the value of the total extracellular fluid volume, 15 liters. Furthermore, it is apparent from Equations 15 and 16 that the volume of distribution varies linearly with fu whether drug is bound in tissue ($fu_R < 1$; $V_R = 27$ liters) or restricted to extracellular space ($V_R = 0$).

The volume of distribution based on unbound drug, Vu, by definition is V/fu. Thus, from Equation 14

★

$$Vu = \frac{7.5}{fu} + 7.5 + \frac{V_R}{fu_R} \qquad\qquad 17$$

Note that the smallest value of Vu possible is 15 liters, a value expected for a drug that is not bound to plasma proteins ($fu = 1$) or tissue components ($fu_R = 1$) and does not enter cells. If it does readily enter cells ($V_R = 27$ liters), but does not bind anywhere, the unbound volume is that of total body water, 42 liters. Increased binding (fu decreased) to plasma proteins increases the unbound volume of distribution. In contrast, increased binding to plasma proteins decreases the volume of distribution based on the total drug concentration in plasma (Eqs. 14 through 16). These changes in V and Vu with fraction unbound are shown in Figure 25–2 for 3 drugs with normal fu values of 0.01, 0.05, and 0.1.

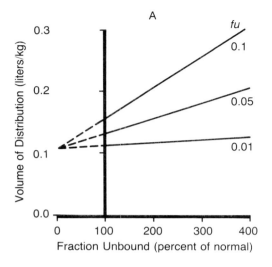

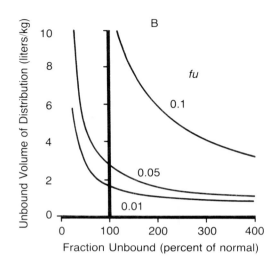

Fig. 25–2. An increase in the fraction unbound in plasma, expressed here as percent of the normal value, has only a minor effect on the (total) volume of distribution (Panel A), but dramatically decreases the unbound volume of distribution (Panel B) for three hypothetical drugs. These drugs bind only to albumin ($fu_R = 1$), distribute throughout body water, and have normal fractions unbound in plasma of 0.1, 0.05 and 0.01. Note that with this model (Eq. 15) the (total) volume of distribution approaches a limiting value of 0.11 liter/kilogram, the apparent volume of distribution of the binding protein albumin as fu approaches zero. On the other hand, the unbound volume of distribution (Eq. 17) approaches a large value as fu approaches zero.

To illustrate the utility of the proposed model, consider the data in Figure 25–3. Shown is a linear relationship between V and fu for a series of cephalosporins. This dependence might have been explained by the general model, $V = V_p + V_{TW} \cdot fu/fu_T$, assuming fu_T does not vary among the cephalosporins. A major problem would have been noticed here, however. The observed volume intercept when fu approaches zero is 0.11 liter/kilogram (7.3 liters/70 kg), a value

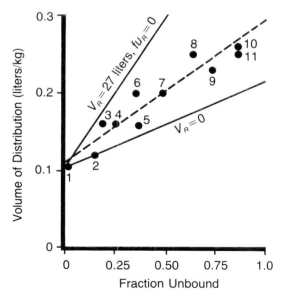

Fig. 25–3. The volumes of distribution of a series of cephalosporin antibiotics increase with the fraction unbound to plasma proteins. The slope of the line of best fit (----) lies between the expected relationships for drugs that do not enter tissue cells, $V_R = 0$ (Eq. 16) and those that do (Eq. 15), but do not bind to tissue components ($fu_R = 1$). The cephalosporins shown are: 1 = cefonicid, 2 = cefazolin, 3 = ceforanide, 4 = cefamandole, 5 = cefotaxitin, 6 = cephalothin, 7 = moxalactam, 8 = cefotaxime, 9 = ceftazidime, 10 = cephalexin, and 11 = cephradine. (Drawn from data compiled by Dudley, M.N. and Nightingale, C.H.: Effects of protein upon activity of cephalosporins: New beta-lactam antibiotics: A review from chemistry to clinical efficacy of the new cephalosporins. Edited by H.C. Neu, Philadelphia, Francis Clark Wood Institute for the History of Medicine, College of Physicians of Philadelphia, 1982, pp. 227–239.)

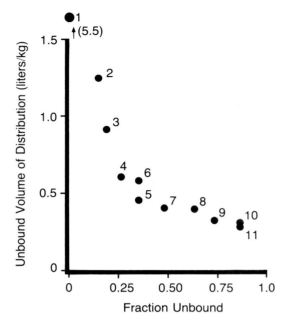

Fig. 25–4. The unbound volumes of distribution of the same cephalosporins shown in Figure 25–3 decrease dramatically with an increase in the fraction unbound. For those cephalosporins with unbound volumes much greater than the extracellular space (V_E = 0.22 liter/kg) or the total body water (0.6 liter/kg), binding to plasma proteins clearly reduces the concentration of the active form for a given dose. (See Figure 25–3 for identification of the cephalosporins and the source of the information.)

much larger than the plasma volume, V_p, of 3 liters. The observations are much better explained by the proposed model. The discrepancy between the two models lies in the distribution of the plasma protein. The proposed model suggests that albumin is the major binding protein for these antibiotics in that those cephalosporins that are tightly bound have distribution characteristics in common with albumin.

The volumes of distribution of the cephalosporins at higher fractions unbound, however, indicate that the drugs must partially enter cells or be bound to some extravascular structures. The extent of this distribution outside the extracellular fluids, on average, must be relatively small in that by extrapolation to $fu = 1$, corresponding to a cephalosporin with no binding to plasma albumin, the volume is 0.29 liter/kilogram (20 liters/70 kg), a value greater than the extracellular volume (15 liters/70 kg), but considerably less than total body water (42 liters/70 kg).

The unbound volumes of distribution within the series of cephalosporins (Fig. 25–4), in contrast to the total volume of distribution, dramatically decrease as the fraction unbound is increased. For those cephalosporins that are highly bound (low fu) the binding protein effectively ties up the drug. The consequence of plasma protein binding here is that a much larger amount of drug must be in the body to give the same antimicrobial effect for those drugs with the same minimum inhibitory unbound concentration.

MODEL APPLICATIONS

The real virtue of this model is in its providing a means of analyzing the distribution of a drug and the plasma protein to which it binds. Representative drugs with volumes of distribution less than 0.2 liter/kilogram and to which this model is potentially applicable are given in Table 25–3.

Table 25–3. Representative Drugs with Volumes of Distribution less than 0.2 liter/kilogram[a]

Acetylsalicylic Acid	Clofibric Acid	Phenylbutazone
Carbenicillin	Dicloxacillin	Piperacillin
Cefamandole	Diflunisal	Probenecid
Cefazolin	Flurbiprofen	Salicylic Acid
Cefonicid	Furosemide	Sulfisoxazole
Ceforanide	Ibuprofen	Tolbutamide
Cefotaxitin	Ketoprofen	Tolmetin
Chlorothiazide	Naproxen	Valproic Acid
Chlorpropamide	Oxyphenbutazone	Warfarin

[a]Binding to albumin is assumed.

Table 25–4. Examples of Conditions in Which the Plasma Concentration of the Two Major Plasma Proteins to Which Drugs Bind are Altered

Plasma Protein	Condition	Change in Concentration of Plasma Protein
Albumin	Cirrhosis	Decrease
	Burn	Decrease
	Nephrotic Syndrome	Decrease
	End-stage Renal Disease	Decrease
	Pregnancy	Decrease
α_1-Acid Glycoprotein	Myocardial Infarction	Increase
	Surgery	Increase
	Crohn's Disease	Increase
	Trauma	Increase
	Rheumatoid Arthritis	Increase

Location of Drug in Body

The fractions of drug in the body that are in plasma (bound and unbound), in or outside extracellular fluids, and bound in plasma or throughout extracellular fluids can be useful pieces of information, particularly with those conditions, examples listed in Table 25–4, in which there are changes in the distribution of plasma proteins. Relationships to calculate these values are given in Table 25–5. The way in which they are derived follows.

The fraction of drug in plasma is simply

$$\text{Fraction in plasma} = \frac{V_P}{V} \qquad 18$$

a relationship previously given (Eq. 8, Chap. 10).

Table 25–5. Relationships and their Approximations for Analyzing Drug Distribution

Fraction of Drug in Body	Relationships	Approximation[a]
In plasma	V_P/V	$3/V$
Unbound in body water	$\dfrac{V_{bw} \cdot fu}{V}$	$\dfrac{42 \cdot fu}{V}$
Unbound in extracellular fluids	$\dfrac{(V_P + V_E) \cdot fu}{V}$	$\dfrac{15 \cdot fu}{V}$
In extracellular fluids	$\dfrac{V_P(1 + R_{Ell}) + fu(V_E - V_P \cdot R_{Ell})}{V}$	$\dfrac{7.5(1 + fu)}{V}$
Outside extracellular fluids	$\dfrac{V - V_P(1 + R_{Ell}) - fu(V_E - V_P \cdot R_{Ell})}{V}$	$\dfrac{V - 7.5(1 + fu)}{V}$
Bound to proteins in plasma	$\dfrac{V_P \cdot (1 - fu)}{V}$	$\dfrac{3(1 - fu)}{V}$
Bound to extracellular proteins	$\dfrac{V_P}{V}(1 - fu)(1 + R_{Ell})$	$\dfrac{7.5(1 - fu)}{V}$
Bound outside the extracellular fluids	$\dfrac{V - V_{bw} \cdot fu - V_P(1 - fu)(1 + R_{Ell})}{V}$	$\dfrac{V - 35 \cdot fu - 7.5}{V}$

[a]Applies to drugs that bind to albumin; assumes that V_P, V_E, and V_R are 3, 12, and 27 liters, respectively; and R_{Ell} equals 1.5.

The fraction of drug in the body unbound in the total body water, V_{bw}, is

$$\frac{(V_P + V_E + V_R)Cu}{V \cdot C} = \frac{V_{bw} \cdot fu}{V} \qquad 19$$

and the fraction of drug unbound in extracellular fluids is

$$\text{Fraction unbound in extracellular fluids} = \frac{(V_P + V_E)}{V} \cdot fu \qquad 20$$

Since

$$
\begin{array}{ccccc}
\text{Amount bound} \\
\text{to extracellular} & = & V \cdot C & - (V_P + V_E)Cu & - V_R \cdot C_R \\
\text{protein} \\
& & \begin{array}{c}\text{Amount} \\ \text{in body}\end{array} & \begin{array}{c}\text{Amount} \\ \text{unbound in} \\ \text{extracellular} \\ \text{fluids}\end{array} & \begin{array}{c}\text{Amount in} \\ \text{remainder} \\ \text{of body}\end{array}
\end{array} \qquad 21
$$

it follows that

$$\begin{array}{c}\text{Fraction of drug in body} \\ \text{bound to extracellular protein}\end{array} = \frac{V \cdot C - (V_P + V_E)Cu - V_R \cdot C_R}{V \cdot C} \qquad 22$$

Knowing that $V_R \cdot C_R = V_R \cdot fu \cdot C/fu_R$, solving Equation 3 for $V_R \cdot C_R$, and substituting these relationships and Equation 11 into Equation 22 gives

$$\text{Fraction bound to extracellular protein} = \frac{V_P(1 - fu)(1 + R_{E/I})}{V} \qquad 23$$

The fraction of drug bound outside the extracellular fluids is 1 minus the sum of the fractions of drug in the total body water (Eq. 19) and bound to extracellular proteins (Eq. 23). That is,

$$\text{Fraction bound outside extracellular fluids} = \frac{V - V_{bw} \cdot fu - V_P(1 - fu)(1 + R_{E/I})}{V} \qquad 24$$

Similar relationships for the fractions inside and outside the extracellular fluids can be derived; they too are listed in Table 25–5.

The relationships summarized in Table 25–5 have a potential utility in identifying, analyzing, and predicting alterations in the apparent volume of distribution of any drug when there is an alteration either in the unbound fraction in plasma or in the unbound fraction outside the extracellular fluids, or when there is a change in the extravascular/intravascular distribution ratio of the binding protein as occurs, for example, in severe burns, after surgery or trauma, in the nephrotic syndrome, and in pregnancy.

Distribution of Protein

When virtually all the drug in the body is bound to a single plasma protein, the apparent volume of distribution of the drug is identical with the apparent volume of distribution of that binding protein. In this situation, Equation 13 simplifies to

★

$$V = V_P(1 + R_{E/I}) \qquad 25$$

If V_P is known or is measured, the value of $R_{E/I}$ can be calculated.

The principles above for distribution of drug and its binding protein may also be applied to other plasma proteins. α_1-Acid glycoprotein, the protein that binds many basic drugs, appears to have an extravascular/intravascular distribution ratio that is the inverse of that of albumin, that is, its value of $R_{E/I}$ is about 0.7 rather than 1.5.

CONSEQUENCES OF LOW VOLUME OF DISTRIBUTION

When the apparent volume of distribution of a drug is large (greater than 50 to 100 liters), the terms $V_P(1 + R_{E/I})$ and $fu(V_E - V_P \cdot R_{E/I})$ in Equation 13 negligibly contribute since the largest possible value of the sum of these terms is 15 liters. The apparent volume of distribution is then approximately

$$V \approx V_R \cdot \frac{fu}{fu_R} \qquad 26$$

which is virtually the same as that predicted by Equation 2. The major area of practical application of the model developed in this chapter, however, is for drugs with small volumes of distribution, that is, with values approaching 7.5

liters/70 kilogram for drug bound to albumin. This utility is demonstrated by the data on clofibric acid shown in Table 25–6.

The half-life of clofibric acid (the active material formed by hydrolysis of the administered ethyl ester, clofibrate) shortens from the usual 16.5 hours to 8.7 hours in patients with the nephrotic syndrome. It is tempting to conclude that metabolism (only 6 percent of clofibric acid is excreted unchanged) had somehow been induced and that dosage requirements may need to be increased in these patients. From a pharmacokinetic point of view, these conclusions are incorrect, as the following shows.

In the nephrotic syndrome there is an extensive loss of plasma proteins into the urine, which results in a twofold drop in serum albumin, as shown in Table 25–6. The influence of this drop in serum albumin on fu can be estimated from rearrangement of Equation 19 (Chap. 10), that is, $Ka = (1 - fu)/(fu \cdot fu_P \cdot P_t)$. The normal serum albumin concentration reported is 4.3 grams/deciliter and for clofibric acid fu is 0.03. Assuming that fu_P, the fraction of available binding sites unoccupied, is equal to 1, the value of Ka is 7.5 deciliters/gram. At a serum albumin concentration of 2.3 grams/deciliter, the calculated fraction unbound in nephrotic patients is then

$$fu = \frac{1}{1 + 7.5 \times 2.3} = 0.055$$

Clofibric acid has a low extraction ratio in that its clearance (calculated from $k \cdot V$) is 0.32 liter/hour in normal patients; a value much smaller than hepatic blood flow, 81 liters/hour. Although one might argue that blood clearance is much larger than plasma clearance (also $C/C_b > 1$), this is impossible. Virtually all the drug in the body is bound to albumin ($V = 0.11$ liter/kg). Thus, the plasma drug concentration can only be greater than the blood drug concentration by a factor of 1.7 [$1/(1 - \text{hematocrit})$; see Appendix E].

With clofibric acid being a low extraction ratio drug, clearance is expected to increase in nephrotic patients. The value of unbound clearance, CL/fu, is 10.7 liters/hour in normal patients. If one assumes the same unbound clearance in nephrotic patients, then clearance, $fu \cdot CLu$, in this group is 0.59 liter/hour.

Table 25–6.   Renal Function Measures, Serum Albumin, Daily Protein Excretion, and Half-life of the Active Form of Clofibrate, Clofibric Acid, in Patients With and Without the Nephrotic Syndrome[a]

	Serum Creatinine (mg/deciliter)[b]	Creatinine Clearance (ml/minute)	Serum Albumin (grams/deciliter)	Clofibric Acid Half-life (hours)	Protein Excretion (grams/day)
Nephrotic group (N = 5)	1.3 ± 0.1	100 ± 24	2.3 ± 0.5	8.7 ± 3.5	13 ± 12
Control group (N = 8)[c]	1.2 ± 0.2	98 ± 20	4.4 ± 0.4	16.5 ± 4.7	0

[a]From Goldberg, A.P., Sherrard, D.J., Haas, L.B., and Brunzell, J.D.: Control of clofibrate toxicity in uremic hypertriglyceridemia. Clin. Pharmacol. Ther., 21:317–325, 1977.

[b]One milligram/deciliter = 88 micromolar.

[c]In healthy subjects, the volume of distribution of clofibric acid is 0.11 liter/kilogram, the fraction unbound in plasma is 0.03, and the fraction excreted unchanged is 0.06. (Data from Appendix II, The Pharmacologic Basis of Therapeutics. 7th ed., Edited by A.G. Gilman, L.S. Goodman, T.W. Rall, and F. Murad, New York, Macmillan Publishing, 1985.)

The volume of distribution of clofibric acid, given in Table 25–6, is 7.7 liters/ 70 kilograms. This value depends little on changes in plasma protein binding (Fig. 25–2A); therefore, Equation 14 can be rearranged and expressed as

$$V = 7.5 + \text{Constant} \cdot fu$$

With an apparent volume of 7.7 liters, the constant is 6.7. If fu is increased to 0.055, then the apparent volume becomes 7.9 liters. The volume unbound (V/fu), however, decreases from 257 to 143 liters. The calculated half-life ($0.693 \cdot V/CL$ or $0.693 \cdot Vu/CLu$) in the nephrotic patients is then about 9.3 hours, a value very close to that observed, 8.7 hours.

The two questions originally posed are now answered. The half-life is shortened in the nephrotic patients because of decreased binding to albumin. The metabolism was not induced. The unbound clearance was not changed, and therefore no change in the usual dosing rate of 1.5 to 2.0 grams/day is needed in nephrotic patients to produce the same average unbound concentration in plasma as achieved in patients with normal serum albumin values. A shorter dosing interval (and correspondingly smaller maintenance dose) might be considered because of the shortened half-life.

Study Problems

(Answers to Study Problems are given in Appendix G.)

1. (a) Given the information in Table 25–7, complete Table 25–8 by replacing dashes.

   (b) For which one of the drugs in Table 25–7 would a twofold increase in the fraction unbound in plasma give the greatest (percent) change in the apparent volume of distribution?

Table 25–7. Distribution Parameters of Selected Drugs[a]

Drug	Volume of Distribution (liters/kg)[b]	Fraction Unbound in Plasma
Valproic Acid	0.13	0.07
Nitrazepam	1.9	0.13
Chlordiazepoxide	0.30	0.035

[a]Appendix II, The Pharmacological Basis of Therapeutics, 7th ed., Edited by A.G. Gilman, L.S. Goodman, T.W. Rall, and F. Murad. New York, Macmillan Publishing, 1985.
[b]Assume unbound drug distributes evenly throughout total body water and albumin is the only protein to which the drugs bind in plasma. The extravascular/intravascular distribution ratio of albumin is 1.5.

Table 25–8. Analysis of the Distribution of Valproic Acid, Nitrazepam, and Chlordiazepoxide[a]

Fraction of Drug in Body	Valproic Acid	Nitrazepam	Chlordiazepoxide
Unbound	0.32	0.04	–
In extracellular fluids	–	0.06	0.37
Outside extracellular fluids	0.12	–	0.63
Bound to protein in plasma	0.31	0.02	–
Bound to plasma protein in extracellular fluids	–	0.05	0.34
Bound intracellularly (in or on tissue cells, including blood cells)	–	–	0.58

[a]Assumes a 70-kilogram person.

2. What effect would a shift of albumin, intravascular to extravascular (as occurs in pregnancy and burns), have on the volume of distribution of nitrazepam? Assume the serum albumin drops from 4.3 grams/deciliter (normal) to 3.2 grams/deciliter and the value of $R_{E/I}$ increases from 1.5 to 2.6. Also assume the drug occupies only a small fraction of available binding sites and intracellular binding is unaffected by the shift of albumin.

3. The information contained in Table 25–9 summarizes the effect of acute viral hepatitis on the disposition of tolbutamide, a drug that is eliminated by hepatic metabolism.

Table 25–9[a]. Effect of Acute Viral Hepatitis on Tolbutamide Disposition

Subjects	Half-life (hours)	Volume of Distribution (liters/kg)	Clearance (ml/hour per kg)	Fraction of Drug in Plasma Unbound
Healthy	5.8	0.15	18	0.06
Acute viral hepatitis	4.0	0.15	26	0.10

[a]From Williams, R.L., Blaschke, T.F., Meffin, P.J., Melmon, K.L., and Rowland, M.: Clin. Pharmacol. Ther., 21: 301–309, 1977.

Explain the apparent differences in tolbutamide disposition between these two groups. What is the cause of the shorter half-life in the subjects with acute viral hepatitis?

DEFINITIONS OF SYMBOLS*

A Amount of drug in body, milligrams or micromoles.

Aa Amount of drug at absorption site remaining to be absorbed, milligrams or micromoles.

Ae Cumulative amount of drug excreted unchanged in the urine, milligrams or micromoles.

$Ae_{\tau,ss}$ Cumulative amount of drug excreted unchanged in the urine during a dosing interval at steady state, milligrams or micromoles.

Ae_∞ Cumulative amount of drug excreted unchanged in the urine to time infinity after a single dose, milligrams or micromoles.

$A(m)$ Amount of metabolite in body, milligrams or micromoles.

A_{min} The minimum amount of drug in body required to obtain a predetermined level of response, milligrams or micromoles.

$A_{N,max}$; $A_{N,min}$ Maximum and minimum amounts of drug in body after the Nth dose of fixed size and given at a fixed dosing interval, milligrams or micromoles.

$A_{N,t}$ Amount of drug in body at time t after the Nth dose, milligrams or micromoles.

ARE Amount of drug remaining to be excreted in urine after a single dose, milligrams or micromoles.

A_{ss} Amount of drug in body at steady state during constant-rate intravenous infusion, milligrams or micromoles.

$A_{ss,av}$ Average amount of drug in body during a dosing interval at steady state, milligrams or micromoles.

$A_{ss,max}$; $A_{ss,min}$ Maximum and minimum amounts of drug in body during a dosing interval at steady state on administering a fixed dose at a fixed dosing interval, milligrams or micromoles.

$A_{ss,t}$ Amount of drug in body at time t within a dosing interval at steady state on administering a fixed dose at a fixed dosing interval, milligrams or micromoles.

AUC Total area under the plasma drug concentration-time curve, milligram-hours/liter or micromolar-hour.

AUC_b Total area under the blood drug concentration time curve, milligram-hours/liter or micromolar-hour.

$AUMC$ Total area under the first moment-time curve, milligram-hours^2/liter or micromolar-hours^2.

C Concentration of drug in plasma, milligrams/liter or micromolar.

C_1; C_2 Coefficients with units of concentration, milligrams/liter or micromolar.

Ca Concentration of drug in fluids at the absorption site, milligrams/liter or micromolar.

C_A Concentration of drug in arterial blood, milligrams/liter or micromolar.

C_b Concentration of drug in blood, milligrams/liter or micromolar.

*Usual units are given.

451

C_{bd} Concentration of bound drug in plasma, milligrams/liter or micromolar.

C_I Concentration of inhibitor of metabolism, milligrams/liter or micromolar.

CL Total clearance of drug from plasma, liters/hour.

CL_b Total clearance of drug from blood, liters/hour.

CL_{bD} Dialysis clearance based on drug concentration in blood, liters/hour.

$CL_{b,H}$ Hepatic clearance of drug from blood, liters/hour.

CL_{cr} Renal clearance of creatinine, milliliters/minute or liters/hour.

CL_D Dialysis clearance based on drug concentration in plasma, liters/hour.

CL_f Clearance associated with formation of a metabolite from a drug, liters/hour.

CL_H Hepatic clearance of drug from plasma, liters/hour.

CL_{int} Intrinsic clearance of drug in organ of elimination, liters/hour.

$CL(m)$ Total clearance of a metabolite, liters/hour.

CL_{PD} Peritoneal dialysis clearance based on drug concentration in plasma, liters/hour.

CL_R Renal clearance of drug, liters/hour.

CLu Clearance of unbound drug, liters/hour.

$C(m)$ Concentration of metabolite in plasma, milligrams/liter or micromolar.

$C(m)_{ss}$ Concentration of a metabolite at steady state during a constant-rate intravenous infusion of drug, milligrams/liter or micromolar.

C_{min} Minimum concentration required to obtain a predetermined intensity of response, milligrams/liter or micromolar.

$C_{N,max}$; $C_{N,min}$ Maximum and minimum concentrations of drug in plasma after the Nth dose on administering a fixed dose at equal dosing intervals, milligrams/liter or micromolar.

C_{PC} Concentration of drug in peritoneal cavity, milligrams/liter or micromolar.

C_{ss} Concentration of drug in plasma at steady state during a constant-rate intravenous infusion, milligrams/liter or micromolar.

$C_{ss,av}$ Average drug concentration in plasma during a dosing interval at steady state on administering a fixed dose at equal dosing intervals, milligrams/liter or micromolar.

$C_{ss,max}$; $C_{ss,min}$ Maximum and minimum concentrations of drug in plasma at steady state on administering a fixed dose at equal dosing intervals, milligrams/liter or micromolar.

C_T Average concentration of drug in fluids outside plasma, milligrams/liter or micromolar.

C_{upper}; C_{lower} Maximum and minimum plasma drug concentrations desired, milligrams/liter or micromolar.

Cu Unbound drug concentration in plasma leaving an organ, milligrams/liter or micromolar.

C_V Concentration of drug in venous blood, milligrams/liter or micromolar.

D_L Loading dose, milligrams or micromoles.

D_M Maintenance dose of a fixed-dose regimen, milligrams or micromoles.

$D_{M,max}$ Maximum maintenance dose to ensure that the plasma drug concentration remains within C_{upper} and C_{lower} limits during a dosing interval at steady state, milligrams or micromoles.

E Extraction ratio, no units.

EC_{50} Concentration giving one-half the maximum effect, milligrams/liter or micromolar.

E_H Hepatic extraction ratio, no units.

E_{max} Maximum effect, units of response measurement.

E_R Renal extraction ratio, no units.

F Availability of drug, no units.

f_{bd} Ratio of bound to total drug concentrations in plasma, no units.

f_D Dialysis clearance as a fraction of total clearance during a dialysis treatment, no units.

fe Fraction of drug systemically available that is excreted unchanged in urine, no units.

F_H Fraction of drug entering the liver that escapes elimination in that organ, no units.

fm Fraction of drug systemically available that is converted to a metabolite, no units.

Fm Fraction of administered dose of drug that enters the general circulation as a metabolite, no units.

fu Ratio of unbound and total drug concentrations in plasma, no units.

fu_b Ratio of unbound concentration in plasma and total drug concentration in blood, no units.

fu_P Ratio of unbound and total sites available for binding on a plasma protein, no units.

fu_T Ratio of unbound and total drug concentrations in tissues (outside plasma), no units.

γ Shape factor in concentration-response relationship, no units.

GFR Glomerular filtration rate, milliliters/minute or liters/hour.

k Elimination rate constant, hour^{-1}.

Ka Association constant for the binding of drug to protein, liters/mole.

ka Absorption rate constant, hour^{-1}.

k_D Elimination rate constant while a patient is on dialysis, hour^{-1}.

ke Urinary excretion rate constant, hour^{-1}.

k_f Rate constant associated with the formation of a metabolite, hour^{-1}.

K_I Inhibition equilibrium constant, milligrams/liter or micromolar.

$k(m)$ Rate constant for the elimination of a metabolite, hour^{-1}.

Km Michaelis-Menten constant, milligrams/liter, micromolar.

Kp Equilibrium distribution ratio of drug between tissue and blood or plasma, no units.

k_T Fractional rate at which drug leaves tissue, hour^{-1}.

k_t Fractional turnover rate, hour^{-1}.

$\lambda_1; \lambda_2$ Exponential coefficients, hour^{-1}.

MRT Mean time a molecule resides in body, hours.

n A unitless number.

N Number of doses, no units.

P Concentration of binding sites on a protein that are unoccupied by drug, micromolar.

P_t Total concentration of sites on a protein available for binding drug, micromolar.

Q Blood flow, liters/minute or liters/hour.

Q_H Hepatic blood flow (portal vein plus hepatic artery), liters/minute or liters/hour.

R_{ac} Accumulation ratio (index), no units.

Rd Ratio of unbound clearance of an individual patient to that of a typical patient, no units.

RF Renal function in an individual patient as a fraction of renal function in a typical patient, no units.

R_o Rate of constant intravenous infusion, milligrams/hour.

R_t Turnover rate, milligrams/hour.

S Salt form factor, no units.

SA Surface area, square meters.

τ Dosing interval, hours.

τ_{max} Maximum dosing interval to remain within C_{upper} and C_{lower} limits, hours.

t_d Duration of effect, hours.

t_{inf} Duration of a constant-rate infusion, hours.

Tm Maximum rate of drug transport (secretion) into renal tubule, milligrams/hour.

$t_{1/2}$ Elimination half-life, hours.

t_t Turnover time, hours.

V Volume of distribution (apparent) based on drug concentration in plasma, liters.

V_b Volume of distribution (apparent) based on drug concentration in blood, liters.

V_B Blood volume, liters.

V_D Volume of dialysate solution collected during a hemodialysis treatment, liters.

V_1 Volume of initial dilution compartment, liters.

Vm Maximum rate of metabolism by an enzymatically mediated reaction, milligrams/hour or micromoles/hour.

V_P Plasma volume, liters.

V_T Physiologic volume outside plasma into which drug distributes, liters.

V_{ss} Volume of distribution (apparent) under steady-state conditions based on drug concentration in plasma, liters.

V_{TW} Aqueous volume outside plasma into which drug distributes, liters.

Vu Volume of distribution (apparent) based on unbound drug concentration in plasma, liters.

SELECTED READING

JOURNALS

Reviews and original scientific articles in pharmacokinetics are found frequently in the following journals:

British Journal of Clinical Pharmacology
Clinical Pharmacokinetics
Clinical Pharmacology and Therapeutics
Drug Metabolism and Disposition
European Journal of Clinical Pharmacology
Journal of Pharmaceutical Sciences
Journal of Pharmacokinetics and Biopharmaceutics
Journal of Pharmacology and Experimental Therapeutics
Journal of Pharmacy and Pharmacology
Pharmaceutical Research
Therapeutic Drug Monitoring

BOOKS AND SPECIFIC ARTICLES

Selected references to monographs and journal articles containing material related to topics of this book follow. The references are listed by topic area. Many of the references could be listed in multiple areas, particularly the general ones that survey the field. To avoid repetition, references are listed in only one category even though they may contain material pertinent to several others.

General

Ames, M.M., Powis, G., and Kovach, J.S.: Pharmacokinetics of Anticancer Agents in Humans. Elsevier, New York, 1983.

Benet, L.Z., Massoud, N., and Gambertoglio, J.G.: Pharmacokinetic Basis for Drug Treatment. Raven Press, New York, 1984.

Benet, L.Z., Levy, G., and Ferraiolo, B.L.: Pharmacokinetics: A Modern View. Plenum Press, New York, 1984.

Blanchard, J., Sawchuk, R.J., and Brodie, B.B.: Principles and Perspectives in Drug Bioavailability. S. Karger, Basel, 1979.

Evans, W.E., Schentag, J.J., and Jusko, W.J. (eds.): Applied Pharmacokinetics, 2nd ed. Applied Therapeutics, San Francisco, 1986.

George, C.F. and Shand, D.G. (eds.): Presystemic Drug Elimination. BIMR Clinical Pharmacology and Therapeutics 1. Butterworths, London, 1982.

Gibaldi, M. and Perrier, D.: Pharmacokinetics, 2nd ed. Marcel Dekker, New York, 1982.

Gibaldi, M. and Prescott, L. (eds.): Handbook of Clinical Pharmacokinetics. ADIS Health Science Press, Balgowlah, New Zealand, 1983.

Gibaldi, M.: Biopharmaceutics and Clinical Pharmacokinetics. Lea & Febiger, Philadelphia, 1984.

Levy, R.H. and Shand, D.G.: Clinical implications of drug-protein binding. Proceedings of a symposium. Clin. Pharmacokin., 9:51–104, 1984.

Rowland, M. and Tucker, G. (eds.): Pharmacokinetics: Theory and Methodology. Pergamon Press, Oxford, 1986.

Stanski, D.R. and Watkins, W.D.: Drug Disposition in Anesthesia. Grune & Stratton, New York, 1982.

Vree, T.B. and Hekster, Y.A.: Clinical Pharmacokinetics of Sulfonamides and their Metabolites: An Encyclopedia. S. Karger, Basel, 1987.

Welling, P.G. and Tse, F.L.S.: Pharmacokinetics of Cardiovascular, Central Nervous System, and Antimicrobial Drugs. Royal Society of Chemistry, London, 1985.

Therapeutic Regimens

DeVane, C.L. and Jusko, W.J.: Dosage regimen design. Pharmacol. Ther., 17:143–164, 1982.

Goodman, L.S. and Gilman, A.: The Pharmacological Basis of Therapeutics, 7th ed. Macmillan Publishing, New York, 1985.

Heilmann, K.: Therapeutic Systems. Rate-controlled Drug Delivery: Concept and Development, 2nd revised ed. Georg Thieme Verlag, Stuttgart-New York. Thieme-Stratton, New York, 1983.

Robinson, J.R. (ed.): Sustained and Controlled Release Drug Delivery Systems. In Drugs and the Pharmaceutical Sciences, Vol. 6. Marcel Dekker, New York, 1978.

Theeuwes, F.: Drug delivery systems. Pharmacol. Ther., 13:149–192, 1981.

Physiologic Concepts and Kinetics

Øie, S., Guentert, T.W., and Tozer, T.N.: Effect of saturable binding on the pharmacokinetics of drugs: A simulation. J. Pharm. Pharmacol., 32:471–477, 1980.

Pond, S.M. and Tozer, T.N.: First-pass elimination: Basic concepts and clinical consequences. Clin. Pharmacokin., 9:1–25, 1984.

Steinberg, I. and Zaske, D.E.: Body composition and pharmacokinetics. Rep. Ross Conf. Med. Res., 6:96–102, 1985.

Tillement, J.-P. and Lindenlaud, E. (eds.): Protein Binding and Drug Transport. Symposia Medica Hoechst, 20. F.K. Schattauer Verlag, Stuttgart-New York, 1986.

Tozer, T.N.: Concepts basic to pharmacokinetics. Pharmacol. Ther., 12:109–132, 1981.

Wilkinson, G.R. and Shand, D.G.: Commentary. A physiological approach to hepatic drug clearance. Clin. Pharmacol. Ther., 18:377–390, 1975.

Individualization

General

Beal, S.L. and Sheiner, L.B.: Methodology of Population Pharmacokinetics. In Drug Fate and Metabolism, Vol. 5:135–183. Edited by E.R. Garrett and J.R. Hirtz. Marcel Dekker, New York, 1985.

Breimer, D.D.: Interindividual variations in drug disposition: Clinical implications and methods of investigation. Clin. Pharmacokin., 8:371–377, 1983.

Rowland, M., Sheiner, L.B., and Steimer, J.-L. (eds.): Variability in Drug Therapy. Raven Press, New York, 1985.

Vessell, E.S. and Penno, M.B.: Assessment of methods of interindividual pharmacokinetic variations. Clin. Pharmacokin., 8:378–409, 1983.

Welling, P.G. and Tse, F.L.S.: Factors contributing to variability in drug pharmacokinetics. I. Absorption. J. Clin. Hosp. Pharm., 9:163–179, 1984.

Wilson, K.: Sex-related differences in drug disposition in man. Clin. Pharmacokin., 9:189–202, 1984.

Genetics

Weber, W.: Acetylator Genes and Drug Response. Oxford University Press, New York, 1987.

Kalow, W., Goedde, W.H., and Agarwal, D.P.: Ethnic Differences in Reactions to Drugs and Xenobiotics. Alan R. Liss, New York, 1986.

Age and Weight

Abernethy, D.R. and Greenblatt, D.J.: Drug disposition in obese humans: An update. Clin. Pharmacokin., 11:199–213, 1986.

Wallace, S.M. and Verbeeck, R.K.: Plasma protein binding of drugs in the elderly. Clin. Pharmacokin., 12:41–72, 1987.

Disease

Barre, J., Houin, G., Brunner, F., Bree, F., and Tillement, J.P.: Disease-induced modifications of drug pharmacokinetics. Int. J. Clin. Pharmacol. Res., 3:215–226, 1983.

Brenner, B.M. and Rector, F.C., Jr. (eds.): The Kidney, I and II. 3rd Ed. W.B. Saunders, Philadelphia, 1986.

Williams, R.L., Brater, D.C., and Mordenti, J. (eds.): Drug Administration in Disease States. Marcel Dekker, New York, 1988.

Interacting Drugs

Aarons, L.: Kinetics of drug-drug interactions. Pharmacol. Ther., 14:321–344, 1981.

Hansten, P.D.: Drug Interactions: Clinical Significance of Drug-Drug Interactions. Lea & Febiger, Philadelphia, 1985.

Shinn, A.F. and Shrewsbury, R.P.: American Pharmaceutical Association, Professional Drug Systems. In Evaluations of Drug Interactions, 3rd ed. C.V. Mosby, St. Louis, 1985.

Stockey, I.H.: Drug Interactions: A Source Book of Adverse Interactions, Their Mechanisms, Clinical Importance and Management. Blackwell Scientific, Oxford-Boston, 1981.

Welling, P.G.: Interactions affecting drug absorption. Clin. Pharmacokin., 9:404–434, 1984.

Monitoring

Burton, M.E., Vasko, M.R., and Brater, D.C.: Comparison of drug dosing methods. Clin. Pharmacokin., 10:1–37, 1985.

Gerson, B.: Essentials of Therapeutic Drug Monitoring. Igaku-Shoin, New York, 1983.

Lin, E.T. and Sadee, W.: Drug Level Monitoring: Analytical Techniques, Metabolism and Pharmacokinetics, II. Wiley & Sons, New York, 1986.

Taylor, W. and Finn, A.: Individualizing Drug Therapy: Practical Applications of Drug Monitoring. Gross, Townsend, Frank, New York, 1981.

Winter, M.E.: Basic Clinical Pharmacokinetics, 2nd ed. Applied Therapeutics, Spokane, 1988.

Selected Topics

Distribution Kinetics

Gibaldi, M. and Perrier, D.: Pharmacokinetics, 2nd ed. Marcel Dekker, New York, 1982.

Riddell, J.G.: A new method for constant plasma concentrations: Application to lidocaine. Ann. Int. Med., 100:25–28, 1982.

Pharmacologic Response

Hennis, P.J. and Stanski, D.R.: Pharmacokinetic and Pharmacodynamic Factors that Govern the Clinical Use of Muscle Relaxants. *In* Seminars in Anesthesia, IV:21–30. Edited by R.L. Katz. Grune and Stratton, New York, 1985.

Holford, N.H.G. and Sheiner, L.B.: Understanding the dose-effect relationship: Clinical application of pharmacokinetic-pharmacodynamic models. Clin. Pharmacokin., 6:429–453, 1981.

Holford, N.H.G. and Sheiner, L.B.: Kinetics of pharmacologic response. Pharmacol. Ther., 16:143–166, 1982.

Tallarida, R.J. and Jacob, L.S.: The Dose-Response Relation in Pharmacology. Springer-Verlag, New York, 1979.

Metabolite Kinetics

Garattini, S.: Active drug metabolites: An overview of their relevance in clinical pharmacokinetics. Clin. Pharmacokin., 19:216–227, 1985.

Houston, J.B.: Drug metabolite kinetics. Pharmacol. Ther., 15:521–552, 1981.

Jenner, P. and Testa, B. (eds.): Concepts in Drug Metabolism, Parts A and B. Marcel Dekker, New York, 1980.

Pang, K.S.: A review of metabolite kinetics. J. Pharmacokin. Biopharm., 13:633–662, 1985.

Dose and Time Dependencies

Dayton, P.G. and Sanders, J.E.: Dose-dependent pharmacokinetics: Emphasis on phase I metabolism. Drug Metab. Rev., 14:347–405, 1983.

Labrecque, G. and Belanger, P.M.: Time-dependency in the Pharmacokinetics and Disposition of Drugs. *In* Topics in Pharmaceutical Sciences, Edited by D.D. Breimer and P. Speiser. Elsevier, Amsterdam, 1985, pp. 167–178.

Levy, R.: Mechanistic Aspects of Time Dependent Phenomena in Pharmacokinetics. *In* Topics in Pharmaceutical Sciences, Edited by D.D. Breimer and P. Speiser. Elsevier, Amsterdam, 1985, pp. 167–178.

Van Rossum, J.M., Van Lingen, G., and Burgers, J.P.T.: Dose-dependent pharmacokinetics. Pharmacol. Ther., 21:77–100, 1983.

Turnover Concepts

Rescigno, A. and Segre, G.: Turnover. Chap. 5. *In* Drug and Tracer Kinetics. Blaisdell, Waltham, MA, 1966.

Shipley, R.A. and Clark, R.E.: Tracer Methods for In Vivo Kinetics: Theory and Applications. Academic Press, New York, 1972.

Dialysis

Bennett, W.M., Aronoff, G.R., Morrison, G., Golper, T.A., Pulliam, J., Wolfson, M., and Singer, I.: Drug prescribing in renal failure: Dosing guidelines for adults. Am. J. Kid. Dis., 3:155–191, 1983.

Gokal, R.: Continuous Ambulatory Peritoneal Dialysis. Churchill Livingstone, Edinburgh, 1986.

Gotch, F.A.: Kinetics of hemodialysis. Art. Org., 10:272–281, 1986.

APPENDIX A

Assessment of Area

Several methods exist for measuring the area under a concentration-time curve. One method, to be discussed here, is the simple numeric estimation of area by the *trapezoidal rule*. The advantage of this method is that it only requires a simple extension of a table of experimental data. Other methods involve either greater numeric complexity or the fitting of an equation to the observations and then calculating the area by integrating the fitted equation.

General Case: Consider the blood concentration-time data, first two columns of Table A–1, obtained following the oral administration of 50 milligrams of a drug. What is the total area under the curve?

Figure A–1 is a plot of the concentration against time after drug administration. If a perpendicular line is drawn from the concentration at 1 hour (7 mg/liter) down to the time-axis, then the area bounded between zero time and 1 hour is a trapezoid whose area is given by the product of the average concentration and the time interval. The average concentration is obtained by adding the concentration at the beginning and end of the time interval and dividing by 2. Since, in the first interval, the respective concentrations are 0 and 7 milligrams/liter and the time interval is 1 hour, it follows that:

$$\text{Area}_1 \quad = \quad \frac{0 + 7}{2} \text{ milligrams/liter} \quad \times \quad 1 \text{ hour}$$

| Area of trapezoid within the first time interval | Average concentration over the first interval | First time interval |

or,

$$\text{Area}_1 = 3.5 \text{ milligrams-hours/liter}$$

Table A–1. Calculation of the Total Area Using the Trapezoidal Rule

Time (hours)	Blood Concentration (mg/liter)	Time Interval (hours)	Average Concentration (mg/liter)	Area (mg · hours/liter)
0	0	–	–	–
1	7	1	3.5	3.5
2	10	1	8.5	8.5
3	5	1	7.5	7.5
4	2.5	1	3.75	3.75
5	1.25	1	1.88	1.88
6	0.6	1	0.93	0.93
7	0.2	1	0.4	0.4
8	0	1	0.1	0.1
			Total Area =	26.60

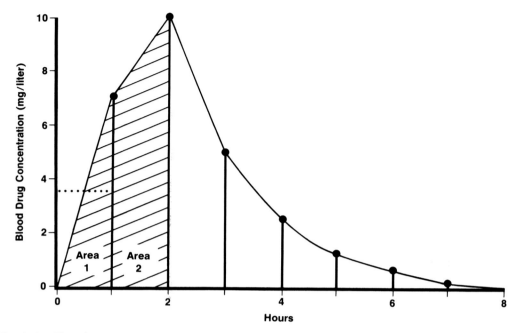

Fig. A–1. Plot of concentration-time data of Table A–1. The dotted line is the average concentration in the first interval.

In this example, the concentration at zero time is 0. Had the drug been given as an intravenous bolus, the concentration at zero time might have been the extrapolated value, C(0).

The area under each time interval can be obtained in an analogous manner to that outlined above. The total area under the concentration-time curve over all times is then simply given by

Total area = Sum of the individual areas

Usually, *total* area means the area under the curve from zero time to infinity. In practice, infinite time is taken as the time beyond which the area is insignificant.

The calculations used to obtain the total area under the curve, displayed in Figure A–1, are shown in Table A–1. In this example the total area is 26.6 milligrams × hours/liter.

SPECIAL CASE

An Intravenous Bolus. When a drug is given as an intravenous bolus and the decline is monoexponential, the total area under the curve is calculated most rapidly by dividing the extrapolated zero-time concentration (C(0)) by the elimination rate constant (k). For example, if C(0) is 100 milligrams/liter and k is 0.1 hour^{-1}, then the total area is 1000 milligrams-hours/liter.

Proof: The total area under the curve is given by

$$\text{Total area} = \int_0^{\infty} C \cdot dt \qquad \qquad 1$$

But $C = C(0) \cdot e^{-kt}$, and since $C(0)$ is a constant it follows that

$$\text{Total area} = C(0) \int_0^{\infty} e^{-kt} \cdot dt \qquad \qquad 2$$

which on integrating between time zero and infinity yields

$$\text{Total area} = \frac{C(0)}{-k} \left[e^{-kt} \right]_0^{\infty} = \frac{C(0)}{-k} [0 - 1] = \frac{C(0)}{k} \qquad \qquad 3$$

When Decline Is Logarithmic. The numeric method used to calculate area by the trapezoid rule assumes a linear relationship between observations. Frequently, especially during the decline of drug concentration, the fall is exponential. Then a more accurate method for calculating area during the decline can be used, the *log trapezoidal rule*, as follows.

Consider, for example, two consecutive observations $C(t_i)$ and $C(t_{i+1})$ at times t_i and t_{i+1}, respectively. These observations are related to each other by

$$C(t_{i+1}) = C(t_i) \cdot e^{-k_i \cdot \Delta t_i} \qquad \qquad 4$$

where k_i is the rate constant that permits the concentration to fall exponentially from $C(t_i)$ to $C(t_{i+1})$ in the time interval $t_{i+1} - t_i$, that is, Δt_i. The value of k_i is given by taking the logarithm on both sides of Equation 4 and rearranging, so that

$$k_i = \frac{\log[C(t_i)/C(t_{i+1})]}{\Delta t_i} \qquad \qquad 5$$

Now the area during the time interval Δt_i, Area_i, is the difference between the total areas from t_i to ∞ and from t_{i+1} to ∞, respectively. It therefore follows from events after an intravenous bolus that

$$\text{Area}_i = \frac{C(t_i) - C(t_{i+1})}{k_i} \qquad \qquad 6$$

and, by appropriately substituting for k_i in Equation 6, one obtains

$$\text{Area}_i = \frac{[C(t_i) - C(t_{i+1})] \cdot \Delta t_i}{\log[C(t_i)/C(t_{i+1})]} \qquad \qquad 7$$

This calculation is then repeated for all observations that lie beyond the peak concentration.

In practice, a significant discrepancy arises between the method above and that using the trapezoidal rule only when consecutive observations differ by more than twofold.

Study Problems

1. The following data (Table A–2) were obtained following the ingestion of 50 milligrams of a drug.

Table A–2.

Time (hours)	0	0.5	1	1.5	2	3	4	6	8	12
Plasma concentration (mg/liter)	0	0.38	0.6	0.73	0.85	0.95	0.94	0.87	0.66	0.37

Estimate the total area under the concentration-time curve. It should be noted that the last sample was taken before the concentration had fallen to an insignificant value. (Hint: To estimate the area beyond the last observation, imagine that this last measurement was the zero-time concentration following an intravenous bolus and that the disposition kinetics of the drug does not change beyond the last observation.)

2. The set of data displayed in Figure A–1 is unusual in that the time between collection of blood samples is constant; in this case, 1 hour. Prove in this special case that

$$\text{Total area} = \frac{\text{Time}}{\text{interval}} \left[\left(\frac{\text{First} + \text{last concentrations}}{2} \right) + \left(\begin{array}{c} \text{Sum of all other} \\ \text{concentrations} \end{array} \right) \right]$$

Use the data in Table A–1 to confirm that this simple method works satisfactorily.

3. The concentration of a drug declines exponentially according to the equation $C(\text{mg/liter}) = 64\, e^{-0.1733t}$ (t in hours). Complete Table A–3 to show the errors, if any, in each of the area calculations over the interval given.

Table A–3.

Time Interval (hours)	Area Within Time Interval		
	Calculated area	Trapezoidal rule	Log trapezoidal rule
	$\dfrac{(64 - C(t))}{k}$		
0–2			
0–4			
0–8			
0–12			

Answers to Study Problems

1. *10.93 milligram-hours/liter.* Using the trapezoidal rule, the area up to 12 hours is 8.21 milligram-hours/liter. The elimination rate constant, obtained from a semilogarithmic plot of the concentration-time data, is 0.136 hour⁻¹. Assuming that the last concentration (0.37 mg/liter) is the zero-time concentration following an intravenous bolus dose, the area beyond this last observation ($C(0)/k$) is 2.72 milligram-hours/liter.

2. Consider a set of n concentration-time values. Let $C(0)$, $C(t_1)$, $C(t_{n-1})$ and $C(t_n)$ be the concentrations at zero time, the first time, the $(n-1)$th time, and the nth time, respectively. Let Δt be the constant interval of time. Using the trapezoidal rule, the total area under the curve is given by

$$\text{Total area} = \text{area}_1 + \text{area}_2 + \ldots \text{area}_{n-1} + \text{area}_n$$

or

$$\text{Total area} = \Delta t \left[\frac{C(0) + C(t_1)}{2} \right] + \Delta t \left[\frac{C(t_1) + C(t_2)}{2} \right] \ldots$$
$$+ \Delta t \left[\frac{C(t_{n-2}) + C(t_{n-1})}{2} \right] + \Delta t \left[\frac{C(t_{n-1}) + C(t_n)}{2} \right]$$

which on expansion and collection of terms reduces to

$$\text{Total area} = \Delta t \left[\frac{C(0)}{2} + C(t_1) + C(t_2) + \ldots C(t_{n-1}) + \frac{C(t_n)}{2} \right]$$

or

$$\text{Total area} = \Delta t \left[\frac{C(0) + C(t_n)}{2} + C(t_1) + C(t_2) + \ldots C(t_{n-1}) \right]$$

3. The completed Table A–3 should list the following values:

Table A–3.

Time Interval (hours)	Area Within Time Interval[a]		
	(calculated area) $(64 - C(t))$ k	(trapezoidal rule)	(log trapezoidal rule)
0–2	108	109	108
0–4	185	192	185
0–8	277	320	277
0–12	323	432	323

[a]Note that up to an interval equal to the half-life, 4 hours, both numeric methods are reasonably accurate. By 3 half-lives the trapezoidal rule is 134 percent of the actual value.

APPENDIX B

Estimation of the Elimination Half-life from Urine Data

Consider the urine data in Table B–1, obtained following a 50-milligram intravenous bolus dose of a drug. These are the same data as presented in Table 3–1. The observations are times of urine collection, volumes collected, and concentrations of unchanged drug in each sample. These data are treated to derive further information. Especially of interest are the rate and the cumulative amount excreted. The amount excreted in each time interval is the product of the volume of urine collected and the concentration, e.g., the amount in Sample 1 is 120 milliliters times 133 micrograms/milliliter or 16 milligrams; therefore, the average rate of excretion over the first 2-hour period is 8 milligrams/hour. The cumulative amount excreted up to any time is the sum of all drug excreted up to that time. By 24 hours, the cumulative amount excreted is 39.1 milligrams, and since 37.2 milligrams was excreted in the first 12 hours and only another 1.9 milligrams was excreted over the next 12 hours, 39.1 milligrams can reasonably be taken to be the maximum amount of drug that will be excreted.

Excretion rate data are occasionally displayed as a bar histogram, but this form of presentation is not as useful as one in which the rate data are plotted against the midpoint of the collection interval on semilogarithmic paper (Fig. B–1). The time for the excretion rate to fall in half (e.g., from 5 mg/hour to 2.5 mg/hour) is the elimination half-life of the drug (2.8 hours). The reason for using midpoint time was given in Chapter 3, namely, the measured urinary excretion rate reflects the average plasma concentration during the collection interval.

Formal proof of the observation of elimination half-life is not difficult to derive.

Table B–1. Urine Data Obtained Following an Intravenous Bolus Dose of Drug

	Observation			Treatment of Data			
Sample	Time of Collection (hours)	Volume of Urine (ml)	Concentration of Unchanged Drug in Urine (micrograms/ml)	Amount Excreted in Time Interval (mg)	Excretion Rate (mg/hour)	Cumulative Amount Excreted (mg)	Amount Remaining to Be Excreted (mg)
0	0		—		—	0	39.1
1	0–2	120	133	16.0	8	16.0	23.1
2	2–4	180	50	9.0	4.5	25.0	14.1
3	4–6	89	63	5.6	2.8	30.6	8.5
4	6–8	340	10	3.4	1.7	34.0	5.1
5	8–12	178	18	3.2	0.8	37.2	1.9
6	12–24	950	2	1.9	0.16	39.1	—

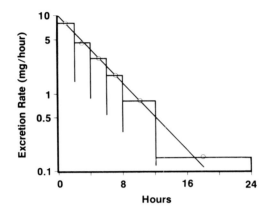

Fig. B–1. Semilogarithmic plot of the rate of excretion against the midpoint time of urine collection. The period over which the average excretion rate was obtained is superimposed. Data from Table B–1.

Re-expressing Equation 20 of Chapter 3 in terms of the amount of drug in the body yields

$$\text{Excretion rate} = \frac{CL_R}{V} \cdot A \qquad 1$$

If $\text{Dose} \cdot e^{-kt}$ is substituted for A,

$$\text{Excretion rate} = \frac{CL_R}{V} \cdot \text{Dose} \cdot e^{-kt} \qquad 2$$

and taking logarithms

$$\log(\text{excretion rate}) = \log\left[\frac{CL_R}{V} \cdot \text{Dose}\right] - k \cdot t \qquad 3$$

The slope of the curve is $-k$.

In practice, the uncertainty of complete bladder emptying and the need to collect urine over short intervals, relative to the elimination half-life of the drug, pose limitations on the quality of excretion rate data. When complete urine recovery of drug is assured, estimates of elimination half-life and elimination rate constant can also be made by analyzing cumulative excretion data. The resultant cumulative excretion plots (Fig. B–2) generally tend to be smoother than the corresponding excretion rate plots.

The cumulative amount excreted up to any time t, Ae_t, is obtained by summing the amount excreted unchanged in each time interval up to that time. For example, by 8 hours, 34.0 milligrams have been excreted. Initially large amounts are excreted, but as the amount of drug in the body falls, so does the excretion rate of drug; by 24 hours, a limiting amount (39.1 mg) has been excreted (Fig. B–2). Small amounts continue to be excreted beyond 24 hours, since theoretically the amount of drug in the body approaches, but never falls to, zero. However, these additional amounts do not substantially alter the 24-hour value. Accordingly, 39.1 milligrams can be taken to be a reasonable estimate of the total amount

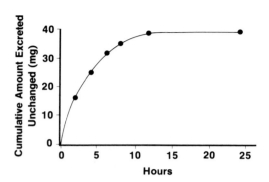

Fig. B–2.   The amount of drug excreted unchanged in the urine accumulates asymptotically toward a limiting value, Ae_x, following an intravenous bolus dose. Half that limiting amount is excreted in one half-life.

of drug to be excreted unchanged (Ae_x). Half this amount (approximately 20 mg) is excreted by 2.6 hours (Fig. B–2). Interestingly, again this is the value for the half-life of this drug, estimated from plasma concentration and urinary excretion rate data. As the following analysis shows, this is more than a mere coincidence.

The rate of excretion at any time is given by

$$\frac{dAe}{dt} = CL_R \cdot C \qquad\qquad 4$$

The amount excreted up to time t is obtained by integrating the rate equation.

$$Ae_t = CL_R \int_0^t C \cdot dt \qquad\qquad 5$$

Since the drug was given as an intravenous bolus, $C = \dfrac{\text{Dose}}{V} \cdot e^{-kt}$, so that

$$Ae_t = \frac{CL_R}{V} \int_0^t \text{Dose} \cdot e^{-kt} \cdot dt \qquad\qquad 6$$

or

$$Ae_t = \frac{CL_R}{V} \cdot \text{Dose} \left[\frac{e^{-kt}}{-k}\right]_0^t \qquad\qquad 7$$

Remembering that $e^{-0} = 1$, the preceding equation reduces to

$$Ae_t = \frac{CL_R \cdot \text{Dose}}{V \cdot k} [1 - e^{-kt}] \qquad\qquad 8$$

but since $e^{-x} = 0$, and $V \cdot k = CL$, the amount excreted by infinite time (Ae_x) must be given by

$$Ae_x = \frac{CL_R \cdot \text{Dose}}{CL} \qquad\qquad 9$$

which when substituted into the preceding equation yields

$$Ae_t = Ae_x(1 - e^{-kt}) \qquad\qquad 10$$

Rearrangement of Equation 10 gives

$$Ae_x - Ae_t = Ae_x \cdot e^{-kt} \qquad\qquad 11$$

and taking the logarithms

$$\log (Ae_x - Ae_t) = \log Ae_x - k \cdot t$$

Thus, a plot of $Ae_\infty - Ae_t$ against time on semilogarithmic paper should give a straight line of slope $-k$.

As the difference, $Ae_\infty - Ae_t$, is the amount remaining to be excreted (ARE), the resulting plot is sometimes called an ARE plot. In practice, the value of ARE at each time is obtained by subtracting the cumulative amount excreted up to that time from the total amount excreted. These values are presented in the last column of Table B–1 and the corresponding semilogarithmic plot of ARE versus time is shown in Figure B–3. The elimination half-life, taken as the time for the ARE to fall by one-half, is 2.8 hours. Hence, $k = 0.25$ hour^{-1}.

Several points should be noted. First, at zero time the value for ARE is Ae_∞. Second, the value of ARE is plotted against the actual time of urine collection, e.g., the time at which 5.1 milligrams remains to be excreted is 8 hours (Table B–1). In this last respect, the ARE plot has a distinct advantage over the excretion rate plot, in which the excretion rate is plotted against the midpoint of the urine collection interval. Recall that the use of the midpoint time was necessary because the excretion rate is an average value over the period of collection.

Although the ARE plot tends to smooth out the data, it is not used as frequently as the excretion rate plot for four reasons: (1) It requires an accurate estimate of Ae_∞, since an underestimation of Ae_∞ tends to grossly underestimate the true ARE values as Ae_t approaches Ae_∞. This means that there has to be complete urine collection for at least four half-lives, which in clinical practice is often difficult to ensure. The rate method does not require urine to be collected until no more drug is excreted. (2) Ae_t values are usually obtained by summing the amount excreted in each collection period. Hence, assay errors are accumulated, while failure to obtain a complete urine collection produces a systematic error in all subsequent estimates of Ae_t. The excretion rate analysis does not contain these sources of error. (3) Smoothing out data can obscure important information. Urinary pH and urine flow fluctuate throughout the day. If the renal clearance of a drug is sensitive to these factors (Chap. 11), it is readily apparent in an excretion rate plot, but tends to be lost in the ARE plot. (4) When the drug is administered extravascularly, e.g., orally, delays in excretion caused by absorp-

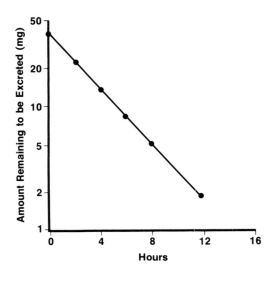

Fig. B–3. The amount remaining to be excreted (ARE), following an intravenous bolus dose of drug, declines exponentially with time. In one half-life, the ARE falls by one-half.

tion produces distortions of the ARE plot, frequently making the analysis difficult. In contrast, the excretion rate plot can be readily analyzed.

Study Problem

1. Swintosky et al. (J. Am. Pharm. Assoc., 46:403–411, 1957) studied the disposition kinetics of the sulfonamide, sulfaethylthiadiazole. Table B–2 contains a list of the amounts of drug excreted unchanged with time following an intravenous bolus dose of 2.0 grams sulfaethylthiadiazole to a subject (weight 81 kg).

Table B–2.

Time interval (hours)	0–3	3–6	6–9	9–12	12–15	15–24	24–48
Amount excreted unchanged (mg)	534	436	181	139	110	202	195

(a) Estimate graphically the elimination half-life of sulfaethylthiadiazole from a semilogarithmic plot of excretion rate against the midpoint time of urine collection.

(b) Calculate the fraction of the dose excreted unchanged.

(c) Estimate the elimination half-life of sulfaethylthiadiazole from cumulative excretion data, and compare the answer with that obtained from the excretion rate data.

Answers to Study Problem

1. (a) Half-life = 6.5 hours. Note scatter in semilogarithmic plot of rate of excretion against midpoint time of urine collection.

   (b) $fe = 0.9$; $fe = Ae_\infty$/Dose = 1800 milligrams/2000 milligrams.

   (c) Half-life = 6.5 hours. Note that the semilogarithmic plot of the amount remaining to be excreted against time of urine collection is much smoother than the excretion rate plot.

APPENDIX C

Estimation of the Absorption Half-life from Plasma Concentration Data

Consider the plasma data in Table C–1, obtained following a 100-milligram oral dose of a drug. Figure C–1 is a semilogarithmic plot of the same data. The half-life, estimated from the linear portion of the decline phase, is 5 hours. Giving the drug intravenously confirmed that this is the elimination half-life of the drug. Hence, disposition rate limits drug elimination.

A graphic procedure to test whether or not absorption is a first-order process and, if so, to determine the absorption half-life, is known as the *method of residuals*. The procedure is simple to follow: (1) Back extrapolate the log linear portion of the decline phase. Let $\overleftarrow{C}$ denote the plasma concentration along this extrapolated line. (2) Subtract the observed plasma concentration (C) from the corresponding extrapolated value at each time point. These calculations are shown in Table C–1. (3) Plot the residuals ($\overleftarrow{C} - C$) against time on the same semilogarithmic graph paper.

If, as in this example, the residual plot is a straight line, then absorption is a first-order process. The absorption half-life, taken as the time for the residual value to diminish by one-half, is 1.3 hours. The corresponding absorption rate constant, ka, is 0.693/1.3 or 0.53 hour^{-1}.

Theoretically, the absorption half-life can also be estimated from urinary excretion data. Assuming that the renal clearance of the drug is constant, the excretion rate parallels the plasma concentration. The method of residuals should, therefore, be equally applicable to excretion rate data. In practice, how-

Table C–1. Plasma Concentration-Time Data Following Oral Administration of a 100-Milligram Dose of a Drug

Observation		Treatment of Data	
Time (hours)	Plasma Concentration C, (mg/liter)	Extrapolated Plasma Concentration $\overleftarrow{C}$, (mg/liter)	Difference in Concentration $\overleftarrow{C} - C$, (mg/liter)
1	0.38	1.90	1.52
2	0.73	1.65	0.92
3	0.91	1.40	0.49
4	0.97	1.23	0.26
5	0.97	1.07	0.10
6	0.92	0.95	0.03
8	0.71	0.71	—
10	0.53	0.53	—
12	0.40	0.40	—
14	0.30	0.30	—

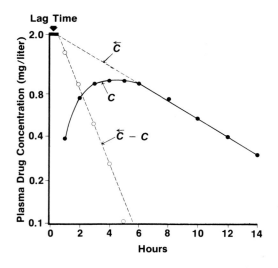

Fig. C–1. By the method of residuals, an estimate can be made of both the absorption half-life and the lag time, following oral administration of a drug.

ever, estimates of absorption half-life from urinary data are usually poor. The half-life of many absorption processes is 30 minutes or less. Incomplete bladder emptying and the inability to collect samples frequently enough to characterize such absorption processes are two major sources of error. Consequently, analysis of plasma data is the preferred method for estimating absorption kinetics.

Let us examine the underlying basis of the method of residuals. At any time the plasma concentration following extravascular administration is given by

$$C = \left(\frac{F \cdot \text{Dose} \cdot ka}{V(ka - k)}\right) (e^{-k \cdot t} - e^{-ka \cdot t}) \qquad 1$$

where all terms are as previously defined in the body of the book. The proof of Equation 1 is involved and is beyond the scope of this book. When (as is most frequently the case) absorption is the more rapid process, the value of $ka \cdot t$ is always greater than $k \cdot t$ and hence $e^{-ka \cdot t}$ approaches zero more rapidly than does $e^{-k \cdot t}$. At some point past the peak plasma concentration, $e^{-ka \cdot t}$ is essentially zero, absorption is over, and the extrapolated line is given by

$$\overleftarrow{C} = \left(\frac{F \cdot \text{Dose} \cdot ka}{V(ka - k)}\right) e^{-k \cdot t} \qquad 2$$

Subtracting C from $\overleftarrow{C}$ therefore yields

$$\overleftarrow{C} - C = \left(\frac{F \cdot \text{Dose} \cdot ka}{V(ka - k)}\right) e^{-ka \cdot t} \qquad 3$$

and taking logarithms

$$\log (\overleftarrow{C} - C) = \log \left(\frac{F \cdot \text{Dose} \cdot ka}{V(ka - k)}\right) - ka \cdot t \qquad 4$$

Hence, if absorption is a first-order process, a semilogarithmic plot of the residual value against time yields a straight line of slope $-ka$. Occasionally, this residual line is not log linear, implying that absorption is not a simple first-order process.

In those instances, other methods are available to calculate how absorption varies with time.

Lag Time: Examination of Equations 2 and 3 suggests a simple graphic method for estimating the lag time, that is, the time between administration and the start of absorption. By definition, absorption begins when the extrapolated and residual curves intersect. This must be so since only at that time, $t = 0$, when $e^{-ka \cdot t} = e^{-kt} = 1$, are the values of the two equations the same, and equal to $(F \cdot Dose \cdot ka)/[V(ka - k)]$. It is seen from Figure C–1 that in the present example the lag time is approximately 30 minutes.

Study Problems

1. The following plasma concentrations (Table C–2) were observed in a patient who took 10 milliliters of an elixir containing 10 milligrams/milliliter of a drug.

Table C–2.

Time (hours)	0.25	0.5	1	2	3	4	6	8	10	12
Plasma concentration (mg/liter)	1.6	2.7	3.7	3.5	2.7	2.0	1.02	0.49	0.26	0.12

(a) Prepare a semilogarithmic plot of the data and determine the rate constants for absorption and elimination.

(b) Estimate when absorption began.

(c) Given that absorption is complete (100 percent), calculate: (1) the clearance of the drug; (2) the volume of distribution of the drug.

2. The absorption kinetics of a drug, known to be acid labile, was studied in two groups: group A, patients with normal gastric function; group B, patients with achlorhydria (a condition in which little or no acid is secreted into the stomach). Each group received the same dose of drug. Analysis of the plasma concentration-time curve yielded the following estimates: group A, $F = 0.30$, $ka = 1.15$ hour^{-1}, group B, $F = 0.90$; $ka = 0.39$ hour^{-1}. The investigators proposed that the longer half-life for absorption of the drug in patients with achlorhydria was caused by a slower gastric emptying in this group. Suggest an alternative proposal that is consistent with all the observations.

Answers to Study Problems

1. (a) $ka = 1.4$ hour^{-1}, $k = 0.35$ hour^{-1}.

(b) Absorption began immediately because there was no lag time.

(c) (1) Clearance $= 5.9$ liters/hour;
Assuming $F = 1$, Clearance $= Dose/Area = 100$ milligrams/(17.05 mg-hours/liter)

(2) V = Clearance/k = 17 liters;

If absorption is the rate-limiting step, then V = 5.9/1.4 = 4.2 liters. This is an unlikely value.

2. Observations can be explained entirely by a competing reaction. With a competing reaction, the observed absorption rate constant ka = ka' + kc, and F = ka'/ka, where ka' is the true rate constant defining the absorption process and kc is the rate constant of the competing reaction. For both groups ka' = $ka \cdot F$ = 0.35 hour^{-1}. Both the lower availability and the apparent faster absorption of the drug in group A are due to more extensive degradation in the acidic gastric contents. Lesson: Be careful in interpreting the value of the absorption rate constant when a competing reaction is likely. For more details see Chapter 9, Absorption.

APPENDIX D

Amount of Drug in the Body on Accumulation to Plateau

Consider the situation in which a dose of drug is given as an intravenous bolus every dosing interval, τ. Recall that after each dose the fraction remaining at time, t, is e^{-kt}. The fraction of drug remaining at the end of a dosing interval τ, therefore, is $e^{-k\tau}$. When time is equal to 2τ, the fraction remaining is $e^{-2k\tau}$. The amount of drug in the body following multiple doses is simply the sum of the amounts remaining from each of the previous doses. The amount of drug in the body just after the next dose is shown in Table D–1 for four successive equal doses given every τ.

It is apparent from the table that the maximum amount of drug in the body just after the fourth dose, $A_{4,max}$, is the fourth dose plus the sum of the amount remaining from each of three previous doses (sum of terms in row 4 of Table D–1). That is, letting $r = e^{-k\tau}$,

$$A_{4,max} = \text{Dose} \ (1 + r + r^2 + r^3) \qquad 1$$

Just after the Nth dose the amount in the body is

$$A_{N,max} = \text{Dose} \ (1 + r + r^2 + r^3 \ldots + r^{N-2} + r^{N-1}) \qquad 2$$

Multiplying by r,

$$A_{N,max} \cdot r = \text{Dose} \ (r + r^2 + r^3 + r^4 \ldots + r^{N-1} + r^N) \qquad 3$$

Subtracting Equation 3 from Equation 2,

$$A_{N,max} \cdot (1 - r) = \text{Dose} \ (1 - r^N) \qquad 4$$

Therefore,

$$A_{N,max} = \text{Dose} \ \frac{(1 - r^N)}{(1 - r)} \qquad 5$$

Table D–1. Drug in Body Just After Each of Four Successive Doses

| Time | Amount Remaining in Body from Each Dose | | | |
	1st Dose	2nd Dose	3rd Dose	4th Dose
0	Dose			
τ	Dose $\cdot \ e^{-k\tau}$	Dose		
2τ	Dose $\cdot \ e^{-2k\tau}$	Dose $\cdot \ e^{-k\tau}$	Dose	
3τ	Dose $\cdot \ e^{-3k\tau}$	Dose $\cdot \ e^{-2k\tau}$	Dose $\cdot \ e^{-k\tau}$	Dose

Hence the amount of drug in the body at any time t during a dosing interval, after the Nth dose, $A_{N,t}$, is

$$A_{N,t} = A_{N,max} \cdot e^{-kt} \qquad\qquad 6$$

At the end of the dosing interval, when $t = \tau$, it follows that the minimum amount in the body after the Nth dose, $A_{N,min}$, is

$$A_{N,min} = A_{N,max} \cdot r = \text{Dose}\,\frac{(1 - r^N) \cdot r}{(1 - r)} \qquad\qquad 7$$

As the number of doses, N, increases, the value of r^N approaches zero, since r is always a value less than 1. The maximum and minimum amounts of drug in the body during each interval each approach a limit. At the limit, the amount lost in each interval equals the amount gained, the dose. For this reason the drug in the body then is said to be at *steady state* or at *plateau*. At steady state, the maximum, $A_{ss,max}$, the minimum, $A_{ss,min}$, and the amount in the body at anytime during the dosing interval, $A_{ss,t}$, are readily obtained by letting $r^N = 0$ in Equations 5 and 7

$$A_{ss,max} = \frac{\text{Dose}}{1 - r} \qquad\qquad 8$$

$$A_{ss,min} = \frac{\text{Dose} \cdot r}{1 - r} = A_{ss,max} - \text{Dose} \qquad\qquad 9$$

$$A_{ss,t} = \frac{\text{Dose}}{1 - r} \cdot e^{-kt} \qquad\qquad 10$$

or expressed in terms of the dose,

$$\frac{A_{ss,max}}{\text{Dose}} = \frac{1}{1 - r} \qquad\qquad 11$$

$$\frac{A_{ss,min}}{\text{Dose}} = \frac{r}{1 - r} = \frac{1}{1 - r} - 1 \qquad\qquad 12$$

and

$$\frac{A_{ss,t}}{\text{Dose}} = \frac{e^{-kt}}{1 - r} \qquad\qquad 13$$

Prove to yourself the identity of the two functions in Equation 12.

Time to Reach Plateau: The time to approach plateau, whether defined with respect to the maximum or minimum amount of drug in the body, depends solely on the half-life of the drug. The proof of this statement is readily apparent by dividing the equations that define the respective amounts after the Nth dose by the equations that define the respective amounts at plateau,

$$\frac{A_{N,max}}{A_{ss,max}} = \frac{A_{N,min}}{A_{ss,min}} = 1 - r^N \qquad\qquad 14$$

As r^N equals $e^{-Nk\tau}$, $N \cdot \tau$ is the time elapsed. Thus, in one half-life, as the fraction remaining equals 0.5, half the plateau value is reached; in two half-lives, three-quarters of the plateau value is reached and so on. A similar conclusion is drawn when relating the average amount during each dosing interval with the average amount at plateau.

Study Problems

The accumulation equations derived in this appendix are applied in the study problems of Chapter 7, Multiple-Dose Regimens.

APPENDIX E

Blood to Plasma Concentration Ratio

The interrelationships among extraction ratio, blood flow, and blood clearance of drugs require the measurement of drug concentration in whole blood. Because plasma is the usual site of measurement, knowledge of how the blood concentration and plasma concentration are related can be useful.

At equilibrium the ratio of blood to plasma concentrations is dependent on plasma protein binding, partitioning into the blood cells, and the volume of the blood cells. This dependence is, perhaps, most readily appreciated from mass balance considerations as follows:

$$C_b \cdot V_B = C \cdot V_P + C_{bc} \cdot V_{bc}$$

| Amount in blood | Amount in plasma | Amount in blood cells | 1 |

where C_b = blood concentration of drug

V_B = blood volume

C = plasma concentration of drug

V_P = plasma volume

C_{bc} = blood cell concentration of drug

V_{bc} = volume of blood cells

The ratio of the concentration in the blood cell to that unbound in plasma, Cu, is a measure of the affinity of the blood cell for the drug. Using ρ for this ratio and since $Cu = fu \cdot C$,

$$C_{bc} = \rho \cdot Cu = \rho \cdot fu \cdot C \qquad 2$$

The volume of blood cells is a function of the hematocrit, H, and the blood volume, that is,

$$V_{bc} = H \cdot V_B \qquad 3$$

The plasma volume is related to the hematocrit by

$$V_P = (1 - H)V_B \qquad 4$$

Substituting Equations 2 to 4 in Equation 1

$$C_b \cdot V_B = (1 - H) \cdot V_B \cdot C + fu \cdot \rho \cdot H \cdot V_B \cdot C \qquad 5$$

Dividing by $V_B \cdot C$, and simplifying,

$$\frac{C_b}{C} = 1 + H[fu \cdot \rho - 1] \qquad 6$$

This relationship clearly shows how the ratio of concentrations, blood/plasma, varies with hematocrit, plasma protein binding, and affinity of the drug for blood cells. The ratio can be calculated if these parameters are known. If the hematocrit and the affinity are constant, a plot of the ratio against *fu* gives a straight line with an intercept of $1 - H$ and a slope of $H \cdot \rho$. This correlation is useful in situations in which the plasma protein binding is variable, such as for certain drugs in uremia, in hypo- and hyperalbuminemic states, and in displacement interactions. In situations in which the plot is not linear, the affinity of the blood cells or the hematocrit is also changing.

If Equation 6 is rearranged to solve for ρ, a useful means of determining the affinity of the blood cells for the drug is obtained, namely,

$$\rho = \frac{H - 1 + (C_b/C)}{fu \cdot H} \qquad 7$$

Determination of ρ requires measurement of the hematocrit, the concentration ratio, and the fraction of drug in plasma unbound to proteins.

Study Problem

1. The ratio of the concentration of a drug in blood to that in plasma usually averages about 2.35 in a typical patient who has an hematocrit of 0.45 and a fraction unbound in plasma of 0.1.

   (a) Calculate the ratio of the concentration in blood cells to that unbound in plasma (ρ).

   (b) In an anemic patient the hematocrit is decreased to 0.27, but the serum concentration of albumin, the protein to which this drug binds, remains normal, 4.3 grams/deciliter. Calculate the expected ratio of the drug concentration in blood to that in plasma in this patient.

   (c) Predict the ratio of plasma and blood clearances in a patient with the nephrotic syndrome in whom the hematocrit is normal but the fraction unbound in plasma is increased to 0.32, a secondary consequence of the loss of plasma proteins into urine.

Answers to Study Problem

1. (a) 40

$$\rho = \frac{H - 1 + (C_b/C)}{fu \cdot H} = \frac{0.45 - 1 + 2.35}{0.1 \times 0.45}$$

   (b) 1.81

$$C_b/C = 1 + H(fu \cdot \rho - 1) = 1 + 0.27 (0.1 \times 40 - 1)$$

The percent change in C_b/C is minor compared to that of the hematocrit. Note that had $fu \cdot \rho$ been equal to 1 (drug concentration in blood cells same as that in plasma), there would have been no change in C_b/C when the hematocrit was altered. Furthermore, if $fu \cdot \rho$ is less than 1, then C_b/C increases with a decrease in H. Finally if $fu \cdot \rho$ is greater than 1, then C_b/C decreases with a decrease in H.

(c) 6.31

$$C_b/C = 1 + H(fu \cdot \rho - 1) = 1 + 0.45 \,(0.32 \times 40 - 1)$$

The increased value of fu, resulting from the lowered plasma albumin concentration, greatly increases the ratio of C_b to C. Had ρ been a small value, the drug would have been largely confined to plasma and changes in fu would have had a minor effect on the ratio of C_b to C.

APPENDIX F

Mean Residence Time

A dose of drug comprises many millions of molecules. For example, even a dose as small as 1 milligram of a drug with a molecular weight of 300 daltons contains close to 2×10^{18} molecules [$(10^{-3}$ grams/300$) \times 6.023 \times 10^{23}$ (Avogadro's number)]. On administration, these drug molecules spend different times within the body. Some are eliminated rapidly, others stay in the body for a long time. A few may stay in our bodies for a lifetime. The result is a distribution of residence times that can be characterized by a mean value.

The *mean residence time (MRT)* is the average time the number of molecules introduced (N) reside in the body, that is,

$$MRT = \sum_{j=1}^{N} t_j/N \qquad\qquad 1$$

where t_j is the residence time of the jth molecule (time between its input and its elimination from the body). Individual molecules cannot be counted, of course, but groups of them can. Letting n_1 be the number of molecules with an average time in the body of t_1, the total residence time accumulated by this group of molecules is $t_1 \cdot n_1$, and the value

$$\frac{(t_1 \cdot n_1) + (t_2 \cdot n_2)}{n_1 + n_2} \qquad\qquad 2$$

is the mean residence time of two such groups of molecules. Extending this concept to account for all molecules administered, the mean residence time becomes

$$MRT = \frac{\sum_{i=1}^{m} t_i \cdot n_i}{\sum_{i=1}^{m} n_i} = \frac{\sum_{i=1}^{m} t_i \cdot n_i}{N} \qquad\qquad 3$$

where n_i is the number of molecules in the ith group; t_i is their average time in the body; m is the number of groups; and the denominator is the total number of molecules introduced.

The mean residence time is determined more readily after an intravenous bolus dose than after any other mode of drug administration. Here all the molecules of the dose start their residence in the body at the same time; thus, for each group, t_i is the time between drug administration and elimination. When the number of molecules eliminated in each group (dn) approaches a relatively small value, the mean residence time can be expressed in integral notation,

$$MRT = \frac{\int_0^N t \cdot dn}{N}$$

4

The limits correspond to the number of molecules eliminated at zero and infinite times. None of the molecules has been eliminated at time zero; at infinite time all have been eliminated. The number of molecules eliminated by all pathways can be expressed in terms of the amounts eliminated, Ael. That is, $Ael = n \cdot$ (molecular weight)/(Avogadro's number). So that

$$MRT = \frac{\int_0^{Ael_\infty} t \cdot dAel}{Ael_\infty}$$

5

The denominator of Equation 5 is the dose of drug administered. Integration of Equation 5, by parts, leads to

$$MRT = \frac{\int_0^\infty (Dose - Ael)\, dt}{Dose}$$

6

where Ael is the amount eliminated up to a given time t.

The MRT after an intravenous bolus dose can be estimated from either urinary excretion or plasma drug concentration data as follows.

Excretion Data: When the fraction excreted unchanged, fe, remains constant with time, the amount of drug excreted unchanged in the urine, Ae, equals $fe \cdot Ael$ and Ae_∞ equals $fe \cdot Dose$. On substituting these values into Equation 6, it is apparent that MRT can be determined from urinary excretion data using the relationship

$$MRT = \frac{\int_0^\infty (Ae_\infty - Ae)\, dt}{Ae_\infty}$$

7

Figure F–1 shows the amount excreted unchanged, Ae, at various times and the amount ultimately excreted unchanged, Ae_∞. The area between these curves (shaded) is the numerator in Equation 7. For a given amount excreted unchanged, it is apparent that the area and, therefore, the mean residence time are increased when the drug remains longer in the body.

Plasma Concentration Data: When clearance is constant with time, the rate of elimination is proportional to the plasma drug concentration, that is, $dAel/dt$ $= CL \cdot C$. Substituting $CL \cdot C \cdot dt$ for $dAel$ and $CL \cdot \int_0^\infty Cdt$ for Ael_∞ in Equation 5 gives

$$MRT = \frac{\int_0^\infty tCdt}{\int_0^\infty Cdt}$$

8

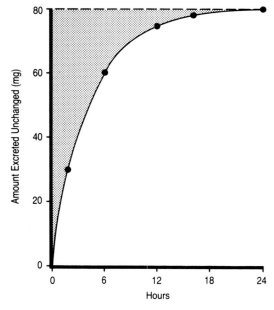

Fig. F–1. The difference between the amount excreted unchanged (solid line) and the amount ultimately excreted (dashed line) is the amount remaining to be excreted. The area under the amount-remaining-to-be-excreted-time curve (shaded), relative to the total amount excreted (Eq. 7 in text), is a measure of the mean residence time of a substance in the body. Data from Table F–1.

The product $t \cdot C$ is called the *first-moment* of the concentration, because concentration is multiplied by time raised to the power of 1. Therefore, the numerator is called the area-under-the-(first)-moment versus time curve *(AUMC)*, whereas the denominator is the area-under-the-concentration versus time curve *(AUC)*. The time course of both the plasma concentration and its first-moment are shown in Figure F–2.

The mean residence time concept is equally applicable to the measurement of the turnover of an endogenous substance, using a tracer, and the determination of the mean time a drug resides in the body. As an example, let us examine the measurement of mean residence time after an intravenous bolus dose of a drug from both the urinary and plasma data contained in Table F–1. The value of *AUC* can be estimated as shown in Appendix A. The value of *AUMC* is calculated

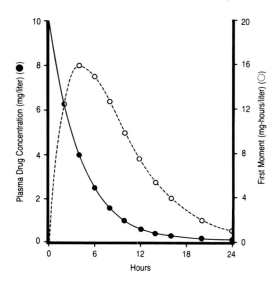

Fig. F–2. After an intravenous bolus dose, the plasma concentration (●) declines with time. The first-moment, (○) product of time and concentration, rises to a peak and declines with time. The area beyond the last sampling time is much greater for the first-moment time curve than for the concentration-time curve. Data from Table F–1.

Table F–1. Plasma Concentration-time, and Urinary Excretion-time Data Following an Intravenous 200-milligram Bolus Dose of a Drug

Time (hours)	Plasma Drug Concentration (mg/liter)	First-moment of Plasma Concentration (mg-hour/liter)	Cumulative Amount Excreted (mg)	Amount Remaining to be Excreted (mg)
0	10[a]	0	0	80[b]
2	6.3	12.6	30	50
4	4.0	16.0	48	32
6	2.5	15.0	60	20
8	1.6	12.8	67	13
10	1.0	10.0	72	8
12	0.63	7.6	75	5
14	0.39	5.5	–	–
16	0.25	4.0	78	2
20	0.10	2.0	–	–
24	0.04	0.96	80	0

[a]Estimated by extrapolation to zero time.
[b]The cumulative amount excreted at infinite time.

from the first-moment (column 3) in a manner similar to that of *AUC*, but the extrapolated area after last point (C_{last} at t_{last}) is different. In this case the area remaining can be shown to be

$$\int_{t_{last}}^{\infty} t \cdot C \cdot dt = \frac{C_{last} \cdot t_{last}}{\lambda_z} + \frac{C_{last}}{\lambda_z^2} \qquad 9$$

where λ_z is the rate constant of the terminal decay of the plasma drug concentration. When the entire concentration-time profile can be described by a sum of exponentials, the area under the first-moment curve can be determined directly from the coefficients and exponential coefficients defining the equation. For example, if $C = C_1 e^{-\lambda_1 t} + C_2 e^{-\lambda_2 t}$, then

$$AUMC = \frac{C_1}{\lambda_1^2} + \frac{C_2}{\lambda_2^2} \qquad 10$$

In the example considered, the calculated areas under the concentration-time curve, the first-moment curve, and the amount-remaining-to-be-excreted versus time curve are 44.2 milligrams-hour/liter, 17.7 milligrams-hour^2/liter, and 340 milligrams-hours, respectively. The areas remaining under the first two curves after the last time point are 0.17 milligram-hour/liter and 4.9 milligrams-hour^2/liter, respectively. Figures F–1 and F–2 contain the data from Table F–1. The calculated mean residence times from Equations 7 (urinary data) and 8 (plasma data) are then 4.25 hours and 4.0 hours, respectively. The simulated value is 4.3 hours. The differences arise from approximations introduced by the use of the trapezoidal rule to calculate area.

The mean residence time, calculated by either Equation 7 or 8, is a measure of the average time a substance spends in the body after an intravenous bolus dose. When a drug is given by a constant-rate intravenous infusion or by an extravascular route, the drug spends additional time in the syringe or at the site of administration (for example, gastrointestinal tract, muscle or subcutaneous tissues). The observed mean residence time, estimated from Equations 7 or 8, is then the sum of the mean times at these sites and in the body. Table F–2 shows the mean input and mean residence times for three common modes of drug input and disposition.

Following extravascular administration, the observed *MRT* is the sum of the mean residence time in the body and the *mean absorption time*. The mean absorption time can be determined from the difference between the mean residence times (calculated from Eq. 7 or Eq. 8), after extravascular and intravenous bolus doses given on separate occasions. After giving a solid dosage form, the mean absorption time includes time for disintegration, deaggregation, dissolution, and movement into the general circulation. Gastric emptying, intestinal motility, and other physiologic and physicochemical factors influence the mean absorption time as well.

Table F–2. Mean Residence Times for Selected Modes[a] of Drug Input

Mode of Administration	Model[b]	Mean Input Time	Observed Mean Residence Time
Single intravenous bolus dose	$\triangledown \overset{k}{\longrightarrow}$	0	$1/k$
Constant-rate intravenous infusion	$\overset{R_o}{\longrightarrow} \bigcirc \overset{k}{\longrightarrow}$	$\tau/2$	$1/k + \tau/2$
Single extravascular dose	$\triangledown \overset{ka}{\longrightarrow} \bigcirc \overset{k}{\longrightarrow}$	$1/ka$	$1/k + 1/ka$

[a]Disposition is assumed to be first-order from a one-compartment model.
[b]The symbol $\triangledown$ denotes a bolus dose into the compartment.

Study Problems

1. Using the definition of mean residence time in Equation 8 and an equation for the time-course of plasma drug concentration after an intravenous bolus dose, prove mathematically that the observed mean residence time given in Table F–2 for this route of administration is correct for a one-compartment model.

2. Prove that the mean time a drug is in a syringe during a constant-rate intravenous infusion is equal to $\tau/2$, where τ is the duration of the infusion.

3. The observed mean residence times in an individual subject, calculated from plasma concentration-time data (Eq. 8) following an intravenous bolus dose, an intravenous infusion, and an oral dose, on separate occasions, were 8, 10, and 12 hours, respectively.

   (a) Assuming a constant-rate input, determine the duration of the infusion.

   (b) Assuming a first-order oral input, determine the absorption half-life.

4. Using Equation 1 in Appendix C and Equation 8 of this appendix, prove mathematically that the calculation of mean residence time (observed value) after extravascular administration depends on neither the dose nor the availability.

Answers to Study Problems

1.

$$MRT = \frac{\int_0^\infty C \cdot t \cdot dt}{\int_0^\infty C \cdot dt} \quad \text{(Equation 8)}$$

$$C = C(0) \cdot e^{-kt}$$

$$MRT = \frac{C(0) \cdot \int_0^\infty e^{-kt} \cdot t \cdot dt}{C(0) \cdot \int_0^\infty e^{-kt} \cdot dt} = \frac{\int_0^\infty t \cdot e^{-kt} \cdot dt}{\int_0^\infty e^{-kt} \cdot dt}$$

$$= \frac{\left[\dfrac{-e^{-kt}}{k^2} (kt + 1) \right]_0^\infty}{\left[\dfrac{-e^{-kt}}{k} \right]_0^\infty} = \frac{1}{k}$$

2.

$$MRT = \frac{\int_0^\tau (\text{Dose} - R \cdot t) dt}{\text{Dose}}$$

Since $R = \text{Dose}/\tau$, then

$$MRT = \frac{\text{Dose} \int_0^\tau \left(1 - \dfrac{t}{\tau} \right) dt}{\text{Dose}}$$

$$= \left[t - \frac{t^2}{2\tau} \right]_0^\tau = \frac{2\tau^2 - \tau^2}{2\tau} = \frac{\tau}{2}$$

3. (a) 4 hours.

   Mean infusion time = 2 hours $(10 - 8) = \dfrac{\tau}{2}$

   Therefore, $\tau = 4$ hours.

   (b) 2.77 hours.
   Mean absorption time = 4 hours $(12 - 8)$.
   If absorption is first-order and obeys single compartment kinetics, mean absorption time = $1/ka$. Therefore, $ka = 0.25$ hour^{-1} and absorption half-life $(0.693/ka) = 2.77$ hours.

4.
$$C = \frac{F \cdot D \cdot ka}{V \cdot (ka - k)} (e^{-kt} - e^{-ka \cdot t}) = I (e^{-kt} - e^{-ka \cdot t})$$

where $I = \dfrac{F \cdot D \cdot ka}{V \cdot (ka - k)}$

$$\text{Observed } MRT = \frac{\int_0^\infty C \cdot t \cdot dt}{\int_0^\infty C \cdot dt} = \frac{I}{I} \left[\frac{\int_0^\infty (e^{-kt} - e^{-ka \cdot t}) \cdot t \cdot dt}{\int_0^\infty (e^{-kt} - e^{-ka \cdot t}) \cdot dt} \right]$$

$$\text{Observed } MRT = \frac{\left[\dfrac{1}{k^2} - \dfrac{1}{ka^2} \right]}{\left[\dfrac{1}{k} - \dfrac{1}{ka} \right]} = \frac{\left[\dfrac{1}{k} + \dfrac{1}{ka} \right] \left[\dfrac{1}{k} - \dfrac{1}{ka} \right]}{\left[\dfrac{1}{k} - \dfrac{1}{ka} \right]} = \frac{1}{k} + \frac{1}{ka}$$

Neither Dose nor F is in the relationship.

APPENDIX G

Answers to Problems

Answers to Study Problems (Chap. 2)

1. Pharmacokinetics—quantitation of the time-course of a drug and its metabolites in the body.

   Intravascular administration—parenteral injection of a drug directly into the blood, either arterial or venous.

   Extravascular administration—administration by any route other than directly into the blood.

   Absorption—process by which a drug proceeds from the site of administration to the site of measurement within the body.

   Disposition—all the processes that occur subsequent to the absorption of a drug.

   Distribution—reversible transfer of a drug to and from the site of measurement.

   Metabolism—irreversible conversion to another chemical species.

   Excretion—irreversible loss of the chemically unchanged drug.

   First-pass effect—a drug must first cross the gastrointestinal membranes and pass through the liver to be absorbed. Removal of drug on this first passage into the general circulation is the *first-pass effect*.

2. (a) It must, since the amount ultimately excreted equals the dose. An exception might be the renal excretion of an unstable metabolite which, during storage of the urine or under assay conditions, reverts back to the original drug. In this case, excretion of unchanged drug is not being measured; the observation is an artifact.

   (b) When the rate of elimination equals the rate of absorption. Prior to that time, the rate of absorption exceeds the rate of elimination, subsequently the converse is true.

   (c) Yes, if the amount of drug in the body and the amount of drug eliminated are both known.

   (d) When the rate of absorption is zero. This is the case following intravascular administration or following extravascular administration when absorption has stopped.

   (e) When the rate of elimination is virtually zero. This condition exists when there is no drug in the body. It occurs initially following extravascular administration and is essentially the case during most of the absorption phase, if absorption is much faster than elimination.

3. No. By measuring radioactivity, no distinction is made between drug and metabolite(s). The drug may have been degraded in the gut lumen, on passage across the gut wall, or in the liver, with the products being fully excreted into the urine. Only specific measurement of unchanged drug permits one to estimate its absorption.

Answers to Study Problems (Chap. 3)

---

1. (a) 1/16 or 6.25 percent. The fraction remaining after 4 half-lives (n = 4) is $(\frac{1}{2})^4$ or $\frac{1}{2} \times \frac{1}{2} \times \frac{1}{2} \times \frac{1}{2}$. Also, the fraction remaining, e^{-kt}, when k = $0.693/t\frac{1}{2}$ and t = $4 \times t\frac{1}{2}$ is $e^{-0.693 \times 4}$.

   (b) Ten percent. Number of half-lives elapsed since administration (n) = 20/6 or 3.3. The value of $(\frac{1}{2})^n$ when n = 3.3 is 0.1. Also, the fraction remaining, e^{-kt}, when k = 0.76 hours and t = 20 hours is $e^{-0.693 \times 20/6}$.

   (c) 4.3 hours. The value of n which gives a value of 0.2 for $(\frac{1}{2})^n$ is 2.32. Hence, the half-life is 10 hours/n or 4.3 hours. Also, if e^{-kt} = 0.2 when t = 10 hours, then k = 0.161 hours^{-1} and $t\frac{1}{2}$ = 0.693/k.

2. (a) Half-life = 27 hours.

   (b) Using the relationship, AUC = $C(0)/k$, AUC = 5.5×10^3 milligrams-hours/liter. Using the trapezoidal rule and remembering that at zero time the concentration is $C(0)$, AUC = 5.7×10^3 milligram-hours/liter. The slightly higher value using the trapezoidal rule arises because, at any time, the concentration along the straight line connecting two data points is always greater than the corresponding concentration on the declining exponential curve.

   (c) Clearance = 33 milliliters/hour.

   (d) Volume of distribution = 1.3 liters. This is a newborn infant of 3.7 kilograms (184 mg divided by 50 mg/kg). Thus, the volume of distribution is 0.35 liter/kilogram.

3. First determine the half-life (0.693/0.347 = 2 hours). Place a datum point of 0.9 milligram/liter at zero time and another point, 0.45 milligram/liter, at the half-life (2 hours). Connect and extend the line joining these two data points.

4. (a) Plot of data on semilogarithmic paper (not shown).

   (b) Half-life = 0.7 hour;

   Total clearance = 1.4×10^2 liters/hour. *Calculated from:*

   $$CL = \frac{Dose}{AUC}.$$ For the intravenous bolus case only: AUC = $C(0)/k$.

   (c) Volume of distribution = 1.9 liters/kilogram.

Answers to Study Problems (Chap. 4)

1.

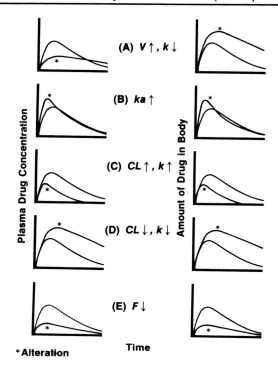

Fig. G-1

2. (a) A delayed esophageal transit profoundly affects the rapidity, but not the extent, of absorption of acetaminophen. The peak concentration is much lower (delayed transit group, 3.9 mg/liter; normal transit group, 6.3 mg/liter) and delayed (90 minutes versus 40 minutes), but the AUC values (715 versus 743 mg-hour/liter) are comparable.

(b) Drug disposition is the rate-limiting step; the declining plasma concentrations for the two groups are parallel. They would be divergent if absorption had been the rate-limiting step.

(c) To ensure rapid absorption, acetaminophen should be taken while upright with plenty of water.

3. (a) From AUC analysis, $F = 0.76$; $F_{rel} = 0.95$
   From Ae_∞ analysis, $F = 0.83$; $F_{rel} = 0.94$

   AUC Analysis

$$F = \frac{[AUC/Dose]_{oral}}{[AUC/Dose]_{iv}} = \frac{[(19.9 \text{ mg} \times \text{hour/liter})/100 \text{ mg}]}{[(13.1 \text{ mg} \times \text{hour/liter})/500 \text{ mg}]}$$

$$F_{rel} = \frac{[AUC/Dose]_2}{[AUC/Dose]_1} = \frac{[(19.9 \text{ mg} \times \text{hour/liter})/1000 \text{ mg}]}{[(20.9 \text{ mg} \times \text{hour/liter})/1000 \text{ mg}]}$$

   Urine Analysis

$$F = \frac{[Ae_\infty/Dose]_{oral}}{[Ae_\infty/Dose]_{iv}} = \frac{(554 \text{ mg}/1000 \text{ mg})}{(332 \text{ mg}/500 \text{ mg})}$$

$$F_{rel} = \frac{[Ae_\infty/Dose]_2}{[Ae_\infty/Dose]_1} = \frac{(554 \text{ mg}/500 \text{ mg})}{(586 \text{ mg}/500 \text{ mg})}$$

Assuumptions made are:

1. Estimates of AUC and Ae_∞ are accurate.

2. CL and fe do not vary between treatments.

(b) Time interval of 48 hours is adequate to ensure a good estimate of Ae_∞. With half-life of about 2.7 hours, 48 hours corresponds to 18 half-lives. The high percent of the dose excreted unchanged (fe = 332 mg/500 mg = 0.66) indicates that urine analysis is appropriate for assessment of availability of procainamide.

(c) CL_R values (Ae_∞/AUC) are 25, 28, and 28 liters/hour for the intravenous, formulation 1 and formulation 2 treatments, respectively. These differences are small.

4. (a) Availability = 1.01.
Using the trapezoid rule (Appendix A),

$$F = \frac{[AUC/Dose]_{im}}{[AUC/Dose]_{iv}} = \frac{[(275.8 \text{ mg} \times \text{hour/liter})/500 \text{ mg}]}{[(136.3 \text{ mg} \times \text{hour/liter})/250 \text{ mg}]}$$

(b) A semilogarithmic plot shows that decline in plasma concentration after intramuscular administration is slower than that following intravenous administration, indicating that absorption from the intramuscular site rate limits the elimination of phenytoin from the body.

(c) Absorption is better described by a first-order process than by a zero-order process after the initial rapid absorption. When plotted on regular graph paper, the amount absorbed does not increase at a constant rate, as expected if absorption was zero-order, but approaches the total amount absorbed asymptotically, as expected if absorption is a first-order process. The first-order nature of the absorption process is confirmed by a semilogarithmic plot of the amount remaining to be absorbed against time; the decline is a straight line, with a half-life of 20 hours.

5. (a) Absorption rate limits griseofulvin elimination for 30 to 40 hours. This time corresponds to the normal transit time of food in the gut. Thereafter unabsorbed drug is expelled from the gut, and the plasma concentration of griseofulvin then falls parallel to that following the intravenous dose.

(b) Griseofulvin is poorly available in this subject. A cursory examination of the data plotted on regular graph paper indicates that, based on AUC corrected for dose, griseofulvin is poorly available (F approximately 0.4). Griseofulvin, sparingly soluble in water (10 mg/liter), is difficult to dissolve.

Answers to Study Problems (Chap. 5)

1. A dose does not take into account the time-course of absorption and disposition of a drug. Concentration in plasma, presumably a reflector of the concentration at the site(s) of action, does take them into account.

2. (a) Presence of active metabolite. Here the response is a function of both drug and metabolite. There is even a possibility that the drug disappears before the active metabolite does. Correlation of response to drug concentration would then be nonsense.

   (b) Tolerance. When tolerance is caused by a change in response at a given amount in the body or at a given plasma concentration, one expects to see a poor concentration-response relationship, unless time is considered.

   (c) Measured response is an indirect effect of drug. There may be a number of steps between the direct action of the drug and the response actually measured, producing time delays and a poor correlation between measured response and concentration.

   (d) Measured response related to duration of exposure. The effect of the drug may be more closely related to the duration of inhibition of a process or to the area under the plasma concentration-time curve than to the concentration at any one time.

3. (a) An all-or-none response is a drug effect that is measured in on/off or yes/no units. Death, induction of sleep, and lowering of blood pressure by 25 millimeters of mercury are examples.

   (b) A graded response is a drug effect that is scaled or graded. Examples here are extent of contraction of a muscle in an *in vitro* preparation, change in heart rate, and increase in urine flow.

   (c) The therapeutic window is the region of plasma drug concentrations within which there is a high probability of achieving therapeutic success.

   (d) A utility curve, as used here, is a curve that incorporates the incidence of both desired and undesired effects and the relative importance of these "good" and "bad" effects, as a function of the plasma drug concentration.

   (e) Tolerance denotes a diminished pharmacologic response to a drug with time.

4. See Table 5–2. The therapeutic windows of these drugs will be referred to again in subsequent chapters.

Answers to Study Problems (Chap. 6)

1. (a) 0.42 of a half-life.

$$(½)^n = \frac{C_{ss} - C}{C_{ss} - C(0)} = \frac{15}{20}$$

$$n = \log(15/20)/\log(0.5).$$

   (b) 4.74 half-lives.

$$(½)^n = \frac{C_{ss} - C}{C_{ss} - C(0)} = \frac{-15}{-400}$$

$$n = \log(15/400)/\log(0.5).$$

2. 2.8 and 28 minutes. At plateau, infusion rate $(R_0) = k \cdot A_{ss}$, or $t_{1/2}$ is given by 0.693 $\cdot A_{ss}/R_0$. For succinylcholine, $A_{ss} = 20$ milligrams, so that when $R_0 = 0.5$ milligram/minute, $t_{1/2} = 28$ minutes and when $R_0 = 5$ milligrams/minute, $t_{1/2} = 2.8$ minutes. The wide range in the half-life of succinylcholine arises from differences in the amount and type of pseudocholinesterase, the enzyme responsible for succinylcholine hydrolysis and inactivation. The longer half-life is only rarely encountered.

3. (a) $CL = 1.2$ liters/minute; $t_{1/2} = 1.6$ hours; $V = 164$ liters. $CL = R_0/C_{ss}$. The half-life is estimated from the slope of a semilogarithmic plot of the declining plasma concentration observed on stopping the infusion. The volume of distribution is obtained by dividing clearance by the elimination rate constant $(0.693/t_{1/2})$.

   (b) Yes. Half the plateau value, 10.5 micrograms/liter, should be reached by 1.6 hours and 14.5 micrograms/liter reached by 2 hours. More precisely, using the equation $C = C_{ss}(1 - e^{-kt})$, the expected values at 1, 2, 4, and 6 hours are 7.4, 12, 17, and 19.6 micrograms/liter, which are in reasonably close agreement with the observed values.

   (c) Plasma concentrations are 14.8, 24, and 42 micrograms/liter. Doubling the infusion rate results in a doubling of the concentration at all times.

   (d) Loading dose = 6.9 milligrams; Dose = $V \cdot C(0) = 164$ liters × 42 micrograms/liter.

4. $V = 25$ liters, $k = 0.1$ hour^{-1}, $t_{1/2} = 7$ hours, and $CL = 2.5$ liters/hour.

$$V = \frac{\text{Dose}}{C(0)} = \frac{250 \text{ milligrams}}{10 \text{ milligrams/liter}} \text{ and } CL = R_0/C_{ss} = (10 \text{ mg/hour})/(4 \text{ mg/liter}).$$

$$k = \frac{CL}{V} = (2.5 \text{ liters/hour})/(25 \text{ liters}).$$

5. $V = 22$ liters, $t_{1/2} = 2.5$ hours, and $CL = 6.25$ liters/hour. From postinfusion data, $t_{1/2} = 2.5$ hours ($k = 0.28$ hour^{-1}). At $t_{1/2}$ during infusion,

$$C = \frac{R_0}{2kV} = \frac{C_{ss}}{2} = 4 \text{ milligrams/liter}$$

$$CL = \frac{R_0}{C_{ss}} = \frac{50 \text{ milligrams/hour}}{8 \text{ milligrams/liter}}$$

$$V = \frac{CL}{k} = \frac{6.25 \text{ liters/hour}}{0.28 \text{ hour}^{-1}}$$

The answers might also have been obtained by estimating clearance from the relationship $CL = \text{Dose}/AUC$, where Dose is 50 milligrams/hour × 7.5 hours and the total area under the curve, calculated by the trapezoidal rule, is 60.4 milligram-hours/liter.

Answers to Study Problems (Chap. 7)

1. (a) True. The process of accumulation always occurs on multiple dosing.

   (b) False. The less frequently a drug is given, the lower its extent of accumulation.

   (c) False. The time to reach plateau depends on the elimination half-life.

   (d) Only true if $F = 1$.

   (e) False. $C_{ss,av}$ is independent of volume of distribution.

   (f) False. $C_{ss,av}$ is independent of the absorption kinetics, unless absorption becomes so protracted as to affect availability.

2. (a) 1. $A_{ss,max} = 100$ milligrams; $A_{ss,min} = 68$ milligrams.

      2. Accumulation ratio $= 3.1$.

      3. $C_{ss,min} = 0.24$ milligram/liter.

      4. Time to reach 50 percent of plateau $= 1.83$ days $(t_{1/2})$.

   (b) **Table G–1.**

Dose	1	2	3	4	5	6	7	∞
$A_{N,max}$ (mg)[a]	32	54	69	79	85	90	93	100
$A_{N,min}$ (mg)[b]	22	37	47	53	58	61	63	68

$$^aA_{N,max} = \frac{F \cdot D(1 - e^{-Nk\tau})}{(1 - e^{-k\tau})}$$

$^bA_{N,min} = A_{N,max} \cdot e^{-k\tau}$

   (c) Sketch should be scaled as follows: Amount to 100 milligrams $(A_{ss,max})$ and time to 7 days (5 half-lives), at least.

   (d) Loading dose $= 150$ milligrams $(A_{ss,max}/F)$.

3. Several possibilities, no single solution. Three 100-milligram tablets to start, then either three 100-milligram tablets every 8 hours or two 200-milligram tablets every 12 hours, if given as a controlled-release product.

   Regimen Design

$$t_{1/2} = \frac{0.693 \cdot V}{CL} = 8.7 \text{ hours}$$

$$t_{max} = 1.44 \cdot t_{1/2} \cdot \log (C_{max}/C_{min}) = 8.7 \text{ hours}$$

$$D_{M,max} = \frac{V}{F} (C_{max} - C_{min}) = \begin{array}{l} 5 \text{ milligrams/kilogram or} \\ 300 \text{ milligrams of theophylline} \end{array}$$

$$\text{Dosing rate} = \frac{D_{M,max}}{\tau_{max}} = \begin{array}{l} 34 \text{ milligrams/hour, 204 milligrams/6 hours,} \\ 272 \text{ milligrams/8 hours, 408 milligrams/12 hours} \end{array}$$

Table G–2.

Possible Maintenance Regimens	$C_{ss,max}$[a]	$C_{ss,min}$[b]	Comment
One 200-milligram tablet every 6 hours[c]	14.9	9.2	under
Two 200-milligram tablets every 8 hours	24	12.7	over
Three 300-milligram tablets every 8 hours	16.1	8.5	under[d]
Two 200-milligram tablets every 12 hours	18	7.1	under

$$^aC_{ss,max} = \frac{F \cdot D}{V(1 - e^{-k\tau})}.$$

$^bC_{ss,min} = C_{ss,max} \cdot e^{-k\tau}.$

[c]One 200-milligram tablet $= 170$ milligrams theophylline.

[d]Probably satisfactory and convenient if orally administered—especially as a controlled-release preparation.

Loading Dose

$$D_L = \frac{V}{F} \cdot C_{ss,max} = \frac{30}{1} \times 17 \text{ milligrams/liter} = 510 \text{ milligrams} = \text{three tablets of 170}$$

milligrams of theophylline (200 mg aminophylline)

4. (a) Oral maintenance dosing rate = 6.2 milligrams/hour

$$F \cdot Dose_{single} = CL \cdot AUC_{single}$$
$$F \cdot D_M/\tau = CL \cdot C_{ss,av}$$
$$\frac{D_M}{\tau} = Dose_{single} \cdot \frac{C_{ss,av}}{AUC_{single}} = 50 \text{ milligrams} \times \frac{10 \text{ milligrams/liter}}{80.6 \text{ milligram-hours/liter}}$$

(b) 1. Maintenance dose = 75 milligrams (12 hours × 6.2 milligrams/hour)

2. At plateau, the trough plasma concentration at 12 hours is 5.4 milligrams/liter. The trough concentration at plateau is the sum of the concentrations at 12, 24, 36, 48, etc., hours after a single dose of 75 milligrams. Concentrations associated with a 75-milligram oral dose are 1.5 times those obtained with a 50-milligram oral dose. At plateau, one can ignore contributions from doses that are given more than 5 half-lives previously, that is, 5 times 8 hours or 40 hours. Hence,

$$C_{ss} (12 \text{ hours}) = 1.5 [C(12) + C(24) + C(36) + C(48)]$$
$$= 1.5 [2.8 + 0.6 + 0.14 + 0.03]$$

Note: Although helpful, it is not essential to know the half-life of the drug. One includes concentration values until they become insignificant, which can be judged directly from the concentration-time curve following the single oral dose.

5. (a) 70 milligrams. Situation analogous to a constant-rate infusion. Amount in formulation = $k \cdot A_{ss} \cdot n$, where n is time desired to maintain A_{ss}. Amount = (0.693/4 hours) × 50 milligrams × 8 hours.

(b) Immediately. Loading dose (50 mg) + sustaining dose (70 mg).

(c) Total dose for day one = 260 milligrams; total dose for day two = 210 milligrams.

(d) **Table G–3. Amount in Body (mg)**

Time (hours):	0	4	8	12	16	20	24	28	32	36
Regimen										
Every 4 hours	0	25	63	81	91	95	98	99	99.5	100
Every 8 hours	0	25	38	44	47	49	49	50	50	50
Every 12 hours	0	25	38	19	34	42	21	36	43	22

6. (a) Relative availability (from AUC) = 0.93 (Eq. 23); relative availability (from urine) = 1.00 (Eq. 25). *Note:* These equations assume a steady state has been reached, which will take a long time if the drug has a long half-life. Procainamide has a short half-life of 2.7 hours.

(b) Renal clearance (Eq. 24) = 29.4 or 31.6 liters/hour. $CL_R = Ae_{0-\tau}/AUC_{0-\tau}$.

Answers to Study Problems (Chap. 8)

1. Passive diffusion—Tendency for molecules to move down a concentration gradient.
   Passive facilitated diffusion—Enhanced tendency to move down a concentration gradient, but showing capacity-limited properties, presumably caused by a limited amount of a "carrier."
   Active transport—A form of facilitated transport in which movement against a concentration gradient, expenditure of energy, as well as a capacity limitation are evident.

2. (a) True. The perfusion limitation exists because, functionally, there is no diffusional barrier.

   (b) False. Permeability is a property of the membrane. The rate of movement through the membrane depends on surface area, permeability, and concentration gradient across the membrane.

   (c) False. Diffusion in both directions continues. Only the net rate of movement is zero.

   (d) False. Carrier-mediated transport may or may not be coupled with an energy consuming reaction.

   (e) False. Permeability is a property of the membrane. Binding in the aqueous phase does not appear to affect this property.

3. The ionized forms of drugs, be they acids or bases, do not appear to cross most membranes readily. If lipophilic, the un-ionized form does penetrate membranes. Thus, the degree of ionization can be a controlling factor in determining the rate of movement across membranes.

4. 0.45 liters/hour.

$$CL \text{ (during treatment)} = \frac{0.693 \times 38.5 \text{ liters}}{36 \text{ hours}} = 0.74 \text{ liter/hour.}$$

$$CL \text{ (no treatment)} = \frac{0.693 \times 38.5 \text{ liters}}{93 \text{ hours}} = 0.29 \text{ liter/hour.}$$

By difference, CL (charcoal treatment) = 0.45 liter/hour.

Answers to Study Problems (Chap. 9)

1. Insufficient time for absorption, competing reactions in the gastrointestinal tract, and extraction during the first pass through the liver.

2. (a) False. If transmembrane movement also rate limits elimination from the body, then this is true.

   (b) True. Gastric emptying of large nondisintegrating tablets or dosage units can be greatly delayed, especially after a heavy meal.

(c) False. In general, this statement applies only to those situations in which a suspension is administered intramuscularly or drug precipitates at the injection site.

3. Surface area, solubility, pH, and stirring.

4. (a) 1. B; 2. C and D; 3. A, B, C, and D; 4. A, B, C, and D; 5. C and D.

(b) 1. Much faster (solubility of solid has greater effect than pH of medium); 2. at essentially the same rate (dissolution relatively insensitive to pH of solution); 3. in divided doses during the day (solubility problem); 4. A (solubility problem).

Answers to Study Problems (Chap. 10)

1. Apparent volume of distribution—Parameter that relates the amount in the body to the plasma concentration.
   Fraction unbound—Ratio of unbound and total concentrations in plasma.
   Tissue-to-blood equilibrium-distribution ratio—Ratio of concentrations in whole tissue and blood when there is no net transfer of drug to or from the tissue. It is best determined under steady-state conditions.
   Perfusion and permeability limitations in drug distribution—Conditions in which the rate of distribution to the tissue from the blood, or the converse, is limited by the flow of blood and the ability to cross cell membranes, respectively.

2. Times (minutes): Lungs, 0.07; Kidneys, 0.7; Heart, 3.5; Liver, 13; and Skin, 347.
   Calculated from:

$$\text{Time to reach 50 percent of equilibrium} = t_{1/2} = \frac{0.693 \cdot K_p}{Q/V_T}$$

3. (a) 0.025 milligram/liter (Dose/V).

   (b) 600 milligrams ($V \cdot C$).

   (c) 99.993 percent [$(V - V_p)/V$].

4. a and b.

5. (a) True. The volume of the liver is 2.3 percent of body weight; therefore at distribution equilibrium, the minimum volume of distribution (consisting only of plasma and liver) = $V_p + 50 \cdot V_T$ = [3 + (50 × 1.6)] liters = 83 liters.

   (b) True. It would take much longer if the drug primarily distributed into poorly perfused tissues.

6. Fraction of digitoxin unbound in tissues is 0.033. *Calculated from:*

$$V \text{ (38 liters)} = V_p \text{ (3 liters)} + \left[\frac{fu \ (0.03) \cdot V_T \text{ (39 liters)}}{fu_T} \right]$$

7. Digitoxin ($fu_T = 0.033$) is more tightly tissue bound than digoxin ($fu_T = 0.055$). *Calculated from:*

$$V \text{ (550 liters)} = V_p \text{ (3 liters)} + \left[\frac{fu \ (0.77) \cdot V_T \text{ (39 liters)}}{fu_T} \right]$$

Answers to Study Problems (Chap. 11)

1. Theophylline (CL_R of 10 ml/minute $< fu \cdot GFR$ of 60 ml/minute) is filtered and reabsorbed; secretion cannot be ruled out. Phenytoin (CL_R of 0.15 ml/minute $= fu \cdot$ (urine flow)) is filtered and reabsorbed to equilibrium if compound is not ionized (with a pKa of 8.3, it is not). Cefonicid (CL_R of 20 ml/minute $> fu \cdot GFR$ of 2.4 ml/minute) is filtered, secreted, and perhaps reabsorbed.

2. (a) 1. No pH sensitivity unless it is reabsorbed.

   2. pKa lies in the range in which the fraction un-ionized varies substantially with changes in urine pH.

   3. Clearance and volume of distribution are independent parameters.

   4. Possible if pKa lies in the range of 3.5 to 7.0 and un-ionized compound is lipophilic. However, changes in urine pH will not affect the total amount of drug excreted unchanged as $fe = 1$.

   (b) 1,3. If polar, it is unlikely to be reabsorbed in the kidneys.

   2. Both tubular reabsorption and excretion of a substantial percent by the route of elimination, especially during intoxication, is essential for diuresis to affect elimination.

   4. This compound is not secreted and not reabsorbed; its unbound clearance equals the renal clearance of creatinine, a measure of GFR.

   (c) 1. Its renal clearance exceeds GFR, even without correcting for fu.

   2. Its renal extraction ratio is 0.4.

   3. Without knowing total clearance as well as renal clearance, an estimate of the importance of renal excretion to total elimination cannot be made unambiguously.

   4. Many drugs highly bound to plasma proteins have a high renal clearance; they are efficiently handled by the secretory transport system.

   (d) 1. Although high renal clearance is likely to be relatively constant, there is no guarantee this will be so.

2. Occurs when equilibrium exists between drug in urine and that in blood. Then renal clearance varies proportionately with changes in urine flow.

3. Renal clearance is constant with time, because a fixed rate of excretion results from a given plasma concentration when a constant fraction of filtered and secreted drug is reabsorbed.

3. (a) Alcohol is reabsorbed in the nephron virtually to the same extent as water.

(b) The excretion rate is calculated from urine flow times urine concentration. Thus, at a given plasma alcohol concentration, the excretion rate is flow dependent. Because of the variability in urine flow, the excretion rate only roughly correlates with the plasma alcohol concentration.

4. (a) 1. *Tocainide.* Only for this drug is the pKa in the correct range and its un-ionized form nonpolar, enabling tubular reabsorption to occur.

2. *Nafcillin.* CL_R $(0.693 \cdot fe \cdot V/t_{1/2})$ = 4.7 liters/hour; the CL_R values of the other drugs are lower.

3. *Nafcillin.* Being polar, it will have great difficulty crossing the placenta to the fetus.

4. *Tocainide.* This drug is extensively reabsorbed in the kidneys (CL_R of 1.46 liters/hour $<$ $fu \cdot GFR$, 6.8 liters/hour), and a substantial fraction is excreted unchanged even under normal conditions (fe = 0.14). This fraction is likely to increase in intoxication owing to saturation of metabolic enzymes, which frequently occurs. Nafcillin is not reabsorbed, and for cyclosporine A, renal excretion is too small a pathway of elimination, even if renal clearance increases markedly during diuresis.

5. *Nafcillin.* It has the smallest volume of distribution.

6. *Tocainide.* It has the lowest clearance (0.693 $V/t_{1/2}$ $-$ 10.4 liters/hour).

(b) 1. *Increase*—because the renal clearance of nafcillin, 4.7 liters/hour, is low compared to either renal blood flow (78 liters/hour, assuming a blood to plasma concentration of one) or renal plasma flow (43 liters/hour, assuming the drug is restricted in blood to plasma).

2. *Alkalinization*—because the drug tocainide is an amine for which tubular reabsorption is likely to be more extensive at higher pH values, at which the fraction un-ionized is greater.

3. *Is not*—because nafcillin would have to have a volume of distribution of 15 liters and be unbound in plasma.

4. *Metabolism*—because fe is very low. Cyclosporine A could be eliminated primarily by biliary excretion, but being nonpolar, this is unlikely and in fact is not the case.

5. *Can*—because a large volume of distribution only indicates that the affinity of tissues for drug is much greater than that of plasma. The value of fu for cyclosporine A is 0.05.

6. *99 percent*—because percent outside plasma $[(V - V_p)/V]$ for tocainide is 98.5 percent.

Answers to Study Problems (Chap. 12)

1. A list of examples of such physiologic variables is contained in Table 12–1.

2. **Table G–4.**

Hepatic Extraction Ratio	Hepatic Blood Flow	Fraction in Blood Unbound	Fraction in Tissue Unbound	Total Clearance[a]	Volume of Distribution[a]	Half-life	Oral Availability
High	↑	↔	↔	↑	↔	↓	↑
High	↔	↓	↔	↔	↓	↓	↑
High	↔	↔	↑	↔	↓	↓	↔
Low	↑	↔	↔	↔	↔	↔	↔
Low	↔	↔	↑	↔	↓	↓	↔
Low	↔	↑	↑	↑	↔	↓	↔

[a]Based on drug concentration in blood.

The key equations used to analyze the changes are

$$CL_H = \frac{Q_H \cdot fu_b \cdot CL_{int}}{Q_H + fu_b \cdot CL_{int}}$$

$$V_b = V_B + V_T \cdot \frac{fu_b}{fu_T}$$

$$t_{1/2} = \frac{0.693 \cdot V_b}{CL_H}$$

$$F_H = 1 - \frac{CL_b}{Q_H}$$

3. (a)

		Before	After
CL (liters/minute)	$= \dfrac{Dose_{i.v.}}{AUC_{i.v.}}$	$\dfrac{800}{1207} = 0.66$	$\dfrac{800}{1405} = 0.57$
F	$= \dfrac{AUC_{p.o.}}{AUC_{i.v.}}$	$\dfrac{142}{1207} = 0.12$	$\dfrac{716}{1405} = 0.51$

(b) The blood clearance is 1.1 liters/hour ($CL \cdot C/C_b$). This value indicates the probability of high first-pass effect. Inhibition of metabolism of 6-mercaptopurine increases availability with only a small decrease in clearance, because of its high extraction ratio.

4. (a) $CL = 154$ liters/hour; $CL_b = 77$ liters/hour; $V_b = 120$ liters; and $t_{1/2} = 1.1$ hours.

$$CL_b = Q_H \cdot E_H = 81 \text{ liters/hour} \times 0.95$$

$$CL = \frac{CL_b \cdot C_b}{C} = 77 \text{ liters/hour} \times 2$$

$$\frac{C_b}{C} = \frac{fu}{fu_b} = \frac{0.01}{0.005} = 2$$

$$V_b = \frac{V}{C_b/C} = \frac{240 \text{ liters}}{2}$$

$$t_{1/2} = \frac{(0.693 \cdot V)}{CL} = \frac{(0.693 \times 240 \text{ liters})}{154 \text{ liters/hour}}$$

(b) Yes; tissue binding is decreased.

$$\frac{fu_T \text{ (uremic)}}{fu_T \text{ (normal)}} = 5.2$$

$$fu_T \text{ (normal)} = \frac{V_T \cdot fu}{V - V_p}$$

$$= \frac{V_T \times 0.01}{240 - 3}$$

$$fu_T \text{ (uremic)} = \frac{V_T \times 0.03}{140 - 3}$$

(c) A sixfold increase. Blood clearance should not change, therefore the total plateau concentration is unaltered, but the unbound concentration increases from 0.5 percent to 3 percent of the total.

5. See Figure G–2.

6. Minimum oral maintenance dose = 220 milligrams.
   The renal clearance is 128 milliliters/minute,

$$CL_R = fe \cdot CL = 0.8 \times 160 \text{ milliliters/minute}$$

The plasma ampicillin concentration when the urine concentration is 50 milligrams/liter is 0.39 milligram/liter,

$$C = \frac{(\text{Urine flow}) \cdot (\text{Urine drug concentration})}{CL_R}$$

$$= \frac{1 \text{ milliliter/minute} \times 50 \text{ milligrams/liter}}{128 \text{ milliliters/minute}}$$

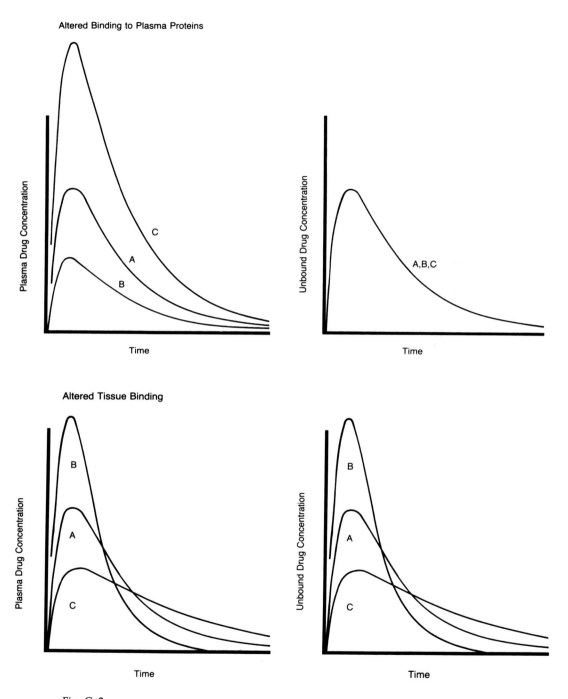

Fig. G–2

The steady-state trough plasma concentration must be 0.39 milligram/liter. The maintenance dose required to achieve this value is 220 milligrams,

$$C_{ss,min} = \frac{F \cdot \text{Dose}}{V} \cdot \frac{e^{-k\tau}}{(1 - e^{-k\tau})}$$

$$\text{Dose} = \frac{C_{ss,min} \cdot V(1 - e^{-k\tau})}{F \cdot e^{-k\tau}}$$

$k = 0.48$ hour^{-1}; $\tau = 6$ hours; $V = 20$ liters; and $F = 0.6$.

Answers to Study Problems (Chap. 13)

1. (a) Any three of the following examples: genetics, disease, age, pharmaceutical formulation, and route of administration.

   (b) See Table 13–2.

2. How much a parameter varies within the population is as important to drug therapy as is its mean value. Information on the distribution of the parameter values helps in deciding the number of dose strengths needed to treat a patient population.

3. Availability, caused by variable hepatic drug extraction on the first pass. Estimates of the ratio CL/F (from Dose/$\tau \cdot C_{av,ss}$) range from 0.25 to 2.5 liters/minute. Therefore either high clearance, low F, or both are responsible. Since nortriptyline is stable in the gastrointestinal tract and lipophilic, high clearance in the liver is the probable explanation. Most variability is in F, as a result of first-pass effect. See Table 9–3.

4. Either the patient population sampled was biased, or this patient represents an extreme of the whole patient population. Recall that the patient was not part of the population from which the population pharmacokinetic values were obtained.

5. Wide differences in hepatic metabolic activity. Alprenolol is highly cleared by the liver. Accordingly, differences in hepatic enzyme activity do not produce much variability in clearance, which is perfusion rate-limited; but these small differences in clearance may cause wide differences in availability ($F_H = 1 - E_H$).

6. (a) Most variable is fu_T, least variable is CLu.

Table G–5.

Subject	1	2	3	4	5	Range
						Mean
CLu^a (liters/hour)	40	42	38	42	40	0.10
fu	0.1	0.15	0.09	0.16	0.11	0.57
$fu_T{}^b$	0.05	0.12	0.18	0.07	0.09	1.27

$^a CLu$ calculated from $\dfrac{R_0}{C_{ss} \cdot fu}$.

$^b fu_T$ calculated from $fu_T = \dfrac{V_T \cdot fu}{V - V_P}$ and $V = \dfrac{CLu \cdot fu}{k}$.

(b) The lack of variability in the unbound clearance means that the unbound concentration and presumably the drug effect at plateau are highly predictable from the rate of administration. There will, however, be differences in the total concentration. Also, the time to achieve the plateau will be variable because of large differences in the half-life, which is primarily a result of variability in tissue binding.

Answers to Study Problems (Chap. 14)

1. Inherited variability in pharmacokinetics is seen with isoniazid and metoprolol. Inherited variability in pharmacodynamics is seen in the resistance to the oral anticoagulant, warfarin, and in drug-induced hemolytic anemia, caused by nitrofurantoin, for example. See Table 14–1 for additional examples.

2. A drug idiosyncrasy is a genetically determined, rare response to a drug. Genetic polymorphism is the occurrence of distinguishable differences in a given characteristic under genetic control. Phenotype is a characteristic expression of an individual.

3. An inherited source of variability in a pharmacokinetic parameter is suggested by a polymodal distribution of the parameter value within the population and by comparative studies between identical and nonidentical twins. It is characterized by familial studies and by correlation studies with other drugs whose pharmacokinetics is known to exhibit genetically determined polymorphism.

4. The poor correlation of atenolol pharmacokinetics with debrisoquine oxidation phenotype is expected; atenolol is primarily excreted unchanged. The strong correlations seen with metoprolol and timolol indicate that they are predominantly eliminated either via a major metabolic pathway or via several pathways that involve the form(s) of cytochrome P-450 concerned with the oxidation of debrisoquine. Propranolol is predominantly metabolized; the weak correlation with this compound suggests that the metabolic pathways involved (e.g., formation of naphthoxylactic acid, p. 354, Chap. 21) are not under the debrisoquine type of control.

5. Frequencies of slow and fast oxidizers are 2.25 percent and 97.75 percent, respectively. Frequency of allele associated with slow oxidation $(p) = 0.15$; frequency of allele associated with fast oxidation $(q) = 0.85$. Hence, the frequency (p^2) of ho-

mozygous slow oxidizers is 0.0225; while 0.9775 ($2pq + q^2$) is the frequency of heterozygous and homozygous fast oxidizers.

Answers to Study Problems (Chap. 15)

1. (a) 24 milligrams (1.6 mg/kg) gentamicin administered intramuscularly every 8 hours. Calculation made using Equation 5. *Note:* The manufacturer's recommended dose of gentamicin for a child is 2 to 2.5 milligrams/kilogram every 8 hours. The age of the adult patient population was not given. If, as likely, those adults with severe infections requiring gentamicin are more elderly, then assuming a mean age of 55 years is reasonable.

   (b) 36 milligrams (0.58 mg/kg) gentamicin administered intramuscularly every 8 hours, or possibly 54 milligrams (0.87 mg/kg) administered every 12 hours, because the half-life will be longer in this elderly patient compared with a 55-year-old patient, both with normal renal function for their age. Calculation made using Equation 5.

   Note: There is a relatively small difference in the maintenance dosing rate (mg/8 hours) between the 4-year-old child in part (a) and in this elderly patient, despite the large difference in body weight.

2. (a) The observations are in broad agreement with the expectations for a drug primarily excreted, which suggests that biliary excretory function follows a trend similar to that of renal function. The low clearance per square meter of body surface area in the neonate and the elder reflects depressed excretory function at both the extremes of life. Between 1 and 20 years, clearance per square meter is expected to be relatively constant; the data in this age range are too few to make a firm conclusion.

   (b) The half-life should be at a minimum at around 2 to 6 years of age, and should be greater than the minimum by a factor of 2 to 3 at the extremes of age. This conclusion is based on the relationship $t_{1/2} = 0.693 \, V/CL$; volume of distribution does not vary much on a weight basis, but clearance per square meter of body surface area is at a maximum between 2 to 6 years of age. As clearance per square meter varies by a factor of 3 (Fig. 15–11), so should half-life.

   (c) Dosing rate needs to be reduced in neonates and in patients over 70 years of age, even when correcting for weight, and perhaps dosing can be less frequent than in the usual adult.

3. (a) The differences among theophylline, digoxin, and diazepam can be explained by the differences in the partition of these drugs into fat. Obese subjects for a given height primarily differ from normal subjects in the much greater preponderance of fat; the body water space is unchanged. Both theophylline and digoxin are poorly lipophilic and so their volume of distribution does not increase with the increase in body fat. In contrast, diazepam is lipophilic and so its volume of distribution increases in the obese subject, both on absolute and weight-corrected bases.

(b) The information has relevance to the loading dose and the degree of fluctuation in plasma concentration on chronic dosing, but not to the maintenance dose requirement, which depends on clearance. No weight correction in the loading dose is needed for either digoxin or theophylline. Diazepam is administered intravenously over 1 to 4 minutes as a sedative, for relief of muscle spasm, and as an anticonvulsant. Under these circumstances, because fat is poorly perfused, there may be little difference in the initial concentrations in plasma and in highly perfused tissues, such as the brain, in obese patients compared with normal weight patients. Accordingly, there may be little need to adjust the intravenous dose of diazepam in the obese patient. A loading dose is not used with oral diazepam regimens. However, associated with the larger volume distribution is a longer half-life of diazepam in the obese patient. Even so, because the half-life of diazepam in normal weight subjects is already long (approximately 40 hours), there should be no need to adjust the usual recommended dosing regimen of diazepam in obese patients, although there will be less fluctuation in the plasma concentration at plateau.

Answers to Study Problems (Chap. 16)

1. Cirrhosis, uremia, congestive cardiac failure, Crohn's disease, thyroid disease, and pneumonia. See Table 16–1 for other examples and brief comments.

2. (a) B > D > C > E > A, calculated from Equation 6 for a typical 55-year-old, 70-kilogram patient.

   (b) B and perhaps C and D.

3. (a) For both pentazocine and meperidine, the blood clearance in control subjects is sufficiently high to expect availabilities $(1 - CL_b/Q_H)$ of about 8 percent and 33 percent, respectively, if elimination occurs only in the liver and the hepatic blood flow is 1.35 liters/minute. For both drugs, cirrhosis appears to decrease clearance by about 35 percent to 37 percent and to increase availability by 278 percent and 81 percent, respectively. Decreased blood flow would explain the decreased clearance, but would not explain the increased availability. Decreased metabolic activity or shunting of portal blood would explain both effects. The latter has been shown to occur in cirrhosis and is probably the major mechanism.

   (b) The availability of pentazocine is more extensively affected by cirrhosis than that of meperidine, because it has the higher hepatic extraction ratio. The higher the extraction ratio, the lower is the availability and the greater is the effect of a decrease in metabolic activity on availability.

4.

Patients:	S.W.	B.J.	D.A.	B.T.
(a) Estimated Creatinine Clearance (ml/minute)[a]:	134	16	10	27
(b) Relative Renal Function:	1.58	0.19	0.12	0.32

[a]See Table 16–2 for equations.

5. (a) $C_{ss,max}$ = 48 milligrams/liter; $C_{ss,min}$ = 12 milligrams/liter

V = 0.4 × 70 = 28 liters

$$C_{ss,max} = \frac{D}{V}\left(\frac{1}{1-e^{-k\tau}}\right)$$

$$= \frac{1000 \text{ milligrams}}{28 \text{ liters}}\left(\frac{1}{1-e^{-12 \times 0.693/6}}\right) = 48 \text{ milligrams/liter}$$

$C_{ss,min} = C_{ss,max} - D/V = 12$ milligrams/liter

(b) Loading dose = 243 milligrams [(17/70) × 1000 milligrams]; Maintenance dose = 100 milligrams/12 hours.

Creatinine clearance in child is

$$\frac{(0.48 \times 108)}{2.7} \times \left(\frac{17}{70}\right)^{0.7} = 7.1 \text{ milliliters/minute}$$

Creatinine clearance in a normal patient (55-year-old) is 85 milliliters/minute

$$RF \text{ (child)} = \frac{7.1 \text{ milliliters/minute}}{85 \text{ milliliters/minute}} = 0.082; \; fe(n) = 0.95$$

$$Rd = RF \cdot fe(n) + [1 - fe(n)]\left[\frac{(140 - \text{Age}) \times \text{Weight}^{0.7}}{1660}\right] = 0.078 + 0.030;$$

Rd = 0.108 (decrease of nine- to tenfold in adult regimen).

Suggest reducing maintenance dose tenfold to achieve a tenfold reduction in dosing rate. It could be 100 milligrams every 12 hours or 200 milligrams every 24 hours. For demonstrative purposes, we have chosen a dosing interval of 12 hours for the subsequent calculations.

(c) Parameters in child: CL = 7.1 milliliters/minute or 0.43 liter/hour, V = 6.8 liters (0.4 liter/kg × 17 kg); k = 0.063 hour^{-1}; and $t_{1/2}$ = 11 hours.

1. Dose: 600 milligrams every 12 hours; regimen adjusted for age and weight only

$$\frac{D_m}{\tau} \text{ (child)} = \frac{(140 - \text{Age}) \times \text{Weight}^{0.7}}{1660} \cdot \frac{D_M}{\tau} \text{ (reference patient)}$$

$$= 0.59 \times 1000 \text{ milligrams/12 hours}$$

$$\approx 600 \text{ milligrams every 12 hours.}$$

2. Dose: 100 milligrams every 12 hours, adjusted for age, weight, and renal function.

$$\frac{D_M \text{ (child)}}{\tau} = Rd \cdot \frac{D_M}{\tau} \text{ (reference patient)}$$

$$= 0.108 \times 1000 \text{ milligrams/12 hours}$$

$$\approx 100 \text{ milligrams/12 hours}$$

3. Table G–6 lists the calculated maximum and minimum amounts in the body

in the child on approach to steady state on giving the maintenance regimen given in 1 and 2. To plot the data the appropriate scales are

Scale time to 4 to 5 half-lives $\approx$ 48 hours.
Scale amount in body to $A_{ss,max}$ on 600 milligrams every 12 hours

$$= 600 \cdot \frac{1}{(1 - e^{-0.063 \times 12})} \approx 1200 \text{ milligrams.}$$

Table G–6. Maintenance Regimen

Time (hours)	0	12	12+[a]	24	24+	36	36+	48
Amount in Body (mg)								
600 milligrams/12 hours	600	282	882	414	1014	476	1076	505
100 milligrams/12 hours	100	47	147	69	169	79	179	84

[a]The plus sign (+) means just after the dose.

Answers to Study Problems (Chap. 17)

1. 100 milligrams initially and either 50 milligrams twice daily or 100 milligrams once daily. The metabolic clearance becomes 20 percent of normal value, which is 80 percent of the normal total clearance value. Renal clearance is 20 percent of the normal total clearance. By summation, the total clearance becomes 36 percent of its normal value. In the presence of the inhibitor, the maintenance dosing rate should, therefore, be adjusted by a factor of 0.36.

2. See Figure G–3.

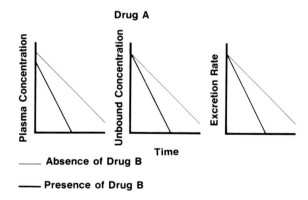

Fig. G–3

3. (a) Drug A is secreted and reabsorbed. Renal clearance/$(fu \cdot GFR)$ is 2.1 in the absence and 0.3 in the presence of Drug B.

   (b) Displacement from plasma and tissue binding sites and either inhibition of tubular secretion or enhanced tubular reabsorption, e.g., by a change in urine pH. The threefold increase in the unbound fraction of Drug A in the presence of Drug B should increase the renal clearance threefold; instead the renal clearance decreased from 1.5 liters/hour to 0.6 liter/hour.

The extrarenal clearance increased approximately threefold. For Drug A alone,

$$CL \text{ (nonrenal)} = \frac{25 \text{ milligrams/hour}}{10 \text{ milligrams/liter}} - 1.5 \text{ liters/hour}$$

$$= 1.0 \text{ liter/hour}$$

and in the presence of Drug B,

$$CL \text{ (nonrenal)} = \frac{25 \text{ milligrams/hour}}{6.7 \text{ milligrams/liter}} - 0.60 \text{ liter/hour}$$

$$= 3.1 \text{ liters/hour}$$

By calculation ($V = 1.44 \cdot CL \cdot t_{1/2}$), the volume of distribution of Drug A, 43 liters, is seen to not change during coadministration with Drug B. As displacement from plasma proteins occurs, so must displacement occur in tissues to keep the volume of distribution unchanged.

(c) The plateau unbound concentration ($fu \cdot C_{ss}$) of Drug A increases from 1 milligram/liter in the absence to 2 milligrams/liter in the presence of Drug B, suggesting that the response produced by Drug A is increased, perhaps excessively. No information is given on A → B.

4. (a) The change in distribution must occur by a decrease in tissue binding ($fu_T \uparrow$). Quinidine decreases the volume of distribution of digoxin, but does not appear to alter plasma protein binding.

(b) If the range of therapeutic plasma concentrations of digoxin remains unchanged in the presence of quinidine, then the digitalizing dose will need to be reduced, on average, about twofold (500/240) to compensate for the change in volume of distribution. To achieve a concentration of 1.5 micrograms/liter requires only 360 micrograms of digoxin intravenously. For digoxin tablets, with an availability of about 0.75, the requirement is about 500 micrograms.

(c) Because of quinidine's relatively short half-life, its accumulation is rapid. By 24 hours it has reached its plateau and, presumably, its maximum effect on the distribution and elimination of digoxin. Associated with the reduction in its volume of distribution, the concentration of digoxin doubles during this period and stays there, since clearance is reduced to one-half of its normal value. The converse occurs when quinidine is discontinued. Because of its relatively short half-life, the plasma concentration of quinidine falls rapidly before much digoxin is eliminated. The fall in quinidine concentration produces a redistribution of digoxin from plasma back into the tissues, with an associated fall in the digoxin concentration in plasma. Then, because the clearance of digoxin returns to its prequinidine value, so does the digoxin concentration.

(d) Yes. Nonrenal clearance (total − renal) in the absence of quinidine is 39 milliliters/minute. In the presence of quinidine it is reduced to 21 milliliters/minute (total clearance of 72 ml/minute minus renal clearance of 51 ml/minute). This change would then require that the dosing rate of digoxin be reduced in a patient with renal insufficiency.

5. **Table G–7.**

		Observation			
	Clearance	Volume of Distribution	Half-life	Fraction Excreted Unchanged	Availability
Drug A	↓	↔	↑	↓	↔
Drug B	↑	↔	↓	↔	↔
Drug C	↔	↔	↔	↔	↔
Drug D	↔	↑	↑	↑	↓
Drug E	↔	↓	↓	↔	↔
Drug F	↑	↑	↔	↔	↔
Drug G	↔	↔	↔	↔	↔

Answers to Study Problems (Chap. 18)

1. The criteria for performing drug concentration monitoring are discussed in the section on Target Concentration Strategy (pp. 278–280).

2. (a) CL = 82 milliliters/minute or 4.9 liters/hour; V = 19 liters; k = 0.26 hour^{-1}; and $t_{1/2}$ = 2.7 hours.

$$CL = CL_{cr} = \frac{(140 - 42) \times 85}{85 \times 1.2} = 82 \text{ milliliters/minute}$$

$$V = 85 \text{ kilograms} \times 0.22 \text{ liter/kilogram}$$

(b) At the time of the first sample, 32 hours has elapsed, i.e., over 10 half-lives. Hence steady-state equations are appropriate. At 45 minutes after end of infusion, C = 5.4 milligrams/liter. Just before the next dose, C = 1.0 milligram/liter.

$$C = \frac{120}{0.75} \times \frac{(1 - e^{-k \cdot t_{inf}})}{4.9} \cdot \frac{1}{(1 - e^{-k \cdot \tau})} \cdot e^{-k(t - t_{inf})}$$

where t_{inf} = 0.75 hour, t_{post} = 0.75 hour, τ = 8 hours, so that at t = 1.5, C = 5.4 milligrams/liter and at t = 8, C = 1.0 milligram/liter.

3. (a) CL = 0.04 × 0.4 × 1.6 × 70 = 1.79 liters/hour; V = 0.5 × 70 = 35 liters; k = 0.051 hour^{-1}, $t_{1/2}$ = 13.5 hours; F = 1.0; and S = 0.85.

(b) 14.9 milligrams/liter.

$$C = (0.85/35) \cdot [400 \cdot e^{-0.051 \times 24} + 200 \cdot e^{-0.051 \times 20}$$
$$+ 300 \cdot e^{-0.051 \times 10} + 300 \cdot e^{-0.051 \times 6}]$$

(c) 14.9 milligrams/liter predicted versus 18 milligrams/liter observed.

(d) Observed and predicted concentrations are fairly close. However, because the sample is obtained at not much more than one half-life after starting therapy and the patient is on an unequal-dose-equal-interval regimen, one has little confidence in revising the parameters. It might be prudent to recommend a lowering of the dose, as the quantity metabolized (amount absorbed minus amount in body) in the 24-hour period is only about 400 milligrams [0.85 × total dose given (400 + 200 + 300 + 300) − amount in body at time of sampling (35 × 18)].

4. (a) *Evaluation.*

    1. *Expected parameter values:*
      CL = 0.27 liter/hour or 6.5 liters/day (0.0037 liter/hour per kg × 74 kg); V = 0.55 liter/kilogram × 74 kilograms = 41 liters; k = 0.0067 hour^{-1} or 0.16 day^{-1}; $t_{1/2}$ = 104 hours or 4.3 days; F = 1; and S = 1.

    2. *Estimation of concentrations at times of sampling:* 30 and 12 milligrams/liter (compliance is assumed, and because $t_{1/2}$ is much greater than τ and the first blood sample is obtained in the middle of the dosing interval after prolonged treatment, the plasma concentration expected at the first sampling time is well approximated by $C_{ss,av}$).

$$C_{ss,av} = F \cdot \frac{Dose}{CL \cdot \tau} = \frac{200 \text{ milligrams}}{\dfrac{0.27 \text{ liter}}{\text{hour}} \times \dfrac{24 \text{ hours}}{\text{day}} \times 1 \text{ day}} = 30 \text{ milligrams/liter}$$

$$C \text{ (6 days later)} = 30 \ e^{-0.16 \text{ day}^{-1} \times 6 \text{ days}} = 12 \text{ milligrams/liter}$$

    3. *Comparison of concentrations (mg/liter):*

Date	Jan. 10	Jan. 16
Predicted	30	12
Observed	56	16

    4. (a) *Estimation of parameter values in individual:*
      Half-life. This parameter is the most accurately estimated one in this case.

$$k = \frac{\log(56/16)}{6 \text{ days}}$$
$$= 0.21 \text{ day}^{-1} \text{ and } t_{1/2} = 3.3 \text{ days.}$$

      Clearance: From k value (greater than expected) and usual volume of distribution,

$$CL = 0.21 \text{ day}^{-1} \times 41 \text{ liters} = 8.6 \text{ liters/day}$$

  (b) *Recommendation.* With an estimated clearance higher than that expected and since a change in volume of distribution cannot explain the high concentration observed (fluctuation is small at steady state for a drug with a 3.3-day half-life), the likely explanation for the 56 milligrams/liter value is that the patient has taken more than prescribed. Phenobarbital therapy should be resumed on January 11.

The following relationship ($F \cdot \dfrac{Dose}{\tau} = CL \cdot C_{ss,av}$) can be used as a guide for dosing.

$$\text{Daily dose} = 8.6 \text{ liters/day} \times \text{Plasma concentration}$$
$$\text{(mg)} \hspace{4cm} \text{(mg/liter)}$$

The clinician can decide whether he wishes to have a steady-state concentration toward the higher or lower end of the therapeutic window, 10 to 30 milligrams/liter. A daily dose of 200 milligrams is expected to give a steady-state concentration in the 20 to 25 milligrams/liter range. Patient education is in order.

5. Using Equation 9 and the expected values of F, S, CL, and k, the predicted plasma theophylline concentrations are 3.4, 11.6, and 14.5 milligrams/liter in the three patients, respectively. Clearly, patient 2 has a lower than average value of clearance and patient 3 has a much higher than average value. By an iterative procedure and using Equation 9, the values of clearance in the three patients are 0.031, 0.016, and 0.107 liter/hour per kilogram, and the values of the half-life are 11, 22, and 3 hours, respectively. In patient 1 the sampling time is so short that one has virtually no confidence in the clearance or half-life estimate; a wide range of clearance values gives essentially the same concentration. In patient 2, the clearance is low, and indeed from the estimated clearance and half-life, the value of 18 is far from the estimated steady-state concentration, 40 milligrams/liter. Clearly, the rate of administration of aminophylline in this patient should be reduced, probably about fourfold. A subsequent sample, obtained about 48 to 72 hours later, would then be appropriate. In patient 3, the estimated value of the half-life is such that a good estimate of clearance is obtained. Here, the rate of administration must be doubled to achieve a concentration within the therapeutic range of 10 to 20 milligrams/liter.

Answers to Study Problems (Chap. 19)

1. Initial Dilution Volume (V_1)—is the volume that the drug appears to occupy initially; its value is given by dividing the intravenous dose by the concentration at zero time, predicted from an equation that fits the plasma concentration-time data.

   Volume of Distribution during Terminal Phase (V)—is the apparent volume of distribution that a drug occupies after distribution equilibrium has been achieved following one or more discrete doses of drug or after stopping an infusion.

   Volume of Distribution at Steady State (V_{ss})—is given by the ratio of the amount of drug in the body at steady state and the corresponding plasma concentration.

2. (a) This is true. The extent of distribution outside of blood may be small and very rapid, in which case frequent sampling at early times after a bolus dose would be needed to observe the kinetics of distribution.

   (b) This is a reasonable assumption for most drugs, as the kidneys and the liver are the major organs of elimination, and both organs are highly perfused. Some drugs are metabolized by many tissues, e.g., nitroglycerin, and for them the assumption that elimination takes place only in the central compartment is questionable.

   (c) This statement is true provided the terminal phase is correctly identified. If the majority of the area under the plasma concentration-time curve is associated with the initial phase, then most of the drug is eliminated before distribution equilibrium is achieved and the terminal phase is reached. In this case, the statement is conservative.

3. (a) Slow acetylator: C_1 = 1.59 milligrams/liter; C_2 = 0.65 milligram/liter; λ_1 = 5.5 hour^{-1}; λ_2 = 0.11 hour^{-1}
   Fast acetylator: C_1 = 1.57 milligram/liter; C_2 = 0.42 milligram/liter; λ_1 = 4.2 hour^{-1}; λ_2 = 0.40 hour^{-1}

   (b) Slow acetylator: CL = 12 liters/hour; V_1 = 33 liters; V = 110 liters
   Fast acetylator: CL = 53 liters/hour; V_1 = 38 liters; V = 132 liters
   The major difference between fast and slow acetylators is in clearance.

   (c) Yes. The initial dilution space (33 and 38 liters) must include some well-perfused tissues.

   (d) Slow acetylator: CL = 12.7 liters/hour; V = 115 liters.
   Fast acetylator: CL = 71 liters/hour; V = 178 liters.
   In addition to differences in clearance, one might have concluded that differences in distribution (V) also existed, which is not so (see 3(b)).

   (e) f_2 = 0.95 (slow acetylator), 0.74 (fast acetylator).

   (f) Yes, since f_2 approaches 1.0 for both subjects, the terminal half-life primarily determines the time for the plasma concentration to reach plateau.

4. (a) V_1 = 18.2 liters; CL = 2.8 liters/hour; V = 295 liters; and V_{ss} = 70.9 liters.

   (b) Only glomerularly filtered.

   $$CLu_R = CL_R/fu = \frac{2.8}{0.37} \text{ liters/hour} = 7.6 \text{ liters/hour} \ (\approx GFR)$$

   and being polar, the drug is not expected to be reabsorbed. Since glomerular filtrate is directly from arterial blood, assuming that elimination occurs from the central compartment only is reasonable.

   (c) $V > V_{ss}$ because elimination of drug from plasma increases the ratio of drug concentration in slowly equilibrating tissue to that in plasma during the terminal phase. The slower the distribution of drug between plasma and the slowly equilibrating tissues, the greater will be the difference between V and V_{ss}.

   (d) f_1 = 0.8; f_2 = 0.2.

   The half-lives of the corresponding exponential coefficients are 3.6 and 73 hours, respectively. The half-lives reflect a composite of distribution and elimination kinetics. In the present case the majority of drug is eliminated before distribution equilibrium is achieved, and so with respect to elimination, the first half-life is of particular importance. Here, the terminal half-life is only of importance if interest lies in the slowly equilibrating tissues. For most drugs, the majority of drug is eliminated during the terminal phase, that is $f_2 > f_1$.

   (e) 1. 5 and 72 hours to reach 50 percent and 90 percent of plateau, respectively. Cannot solve for time explicitly; it is estimated iteratively by successive approximations.

$$\frac{C}{C_{ss}} = f_1 (1 - e^{-\lambda_1 t}) + f_2 (1 - e^{-\lambda_2 t})$$

$$= 0.8 (1 - e^{-0.19t}) + 0.2 (1 - e^{-0.0095t})$$

Table G–8.

Time (hours)	2	4	5	6	12	24	48	72	96
C/C_{ss}	0.26	0.43	≈0.50	0.55	0.74	0.83	0.87	0.90	0.92

Note that 50 percent of the plateau value is reached in approximately one initial half-life (3.8 hours; $0.693/\lambda_1$), but that the rise to the 90 percent value becomes increasingly determined by the long terminal half-life, 73 hours. Under these circumstances, the statement that it takes one half-life to reach 50 percent of plateau and 3.3 half-lives to reach plateau is misleading.

2. A pronounced biexponential curve is observed on stopping the infusion at steady state, because the rate of movement of drug from the slowly equilibrating tissues initially does not match the rapid elimination of drug from plasma. Eventually, decline of drug in plasma becomes controlled by movement of drug out from the slowly equilibrating tissues.

3. Now $f_2 = 0.83$, signifying that distribution equilibrium occurs before much drug is eliminated. Under this circumstance, although there will still be a biexponential fall on stopping the infusion, the first phase will be very shallow because drug rapidly moves from the tissues as it is eliminated from plasma. Given the general inability to distinguish two concentrations that differ by 10 percent and have the usual variation in plasma concentrations, it is unlikely that the first phase will be seen; the postinfusion decay would then appear monoexponential, with rate constant λ_2.

5. The observation in Figure 19–15 is explained by differences in the distribution kinetics of these drugs. For pancuronium, distribution equilibrium is achieved before much drug is eliminated in patients with both normal and impaired renal function; diminished renal clearance then causes a change in the terminal half-life. For d-tubocurarine, most drug is eliminated from the plasma (and the well-stirred pool) before much drug is eliminated in patients with both normal and impaired renal function; the terminal phase in both cases is primarily controlled by slow movement of drug out of the slowly equilibrating tissues. Diminished renal clearance is reflected by a smaller fall in d-tubocurarine concentration before the terminal phase is reached as less drug has been eliminated by that time than in a patient with normal renal function.

6. (a) For halazepam, the fluctuation at plateau primarily reflects a balance between the kinetics of absorption and distribution; the 8-hourly dosing interval is too short to permit distribution equilibrium to be achieved.

   (b) Not well, and certainly not within a dosing interval, which is too short relative to the terminal half-life. Theoretically, the terminal half-life could be measured from the rising trough concentration on approach to plateau, but in practice this measurement has too much error to provide a reliable estimate of terminal half-life. The most reliable estimate is gained on stopping drug administration and following the decline in plasma drug concentration.

Answers to Study Problems (Chap. 20)

1. (a) *F.* Considering even the simplest pharmacokinetic model ($C = (D/V) \cdot e^{-kt}$), for a given end point, with an associated concentration, C_{min}, the duration t_d is proportional to log Dose;

$$t_d = \frac{1}{k} \cdot \log \left[\frac{\text{Dose}}{V \cdot C_{min}} \right]$$

(b) *T.* The concentration always decreases with time. Thus a complete "hysteresis" loop is not possible.

(c) *T.* In the equation, Effect $= E_{max} \cdot C^\gamma/(EC_{50}{}^\gamma + C^\gamma)$, it is apparent that if $C = EC_{50}$, then Effect $= E_{max}/2$, irrespective of the value of γ.

(d) *T.* In this region, where Effect $\simeq (E_{max}/EC_{50}{}^\gamma) \cdot C^\gamma$, the Effect will be directly proportional to C only if $\gamma = 1$.

(e) *T.* Before distribution equilibrium is achieved, interpretation of plasma concentrations is complicated by temporal aspects.

2. $C_{20} = 5.7$ milligrams/liter and $C_{80} = 17.4$ milligrams/liter. On rearrangement of Equation 20–1,

$$C = EC_{50} \cdot \left[\frac{\text{Effect}}{1 - \text{Effect}} \right]^{1/\gamma}$$

where Effect is expressed as a fraction of the maximum response. For $\gamma = 2.5$ and $EC_{50} = 10$ milligrams/liter, $C_{20} = 5.7$ milligrams/liter and $C_{80} = 17.4$ milligrams/liter.

3. (a) $A_{min} = 0.38$ milligram/kilogram, from a plot of t_d versus log dose.

(b) Data consistent; A_{min} still in body when second dose of 1 milligram/kilogram is given; i.e., total effective dose is 1.38 milligrams/kilogram. This total dose, 1.38 milligram/kilogram, on t_d versus log dose graph gives t_d of about 8 minutes.

Same answer by calculation, $t_d = \frac{1}{k} \cdot \log \left(\frac{\text{Dose}}{A_{min}} + 1 \right)$

4. (a) 11.4 hours [$A_{min} = 320$ mg; substitute into equation in (b) above].

(b) 18.3 hours (11.4 hours + half-life).

(c) 1. 22.8 hours and 2. 8.9 hours.

(d) Doubling the dose increases the duration by one half-life. The effect of doubling the half-life depends on the mechanism of the change. A decreased clearance leads to a doubling of the duration of effect, whereas in this example, duration is decreased when the cause of the increased half-life is a doubling of the volume of distribution.

5. Initial dose = 20 milligrams; maintenance dose = 5 milligrams every 12 hours. By interpolation between data in inset of Figure 20–20, 20 milligrams is needed to immediately reduce MAP by 85 millimeters of mercury, and 15 milligrams is needed to reduce MAP by 75 millimeters of mercury. As response wears off at a rate of 10 millimeters of mercury per 12 hours, 20 − 15 milligrams (or 5 milligrams) is needed every 12 hours, to maintain a MAP value between 95 and 105 millimeters of mercury.

6. (a) The increase in duration of action seen after the second, third, and fourth doses of pancuronium is a consequence of distribution kinetics. The effect of the first dose occurs during the distribution phase of the drug. On successive doses, because of a rising tissue concentration, the tendency of drug to move from plasma into tissues decreases, thereby prolonging the time before the plasma concentration reaches the predetermined value.

   (b) No. The duration will reach a limiting value when the amount eliminated during the interval equals the dose of drug administered.

7. (a) $t_{1/2}$ = 2.3 hours. *Calculated from:*
   A linear plot of intensity of effect versus time, the slope $(m \cdot k)$ = 3.5 percent/ hour; given that m = 11.5 percent, then k = 0.3 hour^{-1}.

   (b) 1. 6.3 hours and 2. 7.7 hours.
   After a 20-milligram dose, the effect remains above 15 percent for 4 hours (Table 20–3).

   1. After a 40-milligram dose, the duration is increased one half-life (total of 6.3 hours).

   2. After a 60-milligram dose, the duration is increased an extra 3.7 hours

$$t_d = \frac{\log(60/20)}{k} + 4 = 7.7 \text{ hours}$$

Answers to Study Problems (Chap. 21)

1. Only the clearance associated with the formation of N-acetylprocainamide and the total clearance of N-acetylprocainamide; this follows from the equation $C(m)_{ss,av}/C_{ss,av}$ = $CL_f/CL(m)$. Note that in all patients in whom the ratio is greater than 1.0, the clearance of N-acetylprocainamide must be less than the clearance of procainamide.

2. a only.

   (a) Induction leads to an increase in CL_f.

$$\frac{AUC(m)}{AUC} = \frac{CL_f}{CL(m)}$$

   (b) Ratio independent of V or $V(m)$.

(c) Ratio independent of Dose.

(d) If alternate pathway is reduced, f_m is increased in proportion to decrease in CL, but CL_f is unaffected.

3. The rate of excretion of salicyluric acid can be taken to be its rate of formation from salicylic acid. The rate of elimination of salicyluric acid is limited by, and hence essentially equal to, its rate of formation. However, the rate of elimination of salicyluric acid is its rate of excretion.

4. The gastrointestinal tract plays only a modest role, at best, in the formation of promethazine sulfoxide. This conclusion is based on a dose-corrected AUC ratio of the sulfoxide, oral to intravenous, of 0.8. For significant prehepatic sulfoxide formation to occur, the dose-corrected AUC ratio must be much greater than 1. Note that if drug is completely converted to a metabolite (fm = 1), the dose-corrected AUC ratio for metabolite would be 1, irrespective of the site of its formation, provided that all drug is available to the gastrointestinal tract and all formed metabolite is available systemically.

5. A major fraction of 4-hydroxypropranolol is formed during the absorption of propranolol, which is subject to extensive first-pass hepatic elimination. This metabolite has a shorter half-life than propranolol, and so initially the plasma 4-hydroxypropranolol concentration falls faster than that of propranolol; the terminal decline of metabolite is parallel to that of drug because the elimination of metabolite formed from absorbed propranolol is formation rate-limited. The 4-hydroxypropranolol concentration peaks earlier than that of propranolol because it has the shorter half-life. Recall from Chapter 4, the peak is reached when rate of elimination matches the rate of absorption, and it occurs earlier the shorter the half-life of elimination.

6. (a) Fraction of drug converted to metabolite = 0.90; formation clearance of metabolite = 8.4 liters/hour. Disposition kinetics of metabolite: $t_{1/2}$ = 4.0 hours, $k(m)$ = 0.17 hour^{-1}, $CL(m)$ = 2.9 liters/hour; $V(m)$ = 17 liters.

From a semilogarithmic plot, it can be seen that elimination of metabolite is disposition rate-limited. And, from respective decline phases $t_{1/2}$ (drug) = 1.3 hours, $t_{1/2}$ (metabolite) = 4.0 hours.

For drug

$$(F = 1),\ CL\ (Dose/AUC) = \frac{1000\ \text{milligrams}}{108\ \text{milligram-hours/liter}} = 9.3\ \text{liters/hour}$$

and

$$V\ (\text{from } CL/k) = \frac{9.3\ \text{liters/hour}}{0.53\ \text{hour}^{-1}} = 17\ \text{liters}$$

For metabolite

1. $fm = \dfrac{AUC(m)}{AUC} \cdot \dfrac{CL(m)}{CL}$

And given that $V(m)$ = V, then

$$fm = \frac{AUC(m)}{AUC} \cdot \frac{k(m)}{k}$$

$AUC(m)$ = 319 milligrams metabolite-hours/liter [by trapezoidal rule to 12 hours + $C(m, 12$ hours$)/k(m)$]

= 300 milligrams drug equivalents-hours/liter

Hence

fm = 0.90.

2. $CL_f = fm \cdot CL$ = 8.4 liters/hour.
3. $V(m) = V$ = 17 liters.
4. $CL(m) = V(m) \cdot k(m)$ = 2.9 liters/hour.

(b) 1. $C_{ss,av}$ = 13.5 milligrams/liter; $C(m)_{ss,av}$ = 40 milligrams/liter;

$$C_{ss,av} = \frac{AUC_{single}}{\tau} = \frac{108 \text{ milligram-hours/liter}}{8 \text{ hours}}; \text{ and}$$

$$C(m)_{av,ss} = \frac{AUC(m)_{single}}{\tau} = \frac{319 \text{ milligram-hours/liter}}{8 \text{ hours}}$$

2. **Table G–9.**

Time Within Dosing Interval (hours)	0	1	2	4	6	8
C (mg/liter)	1.2	32	32	9	4	1.2
C(m) (mg/liter)	21.3	39.5	59.0	43.3	32.6	21.3

For both drug and metabolite $C_{ss}(t) = C_1(t) + C_1(t + \tau) \ldots C_1(t + n \cdot \tau)$, where C_1 refers to the concentration after a single dose, and n is a number of doses sufficiently large that the concentration associated with time, $t + n \cdot \tau$, is negligible compared with $C_1(t)$. In practice $n \cdot \tau = 5t_{1/2}$, or n is equal to $5t_{1/2}/\tau$. For drug, n is less than 1. That is, there is negligible accumulation and so the concentrations within a dosing interval, at plateau, are essentially those obtained after a single dose. For metabolite, $n = 2.5$. The concentration at 1 hour after dosing, at plateau, is

$$C_{ss} (1 \text{ hour}) = C_1 (1) + C_1 (9) + C_1 (17) + C_1 (25) + \ldots$$

The values at 9, 17, and 25 hours are calculated from the 8-hour value (16 mg/liter), knowing the elimination rate constant, $k(m)$. Thus $C (9) = C (8)$ $e^{-k(m) \times 1 \text{ hour}}$, $C (17) = C (8) e^{-k(m) \times 9 \text{ hours}}$, and so on. Which gives

$$C_{ss} (1 \text{ hour}) = 22 + 13 + 3.4 + 0.84 + 0.21 + 0.05$$

$$= 39.5 \text{ milligrams}$$

Similarly,

$$C_{ss} (8 \text{ hour}) = C_{ss} (0 \text{ hour}) = C_1 (8) + C_1 (16) + C_1 (24) \ldots$$

$$= 21.3 \text{ milligrams/liter}$$

3. For drug, steady state is reached within one dosing interval. With metabolite, it is reached by 3 dosing intervals.

Answers to Study Problems (Chap. 22)

1. (a) Decrease. The absorption is saturable, and there is a limited transit time for riboflavin and thiamine at the absorption sites within the gastrointestinal tract.

   (b) Decrease. With a hastening of gastric emptying, the absorption sites will be exposed to a higher concentration of the vitamins, thereby increasing the chances of their saturation.

   (c) Increase. Availability will probably increase because the vitamins will stay longer where the transport occurs.

   (d) Decrease. A slower gastric emptying, associated with the full stomach, should lower the concentration at the absorption site, thereby reducing the chances of saturation.

2. (a) I, III, and VI. From the relationship $F \cdot \text{Dose} = CL_b \cdot AUC_b$, it is apparent that either F is increased or CL_b is decreased.

   (b) I and III. At steady state, $R_0 = CL \cdot C_{ss}$. Clearance must decrease with increasing dosing rate.

   (c) I and III. From the relationships $\text{Dose} = V_b \cdot C_b(0)$ and $\text{Dose} = CL_b \cdot AUC_b$ it is evident that volume of distribution is not changed and CL_b is decreased.

   (d) III. From the relationship $CL_{b,R}$ = (excretion rate)/blood concentration, the data show that $CL_{b,R}$ is decreased. No data are available to state how CL_b varies with dosing rate.

   (e) II and VI. The amount excreted unchanged increases disproportionately with increasing oral dose. This could be caused by an increase in either F or CL_R or a decrease in CL_{NR}.

   (f) I, III and VI. From the relationship $F \cdot \text{Dose}/\tau = CL \cdot C_{ss,av}$, it is evident that either F is increased or CL is decreased as dose is increased.

3. Glucose must be actively reabsorbed. At concentrations above 200 milligrams/100 milliliters of plasma, the capacity of the reabsorption system is exceeded.

Table G–10. Glucose Renal Clearance at Various Plasma Glucose Concentrations

Plasma Glucose Concentration (mg/100 ml)	200	301	398	503	605	708	799
Renal Clearance (ml/minute)	2.5	22	38	51	66	73	79

4. Yes. A plot of R_0 (also rate of elimination) against $C_{ss,av}$ shows apparent saturation. Plot of R_0 versus $R_0/C_{ss,av}$ gives Vm = 2600 milligrams/day or 108 milligrams/hour and Km = 1.4 milligrams/liter.

5. Saturable first-pass metabolism produces dose dependence in availability. It occurs by capacity-limited metabolism during the first-pass of an orally administered drug through the intestines and the liver. It can occur without apparent saturable elimination after an equivalent intravenous dose, when the concentration entering the intestines or the liver after the oral dose greatly exceeds that after the intravenous

dose. Factors favoring this condition include rapid absorption and a large volume of distribution.

6. **Table G–11.** **Disposition Kinetics and Total and Unbound Steady-state Blood Drug Concentrations as a Function of Dose Dependency in Each of Several Sources Following Oral and Intravenous Administrations**

Source of Dose Dependency	Direction of Change[a] with Increased Total Daily Dose	Volume of Distribution[b]	Clearance	Half-life	Concentration[c] Rate of Administration Total	Unbound
Oral Administration						
Availability	↓	↔	↔	↔	↓	↓
Absorption Rate Constant	↓	↔	↔	↔[d]	↔	↔
Intravenous Administration						
Fraction Unbound in Blood						
Low extraction ratio drug	↑	↑	↑	↔	↓	↔
High extraction ratio drug	↑	↑	↔	↑	↔	↑
Fraction Unbound in Tissue	↑	↓	↔	↓	↔	↔
Metabolic Clearance	↑	↔	↑	↓	↓	↓
Renal Clearance	↓	↔	↓	↑	↑	↑

[a]Only one example of each direction of change is shown.
[b]A volume of distribution greater than 50 liters.
[c]The average steady-state total and unbound blood drug concentrations relative to the rate of administration.
[d]Unless absorption rate limits elimination of drug, then the terminal half-life will increase.

Answers to Study Problems (Chap. 23)

1. Turnover—The process of renewal of substance in a pool at steady state.
Turnover rate—The rate of input (production and transfer) into a pool.
Turnover time—The time required to bring into a pool an amount equal to that in the pool.
Fractional turnover rate—The ratio of turnover rate and pool size.
Mean residence time—The average time a molecule resides in the body or in a pool.

2. (a) k_t (urea) = 0.105 hour^{-1}; k_t (creatinine) = 0.18 hour^{-1}.

$$k_t = \frac{CL \cdot C}{V \cdot C}$$

$$k_t \text{ (urea)} = \frac{4.2 \text{ liters/hour}}{40 \text{ liters}}$$

$$k_t \text{ (creatinine)} = \frac{7.2 \text{ liters/hour}}{40 \text{ liters}}$$

(b) Urea = 19 hours; creatinine = 11.1 hours. For both compounds the time required is twice the turnover time. In an anephric patient with no elimination of either compound, the rate of increase in plasma concentration is R_t/V and the total increase over time t is $R_t \cdot t/V$.

$$t = \frac{\Delta C \cdot V}{CL \cdot C_{ss}} = \frac{\Delta C}{C_{ss}} \cdot t_t$$

For both urea and creatinine, $\dfrac{\Delta C}{C_{ss}} = 2.$

(c) 15.2 grams. Daily amount excreted in one day ($CL_R \cdot C_{ss} \cdot t$)

$$= \frac{4.2 \text{ liters}}{\text{hour}} \times \frac{24 \text{ hours}}{\text{day}} \times \frac{150 \text{ milligrams}}{\text{liter}} \times 1 \text{ day}.$$

3. No. It depends on the fractional turnover rates of the two enzymes. Enzyme A may have reached its new steady state by 24 hours, while enzyme B may take a week or more to reach its new steady state, which may be more than double its normal value.

4. 2.8 days. The enzyme activity (concentration) will increase to a steady state three times its normal value. The doubling of the concentration (half way between 1 and 3) will occur at one half-life or 0.693 × turnover time.

5. (a) 8 hours. In this anuric patient, the amount of creatinine in the body (and the plasma concentration) doubles in a turnover time. With a rise of 3 milligrams/100 milliliters in 24 hours, the value must have increased by the normal value of 1 milligram/milliliter in 8 hours.

(b) 183 hours. With a normal turnover time of 8 hours, the normal half-life is 5.5 hours ($t_{1/2} = 0.693 \times t_t$). If renal function decreases tenfold, the new half-life is 55 hours. Consequently, it takes 183 hours, or 7.6 days, to reach 90 percent of the full increase to the new steady state.

6. (a) 15.9 days and 0.063 day^{-1}.

$$MRT = \frac{AUMC}{AUC}$$

$$= \frac{\dfrac{1.5}{1.4^2} + \dfrac{1.2}{0.06^2}}{\dfrac{1.5}{1.4} + \dfrac{1.2}{0.06}} = 15.9 \text{ days}$$

$$k_t = 1/t_t = 1/MRT$$

(b) 105 grams and 109 grams.

Intravascular

$$A = V_1 \cdot C(0)$$

$$V_1 = \frac{\text{Dose}}{C(0)^*} = \frac{6.75 \text{ megaBecquerels}}{2.7 \text{ megaBecquerels/liter}} = 2.5 \text{ liters}$$

$$A = 2.5 \text{ liters} \times 42 \text{ grams/liter} = 105 \text{ grams}$$

Total in body

$$A = V_{ss} \cdot C(0)$$

$$V_{ss} = MRT \cdot CL = MRT \cdot \text{Dose}/AUC$$

$$= 15.9 \text{ days} \times$$
$$6.75 \text{ megaBecquerels}/21.07 \text{ megaBecquerel-days/liter} = 5.1 \text{ liters}$$

$$A = 5.1 \text{ liters} \times 42 \text{ grams/liter} = 214 \text{ grams}$$

Amount in extravascular space = Total amount in body
$$\qquad\qquad - \text{ amount in extravascular space}$$
$$\qquad\qquad = 214 - 105 = 109 \text{ grams}$$

(c) 13.5 grams/day.

$$R_t = k_t \cdot A_{ss} = k_t \cdot V_{ss} \cdot C_{ss}$$
$$R_t = 0.063 \text{ day}^{-1} \times 5.1 \text{ liters} \times 42 \text{ grams/liter}$$

7. (a) Plot of S versus time is readily drawn from the data in Table 23–3.

(b) Table G–12 summarizes the data for the synthesis rate of S and the plasma concentration of S. The synthesis rate was calculated from the relationship

$$R_{syn} = \frac{dAs}{dt} + k_s \cdot As$$

which for a small time interval, Δt, is approximated by

$$R_{syn} = \frac{\Delta As}{\Delta t} + k_s \cdot As_{av}$$

where R_{syn} is the average rate of synthesis over Δt;
$\dfrac{\Delta As}{\Delta t}$ is the average rate of change of A_s over Δt; and
As_{av} is the average value of A_s over Δt. Its value is approximated by

$$As_{av} = [As(t_i) + As(t_{i+1})/2$$

and it occurs at the mid-point time,

$$t_{mid} = [t_i + t_{i+1}]/2$$

where t_i and t_{i+1} are the ith and $i+1$ times.

Estimation of k_s. The first 50 percent fall of A_s is the same whether 100 milligrams or 200 milligrams of drug was injected. Hence during this time, inhibition of synthesis must be almost complete ($R_{syn} = 0$), then

$$\frac{dAs}{dt} = -k_s \cdot As$$

Hence k_s is estimated from the slope of the initial straight line when As values are plotted against time on semilogarithmic paper.

Answer. $k_s = 0.170$ hour^{-1} ($t_{1/2} = 4.1$ hours)

therefore, $R_{syn} = k_s \cdot A_s = 17$ percent hour^{-1}.

Table G–12.

Synthesis Rate (percent of normal amount of S in body/hour)	17.0	1.45	1.35	2.2	2.8	4.2	6.0	9.5	12.1	14.9	16.2	16.9
Drug Concentration at Midpoint of Time Interval (mg/liter)	0	7.05	6.4	5.8	5.0	3.7	2.6	1.95	1.2	0.7	0.38	0.21

(c) $EC_{50} = 2$ milligrams/liter; $\gamma = 1.84$.

EC_{50} is concentration at which the synthesis is 50 percent of normal (8.5 percent of normal amount/hour)

The value of γ is obtained by substituting an effect-concentration data pair into the equation.

$$\frac{Effect}{E_{max}} = \frac{C^{\gamma}}{EC_{50}{}^{\gamma} + C^{\gamma}}$$

where $Effect/E_{max}$ is one minus the synthesis rate as a fraction of the normal value, a measure of the degree of inhibition of synthesis. Using a concentration of 5 milligrams/liter and an $Effect/E_{max}$ of 0.844, the value of γ is 1.84.

(d) Bolus = 33 milligrams; infusion rate = 1.65 milligrams/hour.

Desire 30 percent of normal values of As at steady state. This objective is achieved by decreasing the synthesis rate to 30 percent of the normal value, that is, to 0.3×17.3 percent hour^{-1} = 5.2 percent hour^{-1}. From plot in part (b), 3.3 milligrams/liter achieves this objective at steady state. Bolus dose (to produce 3.3 milligrams/liter) = 3.3 milligrams/liter $\times$ 10 liters = 33 milligrams. Infusion rate (to sustain 3.3 milligrams/liter) = $k \cdot V \cdot C_{ss}$ = 0.05 hour^{-1} $\times$ 33 milligrams = 1.65 milligrams/hour.

Answers to Study Problems (Chap. 24)

1. Dialysis—Separation of large from small molecules by the preferential passive movement of small molecules through a semipermeable membrane.
   Hemodialysis—A form of extracorporeal dialysis in which blood and dialysate fluid

each flow past opposite sides of a semipermeable membrane, permitting small molecules to be removed from the body.

Continuous ambulatory peritoneal dialysis—Continuous reinstillation, after a dwell time of 4 to 12 hours, of dialysate fluid into the peritoneal cavity. The peritoneal linings function as a semipermeable membrane, allowing small molecules to be removed from the body.

Dialysis clearance—Rate of removal of a substance in the dialysate relative to its concentration in the plasma under steady-state conditions. Blood dialysis clearance and unbound dialysis clearance are the parameters that relate the rate of removal to the drug concentration in blood and plasma water, respectively.

Dialyzer—A general term for the apparatus by which hemodialysis is carried out.

Dialyzer efficiency—Ratio of the rate of removal of substance to the rate of its presentation to the dialyzer under steady-state conditions.

Clinical dialyzability—A general term for the relative ability of dialysis to remove drug from the body. It is quantified by the ratio of the amount removed during the procedure relative to the amount initially in the body. The value of the ratio is the product of the fraction eliminated by dialysis and the fraction lost by all routes of elimination during the dialysis period.

2. (a) 10.5 milliliters/minute.

$$\int_0^6 C \cdot dt \simeq C_{av} \cdot 6 = 22 \text{ milligram-hours/liter}$$

$$CL_D = \frac{\text{Amount recovered}}{\int_0^6 C \cdot dt} = \frac{14 \text{ milligrams}}{22 \text{ milligram-hours/liter}}$$

$$= 10.5 \text{ milliliters/minute.}$$

(b) 3.5 percent.

$$Q_b = 0.305 \text{ liters/minute} = 18.3 \text{ liters/hour}$$

$$\text{Efficiency} = \frac{V_D \cdot C_D}{Q_b \cdot \int_0^\tau C_{b,in} \cdot dt} = \frac{14 \text{ milligrams}}{18.3 \text{ liters/hour} \times \dfrac{22 \text{ milligram-hours}}{\text{liter}}}$$

(c) No, $C_{b,out}/C_{b,in} = 0.965$.

The ratio of $C_{b,out}$ and $C_{b,in}$ can be calculated from

$$\frac{C_{b,out}}{C_{b,in}} = 1 - \text{Efficiency}$$

The concentrations of the drug in blood entering and leaving the dialyzer are too close to obtain an accurate estimate of their difference. In addition, only minor differences in flow rates in and out, caused by loss of water into dialysate, can make concentration differences smaller or even negative.

(d) 4 percent.

$$\frac{\text{Amount recovered}}{\text{Dose}} = \frac{14 \text{ milligrams}}{350 \text{ milligrams}} = 0.04.$$

(e) Yes. 10.5 milliliters/minute measured versus 11.7 milliliters/minute predicted.

$$CL_D \simeq \frac{\text{Dialysis clearance}}{\text{of creatinine}} \cdot \sqrt{\frac{113}{252}} \times fu$$

$$CL_D \simeq 83 \text{ minutes} \times 0.67 \times 0.21.$$

3. (a) The manner of calculating dialysis clearance after intraperitoneal administration is the principal cause of the difference in the values. The amount that entered the body during the first 4-hour dwell time after intraperitoneal administration is unknown. It certainly is not equal to the dose, as was assumed by the authors.

(b) Clearance, too, is miscalculated following intraperitoneal administration. The AUC is less than that after intravenous administration because of the exchange of dialysate at 4 hours. After intraperitoneal administration,

$$\frac{\text{Dose}}{AUC} = \frac{CL}{F}$$

It is evident that F is approximately equal to 0.6. This is the same factor by which the peritoneal dialysis clearance after intraperitoneal administration was in error.

4. (a) Yes, because 33 percent of initial amount is needed to cancel what is lost by dialysis.

$$\text{Nonrenal clearance} = (1 - fe(n)) \cdot V \cdot 0.693/t_{1/2} \text{ (normal)}$$

$$= 2.64 \text{ liters/hour;}$$

$$\frac{\text{Half-life}}{\text{off dialysis}} = \frac{t_{1/2} \text{ (normal)}}{(1 - fe(n))}$$

$$= 9.2 \text{ hours;}$$

Fraction of amount initially in body eliminated by dialysis (Eq. 12) $= 0.36;$

Fraction of amount initially in body required to cancel the loss by dialysis (Eq. 17) $= 0.33.$

(b) 150 milligrams. For a regimen of 240 milligrams every 6 hours, the average amount of theophylline in the body is 460 milligrams. The supplementary dose is 0.33 × 460 milligrams, or 150 milligrams.

(c) 240 milligrams initially and every 6 hours, with about 150 milligrams at the end of each dialysis treatment. Values should be adjusted to nearest dose strengths.

5. No. The clearance of the drug $(0.693 \cdot V/t_{1/2})$ is 0.16 liter/hour, a value greater than that of dialysis clearance, <0.1 liter/hour. With a usual half-life of 160 hours, one cannot expect the half-life on dialysis to shorten by much. Furthermore, the amount eliminated by dialysis in 24 hours would be minor.

Answers to Study Problems (Chap. 25)

1. (a) Table G–13 is Table 25–7 completed.

Table G–13.

Fraction of Drug in Body[a]	Valproic Acid	Nitrazepam	Chlordiazepoxide
Unbound	0.32	0.04	**0.07**
In extracellular fluids	**0.88**	0.06	0.37
Outside extracellular fluids	0.12	**0.94**	0.63
Bound to protein in plasma	0.31	0.02	**0.14**
Bound to plasma protein in extracellular fluids	**0.77**	0.05	0.34
Bound intracellularly (in or on tissue cells, including blood cells)	**~0**	**0.91**	0.58

[a]70-kilogram person.

(b) Nitrazepam.

Table G–14.

	$\dfrac{V_R{}^b}{fu_R}$	V (liters)[a]		
		Before	After[c]	Percent Increase
Valproic acid	15.4	9.1	10.7	18 percent
Nitrazepam	958	133	258	94 percent
Chlordiazepoxide	378	21	34.5	64 percent

[a]70-kilogram person.
[b]Estimated from

$$V = 7.5 + 7.5 \cdot fu + \frac{V_R}{fu_R} \cdot fu.$$

[c]Value after fu is doubled.

2. Volume of distribution would increase from 21 liters (0.3 liter/kg) to 28.6 liters (0.41 liter/kg).

Step 1. Change in fu to 0.0465.

$$fu \approx \frac{1}{1 + Ka \cdot (P_t)} = 0.035.$$

$$Ka \cdot (P_t) = 27.6 \text{ when } (P_t) = 4.3 \text{ grams/deciliter,}$$

therefore $Ka \cdot (P_t) = 20.5$ when $(P_t) = 3.2$ grams/deciliter, giving fu a value of 0.0465.

Step 2. Change in $R_{E/I}$, 1.5 to 2.6.

Step 3. The value of $\dfrac{V_R}{fu_R}$ is 378 liters (Table G–15).

Using this value, a new volume can be calculated from

$$V = 3\,(1\, +\, R_{E/I})\, +\, fu\, \cdot\, V_P \left[\frac{V_E}{V_P}\, -\, R_{E/I}\right]\, +\, \frac{V_R}{fu_R}\, \cdot\, fu.$$

3. The unbound volume of distribution (V/fu) is decreased from 2.5 to 1.5 liters/kilogram, whereas the unbound clearance shows very little change, 300 to 260 milliliters/hour per kilogram. The drug is unquestionably of low extraction since CL/Q_H is less than 0.02.

   The lack of change in unbound clearance indicates no effect of acute viral hepatitis on metabolic activity. The decrease in the unbound volume is consistent with the change in fraction unbound for a drug with a small volume of distribution. The half-life shortens, because the decrease in binding to plasma proteins decreases the unbound volume, but not the unbound clearance.

INDEX

Page numbers in *italics* refer to illustrations; page numbers followed by a "t" refer to tables. When more than one section is referred to, the major reference is in **boldface type**.